Get Healthy Now!
with Gary Null

GET HEALTHY NOW!

WITH GARY NULL

Senior Project Editor Amy McDonald

A Complete Guide to Prevention, Treatment and Healthy Living

SEVEN STORIES PRESS

New York / Toronto / London

A Seven Stories Press First Edition

In Canada:
Hushion House, 36 Northline Road, Toronto, Ontario M4B 3E2, Canada

In the U.K.:
Turnaround Publisher Services Ltd., Unit 3, Olympia Trading Estate, Coburg Road, Wood Green, London N22 6TZ U.K.

Library of Congress Cataloging-in-Publication Data

Null, Gary.
    Get healthy now! with Gary Null: A complete guide to prevention, treatment, and healthy living. —Seven Stories Press 1st ed.
        p.   cm.
    ISBN: 1-58322-042-9
    1. Alternative medicine—Popular works. I. Title.
R733.N852 1999
615.5—dc21   98-55547
                                                             CIP

9 8 7 6 5 4 3 2 1

Book design by Cindy LaBreacht

Seven Stories Press
140 Watts Street
New York, NY 10013
http://www.sevenstories.com

Printed in the U.S.A.

CONTENTS

PART ONE: Back to the Basics: What is Nutrition?

PART TWO: Taking Charge of Your Health

PART THREE: Mental Health and Psychological Well-Being

PART FOUR: Musculoskeletal Fitness

PART FIVE: Foot and Leg Care

PART SIX: Heart, Blood, and Circulation

PART SEVEN: Allergy, Asthma, and Environmental Illness

PART EIGHT: Cancer Prevention and Treatment

PART NINE: Chronic and Degenerative Conditions

PART TEN: Women's Health

PART ELEVEN: Of Special Concern to Men

PART TWELVE: Aging Well

PART THIRTEEN: Everyday Health for the Whole Family

PART FOURTEEN: Selecting an Alternative Health Practitioner

PART ONE

Back to the Basics: What Is Nutrition?

1

"You Are What You Eat"

It has finally become conventional to associate good nutrition with good health. Mainstream medicine and the public at large now acknowledge that a good diet can not only promote health, but also prevent disease. Today it is customary to talk about how food choices affect our overall well-being and help ward off heart disease, cancer, diabetes, stroke, osteoporosis, and other ailments. Most people also are aware that a healthy diet can decrease the risk of disease by reducing predisposing conditions such as obesity, high blood pressure, and high cholesterol.

Eating a balanced diet is the most effective way to ensure that our bodies receive the nutrients we need. Nutrition experts recommend that the daily diet include a certain number of servings from each of the five major food groups: breads, cereals, rice, and pasta; vegetables; fruits; milk, yogurt, and cheese; and meat, poultry, fish, dried beans and peas, eggs, and nuts. Fats and sugars should be used sparingly.

Unfortunately, the typical American diet does not meet many of the requirements for good health. Part of the problem relates to the types and proportions of foods that people eat. Just as important to our health, however, is how the foods are grown and processed as they make their way to our grocery shelves and kitchen tables.

Because of today's agricultural and manufacturing practices, foods once full of vitamins, minerals, protein, and fiber have indeed become bankrupt. Not only does refining wheat and other grains strip them of their fiber, the wheat grown on today's soils contains only a fraction of the protein content it once had. But this is not the only adverse consequence of modern-day food production. Even with thorough washing, many chemical pesticides are not removed. They penetrate the skin of fruits and vegetables and invade the body's systems.

Food Supply

A half-century ago roughly a third of the grocery store was devoted to natural, fresh produce. Today, it is a small fraction of that, and even what appears to be natural has often been altered. Fruits and vegetables are routinely grown with artificial fertilizers, sprayed with pesticides, treated with chemicals to control the time of ripening, and coated with waxes to give a glossy appearance.

Modern bread fares no better. For thousands of years wheat has been prepared as bread. Known as the staff of life, whole wheat is a rich source of nutrients: complex carbohydrates, protein, oils, roughage, and an excellent balance of vitamins and minerals. When making whole-wheat flour, these ingredients are retained. Refined flour, used to make white bread, is processed in a different way. Rollers flatten and separate the bran and germ, which carry most of wheat's nutrients. Fiber is lost. Chlorine gases are used to bleach out remaining substances. The product is then "enriched" with synthetic versions of some of the nutrients removed earlier in the processing. To increase shelf-life, preservatives are added.

Among the ingredients commonly listed on loaves of bread made from enriched flour are barley malt, ferrous sulfate, niacin, thiamine mononitrate, riboflavin, corn syrup, partially hydrogenated vegetable shortening, yeast, salt, dicalcium phosphate, and calcium propionate. Potassium bromate was a popular additive until its association with cancer in laboratory animals led many countries to ban its use. In 1999, the Center for Science in the Public Interest petitioned the Food and Drug Administration to prohibit the use of bromate in the United States. While many bakers have voluntarily switched to bromate-free processes, many continue to include bromate in their products. Some of the flour additives and processing chemicals that need not be listed on bread packages include oxides of nitrogen, chlorine, nitrosyl chloride, chlorine dioxide, benzoyl peroxide, acetone peroxide, azodicarbonamide, and plaster of Paris.

Let's take a look at meat and poultry. Many of us picture farms as being like those we remember from childhood, or like those we have seen in pictures or on television. We imagine farm animals in their pens, or even roaming around a farmyard. Such farms may exist, but they are not the source of most of the meat and poultry we buy and eat today. Chickens are raised by the tens of thousands in giant buildings where they never see the light of day. They are kept in cages where they cannot move, with conveyor belts bringing them food and water and carrying away their waste. When they do move about, they often slide around on their breasts, as some modern breeds grow too fat for their legs to support them. They are constantly sprayed and their food is doused with chemicals, hormones, and medicines. Attempts also are being made to breed featherless chickens.

Steers spend most of their lives outdoors, but are no less exposed to chemicals in their upbringing. Today a steer is born, taken from its mother and put on a diet of powdered milk, synthetic vitamins, minerals, and antibiotics. It is permitted to eat some pasture grass, but this is supplemented with processed feed that is premixed with antibiotics and growth-promoting drugs. At 6 months, the steer weighs 500 pounds and is ready for the feed lot. Here it is doused with pesticides and then placed in a pen that is lit around the clock to change natural sleep rhythms and encourage continuous feeding. Food consists of grains, urea, carbohydrates, ground-up newspaper, molasses, plastic pellets, and most recently, reprocessed manure, a high protein source. After 4 months in the feed lot, a steer weighs 1,200 pounds. A few more doses of pesticides, antibiotics, and hormones are administered to pretenderize it while it is still alive, and it is ready for slaughter.

As meat takes an especially long time to digest and is essentially fiberless, chemicals are not easily eliminated and can accumulate to cause all sorts of toxic reactions within the body. According to a recent General Accounting Office report, "of the 143 drugs and pesticides identified as likely to leave residues in raw meat and poultry, 42 are known to cause or are suspected of causing cancer, 20 of causing birth defects, and six of causing mutations."

Pesticides

It has been estimated that more than 2.5 billion pounds of pesticides annually invade our nation's lands, fields, and forests. The Environmental Protection Agency (EPA) has licensed more than 400 pesticides for use on America's foods. But how are these pesticides regulated? How much residue is left in our food? How are pesticides affecting our health and the health of our children?

Governmental regulation of pesticides has been ineffective and inconsistent. In 1996, in recognition of the critical need for new standards for pesticide use on food, the Food Quality Protection Act was signed into law. This law mandates that EPA (*finally!*) "consider the public's overall exposure to pesticides (through food, water, and in home environments) when making decisions to set standards for pesticide use on food." More specifically the law requires EPA to address risks to infants and children, to implement a screening program for reproductive and developmental effects, and to set a "single, health-based standard for all pesticide residues in all types of food." It is alarming to know that these basic safeguards are considered part of a new law. By 2006, EPA is required to review all old pesticides to make sure that their use on food meets the "new, tougher safety standard."

Both agribusiness and the government claim that the U.S. food supply is the safest in the world. That simply is not true. Especially when it comes to pro-

duce. In fact, domestic produce has more toxic pesticides than imported produce in two-thirds of the cases. Consumer's Union recently analyzed the
Department of Agricultural data on the amount of pesticides detected in fruits
and vegetables. Of the 27 foods analyzed, seven were found to have a toxicity
score up to hundreds of times higher than the rest. In order of greater to lesser toxicity, these seven foods are peaches, winter squash, apples, green beans,
pears, spinach, and grapes.

Food Additives

Chemical additives in foods have become so prevalent that they now make up a
good portion of our diet. The average American consumes more than 150 pounds
of food additives annually, More than 3,000 substances are currently listed in the
Food and Drug Administration's Everything Added to Food in the United States
(EAFUS) Database. Most of these additives are not put in foods just to preserve
shelf life or retard spoilage, as is usually claimed. Instead, they are there to make
the product look, taste, feel, and nourish more like the real thing.

Manufacturers contend that these chemicals are safe, that they have been
tested and approved by the Food and Drug Administration. Are all these chemicals really safe? The answer is no. Among some of the more questionable and
well-known additives are nitrates, saccharin, monosodium glutamate (MSG),
and artificial colorings (yellow dye no. 6, red dye no. 2). There are hordes more
less-familiar additives that may pose equal dangers to our health.

If food additives can be dangerous, why are we told otherwise? The answer
lies in the complex interrelations of the food industry, media, government, and
medical research. The food industry is very big business, with annual sales well
over $200 billion. Each year, well over $500 million worth of chemicals are
added to foods. The food industry is a major advertiser in consumer magazines
and on television, so magazines and television too often are careful of being
critical. Food industries are major sources of grants for university research
departments. Government agencies have close relationships with the industries
they are supposed to regulate. Many research scientists and government management personnel eventually enter the industry they previously regulated—
and at much higher paying jobs.

Few of the chemicals have been adequately tested. Many that have been
tested have been known to be dangerous for 30 years or more. Industry fights
attempts to ban such chemicals every step of the way. When a ban is finally
achieved, some producers continue to use it anyway. Diethylstilbestrol (DES) is
a case in point. This synthetic hormone used to fatten cattle has been known
for decades to cause cancer. It was banned from use in food-producing animals
in the United States more than 20 years ago. Yet, as recently as January 2000,
the Swiss government reportedly informed the U.S. government that DES had
been found in beef coming from this country.

Agribusiness encourages a way of eating that disrupts our physical health and erodes the sense of fulfillment that comes from preparing and eating real food. A fast-food rationale enters the community and the home, with deleterious effects. Agribusiness also undermines local farmers, who lend economic and ecological stability to the country. And industrialized foods simply do not taste as good as food should. They are dependent upon salt, sugar, chemicals, and billions of dollars in advertising. The fact is, most of us simply have forgotten what real food tastes like.

SUGAR One of the most common additives in processed foods is sugar. The average American consumes 160 pounds of sugar a year. The U.S. Department of Agriculture (UDSA) recommends that a person who eats a 2,000-calorie diet limit added sugars to no more than 10 teaspoons daily. Unfortunately, the average person actually eats about twice this amount.

Sugar is ideal for the processed-food industry because many people like its taste and it is cheap, but primarily because it is addictive. Sugar in large quantities is concealed in many foods; not only in candy, cake, and soft drinks, but in bread, breakfast cereals, cheeses, condiments, and canned or packaged foods. On a food label, sugars include corn syrup, brown sugar, corn sweetener, lactose, maltose, fructose, glucose, molasses. Most processed foods have large amounts of sugar, and those that do not have large amounts of salt.

In 1999, a number of leading health experts and organizations petitioned the Food and Drug Administration (FDA) to require food labels to disclose how much sugar has been added to soft drinks, ice cream, and other foods. Alarmed at surveys showing that sugar consumption increased nearly 30 percent between 1983 and 1999, these experts also asked the FDA to set a maximum daily value of 10 teaspoons (40 grams) of sugar on Nutrition Facts labels.

Genetically Engineered Foods

In genetic engineering, also called genetic modification, a gene from one seed or crop is inserted into another to give it a desired trait. In 1999, genetically engineered crops were grown on an estimated 25 percent of cropland in the United States. Corn and soybeans make up the bulk of the food on the market today. The Food and Drug Administration and the food industry argue that genetically modified foods are no different from other foods and thus don't need to be identified or labeled as such. The one way you can know you are not eating genetically engineered food is if you eat something labeled "organic," because the law does not permit organic food to be genetically engineered.

European and Japanese consumers have expressed strong resistance to genetically modified foods. In the United States, the reaction has been muted.

"American consumers don't really know what they are eating," says Nichols Fox, an independent investigative journalist and author of *Spoiled—The*

Dangerous Truth About the Food Chain Gone Haywire. "I think most of them would be surprised to find that 50, 60, perhaps as much as 70 percent of processed foods in the American supermarket contain some genetically engineered ingredients."

Fox adds, "I think the American consumer has been mislead to think that the FDA is doing thorough testing of these products and that is not true. What they are doing is looking for a substantial equivalency. If it looks like a tomato, if it is chemically similar to a tomato, then that is fine. They ask the companies to look for allergens or toxins that are produced but they go no further than that. If there are long term feeding studies being done with these products, we don't know about them. They are not being required and if the companies are doing it they are not telling us about them. Really we are the test rats for these products."

Fox explains some of the concerns about genetically engineered foods. "Genetic engineering is basically about the art of the impossible. These are genes that would never cross in real life. You could never get a flounder to breed with a tomato in real life. You could only do it in the lab. Now why are these mixes potentially dangerous? Because we have been co-evolving with the environment for a hundred thousand years. We have developed a relationship with these foods that we eat that has taken a great deal of time to establish itself. When we are confronted with these new genetic crosses, our bodies have no experience. Also, there is a common misperception that a gene has one trait and when you transfer that gene you are simply transferring that one trait to the new product. That is not true. A gene can do many things and it can do different things in different situations so when you put it in to a new environment you may have very unexpected consequences."

Genetic engineering of foods is another example of how the multibillion dollar food industry simply ignores public health in its quest for profit. "Consumers have not been out there saying we want a genetically engineered tomato, we want a genetically engineered soybean," Fox says. "What the companies are telling us is that these products will enable farmers to use less pesticides, less herbicides and perhaps have higher yields. That is not necessarily true. For instance, if you have a corn that is resistant to a certain herbicide such as Roundup it is common sense that you are not going to be using less of it, you are going to be using more of it. USDA studies have found that the yields vary: in some places you may have increased yields and in other situations you may have decreased yields, and the same with pesticide and herbicide use. There is no conclusive evidence that these are universally of benefit. So that really needs to be studied a great deal more, but the fact is that no one is doing this for the consumer. This is being done to enhance the profitability of agriculture and of distribution of processing and of marketing. That is why it is being done, not for us."

Water Supply

Most Americans have grown accustomed to an excellent supply of high quality drinking water. For more than a century, treatment of municipal water with chlorine disinfectants has provided protection against disease-causing microorganisms. Private wells are usually tested periodically to assure quality standards.

However, a larger problem is looming: the industrial pollution of drinking-water supplies. Hundreds of thousands of industrial plants discharge grit, asbestos, phosphates, nitrates, mercury, lead, caustic soda, sulfur, sulfuric acid, oils, and petrochemicals into many of the waterways from which we eventually drink. Treatment plants designed to handle human wastes are unable to remove many of these more toxic, chemically complex, and sometimes unstable substances. Ironically, one of the carcinogens identified as occurring in water results when chlorine mixes with organic matter.

Nationwide, more than 700 chemical pollutants have been identified in public water supplies. Many are believed to cause cancer, birth defects, or other toxic effects. More than 20 scientific studies have documented a consistent link between consumption of trace organic chemical contaminants in drinking water and elevated cancer mortality rates. Parallel failures to protect drinking water quality and to regulate massive discharges of nonbiodegradable industrial wastes forecast a grim future. The response to this dual environmental and health dilemma has been woefully inadequate.

The 1996 Safe Drinking Water Act Amendments are the government's attempt to address the issue of water safety. These amendments require that consumers receive more information from water suppliers and state agencies about the quality of their drinking water. The Environmental Protection Agency (EPA) has issued drinking water standards for more than 80 contaminants, and established pollutant-specific minimum testing schedules for public water systems.

Organic Foods

The organic food industry is one of the fastest growing industries in the country. It has grown about 20 percent a year for the past 7 years. Dr. Elson Haas, a practicing integrative medicine physician and director of the Preventive Medical Center in San Rafael, California, tells about the many benefits of organic food.

In several studies, he says, organic foods are shown to have higher levels of nutrients, vitamins, and minerals. Also there is the taste factor; organic foods are more flavorful. By eating organic, we are preventing potential health problems that may be caused by pesticides and other toxic chemicals. "I think also by supporting organics we are basically supporting an industry and saying we don't want so many chemicals in our food, we don't want so many chemicals in our environment. We are helping independent farmers, we are protecting the soil, we are protecting the water quality, and we are protecting the animals. We are protecting our future."

Basic Nutrition

Nutrition is the way the body makes use of foods to meet its needs for growth, repair, and maintenance. There are six major groups of nutrients: carbohydrates, proteins, fats, vitamins, minerals, and water. Along with an understanding of these basic nutrients, you also need to be aware of the air you breathe, the balance of enzymes in your body, and the function of antioxidants in helping your body to combat disease and degenerative processes. Your body needs all of these nutrients every day. How much you need of each depends on your health as well as your energy needs.

Energy may be why we need food, but it isn't necessarily why we eat the way we eat. When it comes to nourishing our bodies, many of us follow the dictates of myths, fads, or bizarre and exotic diets. We all know the proper kind of gas for a car and the best kind of food for our cat or dog. We may know our carburetors and our Siamese, but we don't know ourselves.

Information about good nutrition abounds. Yet many people don't bother to find out more about it. Some simply don't know where to look or whom to trust. The following chapters should help point the way and begin the journey toward a more healthful life.

2

Carbohydrates

Until recently, carbohydrates have gotten bad press. This is because the highly sugared and refined carbohydrates such as candy, soft drinks, and sweetened cereals have been lumped together with the complex carbohydrates such as fruit, nutritious starchy vegetables, whole grains, and tubers.

Carbohydrates are everywhere. In fact, they are one of the most abundant compounds in living things. The nutrient group includes indigestible cellulose (the fibrous material that helps give plants their shape), as well as starches and sugars, two of the storable fuels that supply living things with immediate energy. Each gram of carbohydrates supplies the body with 4 calories of energy. Many carbohydrate-rich foods also contain substantial amounts of amino acids, the building blocks of protein.

We need carbohydrates. They are the most important source of energy for all of our activities. The foods in which they are found are also important sources of vitamins, minerals, and other nutrients.

Types of Carbohydrates

Carbohydrates come in two forms: complex and refined. Complex carbohydrates are starches and fibers in foods such as cereals, legumes, seeds, nuts, vegetables, and tubers. They exist in these foods just as they are found in nature, having undergone minimal or no processing. Refined carbohydrates, on the other hand, have been substantially tampered with. "Refined" may in fact be an overly refined way of putting it. Having been processed by machinery and industry, they are merely skeletons of the complex carbohydrates found in nature.

While the starches and sugars of all carbohydrates supply energy, complex carbohydrates also offer the fiber necessary for good digestive functioning, supply B and C complex and other vitamins, and manufacture protein, the building blocks of our bodies. In addition, our bodies tolerate and absorb complex carbohydrates better and more effectively than refined carbohydrates.

Refinement is a recent innovation in our long history of evolution, food consumption, and food delivery. When carbohydrates are refined, they are stripped of their outer shell (the bran layer that contains most of the fiber), their oil and a B vitamin-rich germ (found at their cores). Refined carbohydrates may also be bleached, milled, baked (bread), puffed (some cereals), or otherwise processed (sugar).

Unfortunately, these refined carbohydrates predominate in our diets. Breakfast cereals generally are made from wheat, corn, oats, or rice. But, with the exception of real oatmeal and a few hot whole-wheat cereals, they are rarely served in their natural forms. Instead they are dried, refined, bleached, steamed, puffed, flaked, or sugared. Occasionally a small percentage of the recommended daily allowance of certain minerals and (usually synthetic) vitamins are added. The cereals can then be labeled "enriched." Most of the nutrients available from such breakfasts come from the milk that people add rather than from the cereal itself.

Our breads, even "rye" and "whole wheat," are usually produced from refined flour and are often loaded with chemical additives. The white rice that graces our plates may look pretty, but it lacks the fiber, vitamins, and minerals found in whole-grain brown rice.

Refined carbohydrates may not be good for us. What's worse, they may harm us. They contain little or no fiber, so over-reliance on them as a source of energy can lead to poor intestinal health and myriad digestive disorders. Also, overconsumption of refined sugar is linked to obesity, diabetes, and other blood-sugar disorders.

Danger: Sweets Can Quickly Sour

We need carbohydrates for energy, especially to fuel the brain. But we don't really need refined sugar. Honey, maple syrup, molasses, white and brown sugar, corn syrups, and other sweeteners fall into this group. These sugars provide a few traces of minerals and calories, but nothing else. Glucose is the body's most important source of energy. But too much glucose in the bloodstream, an aftereffect of a typical high-sugar coffee and doughnut break, for example, may actually worsen fatigue and overburden the vital organs. If we have a well-balanced diet, we should be relying on our livers to send forth new energy to our working muscles, not on candy bars or doughnuts.

Sugar has been implicated in cardiovascular problems and diabetes. The protective functions of our cells are depressed by all forms of sugar, but especially by sucrose (cane sugar). Sugar seems to provoke and worsen skin conditions such as acne. Cutting it out of the diet often results in visible improvement. Omitting refined sugar from meals will also normalize the levels of various acids and other digestive juices in the stomach.

The brain requires a constant supply of glucose so that its "circuits" can communicate and function properly. Hypoglycemia, or low blood sugar, is often exacerbated by overconsumption of refined sugars and flour. This condition can distort perception and alter behavior. If you suspect you have hypoglycemia, don't take this blood sugar disorder lightly. Consult your doctor for the necessary lab tests. Hypoglycemia is associated with abnormal fatigue and hunger, and can lead to diabetes and obesity.

Even naturally occurring or simple sugars can pose problems. Gastrointestinal complaints, for example, can be caused by a sensitivity to the milk-sugar lactose in dairy products. Fructose, the form of sugar predominant in fruits, has been touted recently as being superior to sucrose. Beware: It may be sweeter, so you may use less of it—but a simple sugar is still sugar to your body. Watch out for any simple or concentrated sugar!

How Many Carbohydrates Do You Need?

More than half the calories Americans consume come from carbohydrates. Unfortunately, most of these are refined carbohydrates. The breads most people eat are 55 percent carbohydrate. Most flour cereals are 80 percent refined carbohydrate; our spaghettis and pastas are 75 percent refined carbohydrate. Jams, candies, and some pastries may be 90 percent refined carbohydrate.

In contrast fresh fruit is only 15 percent carbohydrate; dry legumes, even before being doubled in size by the addition of water in cooking, are just 60 percent carbohydrate; and uncooked whole grains, before the absorption of water, are 70 percent carbohydrate. Green leafy vegetables average 8 percent carbohydrate or less. By eating vegetables, grains, legumes, seeds, and some fruits, all of which have moderate to low carbohydrate content, we are actually reducing calories and sugars in our diet.

The American Heart Association and other groups currently recommend that adults get 55 to 60 percent of their daily calories from complex carbohydrates. This means that for a person consuming 2,000 calories a day, carbohydrate intake should be about 300 grams. The ideal diet actually gets about 85 to 90 percent of its calories and protein from complex carbohydrates, and 10 to 15 percent from fats found in nuts, seeds, and oils. This ratio allows complex carbohydrates to be the mainstay of the diet, with fewer calories from fats and animal protein foods.

Despite what our backgrounds, palates, or emotions may tell us, supplying energy remains the number one purpose of food. Carbohydrates yield immediately available energy; if they are oversupplied, the body builds up its muscle and liver glycogen reserves or converts the extra amount into fat. High-protein diets can be dangerous. Protein is mainly a building material, not a primary energy source. It can be burnt up as fuel, but this is an inefficient way to provide energy to our systems; it requires extra energy, and it results in a waste product called urea, which must be eliminated through the kidneys. Over the long term, eating too much protein and burning protein as fuel can overstress and even weaken the kidneys.

Complex Carbohydrates

SOURCES Complex carbohydrates are not hard to find. You just have to know where to look. Basic whole grains, for example, are a good source. These include whole wheat, rye, triticale (a cross between rye and wheat you may be able to tolerate if you are allergic to real whole wheat), corn, barley, brown rice, oats, millet, and buckwheat. These grains can be served as cereals or side dishes, mixed in soups and casseroles, ground into whole grain flour and baked into bread, or rolled into whole grain pastas.

Legumes also contain complex carbohydrates. Among the common varieties are soybeans and soy products such as tofu, tempeh, and miso, as well as mung beans, lentils, azduki beans, split peas, black-eyed peas, kidney beans, navy beans, red beans, pink beans, pinto beans, black beans, turtle beans, fava beans, chick-peas (garbanzos), and peanuts. (See chapter 13 for a complete guide to natural foods.)

Seeds such as sunflower, pumpkin, chia, and sesame are high in both protein and carbohydrates. Alfalfa, chia, and flax seeds (those grown organically for food, not for fabrics, to avoid pesticide contamination) are highly nutritious when sprouted. Most nuts are mainly fat, but almonds, cashews, pistachios, and pine nuts are high in carbohydrates as well.

The entire vegetable family is a rich source of carbohydrates. Those lowest in calories, such as celery, broccoli, and mushrooms, contain mostly water and fiber. The starchier, root vegetables, such as carrots, beets, potatoes, and yams, tend to be higher in unrefined starches and sugars as well as in fiber.

Fruits are excellent sources of complex carbohydrates, natural sugars, minerals, vitamins, and fiber. Choose from apples, pears, peaches, nectarines, plums, grapes, or citrus fruits. Although the sugar content of these fruits is fairly high, it is diluted with water and released relatively slowly into your system as you chew and digest the cellulose-encased cells of the pulp. Your body doesn't get the kind of sudden jolt it receives from refined, pure sugar. Bananas and other tropical fruits should be eaten in moderation by those sensitive to sugar, since their sugar content is higher. Similarly, dried fruits, including figs, prunes, raisins, dates, apricots, pears, and apples contain three times the sugar dose of fresh fruit; like refined sugar, they are highly concentrated carbohydrates, which should be eaten only occasionally.

Eating too much fruit can add extra calories, but as long as you don't eat fatty foods as well, fruit will not make you fat. An apple indeed may contain the equivalent of three teaspoons of sugar and the calories that go with that. But it is much harder to down three whole apples than nine teaspoons of sugar. Some people consume as much sugar in one cup of coffee, one mug of cocoa, or one doughnut—without getting all the beneficial vitamins, minerals, fiber, and enzymes of the apple.

PREPARING COMPLEX CARBOHYDRATE FOODS Grains should be rinsed before use, and the larger legumes—such as beans—should be soaked overnight before cooking. Using pressure cookers can shorten cooking time.

People who eat meat and wish to switch to a more complex-carbohydrate-oriented, vegetarian diet often worry that eating will become a boring, asensual experience, limited in variety and taste. Pilgrims, seek no more. There are vegetarian recipes and menus to satisfy every palate and taste. The vegetarian recipes included in later chapters will provide a sampling of their variety and set you on the right nutritional track.

For those who must restrict their sodium intake, a variety of other herbs and spices are available that are even livelier that salt. They include leeks, dill, oregano, cumin, curry, and chili peppers. Vegetables may be mixed with legumes for stews and casseroles as well as soups; seasoned grains, such as millet (perhaps combined with soy granules or lentils for protein enhancement), are delicious stuffed into peppers, tomatoes, or hollowed-out zucchinis.

Digestion of Carbohydrates

Normally, carbohydrates are digested quickly. The carbohydrates in fruit juice may be digested in as little as 40 minutes; starchy foods, such as beans or grains, may take up to 90 minutes. The more fiber you consume with your meals, the faster the digestion process because fiber absorbs water and stimulates the actions of the digestive tract.

Animal proteins and fats take much longer to digest. If sweet or starchy foods are eaten at the same time as meat and fish, they can remain in the stomach as long as the proteins (up to 6 hours). This can cause gas and indigestion, as the sugar from the carbohydrates may begin to ferment in the warm acid environment of the stomach.

If you begin your meal with a beverage, you can briefly dilute the acid in your stomach and slow digestion. Cold beverages suspend initial digestion for a short time, as the acids and enzymes of the digestive system usually operate at body temperature.

Some people complain that they have trouble digesting beans, and that flatulence is a problem. Partly, this is because these products may ferment in the large intestines, producing gas. Beans should be soaked for at least 15 hours before cooking. Cook them slowly to avoid altering the protein and thoroughly so that their fiber is completely softened. Digestion will then be easier.

Bean sprouts also may be easier to digest than cooked dried beans. Sprouting increases the nutrient content as well as the digestibility of beans, grains, and seeds. Alfalfa and mung beans are two of the most popular types. Alfalfa sprouts are a nutrition powerhouse, containing five times the amount of vitamin C in alfalfa seeds. Two ounces of sprouts a day will supply you with vitamins and live raw enzymes you might not otherwise obtain from your diet, as well as chlorophyll, which is considered an intestine and blood cleanser. Always steam soy bean sprouts briefly before serving them, since the raw beans contain digestion inhibitors, trypsin, and other natural toxins that can only be neutralized by heating.

The typical American dinner, consisting of meat, potatoes, vegetables, perhaps a salad, and dessert, mixes up all four digestive processes at once, weakening them all. The acid from the meat's protein neutralizes the starches into sugars, so starch digestion is limited and extended. When a sugary dessert is added, its simple refined sugars start fermenting, resulting in too much acid in the stomach. If you then take an antacid, this plays additional havoc with the digestive process. Eventually such habits can lead to chronic indigestion and too much stress for the gastrointestinal tract.

It would be best to eat complex carbohydrates at one meal, protein at another, and fruits as snacks between meals. Protein meals take a long time to digest, and can leave you with less energy for several hours after eating. Much of your energy is used just to digest the protein, with blood channeled from other parts of the body to the digestive organs to help with the work. Eating fruit 10 to 15 minutes before a protein-heavy meal can prevent blood-glucose levels from declining during digestion.

What About Fiber?

Fiber, quite simply, is made up of carbohydrates that the human body cannot digest. In the not too distant past, many people thought that because it was indigestible, it served no useful purpose. As most of us now know, fiber acts as a kind of super janitorial service for the intestines. It scrubs the walls of the colon and bowels, hastens digestion and helps eliminate toxins, including some powerful cancer-causing chemicals. Fibrous foods stimulate and exercise the mouth, gums, and facial muscles. Fiber also fills you up, so you don't have to snack so often. Fiber is not found in meats or cheeses, and is found only minimally in refined carbohydrates and highly processed foods. In other words, it is lacking in the typical American diet.

Fiber should be eaten in its natural form. If you are in fairly good health, 40 to 60 grams, or 1 to 2 ounces a day of fiber from natural sources should be adequate. If occasional periods of irregularity are a problem, a few extra tablespoons of untreated, unheated oat germ, wheat bran, or even a tasty variation such as rice or corn bran can be sprinkled over your morning cereal or evening salad. If you prefer to use fruits and salads to meet your roughage requirements, a raw salad for lunch and a partially cooked grain salad such as tabouli for dinner, plus a big puree of fresh fruit in season, are good choices.

All vegetables were not created equal in terms of fiber. Root vegetables such as carrots are at the top of the list: their crunchy quality and hardness indicate a high fiber yield. They also require exercise of your jaws and teeth. Buy produce in season, buy it fresh, and eat it raw when possible. Vegetables can be grated for uncooked salads. But do not neglect the less common tubers: yams, kohlrabi, parsnips, and eggplant. Never peel away any vegetable skin if it isn't essential to your recipe to do so; much of the plant's roughage and nutrients are stored in and near the skin.

The whole legume family deserves special attention. Sprouting peas, chickpeas, mung beans, and lentils rather than cooking them rewards you with the full value of the live food, including minerals, amino acids, and carbohydrate energy. Remember to steam bean sprouts briefly before serving.

A little bran every day will improve your health and regularity, but there's no substitute for a well-balanced diet. And no two fibers are the same. Fiber in fruits and vegetables is different from that in grains. Include them all.

Take, for instance, the fiber in citrus fruits. If you've had a grapefruit or orange for breakfast, you've already had a beneficial two-carbohydrate food factor—protopectin. The pulp of all citrus fruits contains this combination of cellulose plus pectin.

The cellulose in the citrus fruit absorbs fluid from your intestines. So as it enlarges, it quickly pushes along any contents in the intestinal tract. Meanwhile, the pectin becomes gelatinous, and counters the absorbing effects of cellulose. It provides lubrication and ensures smooth passage for the food.

In addition, protopectin helps you get maximum value from the other nutritious foods you eat and enhances your system's use of dietary fats. This, in turn, helps provide some protection against the cardiovascular dangers posed by high cholesterol levels.

3

Fats

Americans get nearly half of their calories from fat. Our overindulgence in fatty foods has taken its toll by contributing to weight gain as well as degeneration of the heart and blood vessels. The American Heart Association recommends that we reduce the amount of saturated fat and cholesterol in our diets to 30 percent of daily calories to decrease blood cholesterol levels, prevent heart disease, and reduce the risk of certain cancers. Some Americans are heeding this call. However, many continue to eat high-fat diets and the number of overweight people continues to rise.

About half of American adults and 20 percent of children are overweight, twice the numbers of just 30 years ago. During the 1990s, the prevalence of obesity in the United States jumped from 12 percent to nearly 18 percent, with the highest increases in the young and well-educated. Fat intake is not the only cause of this bulging of America, but it is certainly a major contributor. In 1996, the U.S. Department of Agriculture (USDA) issued new rules to limit the fat (and cholesterol and sodium) content of school lunches. In 2000, it reported that the share of calories children obtained from total and saturated fats continued to come in at higher than recommended amounts.

We should not avoid fat completely. Fats are essential—albeit overconsumed—elements of a sound diet. *Reducing* the fat in one's diet doesn't mean *eliminating* it. People need not overreact, just act.

Fats serve many important functions. They are a highly concentrated source of energy. They help prevent viral infections. Fats protect the heart, blood vessels, and internal organs. Fats slow down the aging process, and help keep skin healthy. They also are essential for the utilization of nutrients and the production of hormones. In fact, much of the body's chemistry revolves around the proper utilization of fat.

Fat yields 9 calories per gram when it is burned up or oxidized. Proteins and carbohydrates each yield only 4 calories per gram. Therefore, a little bit of fat goes a long way in carrying out normal body functions.

Types of Fats

Fats contain an alcohol called glycerol and fatty acids. Certain fatty acids can be manufactured by the body. Others can only be obtained from foods.

There are two types of fats—saturated and unsaturated. The unsaturated fats are further categorized as polyunsaturated and monounsaturated. All fats are actually combinations of saturated and unsaturated fatty acids, and we need both each day. But primarily, the fats in our diet should be of an unsaturated quality.

SATURATED FATS Saturated fats are found in animal food sources such as meat and dairy products. Technically speaking, fat is saturated if the carbon atom chain that makes it up is also saturated with hydrogen atoms. You can tell if fat is saturated if it turns solid at room temperature. Examples of saturated fats include butter, lard, coconut oil, the fatty part of chicken, fish, veal, lamb, pork, and beef (the actual marbled fat that you can see). Coconut and palm oils are also saturated fats.

The saturated fats have been associated with increased levels of serum cholesterol and an increased risk of developing cardiovascular diseases. But small amounts are needed by the body. The liver needs it, for example, to produce cholesterol. The American Heart Association recommends that we get less than 10 percent of our calories from saturated fats.

UNSATURATED FATS Unsaturated fats are primarily found in grains, legumes, seeds, nuts, and the oils derived from them, including corn oil, safflower oil, sunflower oil, and soy oil. All of these fats are liquid at room temperature. These unsaturated oils should represent the majority of our fat intake. Unsaturated fats should be used because they provide us with the essential fatty acids that the body cannot make on its own. They have several functions: controlling high blood pressure; helping form prostaglandins (important chemicals for a host of bodily functions); and regulating the ability of substances to enter and leave cells.

POLYUNSATURATED FATS

The essential fatty acids are all polyunsaturated. Our systems can make saturated and even some monounsaturated fats from carbohydrates, but not the polyunsaturated ones. So we must supply these substances from our diet.

What are the vital functions for which we need polyunsaturated fatty acids? First, they are an important part of the membranes that interconnect every cell in our body. Almost all of our cells have both inner and outer membranes. Most of the enzymes in the body are strung along the inner cell membranes, which form a physical locus for the performance of our metabolic functions. And how these membranes influence our enzymes depends largely on the fatty acids in them. A membrane with a high proportion of saturated fat will be very stiff. On the other hand, a higher proportion of mono- and polyunsaturated fats will allow it to function in a more balanced, responsive way.

A second function performed by fatty acids is to make a special class of hormones, the prostaglandins. A classic hormone is made in one gland—the thyroid, for example—and travels throughout the body giving various signals to cells. Prostaglandins, on the other hand, are made throughout the body. Every single cell, with the exception of the red blood cells, makes prostaglandin. These hormones don't travel far, though, and tend to be destroyed after one passage through the circulatory system. They regulate the local responses of the body to other stimuli, including other hormones, brain chemicals, and drugs.

There are about 50 different biologically active prostaglandins, and the balance between these hormones can have a profound effect on our bodies' functions. Since prostaglandins are manufactured from various fatty acids, an imbalance in the intake of fatty acids can disturb the balance between prostaglandins and trigger a wide range of disorders. Heart disease, cancer, and AIDS, as well as allergies, asthma, and pre-menstrual syndrome are consistently accompanied by prostaglandin imbalances.

The fats in fish such as tuna steak, salmon, mackerel, and sardines contain omega-3, an essential fatty acid that has been found to reduce the risk of heart disease as well as certain types of cancer. Omega-3 is also found in flaxseed. Omega-6, the polyunsaturated fat in corn and safflower oil, is also essential for the body. Unfortunately, it has become too prevalent in our modern diets (see below). It may actually contribute to heart disease and tumor growth.

MONOUNSATURATED FATS

Canola oil and olive oil are high in monounsaturated fats. Evidence has shown that these fats actually help protect the heart by lowering the blood's level of low-density lipoprotein (the "bad" cholesterol) and raising its level of high-density lipoprotein (the "good" cholesterol). In one 1999 study, diets high in olive oil, peanut oil and peanuts/peanut butter were found to lower LDL cholesterol by as much as 14 percent.

TRANS FATS

Trans fats are created by hydrogenation, the process by which liquid oils are made more solid. What actually occurs is that hydrogen atoms are added to an unsaturated fat molecule, making it partially or completely saturated. Many types of margarine, shortening, pastries, and prepared fried foods contain trans-fatty acids. Trans fat has been found to increase blood cholesterol and therefore the risk of heart disease. Some manufacturers and restaurants have come up with healthier alternatives to trans fats that work just as well.

Cholesterol

Cholesterol is a crystalline substance found in the brain, nerves, liver, blood, and bile.

In the right amounts, it is vital to the body. It helps digest and transport important fats. When blood levels of cholesterol get too high, it can clog the arteries and strain the heart. Low-density lipoproteins (LDLs) are the compounds associated with an increased risk of atherosclerosis, in which the arteries become thickened and blood flow is blocked. High-density lipoproteins (HDLs) assume the opposite role. They clean up cholesterol debris in the blood and help prevent fatty buildup in the arteries.

Safe serum cholesterol levels are generally between 125 and 200 milligrams per deciliter (mg/dL) of blood. For most people with levels above 225, the liver is sluggish or out of balance. When assessing cholesterol, it is also important to look at the ratio of HDL to total serum cholesterol. Ratios of 4:1 or better are desirable. According to the American Heart Association, you may be at increased risk for heart attack and stroke if your total cholesterol is 240 mg/dL or higher and your HDL is less than 35 mg/dL.

Cholesterol is both made by the body and obtained from food. Food sources high in cholesterol include egg yolks, organ meats, poultry, fish, and dairy products. Many of these foods are also high in saturated fats. Plant-based foods such as peanut butter, olives, and beans, even those that are high in fats and oils, do not contain cholesterol.

How Much Fat Do You Need?

There is considerable disagreement regarding how much fat is necessary and appropriate in the diet. Estimates range from 10 to 30 percent of total caloric intake. To be safe, our consumption of calories from fat probably should be limited to 15 to 20 percent of our total calories. A quarter of these could be saturated. The rest should come from the unsaturated fats found in cooking and salad oils or, more beneficially, from those naturally occurring oils in vegetables, grains, legumes, nuts, and seeds. In their natural state—if they are unbleached, unadulterated, and have not been clarified or chemically altered to destroy their nutritional benefits—oils not only provide us with fat that the body can use, but also supply vitamin E, a substance that has powerful antioxidant properties. Antioxidants help neutralize the toxic free radicals roaming our bodies. Vitamin E promotes nerve growth and keeps cells functioning normally.

FATS AND DIETING One of the reasons doctors may prescribe high-fat, high-protein, low-carbohydrate diets is because of the ability of fat and protein to keep you feeling full after a meal, allaying between-meal hunger pangs. If, on the other hand, you eat a complex carbohydrate in the form of a grain or vegetable, it is digested and goes through your system in a matter of 30 to 80 minutes. You benefit from the energy and you're not taxing your digestive system. But it also means there will be a tendency to get hungry sooner.

After all, we tend to gain weight in large part because we get hungry and have snacks between meals. A fatty or high-protein food eaten at mealtime will require 1 to 4 hours of digestion just to empty out the stomach. As long as you have that much food in your stomach, your appetite is suppressed so you do not feel hungry. Snacks usually come in the form of high-sugar, refined carbohydrate foods like candy bars and soft drinks. Bypassing the midmorning, midafternoon, and late evening snack can mean eliminating 400 to 900 calories. In a period of a week you would be able to knock off a pound just by modifying your diet to reduce snacks and increase the protein and fat content.

Essential Fatty Acid Deficiency

As mentioned, the essential fatty acids are those that the body cannot make on its own.

Essential fatty acids include the omega-6 family derived from plant oils (linoleic acid and arachidonic acid) and the omega-3 family derived from fish oils (gamma-linolenic acid, eicosapentaenoic acid and docosahexaenoic acid). Omega-6 is important for blood clotting and constriction of blood vessels. Omega-3 helps regulate blood cholesterol and promotes the health of the immune, cardiovascular, and nervous systems. Dietary changes over the past century have created a fatty acid problem throughout our society. While our grandparents' diets contained small but equal amounts of omega-6 and omega-3 fatty acids, our diets now lean more heavily toward the omega-6s.

Signs of an essential fatty acid deficiency include dry skin, rough skin on the backs of the arms or thighs, brittle fingernails, and dry, unmanageable hair. Another warning sign is excessive thirst, which usually is not accompanied by a corresponding increase in urination. These are not surefire guides, though; vitamin A, B_6, or zinc deficiencies can produce similar symptoms.
Intense menstrual cramps, asthma, eczema, and arthritis may be signs of an excess production of certain prostaglandins. Families with a tendency toward allergies may have an inherited dysfunction in the way their bodies process essential fatty acids, and may require more to offset this problem.

CORRECTING THE DEFICIENCY Americans consume the greatest number of nutritional supplements in the world. But taking in fatty acids as supplements is no magic formula. They have to be utilized in the body, and that requires a balance of vitamins and minerals. Instead of taking oil supplements, we can increase the efficiency with which our bodies use essential fatty acids by taking extra zinc and B vitamins. Many people have a problem absorbing and metabolizing fatty acids, as noted above. But if the basic levels of these substances aren't provided, it is impossible to tell if the problem is metabolic.

The first step, then, is to boost intake of the omega-3 fatty acids. Unfortunately, the nutrients in certain fish that contain omega-3 are removed by the time they are purchased. For example, sardines are usually canned not in their own oil, but in olive or soybean oil. In fact, due to potential spoilage problems, it's illegal to can sardines in their own oil. Fresh sardines, however, and almost any fresh cold water fish, are good sources of omega-3.

Nut butters are also rich in omega-3, particularly those made from walnuts and chestnuts. So are cold-pressed nut oils. "Cold pressed" is actually a misnomer, though, because the process does heat the oil to a degree, resulting in a loss of some of the valuable fatty acids. In the processing of nut butters some oils also are lost or altered through exposure to air during chopping and grinding. These losses, however, are far outweighed by the food value that does remain.

As mentioned, one of the richest sources of omega-3 is food-grade flaxseed (linseed) oil. Whole-grain winter wheat is palatable and practical. Vegetable leaves have fish oil-type fatty acids in high proportion to other types of fat, but have so little total fat that they are not a very efficient way of supplying these oils.

One way to ensure that we get enough essential fatty acids for ideal functioning is to remove foods from our diet that can interfere with their processing. Saturated fats and partially or fully hydrogenated vegetable oils should be avoided. Sugar and alcohol also hamper the efficient metabolizing of fatty acids.

Evening primrose oil is more similar to corn oil than to fish oil in its fatty acids. It has an advantage over corn or safflower oil, though; it bypasses a step in the body's metabolic process that is required to utilize the other oils. People who have an enzyme deficiency that makes it difficult to metabolize essential fatty acids can use evening primrose oil, which doesn't require this enzyme.

Oils lose much of their value when they are used for cooking. Heat destroys much of their fatty acid content. So if you're going to rely on oils as supplements, they should be taken in an uncooked form. You can use the oils as salad dressing or mix them into margarine. In addition, the essential fatty acids in oils oxidize easily, and therefore have a short shelf life. The byproducts of oxidation are dangerous, so as you increase your intake of essential fatty acids it is wise to also take in antioxidants—particularly vitamin A and selenium—to safeguard yourself against oxidation.

All of the substances that supply concentrated essential fatty acids should be used carefully as supplements, as it is possible to "overdose" on essential fatty acid intake. It is also important to be aware of a competitive relationship between some different types of fatty acids in the body's metabolic processes. Taking too much of one type can produce a relative deficiency of the other.

The Hazards of Fat

Many people like deep-fried foods such as french fries, onion rings, fried fish, potato chips, and doughnuts. These are prepared with fatty oils heated to high temperatures that alter the chemical structure of the fat, creating free fatty acids that can have an irritating effect upon the stomach and on the sensitive mucous linings of the intestines. Eating fried foods frequently can set into motion the ultimate dysfunction of your intestine. Colitis, spastic colon, or some other form of irritable intestine condition may be the result.

Heated fats also slow down digestive time. The longer fat is cooked, the more difficult it is for the enzymes in the stomach and the intestine to break it down. Liquid fats are easier to digest. Oils (or unsaturated fats) go through the system much more rapidly than saturated fats.

As mentioned, when you have a lot of fat in your stomach after a meal, you will have less energy. Your energy is being diverted to facilitating the proper digestion, utilization, absorption, and elimination of food—a lengthy process. Blood and oxygen, also are diverted, even from your brain, just for digestion.

Nearly 95 percent of the fat we consume is digested and used by the body. It is fine to have some amount of fat as reserve, but in the absence of regular, daily exercise the muscles begin to atrophy and fat infiltrates into the muscle. Fat then takes the place of unused, atrophied muscles. We lose our strength, endurance, and stamina, and we become more susceptible to body injury, accident, and disease.

4

Protein

A thick, rare steak, a hamburger, a platter of fried chicken—the joys of protein? For many of us, protein equals meat, which equals strength, endurance, growth, and health. We have been misled! Meat is only one of several possible dietary sources of protein. Moreover, not all meats fit the bill. Cured ham has only 16 percent protein. Hot dogs have only 7 percent, less than dried skim milk, which has over 34 percent and sunflower seeds with 27 percent. Lentils have more than 23 percent protein.

Meat has become the predominant and most expensive source of protein in the average American diet. Our image of protein as the one most important nutrient ("protein" is derived from the Greek "protos," meaning first) has led us to eat so much meat that we often consume more protein than we need each day.

On average, Americans eat nearly 100 grams or 6 1/2 ounces of protein daily. All most of us actually need is three-quarters of that. And despite the legends, even athletes are better off increasing their carbohydrate intake rather than their protein consumption if they want to increase their endurance and stamina. Eggs, dairy products, grains, legumes, nuts, and seeds are all excellent sources of protein that can supplement meat or replace it in the diet.

What Are Proteins?

Proteins are the building blocks of life. They are the basic materials from which all our cells, tissues, and organs are constructed. Only water represents a larger percentage of total body weight than protein. Proteins are constantly being replaced, 24 hours a day throughout life, as our bodies use and lose cellular materials. The optimal intake of high-quality proteins allows the body to grow and maintain healthy bones, skin, teeth, muscles, and nerves.

Protein helps maintain the blood count and allow the metabolism—the body's ability to use food sources—to function at its highest level. Hemoglobin, the part of the red blood cells that provides oxygen to the cells, is made primarily of protein.

When we think of protein, we usually think of it as a body-building substance found in muscles. However, only one-third of our body's protein is concentrated in muscle tissue. Protein is part of every living cell in our body, from the hair on our heads to the nails on our toes. Skin, nails, hair, muscles, cartilage, and tendons all have fibrous protein as their main constituent.

At 4 calories per gram, protein is also a source of energy. When carbohydrates and fats are in short supply, protein can be converted to glucose, providing necessary energy to the brain and spinal cord. Protein molecules called enzymes start the metabolic process. They are required for hundreds of necessary chemical reactions and interactions in our bodies. Enzymes allow energy to be stored and released in each cell, and they allow protein, fats, carbohydrates, and cholesterol to be synthesized by the liver. Protein is responsible for keeping blood slightly alkaline, and it is the raw material out of which the antibodies that shield us from infection are created. Hormones, which regulate metabolism, also contain some protein.

THE ESSENTIAL AMINO ACIDS Amino acids are the chief components of protein. Some amino acids can created by the body itself. Eight amino acids cannot be created by the body, and therefore must be obtained from the diet. Known as the essential amino acids, they are threonine, valine, tryptophan, lysine, methionine, histidine, phenylalanine, and isoleucine.

Amino acids are necessary for certain vitamins and minerals to be utilized. The amino acid tryptophan, for example, initiates the production of the B vitamin, niacin. Amino acids help transport fats through the bloodstream by combining with them to form lipoproteins.

All the necessary amino acids must be present simultaneously in sufficient amounts so that cells can make the proteins they need to grow. This means that if any one amino acid is not present, the protein cannot be constructed. Since protein cannot be stored (except, perhaps, by lactating mothers), it is necessary to eat complete proteins at each meal. Complete proteins contain all eight essential amino acids. If you are not eating animal products, you should mix your protein sources to form complete proteins (See below). To provide the body with only some of the amino acids it needs is like being a baker who buys 100 pounds of flour and 100 pounds of shortening, but only 1 ounce of yeast. He can bake only one or two cakes with that amount of yeast. But what happens to all of that flour and shortening? In the body, unused amino acids might be excreted, or broken down and oxidized for energy and other metabolic needs. Protein deficiencies occur when we don't consume enough protein for our body's needs, or when the proteins we do consume lack one or more of the essential amino acids.

Eggs, meat, fowl, fish, grains, legumes, nuts, seeds, vegetables, fruits, and dairy products contain complete proteins. Partially complete proteins may contain all eight, but not in the correct proportions. Thus foods high in partially complete proteins, such as brewer's yeast (also called nutritional yeast), wheat germ, tofu, peanuts, and certain micro-sea algae, should be eaten in combination with other protein foods.

How Much Protein Do We Need?

The recommended amount of protein for most adults is about 55 to 65 grams per day. Pregnant and lactating women may need more. As mentioned, the average American actually gets a lot more. Some, however, do not get enough.

TOO LITTLE PROTEIN Eating an inadequate amount of high-quality protein forces our bodies to break down more tissue than it can build up, resulting in overall deterioration. Some symptoms of protein deficiency are muscle weakness, loss of endurance, fatigue, growth retardation, loss of weight, irritability, lowered immune response, poor healing, and anemia. Pregnant women must be extra careful to avoid this deficiency, since it will not only affect their health but that of their unborn baby. A protein deficiency can promote a miscarriage, premature delivery, or toxemia. Its effects on the baby's development may set the stage for chronic diseases later in life.

The amino acids in grains are high quality and will maintain life and growth. When supplemented with foods containing other amino acids, they may yield even higher quality protein in greater quantities. For example, wheat is a fairly good protein. It can maintain life, and millions of poor people have subsisted on bread or cereal alone for long periods of time. However, wheat alone cannot promote optimal growth, and even adults who restrict their protein to one or two food groups or types of foods (a mono-diet) run the very real risk of lowering their body's immune response. Remember, proteins also are needed for the body's natural disease fighters—the antibodies that combat infections. The poor quality of the hair and skin of those on mono-diets reflects their nutritional deficiencies. Their bodies function much as cars do that run on four cylinders when they were built for six or eight.

TOO MUCH PROTEIN Researchers now agree that American meat eaters and vegetarians alike are getting more protein than they need. A study done by the U.S. Department of Agriculture (USDA) found that the average consumer of animal products gets more than 165 percent of their recommended daily allowance for protein. Children fed by their overcautious—and sometimes protein-fanatical

—parents get a whopping 209 percent. Surprisingly, vegetarians get only 15 percent less protein than their nonvegetarian counterparts do.

When it comes to certain nutrients, the more the merrier. For example, research indicates that water-soluble vitamin C helps fortify our immune system, and in high doses it may even prevent or reverse certain forms of cancer. In the case of protein, however, more does not mean better. In the short run, our bodies can cope with an excess of protein by burning it for energy. This may be inefficient, since protein takes more energy than carbohydrates or fat to metabolize, but it is not harmful. However, over the long run, too much protein can hurt. Ammonium is released when protein is burned in the cells. The ammonium is turned into urea and excreted through the kidneys. Along with the excess of sodium that generally characterizes the animal-protein diet, this stepped-up excretion process taxes the kidneys. Too much animal protein can also lead to localized edema and generalized dehydration, as people on high-protein diets require more water than others do. To process a high-protein diet the body may require up to four times as much water as it would need for a high-carbohydrate diet.

There are numerous other side effects of eating too much protein. Too much protein causes you to lose calcium through the urine, sometimes resulting in a deficiency in that important mineral. High-protein intake has been linked to osteoporosis, a degenerative disease that causes the demineralization and loss of calcium from bones by increasing urinary excretion of calcium. Older women suffer most from this condition.

High-protein diets can be dangerous. For example, 8 ounces of beef supplies more than 500 calories, while it is only 22 percent protein. But it also contains lots of fat and water. High-protein diets provide too much saturated fats, cholesterol, and sodium, all of which are implicated in heart disease.

Statistics show that each year Americans approximately 200 pounds of red meat, 50 pounds of chicken and turkey, 10 pounds of assorted fish, 300 eggs, and 250 pounds of various dairy products. In this country, animal sources of protein often contain large amounts of synthetic hormones, saturated fats, antibiotics, pesticide residues, nitrates, and a host of other potentially harmful ingredients. Although we've heard warnings about the nasty ingredients in those plump "butterball" turkeys, about the effects of charcoal broiling or frying fatty beef, the residues in milk, and the mercury and toxic wastes in fish, we're still buying them.

The Egg Project

It is possible to create complete, or high-quality, proteins by combining foods so that those that are low in some amino acids are eaten together with foods that are high in those same acids. These complementary proteins—all from plant sources—can supply protein needs quite nicely.

More than a dozen years ago, a review of the available literature on protein requirements found that there was an inconsistency between the prevalent beliefs of the scientific community and the personal experiences of many individuals. The people who should have been feeling healthy because they were getting more than adequate amounts of protein in their diets were frequently not receiving the healthful benefits from the protein. There was an escalating incidence of kidney disease in America that had no apparent cause. The prevailing myth was that all of the protein from animal sources was complete, meaning that it contains all the essential amino acids and that the protein plant foods was incomplete—capable of sustaining life, but not of promoting optimum growth and maturation.

Dr. Hillard Fitsky, who has a background in computer sciences, my brother Steven, and I did a computer-assisted analysis of the 110 or so most commonly consumed vegetarian foods. We matched each one of the amino acids in the given food against the food source that is considered to contain the most complete protein, the chicken egg.

As the research progressed, it became clear that many of the assumptions concerning protein and food selection were grossly in error. First, we found that not all animal protein is high quality and complete. Generally, only 40 percent is high quality. Second, we confirmed that not all vegetarian foods are incomplete. To the contrary, the vast majority of vegetarian foods are complete, containing all of the essential amino acids. The bean or legume family in particular tended to have protein in large quantities and of a high quality. This made it easier to understand how the Asian and Indian cultures have been able to sustain themselves and demonstrate remarkable longevity on a limited vegetarian diet.

Taking this logic one step further, we reasoned that if single foods in the grain, legume, and sea vegetable families tended to have remarkably high-quality protein, what would be the result of combining two or three of these together? What we found was that the overall quality of the protein tended to increase tremendously. Not only did specific combinations approximate the completeness of the egg, but some actually exceeded the egg in terms of the amounts of complete, usable protein they provided.

Of the 5,000 combinations computed over a 5-year period, all offered protein of a quality nearer to the egg than the closest animal protein food source, milk. Other animal protein foods, including fish, hamburger, veal, chicken, and cheese all proved to offer far less complete and less usable protein than that available in the right combinations of vegetarian foods. Of course, the plant foods had far fewer calories, none of the cholesterol, the high saturated fat, the toxic growth-stimulating hormones, or the antibiotic residues such as penicillin that we find in the animal products. They offered instead quality protein, abundant fiber, plentiful B vitamins, vitamin A, vitamin C, minerals, and a full spectrum of other nutrients.

Soybeans and Other Legumes

Soybeans not only contain high amounts of protein, but also are a rich source of calcium, iron, zinc, phosphorus, magnesium, B vitamins, omega-3 fatty acids, and fiber. Many of us have known about the health benefits of soy for years. In late 1998, the Food and Drug Administration formally recognized the importance of soy, and announced that 25 grams of soy protein a day as part of a diet that is low in saturated fat and cholesterol may reduce the risk of heart disease. Many studies have shown that soy contains important disease-fighting substances known as phytochemicals. Some of the most important phytochemicals in soy are protease inhibitors, phytates, lecithin, and isoflavones. These substances may help in preventing cancer, reversing osteoporosis, and easing menopause.

Soybeans are low in the amino acid tryptophan but high in lysine. Their biological values can be enhanced by combining them with complementary proteins like nuts, grains, and seeds, which are low in lysine but high in tryptophan. In countless combinations, soybeans can make satisfying, delicious dishes.

Tofu, made by curdling soybean milk and packing the solids in layers of cloth, has a protein value—in terms of completeness, digestibility, and other factors—only slightly less than animal flesh. It can be made even higher in quality by combining it with grains such as brown rice. Soybean sprouts and soy flour can also be used in cooking to enhance the complementary values of other foods.

A 4-ounce serving of dry roasted soy nuts provides 39.6 grams of soy protein. Four ounces of firm tofu offers 15.8 grams. Tempeh, another soy product, provides 19 grams and cooked soybeans give 16.6 grams per 4-ounce serving.

Other legumes, such as chick-peas and lentils, are similarly low in certain amino acids, but high in others. They, too, can be combined with grains, nuts, and seeds to form complementary proteins of high nutritional value. Consider how the rest of the world, which has not had the luxury of high meat diets, subsists. Central American and Caribbean nations use beans and rice as staples. Middle Eastern countries combine sesame paste with chick-peas, while Italians mix lentils, chick-peas, and other beans with pasta.

GRAINS AND CEREALS Grains and cereals make ideal complements to legumes because they are generally high in tryptophan and low in isoleucine and lysine. Grains and cereals supply half the world's protein and are great sources of fiber, too. They do not need to be complemented with meat products to raise the protein values. The myth has been that cereals, grains, and seeds are incomplete, and poor sources of protein even when combined. This is false. Consider breakfast cereals with soy milk, macaroni and cheese, or tofu eggs—or real eggs if you prefer—served with whole grain breads. These combinations work well because they complement each other.

Preparing Protein Foods

Protein digestion is improved by correct cooking practices. Moderate heating of most protein foods increases their digestibility, particularly in the case of beans, grains, and meat. Beans and other legumes contain several toxins (such as trypsin inhibitors) that can inhibit digestion, but they become harmless when they are cooked or sprouted.

Legumes should never be eaten raw: many contain strong toxins that must be neutralized by heat. All grains and some legumes contain phytic acid in their outer husks. In the intestines, these can form phytates. Phytates can bind with zinc, calcium, and other minerals and can cause deficiencies in these minerals. Grains should be sprouted, baked with yeast (unleavened breads contain more phytates than leavened breads), or cooked thoroughly. Vegetarians should supplement their diets with zinc and calcium, or foods containing them. Zinc is present in seafood, peas, corn, egg yolk, carrots, and yeast.

It is also important to cook meat slowly and thoroughly. Pork harbors a parasite that can cause trichinosis if it is not thoroughly cooked. Other meats should be broiled or roasted. Excessive heating of any protein, whether of animal or plant origin, may cause what are known as cross-linkages (the same mechanisms that cause your hair to stay curled after a permanent wave). Cross-linkages make it difficult for protein-digesting enzymes to break protein down into simple amino acids so they can be absorbed. Therefore, it is best to stay away from deep-fried or overdone protein foods. Milk and milk products are especially sensitive to heat, and should not be heated above the boiling point.

If you have trouble digesting milk, you might try yogurt, buttermilk, or other cultured milk products. These contain live, healthy microorganisms that "predigest" lactose, the sugar in milk that many people cannot tolerate, changing it to more easily absorbed lactic acid. Other ideas: sprinkle brewer's yeast (if you are not allergic to it) on your cereal or blend it with milk, combine tofu with algae in salads, add wheat germ to lentil burgers, and spread peanut butter on whole wheat bread.

Protein and Dieting

A 1999 survey published in the *Journal of the American Medical Association* found that more than two-thirds of all adults in the United States are trying to lose or maintain their weight. It is estimated that nearly 80 million Americans in any given year are following a dietary program to shed the pounds. Regrettably, many will be going on one version or another of a high-protein, low-carbohydrate diet, with the misconception that protein is low in calories. In fact, the protein foods recommended on most of these diets are very high in calories.

One gram of protein yields 4 calories. Filet mignon, for example, is nearly 40 to 50 percent fat; a single 10-ounce portion can contain up to 1,400 calories. A certain nutritional sleight of hand makes these diets work for some people. Since meats require 6 to 8 hours to digest, you will probably not be very hungry during digestion. To really control overeating, exercise remains more important than limiting calorie intake, as exercise increases metabolic efficiency.

Many diet doctors claim that high-protein diets melt away fat. When we want to lose weight, they say, we should limit our diets to beef, hard-boiled eggs, chicken, and cottage cheese. But these foods contain substantial amounts of saturated fats and lack carbohydrates. Such low-carbohydrate, high-protein diets create an abnormal biochemical state within the body, resulting in weight loss.

But it is not a healthy weight loss. In effect, these diets prevent proteins from being stored as fat, leading to a buildup of high-calorie compounds called ketones in the bloodstream; this is known as ketosis. Many dieters experience anorexia due to the toxic effects of ketones. They eliminate large amounts of water and salt, which contributes to weight reduction. Under normal conditions, our bodies would not excrete this unburned high-energy compound. Ketosis, therefore, can lead to dehydration, burning or wasting essential body proteins, kidney infection, kidney stones and renal damage. In several cases, it has lead to coma and death. These more dangerous conditions usually occur only during starvation or as a metabolic side effect of diabetes.

Before embarking on the new monthly best-seller's advice, consider the potential long-term health hazards. It is not uncommon for participants in fad diets to experience bleeding gums, depression, lowered resistance to infection, fatigue, weakness, irritability, and dizziness. A high-protein diet has been shown to encourage the onset of degenerative diseases such as arteriosclerosis (hardening of the arteries). Excesses of the amino acid methionine can break down into the nonessential amino acid homocysteine, which can irritate the walls of the arteries, generating fat deposits in these vessels. And if we omit foods with carbohydrates or with fiber, like fruits, grains, and vegetables, we may be inducing vitamin and mineral deficiencies and hurting our digestive systems.

Protein and Athletics

One of the most enduring myths about protein is its connection with athletic prowess. Despite scientific evidence to the contrary, many athletes and trainers alike still equate protein with strength. This false notion is based upon the premise that protein, especially animal protein, is turned into muscle when ingested. But what is really needed during a strenuous workout or competition is a quality source of energy. For this, protein is actually a less efficient source than complex carbohydrates, since carbohydrates have more deliverable calories.

Depending on the athletic training schedule a person follows, some extra protein may be advisable. This can amount to about 10 to 30 more grams of high-quality protein daily, which will be used to replace the nitrogen lost by perspiration and to provide the extra protein needed during periods of accelerated muscle growth. However, after the training period, the athlete only needs more calories than the average person does, not more protein. Such misconceptions get many hungry athletes into trouble each year.

Many trainers are well aware of the scientific void behind the "steak and egg" fortification diets, yet they continue high-protein diets because their athletes believe in them. Yet these athletes are hurting themselves in many ways. As we work, play, or sleep, our systems are maintaining a biochemical balance of amino acids. If we make a habit of consuming more than we need, our bodies may start abnormally increasing the rate of amino acid replacement in our cells. This rapid turnover of cells is believed to accelerate the aging process. A high-protein diet, therefore, may be counterproductive to longevity. Athletes on high-protein diets also run the risk of dehydration. Protein does not give us that extra edge. If anything, complex carbohydrates may.

5

Vitamins

Vitamins act as cofactors or catalysts in enzyme reactions throughout the body. They enable these enzyme reactions to proceed at a faster pace than they would if the vitamin was not present. Different vitamins interact with different enzymes. For instance, vitamin A interacts with enzymes found in the eye. Vitamin K reacts with enzymes in blood cells and helps with blood coagulation. Other functions of vitamins are being still determined.

Vitamins exist in one of two forms: water soluble and fat soluble. If a vitamin is water soluble that means it exists in water, like urine or blood. If a vitamin is fat soluble then it exists in lipid or fatty tissues, such as nerve cell membranes or fat cells. Water-soluble vitamins dissolve quickly and can't be stored in the body. As soon as they are exposed to water or blood they dissolve and then are excreted. But the fat-soluble vitamins are stored in the fatty tissues and don't dissolve. They can accumulate in the body. They do not need to be replenished every day like the water-soluble vitamins do. The downside of fat-soluble vitamins is that they can accumulate into toxic doses in the fat tissues and are harder to get out of the body.

The fat-soluble vitamins are vitamins A, D, E, and K. All the rest are water soluble.

In the United States, there are two standards to define doses of vitamins (as well as other nutrients): the MDR and the RDA. The MDR and RDA are currently being re-evaluated due to a lot of new research. The Minimum Daily Requirement (MDR) is defined as the smallest amount of a vitamin needed to prevent signs and symptoms of deficiency. The Recommended Dietary Allowance (RDA) is the recommended amount that is estimated to cover the nutritional requirements of 97 percent of the population, and is generally two to six times the MDR.

In the late 1990s, a major revision began to update and expand these standards. New values, collectively known as Dietary Reference Intakes (DRIs), are being introduced in stages over the next few years. At least three types of reference values will be determined: estimated average requirement, recommended dietary allowance, and tolerable upper intake level. The new DRIs will also list separate recommendations for adults aged 51 to 70, and those older than 70.

These new values take into account the changes in eating habits, physical activity, use of medications, and overall health that affect us as we age. According to the chairman of the committee overseeing this effort, "The new DRIs represent a major leap forward in nutrition science—from a primary concern for the prevention of deficiency to an emphasis on beneficial effects of healthy eating."

Vitamin A

Vitamin A is a fat-soluble, essential vitamin necessary for bones and teeth, sperm formation, epithelial growth (skin tissue), and vision. It is essential in the maintenance of the body's immune response, which helps the body fight infections. It helps maintain healthy skin and protects the mucous membranes of the lungs, throat, mouth, and nose. It also helps the body secrete the gastric juices necessary for protein digestion, and protects the linings of the digestive tract, kidneys, and bladder.

While abundant in carrots, especially in the form of fresh carrot juice, vitamin A is present in even higher concentrations in green leafy vegetables such as beet greens, spinach, and broccoli. Yellow or orange vegetables are also good sources. Eggs contain vitamin A, as do whole milk and milk products. Animal livers are concentrated sources of vitamin A. Care must be taken, however, when obtaining nutrients from livers because livers also are waste-filtering organs. Any hormone or chemical to which the animal was exposed will be concentrated in the liver.

One of the first symptoms of vitamin A deficiency is night blindness and the inability of the eyes to adjust to darkness. Other signs include male sterility, fatigue, unhealthy skin, loss of appetite, loss of sense of smell, and diarrhea.

The recommended daily intake of vitamin A for men ages 11 to 51+ is 1,000 micrograms RE/day (about 5,000 international units). For women of the same age 800 micrograms RE/day (about 4,000 international units) are recommended. (RE stands for "retinol equivalent," which is the standard measure for vitamin A). It is not difficult to obtain this amount from the foods mentioned above in moderate quantities. During times of disease, trauma, pregnancy, or lactation, supplements may be advisable, but should be administered under a physician's or nutritionist's direction, since megadoses of vitamin A can be harmful. Taking more than 50,000 international units per day can cause peeling skin, dermatitis, hair loss, bone and joint pain, headaches, anorexia, and liver injury.

The B Vitamin Complex

The B vitamin complex consists of an array of different components that have been individually identified through research. These are water-soluble vitamins needed by metabolizing cells throughout body. Sources are nutritional yeast, seeds, eggs, meats, and vegetables. There can be deficiencies in one or all of the B vitamins.

VITAMIN B$_1$ (THIAMINE) Vitamin B$_1$ is essential to normal metabolism and normal nerve function. It converts carbohydrates into glucose, which is the sole source of energy for the brain and nervous system. B$_1$ helps the heart by keeping it firm and resilient. It is found in a variety of foods, including whole grains, legumes, poultry, and fish.

A deficiency of vitamin B$_1$ may result in the degeneration of the insulating protective sheath (myelin) that covers certain nerve fibers. Nerves can become hypersensitive, causing irritability, sluggishness, forgetfulness, and apathy. If such nerve destruction continues, nerves in the legs may become weakened, and pain may develop in the legs and feet. Paralysis may result. A deficiency may also result in constipation, indigestion, anorexia, swelling, and heart trouble caused by increased blood circulation.

Adults need a daily minimum of 1 to 1.5 milligrams of vitamin B$_1$. If you drink tea or coffee, perspire a great deal, are under heavy stress, take antibiotics, or have a fever, your intake of vitamin B$_1$ should increase. Some nutritionists suggest that athletes increase their intake to 10 to 20 milligrams daily. Such quantities are not easily obtained from food alone. Therefore, a low potency, all-natural vitamin may be good insurance.

VITAMIN B$_2$ (RIBOFLAVIN) Vitamin B$_2$ helps promote proper growth and repair of tissues, and enhances a cell's ability to exchange gases such as oxygen and carbon dioxide in the blood. It helps release energy from the foods we eat, and is essential for good digestion, steady nerves, assimilation of iron, and normal vision. It is vital to the health of the entire glandular system, most particularly the adrenal glands, which are involved in stress control.

Dairy products, meat, poultry, fish, nutritional yeast, whole grains, leafy green vegetables, and the nutrient-rich soybean can provide ample supplies of vitamin B$_2$.

Lack of B$_2$ is one deficiency that can be seen readily: the tongue will become purplish red, inflamed, or shiny. Other symptoms are cracking at the corners of the lips, greasy skin, vision problems such as hypersensitivity to light, itchiness, bloodshot eyes or blurred sight, headaches, depression, insomnia, and loss of mental alertness.

A minimum of 1.4 milligrams of vitamin B$_2$ daily for adult males and 1.2 milligrams daily for females is recommended. Two servings of most grains will satisfy this requirement without difficulty.

VITAMIN B$_3$ (NIACIN) Vitamin B$_3$ is essential to every cell in the body. It is the fundamental material of two enzyme systems and helps transform sugar and fat into energy.

Many vital functions in the body's food processing plant would stop without an adequate supply of vitamin B$_3$. Low levels of this vitamin have been linked to mental illness and pellagra, a disease that produces disorders of the skin and intestinal tract.

You can get a reasonable amount of vitamin B$_3$ from green leafy vegetables, wheat germ, brewer's yeast, beans, peas, dried figs, prunes, and dates. Organ meats, salmon, and tuna are also plentiful sources.

Adult males need a minimum of 16 milligrams NE/day, and adult females need 14 milligrams NE daily. (NE stands for niacin equivalent, the standard measurement for vitamin B$_3$). Again, a low-potency vitamin is a worthwhile investment to be sure you are getting sufficient amounts of this nutrient. In too high doses, niacin can cause dilation of blood vessels and a flushing of the skin, as well as diarrhea, nausea, and vomiting. Studies have shown that excessive amounts of B$_3$ can cause glycogen (a starch that helps the body utilize the energy of sugars like glucose) to be consumed hyperactively by the muscles, resulting in the early onset of fatigue.

VITAMIN B$_5$ (PANTOTHENIC ACID) Vitamin B$_5$ also works in all our cells. It converts carbohydrates, fats, and protein to energy, acts as an antistress agent, and manufactures antibodies that fight germs in the blood. B$_5$ is found in many foods including eggs, peanuts, whole grains, beans, and organ meats.

The signs of deficiency include high susceptibility to illness and infection, digestive malfunctions such as abdominal pains and vomiting, muscular and nerve disturbances such as leg cramps, insomnia, and mental depression. For teenagers and adults, 5 milligrams per day are recommended. A low-potency vitamin supplement may be used.

VITAMIN B$_6$ (PYRIDOXINE) Vitamin B$_6$ nourishes the central nervous system, controls sodium/potassium levels in the blood, and assists in the production of red blood cells and hemoglobin. It helps protect against infection, and assists in manufacturing DNA and RNA, the acids that contain the genetic code for cell growth, repair, and multiplication. It is particularly valuable for those involved in endurance sports.

The best sources of B$_6$ are brewer's yeast, brown rice, bananas, and pears. It is also found in beef, pork liver, and fish such as salmon and herring. Kidney stones, polyneuropathy (nerve pain), muscle twitching, and severe dandruff are some of the signs of deficiency. Other signs include irritability, nervousness, weakness, dermatitis and other skin changes, and insomnia.

The official recommended daily amount is 1.2 to 1.7 milligrams per day of vitamin B$_6$. This amount is easily obtained from the food sources listed above. I would recommend up to 50 milligrams daily.

VITAMIN B$_{12}$ (COBALAMIN) This vitamin helps in metabolism of all proteins and amino acids and cell reactions called methylation. All B$_{12}$ is manufactured by microorganisms and is not found in fruits and vegetables. Fermented products, such as tofu or tempeh, and poultry and meat all contain vitamin B$_{12}$. Strict vegetarians who eat only fruit and vegetables need to take vitamin B$_{12}$ supplements. Deficiencies of B$_{12}$ can also be due to poor gastrointestinal absorption, which is measured by a Schilling test. There are two reasons for poor absorption: there is no intrinsic factor in the stomach (intrinsic factor is needed to complex with the vitamin B$_{12}$ for absorption) or there is no receptor in the intestines. The resulting anemia is called pernicious anemia. Deficiency can also result in neuropathy and mouth problems.

A daily minimum of 2.4 micrograms of vitamin B$_{12}$ is recommended. If you are a vegetarian, you should include a low-potency vitamin supplement with your diet.

FOLIC ACID Folic acid works mostly in the brain and nervous system. It is a vital component of spinal and extracellular fluid. It is necessary for the manufacture of DNA and RNA and helps convert amino acids. In recent years, research from around the world has shown that consuming extra folic acid before and during pregnancy can reduce the risk of having a child with a neural tube defect such as spina bifida. Unfortunately, the results of a 1999 study showed that only 13 percent of women aged 18 to 45 knew about folic acid's role in preventing birth defects.

Brewer's yeast, dark green leafy vegetables, wheat germ, oysters, salmon, and chicken all contain folic acid.

The official recommended intake is 400 micrograms daily. This is easily obtained from the food sources listed above. If you are pregnant, elderly, or suffer from any nervous disorder, additional amounts are needed. The Food and Nutrition Board recommends that pregnant women obtain extra folic acid from fortified cereal grains or from a supplement.

PARA-AMINOBENZOIC ACID (PABA) Para-aminobenzoic acid is a component of folic acid, and acts as a coenzyme in the body's metabolism of proteins. It helps manufacture healthy blood cells and can help heal skin disorders. In addition, it protects the skin against sunburn by absorbing the portions of those ultraviolet rays of the sun known to cause burns and even skin cancer.

Eggs, brewer's yeast, molasses, wheat germ, and whole grains are good sources of PABA. Signs of deficiency include digestive trouble, nervous tension, emotional instability, and blotchy skin.

No official daily requirements have been established for PABA. My recommended daily intake would be 400 to 600 international units.

CHOLINE Choline is present in all of our cellular membranes. It works to remove fat. It also helps regulate cholesterol levels and is vital to the liver's functions.

Choline aids in building and maintaining a healthy nervous system. If choline is not present in our system, the liver is unable to process any sort of fat. Fatty deposits in the liver interfere with its normal filtering function. A deficiency can also lead to muscle weakness and excessive muscle scarring.

Choline is found in a variety of foods, including wheat germ and bran, beans, egg yolks, brewer's yeast, whole grains, nuts, lecithin, meat, and fish. The body also produces its own supply of choline, using protein and other B vitamins. A daily intake of 30 micrograms is recommended. In addition to the foods listed above, 2 tablespoons of lecithin granules may be taken as a supplement to help meet these requirements.

INOSITOL Inositol is responsible for breaking down fats. It plays an important role in preventing cholesterol buildup and normalizing fat metabolism. Studies indicate that inositol has an anxiety-reducing effect similar to some tranquilizers.

A good supply of inositol can be found in wheat germ, brewer's yeast, whole grains, oranges, nuts, and molasses. Keeping the intestinal tract healthy may be the best way to make sure you are getting enough inositol. The bacteria or intestinal flora found there are indispensable for making inositol in the body. If you suffer from insomnia, hair loss, high cholesterol levels, or cirrhosis of the liver, you may have a deficiency of inositol.

A minimum daily requirement for inositol has not yet been established. I recommend 500 milligrams daily.

BIOTIN Biotin helps keep hair, skin, bone marrow, and glands healthy and growing. It helps produce and then change into energy fatty acids, carbohydrates, and amino acids. It is vital to the production of glycogen. The body manufactures biotin in the intestinal tract. We can also get it from eggs, cheese, nuts, and many other common foods.

Deficiencies are rare. However, when they occur, symptoms include fatigue, depression, skin disorders, slow healing of wounds, muscular pain, anorexia, sensitivity to cold temperatures, and elevated blood-cholesterol levels.

For adults, the official recommendation is 30 micrograms of biotin per day.

Vitamin C

Vitamin C has many benefits. It strengthens the immune system, keeps cholesterol levels down, combats stress, promotes fertility, protects against cardiovascular disease and various forms of cancer, maintains mental health, and ultimately may prolong life. Its presence is necessary to build collagen, the "cement" that holds together the connective tissue throughout the body. Athletes need more vitamin C for collagen synthesis and tissue repair. Vitamin C combats toxic substances in food, air, and water, and is a natural laxative.

Oranges and other citrus fruits, sprouts, berries, tomatoes, sweet potatoes, and green leafy vegetables are important sources of vitamin C. Symptoms of vitamin C deficiency include bleeding gums, a tendency to bruise easily, short-ness of breath, impaired digestion, nosebleeds, swollen or painful joints, ane-mia, lowered resistance to infection, and slow healing of fractures and wounds.

In 2000, the recommended dietary allowance for vitamin C was raised from 60 milligrams to 75 milligrams for women and 90 milligrams for men. This amount can be obtained easily by eating fresh fruits and vegetables. People with elevated needs for vitamin C are the elderly, dieters, smokers, heavy drinkers, users of certain medications including oral contraceptives, and pregnant and nursing women. The Institute of Medicine has set an upper limit of vitamin C at 2,000 milligrams daily because larger amounts may cause diarrhea and are likely to be excreted by the body unused. As you will learn in later chapters of this book, some nutritionists and doctors believe that much higher doses can help heal serious illnesses and reduce the risk of cancer.

Vitamin D

Vitamin D helps the body utilize calcium and phosphorus, and form strong bones and teeth, and healthy skin. Its action also is vital to the nervous system and kidneys.

A prime source of vitamin D is sunshine, but it may be necessary to get this vitamin from food sources and supplements if sunlight is inaccessible, or if sun-shine is to be avoided for other health reasons. Food sources include fortified milk and butter, egg yolks, fish liver oils, and seafood such as sardines, salmon, tuna, and herring.

The symptoms of deficiency include brittle and fragile bones, pale skin, some forms of arthritis, insomnia, sensitivity to pain, irregular heartbeat, soft bones and teeth, and injuries that take an abnormally long time to heal.
The RDA for vitamin D is 5 to 10 micrograms. People over the age of 70 should get more (15 micrograms). Greater amounts may be necessary to build strong resistance against bone disease. However, megadoses of this oil-soluble vitamin are not recommended. One-half hour of good sunlight per day is the best supplement.

Vitamin E

Vitamin E is basically an antioxidant; that is, it protects our fatty acids from destruction and maintains cellular health and integrity. It is especially impor-tant for promoting the health of our muscles, cells, blood, and skin. It is a pri-mary defense against respiratory infection and disease. Vitamin E also is an excellent first aid tonic for burns. It is believed that vitamin E's antioxidant effects make available larger amounts of fats for metabolism, providing the body with extra energy for muscle contractions as is important for exercise.

Ideal sources of vitamin E are wheat germ and wheat germ oil. Leafy plant foods eaten with cold-pressed oils, whole grains, seeds, nuts, and eggs are also good sources. Some common symptoms of low vitamin E levels are swelling of the face, ankles, or legs, poor skin condition, muscle cramps, abnormal heartbeat, and respiratory difficulties.

In 2000, the official recommended dietary allowance for vitamin E was increased to 15 milligrams a-TE (alpha-tocopherol) per day for adults, up from 10 milligrams per day for men and 8 milligrams per day for women. The upper limit for adult daily consumption was set at 1,000 milligrams. Some nutritionists and doctors recommend higher daily dosages.

Vitamin K

Vitamin K is an oil-soluble substance that helps the blood clot properly and aids in proper bone development and function.

The microorganisms and bacteria that naturally live in the large intestine produce vitamin K. We can help them work by eating yogurt and other fermented dairy and soy products. Other good sources include green leaves of plants like kale and spinach, cauliflower, broccoli, and cabbage. A tendency to bruise easily is a symptom of vitamin K deficiency. It can be the symptom of other nutritional deficiencies as well.

About 60 to 80 micrograms per day are recommended.

Bioflavonoids

Bioflavonoids are a group of water-soluble substances that ensure the strength and proper function of the capillaries. Along with vitamin C, with which they are almost always found in food, the bioflavonoids help manufacture collagen. They also protect the cells against attack and invasion by viruses and bacteria.

Excellent sources of bioflavonoids are grapes, rose hips, prunes, oranges, lemon juice, cherries, black currants, plums, parsley, cabbage, apricots, peppers, papaya, cantaloupe, tomatoes, broccoli, and blackberries. The white pulp inside of a grapefruit is also a rich source.

Symptoms of bioflavonoid deficiency include bleeding gums and easily bruised skin.

Vitamin Supplements

One-quarter to one-third of Americans currently take vitamin supplements. Thousands of different vitamin and mineral supplements are on the market today. Research has shown that supplements can not only help reverse nutritional deficiency, but also maintain physical as well as emotional health.

More and more, we are learning that supplements can help people fight certain illnesses and diseases. In early 2000, a study of more than 5,000 women revealed that high sunlight exposure and vitamin D intake of at least 200 international units per day decreased the risk for developing breast cancer. Vitamin

A has been found to prevent cataracts, heart disease, and cancer. Vitamin E has been shown to boost the immune system, cut the risk of prostate cancer, and lower the risk of heart disease. Vitamin C can prevent the progression of osteoarthritis and has been found to lower blood lead levels in smokers. The list goes on. In later chapters of this book you will find more specific information.

Sorting the Hype from the Science

Sorting out the hype from science about supplements is not always easy for the professional let alone the average person. So many claims have been made by so many different people. Over $3 billion is being spent annually by consumers. It has become a very big business. Sorting our way through this can be challenging.

Vitamin supplements are classified by the Food and Drug Administration as foods rather than drugs. Therefore they not tightly regulated in regard to manufacturing standards, purity standards, ingredient standards, or dosages. As over-the-counter medications the general public is free to take whatever they may believe is healthy without regard to potential toxicity or to potential inter-actions with other medications they may be taking. And there is no consensus right now about what a healthy dose is.

It can be difficult to know whose judgment to trust and what information we need to make our own decisions. Which supplements have undergone extensive research? What reports have been published in scientific medical journals? Dr. Michael Janson is president of the American Preventative Medical Association and author of *The Vitamin Revolution*. He graduated from Boston University School of Medicine and has served as program chairperson of the American College for the Advancement of Medicine.

Dr. Janson has this to say about published reports of supplements. "Quite a few have been reported on in many medical journals. Unfortunately some-times the authors of these published articles found themselves later having trouble getting research grants. It was obvious that a lot of political things were going on. I think it becomes a little clearer when you realize about two-thirds of the pages of these journals are filled with ads from drug companies. You understand just how much of an influence the drug industry has on the way medicine is practiced. I think there is clearly a lot of influence that the drug companies have in suppressing information about supplements that might replace some of their medications.

"The medical profession has taken a stand that if you eat what they call a balanced diet you don't need dietary supplements. We know from the research that that isn't true. But it has been difficult for the medical profession to accept that what they have been saying for 40 years is incorrect. It puts them in a bad light. They are gradually starting to realize that number one the evidence for the value of supplements is overwhelming and number two the public demand is overwhelming. They are gradually starting to change.

Shopping for Supplements

What types of supplements are best and how much should they cost? Dr. Janson has some advice. "There are several guidelines I recommend. One is to shop around, a typical thing that Americans are used to doing. Find different price ranges for different supplements. For instance, find the standardized extract and the number of milligrams of something like ginkgo extract and note the price. Then go to a big chain store or discount place and find the same supplement with the same number of milligrams but at a lower price. If it is too cheap by far it might not be the right substance. Or if the price is too high you might be able to get it at a more reasonable price. Sometimes you can find a good deal on a supplement. Some stores offer a two-for-one special. There is nothing wrong with that.

"Another concern I have is the typical drugstore or the supermarket variety of multivitamins, the type you take one-per-day that is supposed to have everything in it. First of all, generally it doesn't have everything in it. And generally it doesn't have a large enough dose to be therapeutic, based on the research we are seeing today. I recommend that you do not get those. They also frequently have artificial colors, glazes and coatings and things that prevent their dissolving or disintegrating so that your body can use them. What you want to look for is generally a health food store brand that will be a better quality product. This is not always the case but I think it is more reliable to get them from a health food store or from a health food chain mail order company where the product itself is a brand name. The one-per-day types are artificially colored with red or whatever color to make them look nice but it doesn't make them more effective. In fact it probably makes them less effective. So pricing and quality of the supplement is important."

Time Released Vitamins

"People ask about time released vitamins because they reason that the vitamins would last longer in the body," Dr. Janson says. "They know the water-soluble vitamins like vitamin C and the B complex vitamins go into your bloodstream after they get absorbed. They may not last long because they get excreted through the kidneys and out into the urine. There are several problems with some, but not all, of the time released vitamins. For one they may not dissolve early enough in the intestinal tract. Vitamins need to be absorbed at specific locations in the gut and if they don't disintegrate in time you may not get the value of the supplement. Particularly with vitamin C the time release form is a slow dissolving tablet that might gradually get into the bloodstream but never achieves the peak level that you get when you take a plain vitamin C. The plain form of vitamin C is absorbed more rapidly and will create a higher blood level although it lasts for a shorter time. The high blood level itself can be very important for helping kill viruses, enhancing immune function, or helping to detoxify the system. You need to get a high level in the bloodstream to start removing the toxins from your body.

"It is true that when you take a larger dose you may not absorb all of it because not everything will get absorbed. What gets excreted, though, is not a bad thing because when it gets excreted it helps the urinary tract. The kidneys, bladder and the urethra help to prevent infections, cancers, or inflammatory conditions so the vitamins that get excreted can also be beneficial. The time released ones may not give you all the benefits.

"However there are situations where time released forms can be a value. One example is iron. Some people do not tolerate iron supplements very well and get stomach upset or constipation. If they take a time release iron they generally tolerate it better.

"Another supplement I have found of value in time release form is niacin or vitamin B$_3$. Plain niacin can cause flushing of the skin as though you have a mild sunburn because of histamine release. It is not a harmful reaction and although it can be severe it does not last more than 15 or 20 minutes. With the time release form people generally do not get the flush reaction. I give people with low blood sugar 250 milligrams of time released niacin two or three times a day and it does help reduce their hypoglycemia symptoms. And they don't get the flushing reaction. There is also a naturally non-flush niacin form called inositol hexaniacinite or by its brand name No-Flush Niacin. It does not cause the mild histamine reaction."

"I also routinely use time release 3 milligram tablets of melatonin. Your body's melatonin level peaks at 2:00 in the morning. If you take a tablet of melatonin when you go to bed at 10:00 or 11:00, you may not be getting the peak at the time when your body would normally be expecting it. So a time released melatonin might work better for somebody who needs to take melatonin. I give it for a number of reasons, one of which it helps reduce tumor growth in cancer cells."

Other Dietary Supplements

Dr. Janson also tells us about other types of supplements. " I think people should be aware that there are many things besides vitamins and minerals that enhance health. Vitamins and minerals are important but there are also dietary supplements. A nutriceutical is a fancy word for dietary supplements that combines the word nutrition with pharmaceutical. Phytochemicals are sometimes referred to as nutriceuticals. Phytochemicals are found in plants and have many different chemical and biological effects to enhance health, including things like flavonoids, isoflavones, and pigments. We've read of red wine extract or red wine itself or grape seed extract helping with either allergies or heart disease or cholesterol levels or immune function. Flavonoids are extracts of green foods that help with different things for example alfalfa and barley.

"Some people have reported importance in arthritis and many of the herbs contain a lot of these substances and have their therapeutic value because of the substances they contain that are either related to flavonoids or substitutes for them. Some of these things are available, in addition to just the herb itself, but as standardized extracts of the herbs. Again, sometimes people call them nutriceuticals but that doesn't make them much different from other nutritional factors. People should be aware that they shouldn't pay a special price just because something is called a nutriceutical if it is the same thing that can be found in a dietary supplement."

6

Minerals

Minerals serve as building materials for bones, teeth, tissue, muscle, blood, and nerve cells. They help spur many biological reactions in the body and maintain the fragile balance of fluids.

We need minute amounts of minerals. They constitute only 4 or 5 percent of our total body weight. Although we will examine them individually here, understand that the actions of minerals within the body are interrelated. No one mineral can function in isolation.

Calcium

Calcium is the body's chief mineral. It is the principal component of bones and teeth, and a vital component of the liquid that bathes cells. Calcium is one of the raw materials used in the bloodstream. Emotionally, it helps us to cope with stress. An active ingredient of some enzymes, calcium is also an enzyme stimulator, that is, it must be supplied before sugar (glucose) can be stored as glycogen in the muscles. Along with several other minerals, calcium also helps maintain the delicate acid-alkaline balance in blood, protecting it against overacidity.

Without a steady supply of calcium, bones and teeth would not remain hard and durable. The brain would not function properly, and muscles wold not store energy. Digestive, circulatory, and immune systems would suffer. Adequate amounts of calcium are necessary to avoid the many complications of calcium deposits, which occur when calcium that has been removed from the body's reserves lodges in soft tissue. Signs of calcium deficiency include nervousness, depression, headaches, and insomnia.

Milk is one of the best sources of calcium, as are other, more easily absorbed dairy products such as buttermilk, yogurt, acidophilus milk (a healthful bacteria-rich fermented milk product), and kefir (also a milk product). I would suggest not trying to obtain your calcium from dairy. Oatmeal, collard greens, and tempeh are also rich in calcium. Sesame seeds, torula yeast, carob flour, and sea vegetables all contain calcium in smaller quantities.

The body may have difficulty absorbing and utilizing calcium. For example, if there are not enough complete proteins in the diet, the necessary substances that allow calcium to be absorbed by bones won't be available. Also, protein is needed to make collagen. If you eat high-protein foods, you will absorb 15 to 20 percent of the calcium in your food, as opposed to 5 percent if you don't. However, an excessively high protein diet will cause you to lose calcium through the urine. Sugar in the diet (except for lactose or milk sugar) will also antagonize the absorption of calcium.

For a healthy adult, 800 to 1,200 milligrams of calcium daily are sufficient. This is usually obtainable from foods in the diet such as those listed above. For women who are pregnant or breast-feeding, 1,200 milligrams is required. People at risk for osteoporosis should be especially vigilant; 1,000 to 1,300 milligrams daily is recommended. Calcium supplements, ideally in forms like amino acid chelate, might be necessary to fight the onset or severity of osteoporosis.

Recent surveys show that calcium and vitamin D are the nutrients most likely to be deficient in Western diets. On average, children and teens consume about 700 to 800 milligrams per day, significantly less than the daily recommendation of 1,300 milligrams. Adults, too, consume less than recommended amounts.

Chromium

Chromium is important to the heart, liver, brain, and glucose metabolism system. It is vital to the production of protein and to white blood cells. It helps fight bacteria, viruses, toxins, arthritis, cancer, and premature aging. To counteract stress, the adrenal glands must have an adequate supply of chromium.

The best food sources of chromium are whole wheat flour, brewer's yeast, nuts, black pepper, all whole grain cereals except rye and corn, fresh fruit juices, dairy products, root vegetables, legumes, leafy vegetables, and mushrooms.

Without chromium, insulin cannot transport glucose from the bloodstream to the cells, nor can the liver properly remove excess fats from the blood. A deficiency can result in rapid premature aging, since protein production will be seriously impaired. Symptoms of chromium deficiency include fatigue, dizziness, anxiety, insomnia, a craving for alcohol, blurred vision, depression, and panic.

The daily recommendation for chromium is 50 to 200 micrograms. This is usually obtainable from the diet.

Iodine

Iodine is essential to the manufacture of thyroxin, the hormone that controls the speed at which blood takes food from the intestines to the cells where it is used for energy. It is particularly important to the heart and immune system, and for protein synthesis.

Fresh seafood is a good source of iodine, as is garlic. You can enhance the iodine content of your diet by using sea vegetables, such as hijiki, wakame, kelp, or dulse. Dried mushrooms, leafy greens, celery, tomatoes, radishes, carrots, and onions also supply iodine.

Without adequate amounts of iodine, the way cells use energy would be seriously impaired. Proper growth in childhood could not take place, and maintenance of healthy adult tissue could not occur. An iodine deficiency can lower resistance to infection and impair metabolism of fat in the bloodstream. Thyroid malfunctions are a direct result of iodine deficiency. Symptoms of inadequate iodine consumption include sluggishness, bad complexion, and unhealthy-looking hair, teeth, and nails. You need 150 micrograms of iodine daily. Some nutritionists believe that 3 milligrams a day of this trace mineral is necessary to prevent serious thyroid disorders. Sufficient amounts of iodine are generally available in the foods we eat without supplements.

Iron

Without the oxygen-carrier iron, you could not live. The hemoglobin in red blood cells, the myoglobin in muscles, and the enzymes tied in with energy release all depend on iron.

The most concentrated sources of iron are animal livers but as mentioned, the liver is a waste-filtering organ, and any hormone or chemical—including pesticides and antibiotics—to which the animal was exposed will be concentrated there. Egg yolks contain more iron than muscle meats. Other good sources include leafy green vegetables, dried beans, peaches, apricots, dates, prunes, cherries, figs, raisins, and blackstrap molasses.

A deficiency of iron can cause certain types of anemia. Deficiency symptoms include chronic fatigue, shortness of breath, headache, pale skin, and opaque or brittle nails. The daily requirements for iron are 10 milligrams for adult males and 15 milligrams for women. For pregnant women, 30 to 60 milligrams are required. Starting the day with a hot cereal on which you've sprinkled 2 tablespoons of rice bran, torula yeast, or pumpkin-seed meal will go a long way toward satisfying your iron needs. Daily iron supplements are also recommended.

Magnesium

Magnesium is a versatile, tireless worker in the protein production process. In addition, it is one of the body's most important coenzymes. It works with calcium to turn it into something the body can use. It is necessary for the production of hormones, and works in muscles, cells, and blood, as well as the nervous, digestive, reproductive and immune systems.

Leafy green vegetables are one of the best sources for magnesium. Nuts, seeds, avocados, and turnips also contain significant amounts. Whole grains, legumes, organic eggs, and raw milk are excellent sources. Many fruits and natural sweets such as carob, honey, and blackstrap molasses also contain magnesium.

Magnesium deficiency can result in lowered immunity, improper muscle function, and impaired digestion. Without adequate magnesium, nerves become ragged and supersensitive to pain. Bones grow soft and production of new protein is impaired. Without magnesium, we are unable to store energy or synthesize sex hormones. Signs of magnesium deficiency are an irregular heartbeat, hair loss, and easily broken nails.

The recommended daily intake of magnesium is 420 milligrams for adult men and 320 milligrams for adult women, but 800 to 1,200 milligrams may be a more realistic figure for maintaining optimal health. Sufficient amounts of magnesium can be obtained in the diet from the foods listed above.

Manganese

Manganese is a trace mineral active in protein production and essential to the correct structure of bones, teeth, cartilage, and tendons. Vital in the formation of new blood cells in bone marrow, it is also necessary for transmitting nerve impulses in the brain. Manganese plays an important role in the metabolism of blood sugar and fats, and is necessary for the production of sex hormones.

Nuts, seeds, and whole grains are excellent sources of manganese. Leafy green vegetables, if grown organically in mineral-rich soil, can supply manganese. So can rhubarb, broccoli, carrots, potatoes, peas, and beans. Pineapples, blueberries, raisins, cloves, and ginger are also good sources.

Without manganese, a slow deterioration of muscle health—myasthenia gravis—can develop. Protein production and carbohydrate/fat metabolism would be inhibited. Manganese deficiencies can be related to blood-sugar disorders and sexual dysfunction. There is no official recommended daily requirement for manganese, but trace mineral experts suggest up to 7 milligrams daily. In the case of manganese, it is worthwhile to supplement your diet.

Phosphorous

Phosphorous works in bones, teeth, collagen, nerves, muscles, metabolic and cellular systems, brain, liver, digestive and circulatory systems, and eyes. It is an important part of genetic materials and helps maintain the balance of body fluids. It plays a vital role in supplying energy to muscles by burning carbohydrates, making it indispensable to the runner.

Phosphorus is available in nearly every food we eat. If we eat a lot of refined foods, though, we are in danger of getting too much. Protein foods like meat, poultry, fish, eggs, dairy products, whole grains, nuts, and seeds supply phosphorus in abundance. Vegetables that contain phosphorus include legumes, whole grains, celery, cabbage, carrots, cauliflower, string beans, cucumber, chard, and pumpkin. Fruits also contain a healthy supply. Too little phosphorus, although rarely seen, is responsible for certain anemias. It might also affect white blood cells and reduce immunity to bacteria and viruses. The recommended daily intake of phosphorus is 700 milligrams for adults. Pregnant or lactating women need 1,200 milligrams. A well-balanced meal plan should provide you with this requirement.

Potassium

Potassium, in conjunction with sodium, helps form an electrical pump that speeds nutrients into every cell of the body while speeding wastes out. It is vital to the function of all cells, helping maintain the proper acid-alkaline balance of body fluids. Potassium is particularly vital to the workings of the digestive and endocrine systems, muscles, brain, and nerves.

In general, vegetables, fruits, and other plant foods are far richer sources of potassium than animal foods. Leafy green vegetables, bananas, cantaloupes, avocados, dates, prunes, dried apricots, and raisins top the list. Whole grains, beans, legumes, nuts, and seeds are also good sources.

If you find that injuries take a long time to heal, or your skin and other tissues seem "worn out," you may be suffering from a potassium deficiency. Lethargy and insomnia are other early signs of deficiency, along with intestinal spasms, severe constipation, swelling of tissues, thinning of hair, and malfunctioning muscles.

If you eat correctly, you needn't worry about your potassium intake, although studies show that runners can lose extraordinary amounts of potassium through sweating.

The recommended amount of potassium for adults is 2,000 milligrams per day. You can easily consume most of what you need to replace the amount normally lost in your urine. A variety of grains and legumes will meet this requirement. Runners can eat extra amounts of potassium-rich foods during times of heavy training. I suggest four medium soy pancakes or two potato fritters as a potassium-rich treat.

People taking diuretics to combat hypertension and other medications also require extra amounts of potassium to replace lost minerals. However, potassium supplements should not be taken without a doctor's advice.

Selenium

Selenium's primary function is as an antioxidant, protecting cells from being destroyed. It plays a vital role in the enzyme system and is necessary for the manufacture of prostaglandins, which control blood pressure and clotting. Selenium protects eyes against cataracts, contributes to protein production, and protects the artery walls from plaque buildup. Animal foods tend to have more selenium than plants. Whole grains, mushrooms, asparagus, broccoli, onions, and tomatoes are the best vegetable sources. Eggs are excellent sources of selenium; they also contain sulphur, which helps the body absorb and utilize selenium.

Signs of selenium deficiency include lack of energy, accelerated angina, and the development of degenerative diseases. Deficiencies have been implicated in blood sugar disorders, liver necrosis, arthritis, anemia, heavy metal poisoning, muscular dystrophy, and cancer.

The recommended daily amount for selenium is 55 micrograms for adult men and women. Many nutritionists and doctors recommend higher amounts. A1996 study found that 200 micrograms of selenium daily reduced the risk of prostate, lung, and colon cancer.

Sodium (Salt)

Sodium, along with potassium, pumps nutrients into cells and waste products out of them. It also regulates fluid pressure in the cells, thus affecting blood pressure. With other nutrients, it helps control the acid-alkaline blood levels in the body. Sodium is vital to the ability of nerves to transmit impulses to muscles and to the muscles' ability to contract. It also helps pump glucose into the bloodstream, produces hydrochloric acid for digestion, and keeps calcium suspended in the bloodstream ready for use. Sodium is available in almost every food we eat, including water. Refined foods contain enormous quantities of sodium.

Sodium deficiency is uncommon. When it does occur, it is usually caused by stressful situations such as exposure to toxic chemicals, infections, digestive difficulties, allergies, and injuries. Symptoms of deficiency include wrinkles, sunken eyes, flatulence, diarrhea, nausea, vomiting, confusion, fatigue, low blood pressure, irritability, difficulty breathing, and heightened allergies.

The body needs 55 to 440 milligrams of sodium daily to perform its functions. Under normal conditions, obtaining sufficient quantities is not a problem. Many people consume between 7,000 and 20,000 milligrams daily. Too much sodium can result in serious health problems, including hypertension, stress, liver damage, muscle weakness, and pancreatic disease.

Zinc

Zinc plays an important role in the body's production of growth and sex hormones, and in its utilization of insulin. As a coenzyme, zinc helps start many important activities and sparks energy sources. It is an important element in the body's ability to remain in a state of balance, keeping blood at a proper acidity, producing necessary histamines, removing excess toxic metals, and helping kidneys maintain a healthy equilibrium of minerals. Zinc works in the protein production system, blood cells, circulatory system, and nerves.

Eggs, poultry, and seafood contain sizable amounts of zinc, as do organ meats. Excellent vegetable sources include peas, soybeans, mushrooms, whole grains, most nuts, and seeds, especially pumpkin.

Lack of taste or smell is a sign of zinc deficiency. Skin problems also may indicate zinc deficiencies. Stretch marks are an indication that elastin, the fibers that make skin springy and smooth, are not incorporating enough zinc to keep skin healthy. Acne and psoriasis can result from zinc deficiency, as can an abnormal wearing away of tooth enamel. Other signs of zinc deficiency include opaque fingernails, brittle hair, and bleeding gums.

The daily zinc requirement for adults is 15 milligrams for men and 12 milligrams for women. Most zinc can be obtained from the diet.

7

Water, Air, Enzymes, and Antioxidants

The environment from which we gain sustenance can also have an adverse effect on us. Consider the life-giving and life-supporting elements of the world around us. Although it comprises 50 to 70 percent of our body weight, water is too often overlooked or taken for granted when we consider amounts of water needed and proper balance of nutrients necessary for good health. Similarly, we pay little attention to the quality of air we breathe and the very activity of breathing itself. By not taking seriously the impact of our environment on the enzymes and antioxidants in our bodies, we place our health in danger. We must be as aware of the air we breathe and the water we drink as we are of the food we eat.

Water

You can go days without food, but only a few days without water, the sixth of the major nutrients. Of all the components necessary for life, water is second only to oxygen in importance. It is present in all tissues, including teeth, fat, bone, and muscle. It is the medium of all body fluids, such as blood, digestive juices, lymph, urine, and perspiration. It is a lubricant for the saliva, the mucous membranes, and the fluid that bathes the joints. And it regulates body temperature. Water also prevents dehydration, flushes out toxins and wastes, supplies the body with oxygen and nutrients, and aids muscle cells in producing energy.

The average body contains 40 to 50 quarts of water, with 40 percent of that water inside cells. Lean people have a higher percentage of body water than heavier people do, men have a higher percentage than women, and children have a higher percentage than adults. Water is our life's blood. Indeed, 83 percent of our blood is water. With a loss of 5 percent of body water, skin shrinks and muscles become weak. The loss of less than a fifth of body water is fatal.

How Much Water Do You Need?

Although water occurs naturally in most foods, it must be consciously included in our daily diets. Include 8 glasses, 8 to 10 ounces each, every day. To rehydrate after exercise, drink one glass of water every 20 minutes for the first hour, then one glass for several hours afterward. Your body will determine how much it needs; it will absorb water at a particular rate and eliminate whatever is excess.

Eating a high-protein diet results in the body eliminating water. If you are not a vegetarian, it's especially crucial to keep careful track of water consumption to replenish the water lost in the excretion of animal-protein wastes. If you are concerned or uncertain about pollutants in your tap water, buy pure spring water, not distilled water. Be sure to read the label, even on spring water jugs.

Despite popular theories and practices to the contrary, fruit juice, soda pop, and Gatorade-type drinks—ones that mix sugar and water—will not aid in athletic performance. A Rube Goldberg-type series of reactions occur instead. The sugar in these drinks triggers the release of insulin into the blood. The insulin inhibits epinephrine, which is needed to release free fatty acids, substances needed for fuel. The insulin also lowers blood sugar levels, which causes glycogen stored in the muscles to leave the muscles and enter the blood. This reduces the store of energy needed for exercise. Drinking such sugar drinks 30 to 60 minutes before exercise, therefore, has a negative effect on athletic performance. Also, concentrations of too much sugar force the body to take water from other cells to help dilute and digest the sugar. This leads toward dehydration.

Beer, wine, and other alcoholic beverages can cause fatigue and dehydration through their diuretic actions. (Some recent studies support moderate amounts of these beverages for cardiovascular health). Caffeine drinks like coffee and iced tea also act as diuretics, resulting in dehydration.

Drinking during meals, in a sense, can "drown" your enzymes, reducing their strength. When foods are dry, it is better to allow extra salivation prior to swallowing, to moisten them, rather than washing them down with liquids. Eating green and succulent vegetables with a meal also will help provide natural water or lubricate dry foods.

Air and Breathing

The first and last thing we do on this planet is breathe. But too often we go through life almost ignoring this vital process. Oxygen enters the body through the food we eat and the water we drink as well as the air we breathe. Our bodies have elaborately designed mechanisms for taking in, absorbing, distributing, and utilizing this oxygen.

Disciplined breathing exercises, such as those performed in yoga, are designed to control the vital energy represented by breath. Some people believe you can tune into the larger energies of the universe by working on proper breathing techniques. Breath and thought are integrally related: calm one and you calm the other. It is known that deep breathing can reduce stress and tension and regularize body rhythms.

Enzymes

Enzymes are natural substances that stimulate some of the internal reactions necessary for life. Our bodies contain more than 700 types of enzymes, each one responsible for a different task. A shortage of even one type can dramatically affect health. Enzymes are found throughout the body, with the most vital ones in the salivary glands, pancreas, stomach walls, intestines, and liver.

Without enzymes, food could not be digested. Enzymes help transform food products into muscles, nerves, bones, and glands. They assist in storing excess nutrients in the muscles and liver for future access, help create urea to be excreted in the urine, and facilitate the departure of carbon dioxide from the lungs. Enzymes also help stop bleeding and serve to decompose poisonous hydrogen peroxide to liberate needed oxygen. They help us breathe and attack poisons in the blood.

Enzymes are abundant in fresh, raw foods. However, they cannot survive at temperatures higher than 122 degrees Fahrenheit, which means that they won't exist in cooked foods. The best sources of enzymes are fruits and vegetables, which should be eaten in season and fresh. When cooking vegetables, use as little water as possible to conserve the enzyme content as well as the vitamin content. Cook vegetables only until tender, in a tightly covered pot. Do not soak most fresh foods; the water can destroy enzymes.

The enzyme that begins the entire digestive process is found in the saliva. Proper chewing is necessary to make that enzyme best perform its work. Food that is not chewed well enters the digestive canal only partially prepared. Digestion is therefore less nutritious.

Mental strain or worry also has a deleterious effect on enzyme actions. It is better to avoid large meals during such times, since stressful situations tend to inhibit the flow of enzymes and interfere with the actions of the digestive tract.

To perform their life-sustaining tasks, enzymes must be continually replaced. Unnatural environmental components such as pollution, food additives, and stress all negatively affect the makeup of cells and increase the need for health-promoting enzymes. To get enough of these fragile chemicals, it would be best to avoid processed, refined foods as much as possible.

Antioxidants

Antioxidants oppose the oxidation of substances within the body. They have been identified as important factors in helping us live longer, fight heart disease and lung problems, and combat cancer. They work, in part, by battling the degenerative processes associated with free radicals.

Free radicals are the toxic agents produced by the processing of oxygen. They can damage a cell's DNA and have been linked to certain symptoms of aging. The presence of chemical pollutants found in water, air, food, tobacco smoke, and many cancer-causing agents can cause the release of free radicals. Radiation exposure is another cause.

Antioxidants protect the body by trapping free radicals and preventing the degenerative processes associated with their reactions. Vitamin E is the most common antioxidant. Vitamins A, C, and D are less powerful antioxidants, as are selenium and sulfur-containing amino acids.

Pollution can have a serious effect on a variety of body processes. Environmental pollution, for example, seems to defeat or otherwise interfere with the beneficial effects of antioxidants. Much of our fish comes from rivers, lakes, and waterways poisoned by sewage, chemicals, and a host of other pollutants. Shellfish, particularly, are prone to feed on this sewage and absorb it into their bodies. Fatty fish, as well, are more prone to absorb chemical pollutants and then pass them on to the humans who eat them.

In addition to the obvious stresses environmental pollution causes, it also depletes our vitamin E supplies. Vitamin E is our major hedge against environmental stress. It helps dilute the harmful effects of drinking water containing lead, excess minerals such as sodium, or an otherwise unbalanced mineral content. Vitamin E as an antioxidant protects us from many types of contaminants simply by impeding the formation of compounds that lead to cellular destruction.

Wheat germ and wheat germ oil are superior sources of vitamin E. Whole grains, unrefined cereals, seeds, nuts, bran, and organic eggs are also excellent sources. Vegetable oils such as safflower oil are likely to have vitamin E if they have been refined only minimally. The best source for such scarcely refined oils—so-called cold-pressed oils—is natural foods from health food stores.

The active chemical ingredient in vitamin E is pure alpha-tocopherol. If you're seeking a supplement, get natural vitamin E. There is some indication that the natural form is more active and therefore more useful than the synthetic variety.

Since environmental pollution and other factors seem to have a negative effect on antioxidants, it may be necessary to supplement your intake of nutrients to help make more antioxidants for possible use.

8

Diet and Digestion

The digestive system is composed of intricately interconnected parts that set into motion an incredibly complicated process. Every time you put food into your mouth, you unleash a nearly infinite number of clockworklike reactions and interactions. Although it is possible to track and understand this process to some extent, many aspects remain a mystery. Digestion and absorption of nutrients occur harmoniously and simultaneously.

How Foods are Broken Down

The digestive system begins with the mouth and runs some 30 feet to the anus. It is essentially a long, hollow canal that mechanically chops, grinds, and transports food while chemically breaking it down into molecules for absorption into the blood and cells. The teeth and various internal muscular systems provide the mechanical action. The pancreas and liver are the major contributors of the digestive juices necessary for chemical processing.

All foods are broken down into four elements. Three of them—carbon, hydrogen, and oxygen—are derived from foods containing fats and carbohydrates. The fourth—nitrogen—is obtained from foods containing protein. These four units are metabolized through different body tissues and are made available for the body's maintenance and physiological functioning at the cellular level.

Chewing constitutes the first stage of digestion. The way you masticate food is critical to the sort of nutritional benefit you will receive from the food you ingest. If you do not chew slowly to break down food thoroughly, the saliva secreted in your mouth will not mix sufficiently with the food. Improper chewing also leaves food in chunks that are too large to pass easily through the esophagus and into the stomach for the next stage of digestion.

When food is not broken down properly, it creates an excess secretion of digestive enzymes. Extra stomach acids such as hydrochloric acid must be produced to break down oversized food particles. This means subjecting the inner wall linings of the stomach and intestinal tract to a higher and more sustained acid level. Over the long term, this can be quite damaging because digestive acids are extremely corrosive, aggravate ulcers, and cause heartburn and indigestion. Most important, it upsets the digestive process and internal chemical balance, leaving you susceptible to disease.

When food is not broken down into small enough bits, it can enter the bloodstream as oversized particles. These particles cannot be utilized at the cellular level, and so they are carried along until they eventually pass out through the kidneys. But during their prolonged stay in the blood they are likely to activate antibodies that do not recognize them as being compatible with the body's needs. Thus, improper chewing can lead to heightened levels of stomach acid and overstimulation of the immune response.

Fluids do not require chewing, but they have a significant impact on the digestive process. Drinking large amounts of fluids while you eat can create another problem. Fluids dilute both saliva and digestive acids, interfering with their ability to break down food. To make matters worse, drinking while eating encourages you to gulp down food chunks that you would otherwise have to chew more thoroughly. You may tend to do this if you are in a hurry or if you are impatient with the chewing required by certain foods. "Washing food down" with liquids not only hampers digestion, it is also dangerous. It makes it too easy to get large chunks of food stuck in the throat.

Foods that Facilitate Digestion

In selecting food, make sure to choose items that facilitate digestion and thereby work with your body, and not against it. Look for foods that do not cause allergic reactions or sensitivities; wholesome, natural foods instead of processed, chemically altered, or denatured foods; and foods that contain bulk, with a low density and fat content. Basically this means that you will be selecting many more complex carbohydrates—potatoes, rices, and vegetables—than fats and proteins. If you cannot avoid prepared foods, at least try to find those that are as close as possible to their natural state. Frozen peas, for instance, are much closer to the natural, raw state than peas that have been boiled and canned.

Avoid irradiated produce; while it does not spoil as quickly as raw produce, its essential chemical structure has been so altered that it is hardly the same food anymore.

Be aware that produce often is doused with pesticides and chemicals or is dirty. Some has been waxed. Wash these foods thoroughly or even peel them.

Better yet, don't buy them unless they have been organically grown, that is, grown without pesticides and potentially poisonous chemical fertilizers.

In preparing foods, try to maximize their digestibility without altering their essential integrity and cellular structure, since these are critical to facilitating digestion and keeping the colon and upper gastrointestinal track clear of food mass and toxic buildup. For instance, plant foods with a lot of cellulose (the cellular structure of plants) need to be softened for easier digestion so that the benefits received from the cellulose can be optimized. Celery can be soaked; cauliflower, carrots, and even sprouts can be steamed; and beans and corn can be mashed.

Take care not to overcook your food as it can eliminate the fibrous structure that aids in digestion and provides the vitamin and mineral contents. Steaming is generally preferable to boiling. Boiling in 1 inch of water may be better than boiling in 6 inches, and boiling for 5 minutes is usually preferable to boiling for 20 minutes.

Stress is another integral part of the digestive process. Don't eat when you are tense, upset, or in a hurry. Wait until you have relaxed. If you come home from work and are worried about something that happened at the office or if you are upset because a friend is sick, take some time to get your emotions in order before you eat. Otherwise you will not digest your food properly. The digestive mechanism is interrupted by stress, and if you are nervous or anxious or hurried, you may not chew your food well to begin with.

The Process of Digestion

Many different chemicals and chemical processes are involved in digestion. The most important substance in saliva is protein, including many free-state proteins and amino acids. Besides digesting starch, saliva keeps the mucous membrane of the mouth moist, and its constant flow helps keep teeth and gums clean and free of food particles. Without adequate salivation, you will have dryness of the mouth, bacterial overgrowth, buildup of food particles and dead cells, and loss of the ability to taste.

Enzymes are complex organic compounds, usually proteins, which are task-specific. That is, they work in a specific manner on particular foods. Enzymes that catalyze reactions leading to the breakdown of carbohydrates, for instance, have no effect on fat or protein digestion. Complementary sets of enzymes ensure that the cells get sufficient amounts of the specific foods on which they act.

Carbohydrate Digestion

Carbohydrate digestion is the most important in relation to the energy requirements of the body. Plants, grains, legumes, vegetables, fruits, nuts, and seeds— all carbohydrates—offer the greatest sources of energy for proper physiological functioning.

All carbohydrates are broken down into one type of sugar or another. In fact, carbohydrates are composed primarily of sugars, but also fiber, essential fatty acids, and amino acids. They are classified according to how many glucose or sugar units are present in each molecule. Glucose, which produces most of the complex sugars, is the main form of carbohydrate that goes into the bloodstream and enters the cells in the presence of insulin. It plays a critical role in normal brain functioning and is the chief source of energy for the nervous system.

Carbohydrates may contain either complex or simple sugars. Glucose and fructose are monosaccharides or single-unit, simple sugars. Starch is a polysaccharide, or complex sugar. Some carbohydrates are indigestible and merely pass through the digestive system to be excreted with other waste products in their original, unaltered state. These are the fibers, and even though they are not digested, their action while passing through the digestive system is extremely important. They stimulate peristalsis—the wavelike alternating contractions that move food and waste through the digestion and elimination systems. They further enhance the elimination of toxic wastes by absorbing excess water and joining with other residue to create bulk matter, which passes more readily out of the system. Fiber, then, while indigestible and containing no nutrients, plays a major role in digestion through its stimulating, cleansing, and detoxifying action.

The carbohydrates that are digestible go through various processes. The simple sugars can enter the blood system almost immediately upon ingestion, even before they are swallowed. The multiple-unit sugars are partially digested in the mouth by salivary enzymes. They are moved along until they reach the stomach, where they are passed into the large intestine. This is where the greatest amount of carbohydrate digestion takes place. The sugars are broken down into glucose in the small intestine and are finally ready to pass into the blood in that form. Once in the blood, they are absorbed into the cells and used as a form of energy for the brain and the nervous system.

Protein Digestion

Proteins are far more complicated than carbohydrates, and they vary greatly in their function. All proteins are made up of chains of amino acids, the so-called building blocks of life, which make up part of every living cell in the body.

While there is a great deal that is not known about protein digestion, it is known that proteins are far more difficult to digest than carbohydrates. To be reduced, proteins must have their bonding peptide linkages broken down by the gastric juices.

Some peptides are more difficult to reduce than others are. Those with a lot of fat surrounding them, such as those in meat, are difficult to digest, but not nearly as difficult as deep-fried or charcoal-broiled foods, which form strongly bound molecules that are extremely difficult to separate. When proteins that are hard to digest (e.g., meats) are made even more resistant (e.g., by deep frying), they remain undigested longer. In trying to digest them, the body continues to produce gastric juices so highly acidic that if not properly buffered, they can eat a hole (a penetrating ulcer) through the stomach lining.

Digesting proteins is obviously quite different from digesting carbohydrates. Of course, both proteins and carbohydrates provide the body with essential nutrients, and both are sources of energy. There is a substantial difference in the kinds of energy they produce. It is often thought that proteins are synonymous with high energy, and for that reason people with hypoglycemia, or low blood sugar, are frequently fed high-protein diets. But if one looks at the way these two types of foods are digested, one sees that a high-protein diet may not be a good idea in the case of hypoglycemia.

If a person feels weak because of low blood sugar and eats a piece of fruit, 30 or 40 minutes later the fruit is digested and glucose enters the bloodstream to restore energy. If a person with hypoglycemia eats a lean steak instead, he or she will have to wait 1 to 4 hours for the meal to leave the stomach, depending upon how much is eaten, how it was prepared, and the state of the digestive system. It will take even longer for the amino acids derived from the meat to be converted into usable energy. The protein meal will feel satisfying because of its saturated, high-density fat, which is very slow to digest and therefore delays the hunger mechanism for a long time. In comparison, a carbohydrate meal—fruits, vegetables, pastas, etc.—will pass through all the stages of digestion quickly, and the person may be hungry again an hour later. But carbohydrates deliver the required energy rapidly and efficiently. Protein, on the other hand, not only takes longer in getting energy into the cells but also saps energy in the process so as keep the gastric juices flowing.

The Right Diet for You

It is difficult to separate the fats from the proteins from the carbohydrates. You may be eating too much of one to get some of the other, or you may be cutting down on one to reduce the other. Understanding a little about why you do and don't need each one will help you formulate a sensible diet for your particular needs.

Diets should be individual matters. Not everybody requires the same amounts or proportions of proteins, fats, or carbohydrates. Your body chemistry or lifestyle may indicate that you need to slant your diet a little bit toward this or away from that. What's good for your friend may not be the best for you. Men, women, and children have different requirements. Adults at different ages have varying dietary needs. Don't eat what everyone around you is eating or simply what the latest best-selling book suggests. You'll see in chapter 18 why some of the more popular diets are not recommended. Tailor your diet to your specific needs, which may include your particular health problems. It is best to work with a nutritionist or a physician who is knowledgeable about nutrition in drafting the right program.

PART TWO

Taking Charge of Your Health

9

Detoxification

Toxic substances abound in our air, water, soil, and food. A healthy person can often eliminate harmful substances through the liver and other organs. But a person whose health is compromised, or on a diet that is too high in fats, processed proteins, sodium, refined sugars, and other refined foods has a reduced capacity to rid the body of toxins. When this happens, the toxins accumulate.

Frances Taylor, co-author of *The Whole Way to Natural Detoxification*, tells us more: "As we journey through life the way most people do, we become overloaded with the toxins that absorb in the body. Unless we do something to get rid of these things our bodies become overloaded and our health suffers. We develop symptoms like headache, digestive problems, sluggishness, after-meals fatigue. Many health benefits can be obtained by simply detoxifying the body."

Elimination of external toxins is just one component of detoxification. "We also have to detoxify the normal natural chemicals that are made within the body so that we don't get an excess of these," Taylor says.

Why Detoxification is Necessary

Toxic substances can severely depress the immune system. In the past half-century, with the increase in environmental pollution and dependence on processed foods, we have seen an increase in diseases like cancer, heart disease, and arthritis. People in polluted urban or suburban areas may say they have little control over toxic exposure. But there are things we all can do. We can stop smoking, drinking liquor, using drugs, and eating processed foods. We can start using fresh, untreated foods, raw foods, and fresh juices, whose nutrients are more easily available to the body than packaged foods. We can help restore and reactivate our depressed immune systems and eliminate many toxins from our bodies.

Toxins in food may not all be poisons in the classic sense. They often do their damage more insidiously by inhibiting the actions of enzymes. Enzymes are important activators of almost every digestive or energy-producing activity in the body. Many things can go wrong if enzymes don't do their work properly. Our digestive systems can become sluggish and slow down, causing fat digestion to become difficult and protein digestion inefficient. Our kidneys and liver then become overloaded and fat may be deposited in our arteries. Cardiovascular and other degenerative diseases can result.

Foods that are commercially fertilized may also be denuded of their proper mineral levels. Potassium, for example—the most important activator of enzyme actions in the body—is one of the most vital minerals to be lost in this way. Without the right amounts of potassium, the natural chemicals and enzymes that make digestion efficient could not function. Yet potassium is reduced—and sodium added—in many of our processed foods and toxins often deplete potassium supplies. This changes our basic metabolic balance, opening the door for a host of potential problems. The detoxification process will often depend on rebuilding potassium supplies in the body by including fresh fruits and vegetables in the daily diet.

The solution is to offer the body the right nutrients. Allow the body to open up the eliminative processes, in which the liver and digestive tract play key roles. Start to detoxify by getting used to natural juices, natural mineral sources, and other organic substances, sometimes supplemented by enema or medically supervised, short-duration fasts. The process may be a slow one at the start. When toxins have had so long to build up, their breakdown also will take time.

Determining Your Health Profile

Once you have decided to make a change in your diet and lifestyle, you may want to undergo some simple inexpensive tests to ascertain whether there are specific aspects of your health that should be taken into consideration. These tests are particularly appropriate if your decision to be tested is prompted by health problems or complaints such as generalized fatigue. But very often a state of imbalance may be present long before symptoms appear. The best care is prevention, correcting the imbalance nutritionally before it has developed into a symptomatic disease state.

Personal Medical History

Every individual is biologically unique. This should be reflected in the health profile. Testing should always be preceded by a proper medical history taken by a physician. By taking a history, symptoms begin to stand out. Some of these symptoms are early warning signals of what later may become a toxic or imbalanced state.

Some symptoms that appear during a personal history have not always been duly appreciated by physicians as indicators of an imbalanced or toxic state. For example, problems on the surface of the skin may signify underlying toxicities requiring attention and treatment. The skin, after all, is not just a covering on the body like a coat. It is a living part of our bodies, our largest organ, and has a great deal to do with our internal health. It provides one of the routes to eliminating toxins. Many early warnings of toxicities often appear as minor skin problems, even as simple blemishes on the face. Acne, for example, can be a manifestation of an internal hormonal toxicity. Red, blotchy skin may provide a warning that the liver, kidneys, or lungs are malfunctioning by not removing toxins properly.

Headaches also provide clues. Many headaches are responses to stress or tension. But other headaches may signal a toxic condition. Generalized fatigue may also be caused by a toxic state. Premenstrual syndrome (PMS) and cystic breasts in women may reflect a state of hormonal toxicity. Osteoarthritis may reflect a calcium imbalance associated with toxicity.

GLUCOSE TOLERANCE TEST The glucose tolerance test (also called the GTT, blood-sugar, or glucose test) measures the blood level of glucose, the most important sugar in the body. Glucose is usually maintained at a constant level by means of insulin and other hormones so that when a person fasts, for example, the body produces glucose from its stores of fat and protein. Normally, blood glucose is obtained from the digestion of carbohydrates in the diet.

There are certain imbalanced states, however, where the glucose level is either too high or too low. Lethargy, dizziness, or irritability may be caused by an abnormally low blood-sugar level, or hypoglycemia. Hypoglycemia can occur without a clearly identifiable cause or as the result of excessive use of alcohol or strenuous exercise. At the other extreme, an abnormally high glucose level may cause frequent urination and chronic infections.

The glucose tolerance test requires that you eat adequate carbohydrates for several days prior to being tested, and then fast 12 hours immediately beforehand. Blood and urine samples are taken prior, during, and at the termination of the test, during which glucose is administered either orally as a syrup or intravenously.

Other tests to measure glucose in the blood include the hemoglobin, A1C test, also called the glycosylated hemoglobin test. This test measures the glucose in the red blood cells and may be performed during routine blood tests. It obtains average glucose levels over many weeks, rather than minute-to-minute glucose levels as in the glucose tolerance test.

Tests of pancreatic function, adrenal gland function, and liver function may also be used to measure the glucose levels. Ultimately glucose is controlled by those three parts of the body. The pancreas, for example, is in charge of insulin production. If the pancreas does not create enough insulin, high glucose levels result. If insulin is excessive, low glucose levels appear. Chromium levels are also important in any glucose test because they control how cells actually absorb or use glucose. The presence of chromium can be determined via inexpensive hair analysis or blood analysis methods.

HAIR ANALYSIS Hair analysis is useful in showing when the body is not efficiently absorbing minerals such as calcium, magnesium, zinc, manganese, and chromium. It also is useful in revealing the presence of toxic metals such as lead, mercury, cadmium, arsenic, and aluminum. When you examine just 3 inches of hair, you're observing growth over a period of 3 to 4 months. You therefore can obtain the average level of the body's status over a several-month period. When examining hair, you're looking at a relatively stable part of the body as opposed to the blood, which is constantly in flux.

In the case of exposure to mercury through a silver amalgam mercury, for example, the blood level of the mercury may rise for 12 to 24 hours after exposure. After a day or so, the mercury leaves the bloodstream. But hair analysis will show mercury's impact over days, weeks, or months. In the case of exposure to lead in a work environment, blood levels will rise during the exposure but within 12 to 24 hours decrease to the point that they will not be detectable. Hair analysis, however, will continue to show evidence of the change.

The cost of hair analysis is relatively modest compared to other tests. There are some concerns about the proper interpretation of the results as many labs overemphasize data of minor importance.

THE CLASSIC BLOOD TEST—SMA-24 The standard blood test provides a lot of data, some of which can serve as an early warning and some of which, unfortunately, is already a late warning. Commonly called the SMA-24, or the SMA-12 when abridged, the test is relatively complete and reasonably inexpensive. It should be performed as part of a 6-month or yearly examination.

A patient should always be tested on an empty stomach, that is, after not having eaten for 6 to 8 hours. If you've eaten within 4 hours of the test, it is very difficult to interpret the glucose and triglyceride levels on the blood specimen.

The first item on an SMA-24 is the *glucose level*. In a fasting person, glucose should be between 75 and 100 milligrams per deciliter. A glucose level below 75 is evidence of a possible hypoglycemic (low blood sugar) tendency. A level above 100 is too high. Does that mean you have diabetes? The answer is *maybe*. A high glucose level serves as an early warning sign. The next step is to look into whether the cause is a glucose "thermostat" imbalance or a malfunctioning of the pancreas, the adrenal glands, or the liver. Chromium levels should be considered as a related aspect. A glucose imbalance may mean that something is going to go wrong in the future and is deserving of more attention now.

Next on the SMA-24 are the *sodium levels*. Occasionally sodium is too low. An important aspect rarely appreciated by traditional physicians is that low sodium may indicate an adrenal malfunction. The adrenal gland may be sluggish, not making enough aldosterone, which is the sodium-retaining hormone.

Potassium is a potential problem if it is too low. This may happen when people take blood pressure medicines, and are told to remove salt. One can remove too much potassium.

Carbon dioxide is usually tested on the SMA-24. An elevation of carbon dioxide is a reflection of an alkaline state. The most common cause of an excessively alkaline state is a diminished flow or amount of stomach acids.

Next is *blood urea/nitrogen*. If the urea/nitrogen levels are elevated, the body is experiencing urea toxicity. One should then look at whether the kidneys are working properly, or whether one is protein toxic. Too much protein can eventually lead to excessive urea.

Creatinine is a kidney-related enzyme. Its elevation is kidney related, so one has to go beyond the blood levels themselves.

Blood calcium may be normal and appear normal on the test, even if a person's true calcium status is not. Here's an example where one has to intelligently analyze the blood and not assume that the calcium level overall is correctly balanced just because the blood level is. In about one person in five with a severe calcium imbalance, the blood will show too-low calcium levels. On the other hand, in four out of five people, the calcium may be off without the imbalance appearing on the blood test.

Phosphorous. When phosphorous is too high, it can adversely affect calcium levels.

Uric acid. Elevation of uric acid indicates a gout condition. Many people have gout early on. Even then, uric acid levels may not appear over the upper end of the range. But high uric acid can be a warning of gout that will develop later on, so one has to monitor the uric acid level. In such cases, the physician may also need to take a family history to determine whether gout runs in the family.

Alkaline phosphatase is a complex part of the blood. If elevated, it may reflect a liver imbalance or bone problem.

The *total protein* in the blood may occasionally be low and may indicate a malabsorption of protein.

Albumin in the blood relates to its protein component as do *globulin* levels.

The measurement of *SGOT and SGPT* in most SMA-24s are measures of liver-related enzymes. Elevation of either may indicate that the liver is out of balance. If the liver is even slightly off balance, it can cause a variety of health problems. Such an imbalance should be dealt with nutritionally.

Bilirubin levels also are potentially liver related. Elevation of bilirubin may have other meanings that require further testing.

The *cholesterol* level in the blood should be determined. One also has to look at the HDL (high-density lipoproteins, or "good" cholesterol) verses the total serum cholesterol levels. Ratios of four to one (of total cholesterol to HDL) or better are desirable. For almost all people with serum cholesterol levels above 225 milligrams per deciliter the liver is sluggish or out of balance. This problem plays a major role in cholesterol elevation.

One should always also ask for a *triglyceride level* as part of the SMA-24 test results. Triglyceride levels are almost as important as cholesterol levels. An elevated level is usually due to malfunctioning of either the liver or the pancreas. Triglycerides are dangerous because they are blood fats and may play some part in clogging arteries with harmful plaque.

THE COMPLETE BLOOD COUNT (CBC) The CBC is an inexpensive test that provides valuable information. It examines the white blood cell components and the red blood cell components.

WHITE BLOOD CELLS

A white blood count (WBC) between 4.8 and 10.8 is considered normal. If you fall below 4.8, it probably indicates that your immune system is not working properly. Even just slightly below the 4.8 level is an early warning sign that your immunity is not at 100 percent. A high WBC is usually indicative of an internal infection. The elevation of the white blood cells represents the body's attempt to deal with the invasion of a foreign substance or agent.

It is also important to go beyond the total number of white cells and look at the different types. The basic types of white blood cells are the neutrophils or the polymorphonuclear white blood cells, the lymphocytes, the monocytes, the eosinophils, and the basophils.

The neutrophils tend to make up between 50 and 70 percent of the total white cells. The lymphocytes comprise between 20 and 40 percent. There are fewer eosinophils, monocytes, and basophils.

If a person has more lymphocytes than neutrophils, an inversion of the usual ratio, a viral illness either recently or at the time of testing may explain the imbalance. In the absence of a viral infection, the possibility of an immune system imbalance should be examined further.

RED BLOOD CELLS

Basically one issue concerns red blood cells—anemia. Anemia is a disorder caused by a deficiency in the number of red blood cells, their hemoglobin content, or both. (Hemoglobin is the iron-containing pigment of the red blood cells.)

There are two types of anemia, depending on the size of the red blood cells. If the cells are too small, small-cell or iron-deficiency anemia may be the cause. This condition is almost always related to an iron deficiency, where the body doesn't have enough iron or isn't properly handling the iron it does have. Since the body can't make enough cells without the necessary quantities of iron, it produces smaller and fewer cells.

In the second type of anemia, the cells are too large. The most common reason for this abnormality is a vitamin B_{12} deficient anemia. Treatment is different for each type of anemia. (See chapter 33.)

SEDIMENTATION RATE People should also be tested on a routine basis to determine sedimentation rate. The sedimentation rate is an inexpensive test. In women, a sedimentation rate above 20 millimeters per hour indicates that some inflammatory process exists or is developing. If there is no cold, sore throat, or other obvious infection, one has to seek out other possible causes. In men, a sedimentation rate above 15 is considered abnormal.

THYROID TESTING Thyroid testing is important, although it can pose special difficulties. For example, thyroxin is the hormone that allows the thyroid gland to carry out its function. You can have normal thyroxin levels and normal blood iodine levels at the same time that a food sensitivity to the thyroid gland is causing your metabolism to slow down, causing you to gain weight at an abnormal rate. Chronic fatigue may also be caused by malfunctioning of the thyroid gland. A standard blood test for thyroxin would not detect either the food sensitivity or the chronic fatigue.

Detoxifying and Rebuilding with Foods

After determining your own biochemical profile, you can then tailor your food intake to meet your individual needs. Following are some foods that can help build good health.

SPROUTS A good place to start is with sprouts. Sprouts, quite simply, are one of the most nutrient-rich, powerful, health-building foods in nature. They will help cleanse and rebuild your entire system.

What kind of sprouts should you try? Don't stop with just common sprouts like alfalfa or mung beans. Expand your cuisine. Try high-protein buckwheat sprouts; the sweet sunflower sprout; the aromatic fenugreek sprout; clover sprout; and for a little bite and pinch, try a radish sprout. A mustard sprout tastes as good as mustard, and yet it has that nice salad feel to it.

More than 15 different seeds for sprouting are available commercially. They're inexpensive and versatile. You can make salads out of them, put them into pita bread, use them in casseroles, and put them in soups.

MISO Miso should also be on the list of detoxifying and rebuilding foods. For over 3,000 years, this nutritionally superior food has been helping people build better health. Miso is a fermented product. Like yogurt, its bacteria work well in the intestines. Miso should be used sparingly, however, because it does have a high sodium content.

VEGETABLE JUICES Vegetable juices are an important detoxifier. Generally speaking, drink no more than one glass of carrot juice per day. Beta carotene is a precursor of vitamin A in the body. If you drink too much carrot juice, you'll be overloading the liver with vitamin A and your skin may turn yellow. One glass will give you all the benefits of the vitamin. Celery, cucumber, cabbage, parsley, and sprouts can be added. For people who've never really enjoyed vegetables, juices are another way to get good-tasting, high-quality nutrition into the diet.

GRAINS Grains are another group of foods that help the body cleanse itself and rebuild its strength. It is unfortunate that most Americans never taste whole grain. They eat refined carbohydrates in white bread or white rice, but never eat brown rice or whole grain bread. Whole grains are loaded with far more nutrition than their refined counterparts. The grain family includes rice, corn, buckwheat, rye, oats, and millet, as well as less well-known, newly available grains like triticale, amaranth, and quinoa (pronounced keen-wa), a light, fast-cooking grain from South America.

SEA VEGETABLES The next group of foods to include as part of your health-rebuilding program is the sea family of vegetables. These include hijiki, a form of seaweed that tastes salty like fish. You can buy seaweed dry and store it for months. There are many types, including kombu, wakami, and nori. You can cut it into pieces, flake it, or put it into casseroles or soups. Include seaweed in your miso soup to increase its nutritional value. You can wrap up seaweed like grape leaves. Seaweed is so versatile that entire books are devoted to its use in cookery.

Seaweed is loaded with minerals. By dry weight, hijiki has 10 times more available calcium than cow's milk.

BEANS Beans, or legumes, are a group of healthy, detoxifying foods that many Americans deliberately avoid. Why do people leave the room when Aunt Gertrude helps herself to beans? The main reason we have kept ourselves away from one of nature's most important sources of vitamins, minerals, and fiber is that we have never really understood how to cook it. Most people, and most restaurants, do not soak beans overnight. This slows the digestive process. During digestion, gas forms in the colon, causing indigestion and flatulence. That uncomfortable feeling needn't be. All you have to do is soak beans overnight and then boil them for 1 or 2 hours. That usually takes care of most gas-producing properties. Then be sure to combine them with the right foods: Don't eat fruit or sugary foods with a bean meal.

Legumes have more protein than grains or seeds. They are also high in here are more than 60 different legumes.

JUICE FASTING Juice fasting gives the digestive system a rest and speeds up the growth of new cells, which promotes healing. (If you have any medical problems, do not fast without medical approval and supervision.)

On a juice fast, a person abstains from solid foods and drinks juice, water, and herbal teas throughout the day. "We should be drinking every half hour to an hour," advises Susan Lombardi, founder and president of the We Care Health Center in Palm Springs, California, and author of *Ten Easy Steps for Complete Wellness*. "If we go for long periods of time without drinking anything, then a little glass of juice will not be able to sustain us. But if we are constantly drinking, the day will go by very smoothly." Lombardi recommends a combination of the following:

CARROT JUICE.

High in the antioxidant beta carotene and full of wonderful enzymes.

CELERY JUICE.

High in sodium—not the artificial type poured from the saltshaker, which is bad for you, but the good, natural kind that promotes tissue flexibility.

BEET JUICE.

Beets nourish the liver, one of the most important organs in the body, with hundreds of different functions. If your liver is functioning well, most likely everything else in your body will be too.

CABBAGE JUICE.

Cabbage juice is high in vitamin C.

Mix the juice from each vegetable in equal proportion and drink this combination throughout the day. A little cayenne, which increases circulation, sending blood to every corner of the body to promote healing, can be added for flavor. Lemon juice in water and different herbal teas—some good ones are parsley and dandelion tea for the liver and kidneys and pau d'arco for blood purification—can be added for variety. "Any herbal tea free of caffeine will be good," Lombardi says. "Since you need to drink on an hourly basis, you don't want to drink the same thing over and over."

Chelation Therapy

During the chelation process, many beneficial changes occur at the cellular level. A synthetic amino acid called EDTA is administered to the patient via intravenous drip. Once in the bloodstream, EDTA attaches itself to heavy metals such as lead, cadmium, and mercury and holds onto those toxic substances until they exit the body through the urine. Dr. Martin Dayton, who is board-certified in family medicine, chelation therapy, and clinical nutrition explains why removal of these substances is vital to good health: "The toxic material prevents normal function and repair. For example, lead prevents normal enzymatic processes so that the body cannot function properly and repair itself. This leads to premature aging and the premature development of disease. Removal of toxic material through chelation keeps the body functioning optimally."

Dr. Dayton notes that an excess even of iron, which is necessary for life, accelerates free radical production and causes harm. "Periodic purging of iron from the body via menstrual bleeding is thought to protect women from hardening of the arteries. However, this protection is lost at menopause with the cessation of menstruation. At this time, arterial clogging accelerates. Chelation removes this excess iron."

Dr. Dayton recommends chelation therapy for anyone over 30. "Lead is found everywhere, in the air we breathe, the water we drink, the food supply. It is even found at the North Pole. Lead and other toxic pollutants are hard to avoid in today's world. As a matter of fact, the concentration of lead found in the human skeleton now is several hundred times greater than that found in our pre–industrial revolution ancestors. In one study, where lead was thought to be involved, 18 years following chelation therapy a 10-fold decrease in cancer death rate was found for those who had the treatment versus those who had nothing."

Colon Cleansing

Colon cleansing is an ancient and time-honored health practice for rejuvenating the system; it was used in Egypt over 4,000 years ago. Later, Hippocrates taught these procedures in his health care system. The large intestine, or colon, is healed, rebuilt, and finally restored to its natural size, normal shape, and correct function.

Colon therapist Anita Lotson explains the procedure and some of its physical and psychological benefits: "There are several stages of therapy. The first segment involves cleansing, a thorough washing of the large intestine. The colon is irrigated by a technique whereby water is gently infused into the large bowel, flowing in and out at steady intervals. Through this method, water is allowed to travel the entire length of the colon, all the way around to the cecum area. The walls of the colon are washed and old encrustations and fecal material are loosened, dislodged, and swept away. This toxic waste material has often been attached to the bowel walls for many, many years. It is laden with millions of bacteria, which set up the perfect environment for disease to take root and entrench itself in the system, wreaking havoc. As this body pollution is eliminated, many conditions—from severe skin disorders to breathing difficulties, depression, chronic fatigue, nervousness, severe constipation, and arthritis—are reduced in severity, providing great relief, especially when augmented with dietary changes and other treatment modalities.

"The next phases are healing, rebuilding, and finally restoration of a healthy colon, functioning at maximum efficiency for the final absorption of nutrients, and the total and timely elimination of all remaining waste materials. During the healing phase, we begin to infuse materials into the bowel that will cool inflamed areas and strengthen weak sections of the colon wall. Flaxseed tea, white oak bark, and slippery elm bark all soothe, lubricate, and introduce powerful healing agents directly into the large intestine. These herbal teas may be taken orally as well. Simple dietary changes have been made by now, such as the addition of water. This simple measure spells the difference between success and failure in alleviating many bowel conditions. I ask all my clients to double their intake of water.

"I love to see people's change in attitude from the time they come in to the time that they leave. Sometimes people are very irritable when their bowels are backed up. They're often depressed, and sometimes nasty. By the time they leave, you can see a smile and a bounce in their step. It's a different person altogether."

An excellent formula for colon cleansing is a drink made from ground flaxseeds, psyllium seeds, and bentonite, which is a liquid clay. "Clay absorbs toxins," says Lombardi. "The seeds expand in the water and become like a brush. They brush the interior tubing, our pipe system. When the pipe system is completely clean, foods are absorbed through our digestive system."

A Home Detoxification Program

Some people are fortunate enough to have access to a formal program where they can go to an establishment, undergo appropriate testing, and participate in a detoxification program. Many, however, do not have the time, resources, or opportunity to engage in such activity.

Frances Taylor, co-author of *The Whole Way to Natural Detoxification*, says there are many ways to detoxify at home. Her guidelines are presented below.

WATER One of the first things that people need to do is make sure they consume enough water. Taylor says, "Some people do reasonably well with city water, tap water, which of course contains a number of additives. Most people will do considerably better if they use some type of filtered water or ionized water or reverse osmosis water."

DETOX BATH "We use a lot of detox baths with our patients," Taylor says. "We jokingly refer to detox baths as a poor man's sauna. Hot water increases the blood flow in the capillary action near the surface of the skin and causes a faster release of toxins."

Anybody who has a bathtub can do a detox bath. Taylor explains the procedure. "First of all you need to start off with an absolutely clean bathtub. You wash your body thoroughly before you take your bath. Then you fill the bathtub with water as hot as you can tolerate it without burning your skin. You need to cover the overflow valve so the water will be high enough for you to immerse your body up to your neck.

"This next step is very important. You begin with a 5-minute soak in the hot water. Some people say 'oh gee, it felt so good I stayed in for 15 minutes.' These people frequently cannot get out of bed the next day because their body releases toxins more rapidly than the liver can detoxify them and so they don't feel well. So, it's very important that you stay in the plain hot water bath for 5 minutes only the first time."

"After your bath you must take a shower and scrub every square inch of your skin to get off any toxins that may have been released. If you don't do this, these [toxins] will be reabsorbed into your body."

If you don't have any symptoms after the 5-minute bath, increase bath time by 5 minutes more the next day. Gradually increase your time until you can sit in the plain hot water for 30 minutes. Most people need to do a detox bath only about three times a week. It's a good idea to an 8-ounce glass of water during your bath because you are going to be sweating. You can even take some vitamin C both before and after your bath because this will help your body remove the toxins that are released into your bloodstream.

Taylor recommends the use of Epsom salts in the bath. "The sulfur component in Epsom salts helps detoxify," she says. "It works as a counter irritant on the skin to increase the blood supply and it changes the pH of the skin surface. Begin with only a fourth of a cup of Epsom salts and gradually increase it over time until you are using about 4 cups per tub of clean hot water."

Again you want to do things very gradually so your body won't detoxify too rapidly. You don't want to exceed the capacity of your liver and your detox system to get rid of the toxins.

Apple cider vinegar, baking soda, clay, and herbal teas also may be added to a detox bath, following the same principles as Epsom salts. With apple cider vinegar, Taylor says to start with the plain hot water bath first, then add a fourth of a cup of apple cider vinegar, and over a period of time increase this to 1 cup. Baking soda baths are particularly beneficial for people with weeping open sores. Combining baking soda and salt is effective if you have had an x-ray or been exposed to radiation. "We routinely have our patients take a salt and soda bath if they have to have any x-rays done," Taylor says. "You will use equal amounts of the soda and noniodized sea salt and you build up until you use a pound of each."

For clay baths, Taylor recommends a cup of clay to a tub of water. Clays can be purchased at many health food stores.

Among the herbal teas that can be used in a detox bath are catnip, peppermint, blessed thistle, and horsetail. Use 1 cup of brewed tea per tub of hot clean water. Taylor says use only one of these teas per bath. In addition, "some sensitive people may not tolerate the tea."

DIET Some dietary suggestions were discussed earlier in this chapter. Taylor adds, "You want to eat clean food. Food that has not been pesticided, has not been dyed, doesn't have a wax coating on it. If you have food allergies, of course, you don't want to eat your food allergens. Rotation diets will help people with allergies. Some people even find that fasting is helpful. One word of caution about fasting and that is if you do have numerous food allergies and you start fasting you could have withdrawal symptoms because people are allergic to the foods or they are addicted to the foods to which they are allergic. If a person has a very heavy load of food allergens they may not feel very well if they try a fast."

NUTRITIONAL SUPPLEMENTS "We encourage our patients to take bowel tolerance vitamin C," Taylor says. "I'm talking about a vitamin C that is a clean, pure vitamin C that is free of the common allergens such as wheat, yeast, corn, soy and sugar.

Taylor explains the procedure. "To do bowel tolerance vitamin C you start off with a gram, which is 1,000 milligrams, with each meal, and at bedtime. The next day you would add one at breakfast. Then the next day you would add a second one at lunch. The next day you would add a second one at bedtime and so on. The way you tell when you reach bowel tolerance is you take your dose of vitamin C and then you develop diarrhea. Most people can take much larger amounts of vitamin C than they would ever imagine. If a person is very, very toxic or has a lot of allergies they may be able to take 10 to 20 grams, that is 10,000 to 20,000 milligrams, of vitamin C a day. Between meals we encourage people to take buffered C, which is an ascorbic acid to which calcium and magnesium carbonate and potassium bicarbonate have been added. This helps with detox but also helps with digestion. You would continue adding vitamin C a gram a day until you develop diarrhea and then you would back up 1 gram and that is the amount you would take in divided doses all through out the day."

Other nutrients are important for detoxification. These include the B vitamins. "You need to take a multi-mineral also because detoxification in the body is an enzymatic process and all of the enzymes require a metal to make them work," Taylor says. "Organic germanium is also good because it helps the body oxygenate at the cellular level. It is a little expensive but is very, very worthwhile."

EXERCISE Exercise also helps in detoxification. Taylor says, "Even if you do a fairly mild exercise, it increases your circulation, it helps get the toxins moving in the body. Any activity that makes you sweat will help you detoxify." Walking, running, cross-country skiing, aerobics, and dance are just some of the exercises that fall into this category.

BREATHING Deep breathing also aids in detoxification. "Dr. Andrew Weil teaches his patients a breathing technique that is very helpful," Taylor remarks. "Not only does it help you learn to breathe deeply but also it will help you release stress and anxiety. He tells you to put your tongue on the hump of tissue behind your upper front teeth, breathe in through your nose to the count of four, hold your breath to the count of seven and exhale through your mouth making a noise to the count of eight. It doesn't matter how rapidly or how slowly you go as long as you keep this ratio four, seven, eight. It has many benefits. Not only will it help your breathing technique but it will help relieve stress. This is something that you can do anywhere. You are supposed to do it in cycles of four and the results of it are just absolutely amazing."

BODYWORK Bodywork can help facilitate the release of toxins. There are many different types of bodywork, including therapeutic massage, deep tissue manipulation, reflexology, Rolfing, Hellerwork, and acupressure.

10

Exercise and Weight Management

A whopping 50 percent of American adults and 20 percent of children are overweight. According to *Healthy People 2010*, the public health plan unveiled in 2000, half of these people (23 percent of adults and 11 percent of children) are not just a couple of pounds over their desired weights, but actually are considered "obese." Obesity is defined as having a body mass index—a measure of weight in relation to height—of 30 or more.

With all these extra pounds, more Americans than ever before are worried about their weight. At least two-thirds of all adults in the United States report that they are trying to lose or maintain their weight. Nearly 80 million Americans in any given year are following a dietary program to shed pounds. All this comes at a high cost: Consumers spend $33 billion annually for weight loss products and services. There are virtually hundreds of diet programs available today. Many are based on high-protein, low-calorie regimens, or involve products that are supposed to melt away fat, change the metabolism, or stimulate muscle development. Before embarking upon any of these, you should first examine the notion of what is proper weight, making sure your perception of what constitutes an ideal weight is not mistaken.

It requires from 2 to 4 years of being overfat to actually become overweight. Excess fat will first infiltrate the muscle tissue before it spills out as subcutaneous tissue, that which you can see underneath the folds of skin. By the time the fat is visible on your arms and face, the problem has already reached the advanced stages, and the buttocks, thighs, belly, upper arms, and back have already been saturated. To assume that a crash diet based on fasting or calorie restriction is going to reverse this process can be a dangerous assumption to make. The end result of easy solutions may only be repeated failures. The key to weight management, and ideal weight control, is not diet alone but exercise in combination with diet.

Exercise is more important in maintaining proper weight than counting calories. You may have heard that for every 3,500 calories in excess of your body's metabolic requirements you will gain a pound, while for every 3,500 calories under that requirement you will lose a pound. These are both cumulative figures. So that, for example, if you were eating one extra slice of bread per day, you would have gained over 10 pounds by the year's end, at the rate of 70 extra calories per slice, 490 calories per week. But this represents a gross misunderstanding of how our bodies work. Diets based on such a seemingly rational, logical, though mechanistic view of the body sound simple. Yet they don't work—because the body does not work that way—rationally, logically, or mechanically. Look at all the thin people who eat great quantities of food and never gain an ounce. Look at all the fat people who just have to think about food, or smell food, and gain pounds.

We need to determine what causes weight problems and treat the causes, not the symptoms. The way to do this is to understand how the body works, and then use its own natural mechanisms to produce the desired results.

The Setpoint: A Body's "Fat Thermostat"

Primitive man gorged when food was available and starved when there was none. His body had built-in survival mechanisms that stored fat during the good times and conserved energy during the lean times. The conservation mechanism slowed down his metabolism, making use only of enough energy to keep him alive and functioning. That mechanism is still with us and still working. Decreasing our caloric intake, skipping a meal, or even eating irregularly may trigger the starvation mechanism. The body's protective response is to go into its conservation mode—to conserve energy and preserve the fat, just in case starvation is really imminent. When the body gets food, it puts it in a "band," to ensure against any possible further deprivation. Each of our bodies seems to have a certain natural level, or *setpoint*, that it strives to maintain to keep itself functioning.

What are the causes of weight gain? The answer seems to lie in a weight-regulating mechanism located in a control center in the brain called the hypothalamus. It determines the level of fat that it considers ideal for the body. It proceeds to maintain that level, come what may. That level, selected by the weight-regulating mechanism, then becomes the setpoint. The setpoint is analogous to a thermostat. A thermostat set at 70 degrees activates the heating system when the temperature falls below 70 degrees. Similarly, a setpoint of 140 pounds activates the weight-regulating mechanism to store more fat if the body weight falls below that 140-pound level. In its effort to maintain the setpoint, the weight-regulating mechanism works in two ways: it controls the appetite, and it regulates metabolism and the storage of energy.

Appetite control determines when we feel hungry. It sends a message to eat. We may have no control over the urge to eat—the hypothalamus makes sure of that—but we do have complete control over our response. We can choose when and how to respond. What we eat and how much we eat are totally up to us. The hypothalamus will continue to stimulate the feeding mechanism and we will continue to feel hungry and eat until the desired setpoint level is achieved

A weight-regulating mechanism signals the body when it needs to conserve energy and store it, and when it needs to use it up. If we eat a large amount of food, it increases the rate at which the body burns calories. If we eat a small amount, the body decreases the rate. In each case, the goal is to preserve the setpoint. This explains why people on diets may lose weight temporarily but ultimately regain it and then keep their weight closer to the former, albeit unsatisfactory, level. It's called the yo-yo syndrome, and every dieter is familiar with it. Usually one's weight has been typical for them for many years. It is their setpoint. The body is accustomed to it, feels safe and secure at that level, and consequently does what it can to maintain it. People who are overweight commonly observe that they don't really eat that much. Indeed, studies have confirmed that underweight people commonly eat more than overweight people do.

What we distill from this is that overweight people may have body chemistries geared to making fat even from a low-calorie diet. It seems that they are just better at storing fat than burning fat. Their bodies are programmed to make fat and protect their setpoints. This also explains why other people never seem to gain weight. Their setpoints are low, their ability to use energy is efficient, and so they don't store fat. We can, however, change the setpoint, but only through aerobic exercise.

Reprogramming the Setpoint Through Aerobic Exercise

Lean body mass increases when intramuscular fat is replaced with muscle. Muscles have special enzymes that burn calories during exercise. The more muscle we have, the more enzymes we have that burn calories. As the amount of muscle increases, the amount of fat decreases, and the capacity for burning more calories is further enhanced. So when muscles move, they burn calories and increase lean body mass. It's a new cycle, but this time it's not vicious!

Although there probably are genetic tendencies that predetermine setpoints, it is still possible for most people to "reset" their fat thermostats. The key to reprogramming lies in understanding and acting on the relationship between the kind and amount of exercise we do (your energy output) and the kind and amount of food we eat (your energy input). The trick lies in changing from a fat cycle to a fit cycle.

Running and other aerobic exercises can help us enter the fit cycle. Aerobic exercises use large muscles in a repetitive rhythmic pattern. During aerobic exercise, the body is fueled primarily by free fatty acids and secondarily by glycogen. While exercising, you do not use many calories. For example, you would have to walk 11 1/2 miles to burn up 3,500 calories or 1 pound. Weight loss is the effect of a cumulative process in which calories are being used on a more regular and frequent basis. This cumulative use of calories produces ongoing changes in the body's chemistry, lowering the setpoint, increasing the lean muscle mass with its fat-burning enzymes, and increasing the metabolism so the body burns calories at a higher rate. For hours following the exercise period, the body continues to burn calories at a higher rate. The effects of exercise on the body last long after the exercise period has ended. This will be true as long as you continue to do aerobic exercise at least 3 days a week. Remember, duration is more important than distance or intensity.

Your individual exercise program will start the same way whether your goal is overall fitness or weight management. If you step on the scale after a few weeks of exercising, you may notice an increase in pounds. Don't be dismayed. That is a good sign. It means you are increasing muscle in relation to intramuscular fat (muscle weighs more than fat). Interpret the increase as getting better and stronger, not heavier. Then throw away the scale. Pounds do not measure fitness. Your tape measure and your clothes are better indicators of changes in your body. You will lose inches, usually in the right places.

The Aging Factor

From the age of 30 on, our metabolism decelerates about 5 percent every 7 years. In other words, if we eat the same number of calories at 50 years of age that we ate at 30, we would be gaining several pounds every year. But weight itself is not an indication of optimal body health. A person weighing 200 pounds who lifts weights and exercises may have only 3 to 4 percent body fat. Many football players, for example, would fall into this category. But if these individuals stopped all their physical activity, and a year later they weighed the same, their entire body structure would be different. They would look and feel obese, because their muscle would have turned to fat. Muscle that is not used atrophies.

Weight itself should not be taken as the primary indicator of health. What is important is the percentage of lean muscle tissue and the percentage of fat to total body mass. Ideally, most men should be approximately 15 percent body fat, most women no more than 18 to 20 percent. However, studies indicate that most men are between 22 and 24 percent body fat, most women between 26 and 34 percent.

Eating Plans

Counting calories is not as important as thoughtfully choosing the kinds and amounts of food you eat. The typical American diet needs to be adjusted to include more complex carbohydrates, fewer proteins, and less fat. Begin your new eating plan by eliminating the three whites from your diet: white sugar, white flour, and salt. Then eliminate processed food including most canned, frozen, or prepared convenience foods. Read labels and do not eat anything you can't pronounce.

The best eating plan is to eat more frequently—smaller meals, every 4 to 6 hours, so that both hunger and satiety can be experienced. Do eat breakfast, just keep down fat and sugar consumption. More people who skip breakfast are overweight than underweight. Get in touch with your eating drives. Keep lunch light, preferably eating complex carbohydrates, which are low in calories and high in satiety. Soup is a satisfying lunch, especially a water-based soup full of vegetables, grains, and legumes. Salads are good for lunch, but after eating one you could feel hungry again quite soon. Add whole grain bread to complement it. Beware of salad dressings; most are high in fat, sugar, and calories. Eat enough breakfast and lunch to take away the strong hunger drive, but not enough to feel full. If you are hungry before the next meal, have a snack. Eat only in response to hunger, not for entertainment. The 4-day rotation weight management diet described in the next chapter is a good place to begin.

The weight you eventually reach may not necessarily be the weight you desire. Be realistic and philosophical. The genetic determinants of your set-point may limit what you can realistically accomplish. If you follow the principles of exercise and diet for a reasonable period of time, and your weight stabilizes at a point higher than your fantasy weight, accept it and enjoy being yourself, as you are.

If you continue to exercise aerobically and eat a healthful diet, your weight-regulating mechanism will stabilize your weight and keep it at the new setpoint. Eating and exercising in this way will soon become a natural way of living for you. You won't need a maintenance diet or some other interim discipline to follow. Once you've set your own course, there will be no other course to follow and no need for fad approaches to dieting.

General Guidelines for Aerobic Exercise

Exercise is important not only to weight management but also to overall good health. Doing the same exact exercises all the time, however, develops certain muscles to the exclusion of others. Runners, for example, typically have very healthy internal body systems and well-developed legs, but they lack proportional upper-body strength. Combining different forms of exercise can help achieve a good balance of muscle activity throughout the body.

For maximum benefit, aerobic exercise should be done three or four times a week for at least 20 minutes. Start slowly, increasing the amount of time and intensity by about 10 percent every 2 weeks. Use good quality equipment, including proper foot gear. All sports require both pre- and post-game stretching.

MONITORING HEART RATE To measure the effects of aerobic exercise on the body we need to "watch"—or more appropriately "feel"—our heart rate, by measuring our pulse. There are three different heart rates to monitor.

RESTING HEART RATE The resting heart rate is the rate at which the heart has been pumping after we sit quietly for at least 15 minutes. It is usually 5 to 10 beats per minute slower than the "normal" heart rate.

Measure resting heart rate by taking the pulse for 10 or 20 seconds and then multiplying the result by 6 or 3, respectively. The average resting heart rate for men is 72 to 78 beats per minute, for women it's faster: 78 to 84. The better your aerobic circulation, the lower this rate will be. Athletic training enlarges the heart and slows the heartbeat. Many well-trained athletes have resting rates from 40 to 60 beats per minute. People with high resting heart rates have a greater risk of heart attack.

TARGET HEART RATE To produce a beneficial cardiovascular effort during exercise, heart rate should be elevated sufficiently to strengthen heart muscles while at the same time avoiding any damage to the heart or cardiovascular system.

Take your pulse throughout your aerobic workout to make sure you are neither under- nor over-exerting yourself. Your target zone is 50 to 75 percent of your maximum heart rate (the fastest your heart can beat). Generally, target rate is determined by taking 220 and subtracting your age and then multiplying the result by 70 percent. Whatever you do, you should not exceed 140 beats per minute when you're just starting an aerobic exercise program.

To achieve a training effect on cardiovascular functioning or to lower the setpoint toward "thinness," you must do the exercise continuously for at least 20 minutes at your target heart rate at least three times a week.

RECOVERY HEART RATE The recovery heart rate is measured 5 minutes after cessation of exercise. It gives some indication of whether you have gone too far. If this rate is 120 beats per minute (150 in those over 50 years of age), you need to cut back during your next workout.

AFTER YOU EXERCISE After completing any aerobic exercise you should:
➤Check your pulse. See if you have achieved your target heart rate. If you haven't, exercise a bit harder next time.
➤Avoid hot showers, saunas, or whirlpools. Heat keeps the peripheral capillaries dilated, making it difficult for your blood to return to your heart right after exercise.

➤Avoid strength exercises like weightlifting after doing aerobics. Weightlifting constricts blood capillaries so the blood does not return to your heart. Do them before the aerobic exercises or at another time.

➤Rehydrate yourself, replacing body fluids lost doing exercise.

Specific Aerobic Exercise Regimens

WALKING Walking can be done by almost anyone, almost anywhere. For some people, including those who are elderly, pregnant, suffering from arthritis or heart disease, it is the only form of reasonable cardiovascular exercise. All you need is some comfortable old clothes, a good pair of running (or walking) shoes, and a hat to protect you if the weather is hot and sunny or cold and windy.

Walking is a low-intensity exercise, so you have to do it for a longer time than a sport like running to get maximum cardiovascular conditioning. About 1 1/2 hours of walking will give you the same aerobic effect as 30 minutes of running.

Walk with an even, rhythmic heal-to-toe gait; swing your arms from side to side in a natural way. Don't keep them pressed tightly against your body or in your pockets. Try not to carry anything since it will weigh you down and upset your balance.Start by taking your pulse and doing warm-up exercises. For the first 2 to 3 weeks, walk 20 to 30 minutes a day. Increase that to 1 1/2 hours a day in 10 percent increments every 2 or 3 weeks. Begin each session by walking slowly, building up to your target heart rate, and then tapering off to a slow pace. Check your pulse every 10 minutes. If you feel tired, slow down or stop altogether until you recover. Then start slowly and build up your speed and heart rate again.

You can walk anywhere. Your first choice, and the most fun, should be outdoors on a soft surface of grass or earth. If you walk in the street, be sure to face the traffic by walking on the left side. If the weather or your health do not permit you to go outdoors, walk on a treadmill, up and down the hallway in your apartment building, or snake in and around the rooms in your home. (In chapter 28 you will find a complete walking program as well as other information on keeping your feet and legs healthy.)

SWIMMING Swimming is an outstanding cardiovascular exercise. It is rhythmic, uses all the major muscle groups, stretches the muscles, and keeps you limber. The water's buoyancy reduces the pressure on bones and joints, pressure that can cause injuries in other sports. As a result, people unable to walk or jog because of a skeletal or structural problem often can still take up swimming.

If you are not a swimmer, you can still participate in a water sport. Begin by taking your pulse while walking back and forth slowly in the waist-deep area of a pool. Swing your arms naturally when walking. Build up the intensity of this regime to reach and maintain your target heart rate.

If you are a swimmer, take your pulse and do warm-up exercises. Once in the pool, start slowly and easily with a restful stroke, like the breaststroke or the sidestroke. Build up slowly until you reach your target heart rate. You may eventually change to more intense strokes, such as the crawl or butterfly.

As with other aerobic exercises, swim for 20 to 30 minutes, three to four times a week. But be careful; daily swimming can lead to strained or pulled muscles. Skip a day to allow your body to recover. Periodically, try to increase your swimming speed by sprinting for up to 30 seconds at a time. As soon as you feel yourself winded, return to your normal pace. Repeat this three to five times in a row with a 30-second recovery interval between sprints. This type of interval training can enhance your cardiovascular conditioning.

Swimming builds powerful shoulders and arm muscles, as well as rear leg muscles. After swimming, stretch your rear leg muscles. And since the backstroke uses the anterior leg muscles more, they may also require additional stretching afterwards.

Wear a comfortable suit that will stay on without constant fuss and attention. The ideal pool water temperature is 77 to 81 degrees. Warmer water makes it difficult for the body to eliminate heat; colder water makes it difficult to warm up muscles.

There are some drawbacks to swimming. The biggest problem may be finding a pool. If you choose swimming, choose an alternate sport as well, for those times when a pool is not available. Another disadvantage is the possibility of getting conjunctivitis or ear infections. You can protect yourself against both by wearing goggles and either a bathing cap or earplugs. Select only good goggles—the cheap varieties are ineffective. Be sure not to use a nose plug if your nose is inflamed in any way, since that condition actually is better served by allowing the free circulation of moisture. Some people react badly to the chlorine in the water, especially, as is often the case, if the concentration is high.

BICYCLING Bicycling is another good exercise. Whether you use a 3-speed or a 20-speed bicycle does not really matter. What does matter is that the bike is sturdy, that the frame is suited to your size, and that it is kept in safe operating condition. Structurally, men's bikes are often sounder than women's, and for this reason many women buy them. Adjust the seat height so that you can pedal. Your knee should be almost straight when the pedal is closest to the ground, but even at that position, the leg should be slightly bent. Use pant clips or rubber bands to keep your pants from tangling in the chain. At night, dress so that you can be seen. A red leg light provides a moving signal of your presence on the road.

For exercising, you might want to use a bike with handlebars tilted upward, so you can sit up straight. Your bones will be in alignment, and such bikes are friendlier to your lower back than bikes with racing handles. For distance or racing, you will want to use downward-tilted handlebars.

Riding indoors on a stationary bicycle is also beneficial. The same basic principles apply. The more interesting the exercise bicycle is (for example, with built-in computers), the more the exercise will help hold your interest, reducing some of the boredom that you might otherwise experience.

Anybody who is able to ride a bicycle and at the same time read a novel or a magazine is not riding the bicycle hard enough to gain a cardiovascular benefit. Your concentration should always be on the sport itself.

If you ride a bicycle very slowly, you need more time on it to gain proper cardiovascular conditioning. At the same time, if you sprint all the time you will lose any aerobic benefit as well, so never try to ride a bicycle to the point that you are exercising at over 80 percent of your maximum heart rate. However, you can do interval training, much like swimming, while you bike ride. Ride the bicycle as fast as you can for 30 seconds at a time. Then rest for 30 seconds by riding at a normal pace. Do this three to five times in a row. Such interval training will help increase your aerobic capacity and stamina.

Remember to stretch out properly after bike riding. It is best to wear good biking shoes, since they transmit force to the pedals more efficiently. Walking and running shoes will do well if you can't find biking shoes. You should use foot clips to secure your shoes to the pedals.

Bicycling causes less trauma to the joints and muscles than jogging or running. Still, problems can occur. In addition to collisions, the most common injuries are outer calf pain, knee pain, and chronic soreness of the hands.

JUMPING ROPE Jumping rope, or jumping without a rope, gives you cardiovascular conditioning with a bonus: you can burn more calories per minute jumping rope than running, swimming, or bike riding. If not done properly, however, jumping rope can have a disastrous effect on the legs and lower back. It's especially important to build up your regimen slowly. In the beginning, even a few minutes of jumping rope can be too long.

To begin properly, run in place or walk in place faster and faster, until your legs are coming off the ground at a very fast rate. Stay light on your feet. Avoid pounding them into the ground. Then, for a period of 10 to 20 seconds, start to jump very lightly on both feet at the same time. It is not necessary to jump high. Just keep jumping. After 30 seconds (with or without a rope), start walking or jogging in place again. Do this for a minute or two. As soon as you feel your breath return, start jumping again. Spend no more than 2 to 3 minutes jumping the first day. The older or heavier you are, the less you should do the first few times.

Never jump rope on a daily basis. It can just be too stressful for the body. Increase your jumping time by about 10 percent every 2 weeks. This will allow your bones and musculature to develop proper stress buildup, as opposed to the overstress that would likely be caused by a too rapid increase, leading not only to calf pain and lower back pain, but to stress fractures of the bones in the leg and foot. Your ultimate aim is to jump for 20 to 30 minutes continuously.

Interval training can be used with jumping rope, in much the same way described for swimming or bicycling.

Rope jumping can be done in a small space, like a patio or small yard. In inclement weather, it can be done in a garage, basement, or any room with a ceiling high enough for a rope to clear. A jump rope travels well; it packs easily and permits a workout almost anywhere.

OTHER AEROBIC ALTERNATIVES Other aerobic exercise alternatives include rowing (using a boat or rowing machine), rollerskating or rollerblading, aerobic dancing, and minitrampolining (or rebound jogging). You can also get aerobic effects from tennis, handball, racquetball, squash, and basketball.

Cross-country skiing is another option. Since weather or location may make this alternative difficult, indoor cross-country machines are available and can be used year round. Some experts even think that cross-country skiing is better aerobically than running because you use more muscles. The more muscles involved in exercise, the better the aerobic effect you get.

Specific Anaerobic Exercise Regimens

Anaerobic exercises, which require explosive bursts of energy followed by longer periods of lower energy output or rest, build strength, power, endurance, or the skill of specific muscles or muscle groups.

WEIGHT TRAINING If you're interested in weight training, start with low weights that are easy to lift. Do three sets of 8 to 12 repetitions. The last two repetitions should be difficult; your muscles strengthen only when they fatigue. The initial repetitions—or reps—result in muscle tone, the final reps give muscle strength. As soon as the last two reps become easy, it is time to increase the weights by a minimum of 2 1/2 pounds to a maximum of 10 pounds.

To build muscle mass, or "beach" muscles, use heavy weights and do fewer reps, about 8 to 10. To improve tone, use light weights and do more reps, about 12 to 15 per set.

Weight training actually breaks down muscle. For this reason, you need to allow a full 48 hours between weight-training sessions for the muscles to repair and heal. Many weight trainers think they need to eat huge amounts of protein to rebuild and repair the muscle tissue broken down by exercise. In fact, athletes typically eat too much protein and not enough complex carbohydrates.

Different forms of weight training are available: free weights, universal machines, and isokinetic, or nautilus-type, training procedures. All three systems basically do the same thing. They help muscle become completely fatigued and so increase the size of the muscle fibers.

Free weights can be used at home as well as in an athletic club. But since it takes some time to prepare for each of the different exercises, it may seem to take a long time to get the effect you want. Free weights have to be used very carefully; they pose the most risks of all weight-training procedures.

Weight training can provide an excellent way for a runner to maintain strength and flexibility. By increasing the strength of all the muscles, not just those in the legs, these athletes are better able to withstand the stresses of long distance running.

RACKET SPORTS Tennis, racquetball, squash, paddleball, and handball are basically discontinuous, stop-and-go sports. Players need power for explosive bursts of energy and stamina to run around the court. They come closest to aerobic activity when there are long volleys that result in the continuous use of large muscles.

Racket sports are very popular. Indoor and outdoor courts are abundant and many are accessible year round. To begin, find a good place to play and a good instructor who will guide you on proper technique, equipment, and clothing.

Try to play with people who are at your level to avoid unnecessary tension and embarrassment. Remember, exercise is supposed to benefit you—physically and spiritually.

GOLF Golfers need good neuromuscular coordination and focused concentration. The game is characterized by short bursts of energy interspersed with longer periods of slow activity or rest. Unfortunately, a good deal of stress builds up around each shot. Your caloric expenditure will depend totally on whether you walk (how far and how fast) or ride an electric cart around the 5- or 6-mile golf course. If you walk briskly between holes, you can obtain some aerobic conditioning for brief periods of time.

To start, find a golf instructor who will guide you on appropriate equipment and clothing. It is best to learn proper stance and movement from the beginning, rather than later having to unlearn improper techniques.

If you are playing golf for exercise and pleasure, it can give you both. Golfing in hot or humid weather can lead to dehydration. Drinking water before, during, and after play therefore becomes essential.

Exercise and Nutrition

When you exercise regularly, your body burns a higher than normal percentage of fats. This occurs throughout the day, even when you're not exercising, even while you sleep.

To give your body an adequate supply of essential fatty acids, avoid animal fats and eat extra oils selected from a variety of available vegetable sources. Rely primarily on unrefined oils found in foods such as raw seeds, raw nuts, avocados, and grains. Refined oils increase your risk of consuming too many free radicals —unstable molecules that can attack your cells, speed up the aging process, and weaken your body.

Protein is digested slowly and tends to dehydrate your body by using lots of water for its digestion and elimination. Under normal circumstances, you can only digest and utilize 3 ounces of food at a time, so regulate your protein intake to avoid the taxing waste of energy that follows overconsumption. Complex carbohydrates are much more efficient and should serve as your key foods for replenishing glycogen, the energy fuel.

If you are serious about exercise, dinner should be your smallest meal of the day. In the late afternoon or early evening, your body is in a state of recuperation and repair from exercise. Burdening it with a heavy meal hampers this process.

You shouldn't eat anything substantial for at least 2 hours before you go to sleep because little will leave your stomach within an hour after eating. Once you're in a prone position, whatever is in your stomach has difficulty moving into the intestine. If you are hungry late in the evening, try a light food such as fruit, or have a liquid refreshment like an herbal tea.

Before you exercise, eat enough so as not to feel hungry during the event. Eat modest amounts of complex carbohydrates up to 2 1/2 hours before exercising. Stay away from fat and protein. Avoid salty or spicy foods, simple sugars, and unfamiliar foods that could irritate or upset you. Allow time for your stomach and small intestines to empty. Drink water or diluted fruit juice until 1 hour before the event, then continue to drink water only.

CARBOHYDRATE LOADING Carbohydrate loading is an eating regimen followed by some athletes in preparation for a long competition, such as a running marathon. A typical schedule for a runner begins 7 days before the event with an exhausting bout of exercise, depleting the stores of glycogen in the body. To further aid the glycogen depletion, the runner eats a low-carbohydrate, high-protein, and high-fat diet. Three days before the event, he packs in as many carbohydrates as possible to replenish the glycogen, keeping protein and fat at moderate levels. The body is stressed by this deprivation of carbohydrate fuel and it responds to that stress by overcompensating and storing extra supplies of glycogen in the muscles. Thus, the marathon runner has more energy and can run longer before tiring.

One modification of this classic loading technique is to substitute tapered rest for the exhaustive bout of exercise during the week preceding the event. Also, the last week might feature a high complex carbohydrate diet. A further modification sometimes suggested is for the runner to rest and eat a high complex carbohydrate diet 48 to 72 hours before the event.

SUPPLEMENTS In general, people who eat well-balanced diets do not need vitamin or mineral supplements for their exercise needs. However, people with poor diets, food sensitivities, poor absorption, chemical imbalances, and other problems may need supplements to maintain good health.

Exercise stresses the body, with B complex vitamins in particular burned off by stress. B complex vitamins as well as vitamin A, which help stimulate the immune system, may be recommended in conjunction with an exercise regimen. The antioxidants, vitamins C and E, and selenium, also may be recommended before and after exercise. Calcium and magnesium, in a 1:1 ratio, are commonly used to benefit muscles, as are coenzyme Q10 (100-200 milligrams) and l-carnitine (500-1,000 milligrams). Iron deficiency is common among women and athletes, and runners should be tested for iron deficiency before training begins.

A common misconception is that your body loses salt through perspiration during and after exercise. In fact, it loses only water, leaving the body's salt in higher concentrations than before. You need more water after exercise, not more salt, to help prevent fatigue, irritability, and exhaustion. Salt pills are not recommended.

AFTER YOU EXERCISE During exercise, you use up water and fuel. You need to replenish them—in that order. Water, the recommended beverage, helps alleviate feelings of exhaustion. Give your body an opportunity to return to normal before eating.

Even if you are not consciously thirsty, drink an 8- to 10-ounce glass of water after exercising, and again at 20-minute intervals for the next hour. You cannot restore the water you lost in exercise simply by drinking a lot at one time. Your body's tissues, after all, can only absorb water at a certain rate; the rest is eliminated. The average water consumption per day for a healthy adult who exercises is eight 8- to 10-ounce glasses. What you do not use, the body will eliminate.

If you are ravenous after exercising, it may mean you have run out of fuel. You have depleted your supply of glucose and/or glycogen and your body wants to start replenishing it immediately. In this case, pay attention to eating more as a part of your regular diet to build up glycogen levels.

While pre-exercise nutrition should consist of a high complex-carbohydrate diet, postexercise meals should include protein as well, since you will need protein to rebuild or repair muscles and other tissues.

A 28-Day Exercise Plan for Runners and Other Serious Exercisers

This comprehensive exercise program is designed for the runner or anyone serious about regular exercise that wants to develop and maintain good health. But for it to work, you must be willing to make a commitment to incorporate this gentle, realistic, exercise routine into your lifestyle. Exercise should be viewed in the same way as brushing your teeth, a daily habit whose importance you recognize. Don't regard it as something extra you'll do if you have time after you do everything else. Exercise is part of everything else. Yet also understand it's okay if you miss a day.

The basic 28-day exercise plan calls for your choice of running or some other aerobic exercise on days 1, 3, and 5. For the first 4 weeks, do the exercise for 20 minutes. Increase the duration by 10 percent every 2 weeks if you are younger than 35 years of age and have no history of heart disease. Increase the duration by 10 percent every 4 weeks if you are over 35 or have a history of heart disease.

These exercise plans are designed in 1-week cycles, since most people plan their time that way. Day 1 of the exercise plan may be any day of the week. The sequence is what matters.

To be viable, your exercise program needs to reflect your goals, attitudes, strengths, weaknesses, and lifestyle. Use these suggested plans as guidelines; feel free to alter them to suit your individual requirements.

When choosing aerobic alternatives, use both sides of your brain. Use the left side to choose activities that will enable you to get and keep your body functioning at your target heart rate for 20 to 30 minutes at least 3 days a week. Also be realistic in your expectations. So use the right side of your brain to evaluate activities that appeal to you.

Different exercises affect different muscles. You can combine two complementary exercises in your total program and rotate them according to whim or weather. You could have one indoor and one outdoor choice. For example, skiing and biking build up the anterior leg muscles while providing good aerobic conditioning. If you run outdoors and use a stationary bicycle indoors, you have come up with a set of complementary exercises good for all seasons. Either one could also be combined with swimming. There are outdoor and indoor pools. Weight training is a beneficial form of anaerobic exercise that augments any aerobic exercise. As mentioned, it can be done with free weights or an isokinetic machine, like nautilus equipment.

BEFORE YOU BEGIN Prior to starting any serious exercise or conditioning program, most people should have a complete physical exam. Some people need a stress test. During a cardiovascular stress test, your heart and blood pressure are monitored as you walk or run on a treadmill. The workload is increased at regular intervals. The results can indicate hidden or small conditions that could lead to trouble. Stress tests are done in various centers, hospitals, and some cardiologists' offices. If you are under 35 years of age, not overweight, and have no family history of heart disease, you probably do not need a stress test. A routine physical examination will do.

What time of day is best for exercise? Most people are more flexible and looser (also more fatigued after a day's work) at about 6 p.m. So exercising in late afternoon takes advantage of the flexibility, pumps up energy to revitalize a tired body, and reduces the tensions of the day. Exercising in early morning, on the other hand, takes advantage of a well-rested and fresh state of mind. Each person needs to be in tune with his or her own body, following the monthly rhythms that seem to affect intellect, mood, and physical energy levels. Do it when it feels good. The right time for exercise is any time you manage to find in your busy schedule

It is important to start your routine and proceed very slowly. If any unusual signs manifest themselves, stop right away and check them out immediately with your doctor. If you feel exhausted, reduce the intensity and duration of any exercise by 50 percent. Your body is talking·to you. Listen to it. That's good preventive sports medicine.

Relaxation, warm-ups and cool-down exercise should be used with all types of exercise: physical activity, aerobic, anaerobic, and all those in between. They maintain flexibility in muscles, tendons, ligaments, and joints, and help to prevent injury.Too much, too fast, and too soon are the most common reasons for sport injuries. Do not overdo. Less is better—at the beginning—at least until your body adapts.

The basic 28-day plan described below is good for the rest of your life. The exercises will work for you as long as you do them. There is a variation of the basic plan presented here if you wish to go beyond good health toward excellence, or have special fitness goals. Option A provides an opportunity for anaerobic exercise or sports. Option B adds interval training to aerobic exercise.

THE BASIC 28-DAY PLAN *Steps 1 through 5* are the warm-up sequence: relaxation, nonspecific warm-up, joint warm-up, presport stretching, specific warm-up. *Steps 7 and 8* are postsport stretching and cool-down, respectively. Steps 1 through 5, 7 and 8 should be done every day to maintain good flexibility, circulation, balance, and sense of well-being. *Step 6* is the slot in which you should put your running or chosen aerobic alternative. It is the one part of the sequence that will change from day to day, or from time to time, as your needs and goals change.

(WEEKS 1–4)

DAY	STEPS	TIME
1	warm-ups (#1–5)	20 min.
	choice of aerobic exercise (#6)	
	cool-downs (#7-8)	
2	#1–5 & #7–8	
3	#1–8	
4	#1–5 & #7–8	
5	#1–8	
6	#1–5 & #7–8	
7	#1–5 & #7–8	

Repeat the 7-day sequence four times for a total of 28 days. Beginning on Day 1 of the fifth week (roughly the beginning of the second month), increase the time you exercise by 10 percent. Instead of 20 minutes, exercise aerobically for 22 minutes. Follow the increment schedule as described above until you reach the time limits listed below:

EXERCISE	TIME LIMIT
Walking	1 1/2 hours
Running	30 minutes (unless you want to compete)
Swimming	45 minutes to 1 hour
Bicycling	30 minutes (unless you want to compete)
Jumping	30 minutes (due to high intensity of jumping, it is detrimental to go beyond this limit)

Monitor your pulse to be certain you are exercising within your target heart range. As you become more fit and your body handles the stress of exercise more efficiently, you will have to work harder to get up to and stay at your target heart rate. Do this first by increasing duration until you reach the defined time limit, then by increasing intensity as measured by your heart rate.

This is a lifetime exercise plan. As such, it accommodates itself to you each year. On your birthday, recalculate your target heart range. The formula is 220 minus your age times 70 percent.

If, for reasons of your own, you desire a more demanding schedule, do step 6, your aerobic exercise, a fourth time during each week. A good choice is day 6 or day 7. If you decide to train for a marathon, you could train 3 days, rest one, train 3 days, and then rest one.

OPTION A Option A begins in week 5. For weeks 1 through 4, follow the basic plan. Then you'll choose an anaerobic exercise or sport to alternate with your aerobic exercise. Step 6 will be an aerobic exercise or sport one day a week. Option A is designed for people who enjoy a particular sport, like tennis or golf, and want to incorporate it into their exercise regimen. It will also appeal to people who want to develop stronger and more balanced musculature through weight training or calisthenics.

If you are enthusiastic about your sport and want to play twice a week, below is a suggested schedule to accommodate that. Remember, you need to space bouts of anaerobic exercise at least 48 hours apart. The intensity of such exercise breaks down tissue and it takes 2 full days to repair and recover from that stress. The basic plan is sufficient to achieve and maintain optimal conditioning. Option A is only for those who want more.

Option A suggests an anaerobic exercise or sport on days 2 and 5 (or only 1 day if you prefer). This allows you to include tennis or any other racket sport, golf, or weight training. You may choose to do calisthenics: (1) push-ups for the arms, shoulders, back, stomach, and most of the body; (2) bent-knee sit-ups for the abdominal muscles; and (3) jumping jacks for the legs and shoulders. Start with a few of each and build up. Use proper form and technique with every repetition. If you get sloppy, you will get tired and then quit.

Begin here on day 1 of week 5. Notice that on days 2 and 5, step 6 is anaerobic. On days 1 and 3 continue your usual aerobic exercise—this time for 22 minutes each session.

OPTION A
(WEEK 5)

DAY	STEPS	TIME
1	warm-ups (#1–5)	22 mins.
	choice of aerobic exercise (#6)	
	cool-downs (#7–8)	
2	#1–8	
	#6 anaerobic	
3	#1–8	
	#6 anaerobic	
4	#1–5 & #7–8	
5	#1–8	
	#6 anaerobic	
6	#1–5 & #7–8	
7	#1–5 & #7–8	

Repeat above for days 8–14 (week 6). Thereafter increase time by 10 percent every 2 weeks until you reach the time limit for that particular exercise as listed under the basic plan. If you feel like having a heavy workout, you may do your aerobic exercise after your anaerobic exercise or sport. For example, you may want to swim after tennis. That's fine. But do not do anaerobic after aerobic. If interferes with the body's ability to recover properly.

If you reach a plateau, or a point in your regimen you cannot get past yet you feel you have not reached your physiological limit, seek professional guidance. Something you are doing (or not doing properly) could be imposing a limitation. You could be getting in your own way. Or it may just be that your body can't work any harder.

OPTION B Option B also begins in week 5. Option B adds interval training 1 or 2 days a week to the aerobic exercise in step 6 of the basic 28-day plan. This option is for those who strive for excellence in cardiovascular fitness, beyond what it takes to stay in good physical condition. This is not training for marathoners, but for those who want to do a bit more to improve their stamina, endurance, and conditioning.

Interval training can be done with any aerobic exercise. For example, if you were running, you would run at your target heart rate for 10 minutes. Then run to get your pulse to beat as close to your maximum heart rate as possible (220 minus age times 85 percent) for 30 seconds. Next, run at your target heart rate (220 minus age times 70 percent) for 30 seconds. Repeat four consecutive times during one exercise period. Increase by one repetition every month to a limit of 10 times.

There are cautions to be observed in interval training. The high-intensity nature of this kind of training can lead to injury, and it is not recommended for people who have heart disease or other serious medical problems unless they have a doctor's approval. Interval training is anaerobic, so the cautions regarding anaerobic exercise hold. A full 48 hours is required between anaerobic exercise periods to allow for recovery from the stress it causes.

This kind of conditioning is recommended once a week. If you have specific fitness goals, you may choose to do interval training twice a week. The plan schedules it twice to demonstrate the ideal spacing. Four sets are enough to fatigue most people. A set consists of a 30-second sprint plus a 30-second rest.

Do not attempt to combine the basic plan with option A and option B. It is too much to add both anaerobic and interval training to aerobic exercise without professional guidance.

OPTION B
(WEEK 5)

DAY	STEPS	TIME
1	warm-ups (#1–5)	22 mins.
	choice of aerobic exercise (#6)	
	cool-downs (#7–8)	
2	#1–5 & #7–8	
3	#1–8 with interval	
4	#1–5 & #7–8	
5	#1–8 without interval	
6	#1–8 without interval	
7	#1–5 & #7–8	

Repeat above for days 8–14 (week 6). Thereafter increase time by 10 percent every 2 weeks until you reach the time limit for that particular exercise as listed under the basic plan.

Running a Marathon

If you are really serious about exercise and about running in particular, you may decide to train to run a marathon. Here are a few sensible and practical tips for those who want to go that extra distance.

Top marathon runners seem to follow training routines in which they run 110 to 150 miles a week. This does not constitute normal training. If the average runner attempted this kind of regimen, it would probably end up totally wrecking his or her body.

The best way to train for a marathon is to do it gradually. Start with 3 miles, 5 days a week for the first month. Increase it 1 mile a day for the next 3 months, take off 1 day and add a longer run on Sunday. Increase until you are able to do 6 miles a day, let's say, Tuesday, Wednesday, Thursday, and Friday. Then rest on Saturday, and do 12 miles on Sunday. The total will be 36 miles for the week. Continue to increase your mileage in this manner until you reach your goal. If one of the days during the week is for interval training (faster training), you will enhance both speed and endurance.

Consistency is important when you train. So is getting enough rest. If you run 7 days a week, your body never gets a chance to recuperate. If, on the other hand, you do a 20-mile run on Sunday, rest on Monday, loosen up with 4 miles on Tuesday, do 8 miles on Wednesday, skip Thursday, run 10 miles on Friday, and skip Saturday, you would be doing the same mileage with 3 day's rest. You should definitely rest the day before a marathon. Remember you will also need about 1 day of rest for every mile after you race.

It's also important to keep a diary while you train. There are many factors that will impact your performance, including biorhythms and circadian rhythms, and keeping track of the way you feel can help you understand these subtle cycles.

PACING Try to focus on your pacing. Keep a stopwatch so that you know, within 2 or 3 seconds every mile, how well you're doing. Shifting pace throughout a long race can be very stressful on the body. If you start out slower and get faster in 6-mile increments, you will be doing much better. Because of changes in blood and brain chemistry, proper pacing will improve the way you feel during a long run.

A marathon is tricky. You may feel like you have energy right up to the 23rd mile, and then suddenly it's gone. Your muscles are tight, and you feel lucky even to be able to walk. Suddenly at the 24-mile mark your legs "quit" and you find yourself, with thousands of others, starting to walk. It happens because these people, in all likelihood, didn't eat properly, didn't pace themselves in their training, or didn't build up their exercise program gradually. Another problem may be that they peaked weeks before the race.

WATER It is crucial to properly hydrate yourself before, during, and after a marathon. Drink at least a pint of water before the race. During a marathon, you need to have water every mile.

The best thing to do is have a plastic water container with a sipper in it. When you pick it up, you can sip it as you run for a mile. People who run races in areas where they have friends generally have two or three people throughout the course of the race helping them with water.

Diluted grape juice in water gives you extra glucose, so that you're delaying the time that your body will have to rely upon the extra glycogen it has stored up. In effect, you're always keeping your reserve in reserve. When other people hit the 20-mile mark and their glycogen and glucose are gone, they're out of energy. You don't want this to happen to you.

FORM Keep your head high, breathe through your mouth, and keep your shoulders loose. Your hands and arms should not be swinging; the wrist bone should be at the level of the hipbone. If you hold your arms higher, you'll cause a muscle contraction that will cause fatigue in that muscle group. When muscle fatigue in the shoulders causes the arms to be raised higher, the shoulders slump forward, and the neck drops down. You get less air and your cells get less oxygen. Try to keep your feet close to the ground, almost in a shuffle motion, with your knees slightly bent. You don't want to be running stiff-legged because that can jar the knees. Your body should be slightly bent forward at the waist. When you're running uphill, elbows should be elevated slightly behind you; run more toward the ball of the foot and take shorter steps. Again, your knees should be bent. Your shoulders should be forward to take advantage of the momentum you'll get coming down.

GEAR Most runners tend to wear a pair of running shoes longer than the shoes are able to provide good support. Run-down heels can lead to the displacement of musculoskeletal structure and subsequent hip problems, tendinitis, and strains. Yet they are not the only sign of the end of a shoe's serviceability. A good athletic supply store can help determine the condition of your running shoes.

Make sure that the back lip of the shoe, where the heel is, has been cut off. It serves no purpose, and it can actually dig into the Achilles tendon every time you move, causing it to bruise.

It's a god idea to wear tight, thin socks. Heavy socks tend to bunch up because of sweat; this can lead to painful blisters. Put Vaseline around all your toes, around the ball of your foot, and around the heel. Also put Vaseline in your crotch area, around your breasts, and under your armpits.

In cold weather, it's important to avoid overdressing because trapped perspiration can lead to severe chills. In warmer weather, wear clothes that permit free perspiration. Never wear sweat suits.

DIET On the sixth, fifth, and fourth days before a marathon, you should eat only protein, three times a day. Animal protein is not recommended. Try soybean powder, or protein powder, or tofu—in other words, a high-quality protein.

On the 3 days immediately prior to the race, you should have no protein, just complex carbohydrates. On the day before the race, cut out fruits and salads. Try to eat something that will be only partially through your intestines during the race. That night, have something about an hour before you go to sleep. Try to retire around midnight. This will be a major meal because you want to really saturate your body with glycogen. You could have buckwheat pasta or brown rice, and if you're not allergic to wheat, you could have whole grain pasta or whole grain bread. Avoid greasy, highly seasoned, and sugary foods.

In the morning, if it's at least 4 hours before the race, you could blend two bananas with grape juice. This will give you additional carbohydrates that will help you through the race. Do not eat any solid food before the race. Your body's system will be too nervous. When you're nervous and anxious, your body doesn't digest food normally. Electrolyte replacers are very important. Try to have two of the electrolytes (like potassium or magnesium) prior to a marathon, one every 5 miles during the race, and two at the end.

BEFORE AND AFTER Try to have a full-body massage, a shiatsu massage, or a reflexology massage the day before the marathon. It's also important to float, if possible. Do an isolation tank float one or two times during the week before the marathon, preferably the day before, along with guided imagery.

When you've finished your race, take at least 12 minutes to cool down by going from your running pace to a jog, a slower jog, and then a brisk walk. Never go directly into a sauna, hot tub, hot bath, or hot shower.

11

A Beginner's Weight Management Diet

'*ve been on every ridiculous diet that one can think of. At my age, or any other age, it's not healthy to be doing that. It worries me that I weigh so much. I am really serious about learning to diet right, and I am determined to lose the weight. But where do I start?—Joyce, age 55*

For as long as I can remember I've been about 10 to 15 pounds overweight. Nothing I do seems to get rid of that excess weight. I can lose weight temporarily, but I've tried everything from grapefruit to horseradish, and nothing really seems to help me get my weight down and keep it down. What can I do?—Steve, age 40

I've always been about 20 to 25 pounds overweight. A couple of times in my life I've gone on crash diets. I've lost all the weight I wanted to and felt great for two weeks. But I also have these terrible junk food habits with midnight binges. I think I'm ready to change my entire way of looking at the way I eat food, because what I've been doing is obviously not helping me.—Barbara, age 25

There is no need to upset your whole system and your life in the process of losing weight. In our society, most people don't really eat right for total health. Are you like most Americans? Do you tend to eat too much of foods that undermine your health: animal proteins, saturated fats, fried foods, overly spicy foods, and foods made of refined carbohydrates, such as pizzas, french fries, and different types of confections? Do you indulge, all too often, in bagels, donuts, white bread products, and preserved, pickled or processed foods? These foods have been denatured. That is, much of their vitamins and minerals have been destroyed. And after eating these foods, man-made chemicals end up in your lean muscle and fat tissues. They don't belong there. They can't be utilized for energy, for repair or growth of your body. On the contrary, they disrupt your normal biochemical processes.

The first step in proper eating is to detoxify and rebalance the body (see chapter 9). You can't just repaint an old house whose wood is rotted and deteriorated. You first have to repair it. Otherwise the decay continues, hidden under that fresh coat of paint. The rewards of detoxification are substantial. You will feel better, have more energy, feel lighter, and have an easier time maintaining a normal weight. You will have more endurance. Your body will no longer feel sluggish, and you will probably need less sleep.

The next step if you're looking to lose weight is a rotation diet such as the one described below.

The 4-Day Rotation Diet

Let's look at what we can do to incorporate what we know about good nutrition into a 14-day eating program. Keep in mind that the 14 days could be 1,400 days, 14 years, or the rest of your life. But here is a menu for 2 weeks to help get you started. Let's begin on Monday. We're going to take this on a 4-day rotational basis. The reason will be explained later in the chapter. Take only small quantities of each food. On this eating program, you won't be eating until you're full, but only approximately 3 to 4 ounces of a given food. The idea is to space your food over the day rather than eat a lot at one time.

By spacing your food, you will provide your body with energy, protein, carbohydrates, vitamins, and minerals throughout the day. After all, your body needs these nutrients 24 hours a day. People who skip breakfast, skimp on lunch, and then have the entire kitchen sink for dinner are only—after all is said and done—utilizing about 12 ounces of the food they eat. They're only able to use a small percentage of the protein they're taking in; the rest becomes fat. When you eat small amounts of food, several times throughout the day, very little becomes fat because your body is using it for energy throughout the day. This is a very important lesson if you want to lose weight and stay healthy.

Another important rule: Never eat dessert right after a meal. You do not want to combine a protein food, such as fish, which may take 1 to 3 hours to digest, with a simple sugar food that might have honey or fruit in it and may take only a half hour to digest. Combining sugary foods with protein or fat in the same meal leads to acid indigestion.

DAY 1

BREAKFAST: Start your day with a hot cereal breakfast. Today the hot cereal can be oatmeal.

SNACK: For a midmorning snack you can have a piece of fruit if you do not have hypoglycemia or severe diabetes. If you do, you may want to have a food such as non-dairy cottage cheese or yogurt.

LUNCH: Help yourself to a sardine salad, an egg salad, or a tofu salad. Or you can have a regular salad with a side order of any vegetables you like. You can choose steamed or stir-fried vegetables, and eat them with a grain, such as brown rice. If you are eating a salad, you might want to try serving your rice cold, the way the Japanese sometimes do. But remember—brown rice is preferable to white.

SNACK: For your midafternoon break, let's say between 2:00 and 4:00, have a juice, a fruit, or perhaps some marinated vegetable sticks. If you marinate them the night before in a vinaigrette sauce, you will find that your vegetables have a nice tangy quality to them.

DINNER: For dinner, start off with soup. Try split pea soup with an appetizer of seaweed. There are many recipes for either cold or warm seaweed.

As a main entree, have a soy food over rice. In this way you combine a grain (rice) with a legume, soy beans in this case, in the form of either tofu or tempeh. By the way, if you like the taste of chicken, tempeh is a great alternative. It contains no cholesterol and is made from soybeans. It tastes like chicken, has as much protein, is low in calories, and high in calcium.

Finally, you can enjoy a salad at dinner. It should be a sprout salad on Monday. Make yourself a dressing without oil. There are many recipes for oilless dressings. There are also already-prepared mixes to which you need only add water, vinegar, or lemon juice.

BEFORE BEDTIME: If you feel hungry before bed, drink some carbonated water with a pinch of lime or lemon in it.

Let's take a look at what Monday's foods will do for you. You will have eaten foods that are low on the food chain, meaning that they contain lower concentrations of pesticides and other chemicals than animal protein. You've eaten plenty of fiber. Not only are high-fiber foods low in calories, they will also improve your digestion. You have eaten plenty of calcium and moderate amounts of protein. You've consumed no refined sugar or starch. You've eaten modest amounts of foods that are easily digested, therefore ones that don't overtax your digestive systems, taking away the oxygen and blood that you need in your brain. You've eaten foods from which nutrients are readily and easily available for absorption. Also, because so much chewing is necessary with these foods, you've been helping your jaws and lowering your appetite. The more you chew, the more quickly your appetite is satisfied. Chewing each bite will prevent you from gorging.

DAY 2

Hopefully, you are starting off your day with exercise. Fifteen minutes of aerobic exercise will improve your metabolism and stimulate the cells to burn more fatty acids, reducing overall body fat content and improving muscle tone as well as your overall sense of well-being.

BREAKFAST: For breakfast, begin with a glass of fruit juice. Fresh fruit juice is preferable to frozen or canned juices. Try making yourself fresh-squeezed grape juice. If you do, dilute it with some water, because grape juice is sweet.

Then enjoy a different hot cereal. Today, try millet, an alkalinizing cereal. With the millet, you can puree in a banana and add a sprinkle of cinnamon or nutmeg. Add just a little soy milk, fruit juice, or regular milk.

SNACK: For a midmorning snack, carry a little extra millet with you in a plastic container, and eat four or five tablespoons when you get hungry.

LUNCH: For lunch today, try a three-bean salad of black beans, kidney beans, and lentils. These beans supply protein, fiber, vitamins, and minerals galore. Also, try a salad of vegetables different from those eaten on Monday. For instance, if on Monday you ate watercress, arugula and spinach, then on Tuesday take chicory, romaine, or Boston lettuce. You might have soup as well. This would be a good opportunity for a black bean soup with a slice of whole grain bread. No butter, no margarine. Just moist, chewy whole grain bread.

SNACK: For a midafternoon snack, have a piece of fruit, perhaps with another piece of whole grain bread. Whole grain bread has about 100 calories and plenty of fiber. It will be digested easily and quickly.

DINNER: For dinner on Tuesday, try stir-fried hot millet. Add a salad and a different soup, perhaps kidney bean or great northern bean.

For your main dish, eat fish. Salmon is a good choice. Fish not only gives you quality protein, but also essential fatty acids that your body needs. Omega-3 fatty acids—the kind found in many fish—have been shown to help the heart by lowering cholesterol levels.

SNACK: If you're hungry later in the evening, have a banana. Try freezing it and then putting it into a blender or food processor. Whip it up, and it tastes like banana custard. For a special treat, take frozen cherries and frozen bananas and whip them together in a blender. You will be rewarded with a delicious, nutritious, and tasty dessert, low in calories, and high in complex carbohydrates, vitamins, and minerals. It is also very filling.

Thanks to your banana dessert late in the evening, and your fish, salad, soup, and millet earlier, you will feel full without having consumed too many calories. That's eating right for total health.

DAY 3

BREAKFAST: On Wednesday, begin with a hot rye cereal. Add a fruit of your choice. Make it a fruit you have not eaten on either Monday or Tuesday. Take your cereal with some juice, rice milk, or soy milk.

SNACK: Later in the morning, eat a bit more of the morning cereal cold.

LUNCH: For lunch, enjoy a salad. Use different vegetables and sprouts than you used on Monday and Tuesday. Toss a handful of garbanzo beans into the salad. Garbanzo beans are loaded with protein and are very nutritious. Mix some black-eyed peas or great northern beans in with the garbanzo beans to enhance the protein value. Then enjoy soup made from any legume you didn't already eat on Monday or Tuesday. For example, you might want an aduki bean soup for lunch today.

SNACK: Later in the day, have some fruit or a vegetable if you're hungry

DINNER: For dinner, start with miso soup. Then try a guacamole or avocado salad made with mashed avocado, tomatoes, and lemon. Avocado is the fattiest fruit, so use only a quarter of an avocado for your guacamole. If you don't want guacamole, try another nutritious appetizer, baba ghanoush. This is a dish made from eggplant, garlic, and lemon juice. Anyone who's enjoyed Middle Eastern foods knows the joy of baba ghanoush.For your main course turn again to fish, this time filet of sole. You can also have a side dish of vegetables, such as peas and kale. In a salad, try such vegetables as marinated asparagus tips, broccoli, and cauliflower. That gives you a lot to eat and you'll feel full but not filled out, having kept your calories low but nutrients high.

DAY 4

BREAKFAST: Start off your day with a juice but, as before, make it different from the juice you had earlier in the week. Then enjoy a steaming bowl of wheatena or cream of wheat. These cereals are available everywhere. They are loaded with nutrition and high in fiber. To get even more fiber and help cleanse your system, eat a bran muffin as well and be sure it's unsweetened.

SNACK: For a midmorning snack, have another bran muffin, since it contains only 70 calories. The muffin will help fill you up, but will also pass easily through your system.

LUNCH: For lunch, start off with some navy bean soup. Have salad, this time a marinated salad, like a cold salad or a seaweed salad. For your main entree have eggs, sardines, or tuna, whichever you didn't have on Monday.

SNACK: Later in the day, enjoy a fruit or vegetable that you haven't eaten on the other days.

DINNER: For dinner, begin with a vegetable soup. Then enjoy a tabouli salad made with wheat and chopped parsley. As your main entree, try either sea bass or blue fish served with hot seaweed. For your vegetable, have some red potatoes. This meal supplies complex carbohydrates, complete proteins, and plenty of fiber, along with chlorophyll, vitamins and minerals.

SNACK: Later at night have a piece of fruit or juice, if you feel the need.

The Benefits of Rotation

Why a rotational diet? Because very often people's headaches, mood swings, fatigue, musculoskeletal aches and pains, indigestion, postnasal drip, puffy eyes, and other symptoms of not-quite-perfect health are exacerbated or caused by food sensitivities. We can become sensitive or allergic to any food we eat too frequently, including wheat, dairy, beef, chicken, corn, citrus fruits, peanuts, chocolate, and soy.

If you generally eat one or all these foods every day, you are likely to be food sensitive. This list includes the foods that clinical ecologists and allergists have found most likely to cause allergic reactions, as they predominate in the typical American diet.Most people are familiar with the kind of allergies in which a person gets a skin rash immediately after eating something, such as strawberries. But other kinds of allergies can exist that contribute to a child's inability to pay attention in class or to an adult's lethargy after eating lunch. The allergies that cause these symptoms are very often caused by food sensitivities and can also lead to unnecessary pounds.

Studies have shown that when we are allergic to a food, we frequently have a faulty metabolism and gain weight above normal. One of the fastest ways to lose weight healthfully is to go on a 4-day rotational diet and eliminate those foods to which we are allergic, or rotate them so that we don't have any one of them more frequently than every fourth day. For example, if on Monday we ate oats, rice, split peas, the seaweed hijiki, and soy foods such as tofu or miso, we wouldn't have them again until Friday. Virtually all of the environmental medicine experts (also known as clinical ecologists) believe that our bodies need 4 days to recuperate after exposure to a food to which we are sensitive.

By now it should be clear how to turn a 4-day rotation into a 14-day eating program. You simply continue the same eating plan for 14 days. In other words, every fourth day you would start from the beginning. You can change your recipes, adding any vegetables or fish you haven't eaten for at least 4 days or longer. Give yourself 2 weeks to see the effects of combining exercise with a rotational eating plan, 14 days of eating wholesome, nourishing foods. If you've been allergic to foods, weaning yourself off them will frequently assist weight loss. You will also feel much better, and this will help inspire you to eat right from then on. The rotational diet can be used as the basis for a maintenance dietary program. It's easy, it's inexpensive, and the rewards of eating right for a lifetime will pay off a thousandfold.

This program doesn't just address the problem of weight loss. Excess weight is a symptom of a larger problem, one that can't be solved by going on a crash diet, even if you do lose 10 pounds in a week. This program is not an instant solution but it offers you the chance to revitalize yourself in many areas of health. Weight loss is only one benefit. If you follow these guidelines, you'll feel more energetic and less stressed, and you'll probably live longer. In short, the quality of your life will improve.

If this diet seems to work for you, after 2 weeks try moving on to a vegetarian food diet (see chapter 12). Begin by extending your original 14-day program into a 21-day program, using only vegetarian foods during the final week. Then try staying on the vegetarian diet alone.

12

Vegetarian Rotation Diet and Recipes

I s it possible to eat without partaking of the tainted fruits of technology? A natural food diet, which relies on unrefined grains, legumes, seeds, nuts, and fresh produce and steers clear of unnatural additives, is a step in the right direction (see chapter 13). A diet that also cuts down on or eliminates meat is even closer to an unadulterated, healthful ideal.

There is abundant scientific evidence that proves the adequacy and, in fact, the superiority of a vegetarian diet. The medical literature is filled with studies indicating that plant foods can protect against many common degenerative diseases. More important, modern medicine is discovering that many of these diseases are directly linked to animal product consumption.

More people than ever before now are vegetarians. As of 2000, some 20 million Americans placed themselves in this category. Being a vegetarian offers a wide variety of benefits. To fully grasp this dietary option it is useful to understand that there are a number of diets included under the broad term "vegetarianism."

VEGANS, the strictest of the vegetarians, eat solely on plant foods, specifically vegetables, fruits, nuts, seeds, grains, and legumes. This regimen omits all animal foods, including meat, poultry, and fish, as well as eggs, dairy products, and honey.

LACTO-VEGETARIANS eat milk and milk products in addition to vegetable foods.

LACTO-OVO-VEGETARIANS consume eggs along with milk products and vegetables. This basically is a nonflesh diet.

PESCOVEGETARIANS eat fish in addition to the plant sources. In Asia, hundreds of millions of people follow this type of diet, living on staples of rice and fish.

POLLOVEGETARIANS omit red meat from their diets but eat poultry.

All of the vegetarian diets include an abundance of complex carbohydrates, naturally occurring vitamins and minerals, polyunsaturated fats, fiber, and easily digestible quantities of protein.

Reasons for Choosing Vegetarianism

Underlying any scientific evaluation of vegetarianism is evidence that humans are not biochemically suited to eat meat. Indeed, we possess all of the features of a strictly herbivorous animal. Our flat teeth are not sharp enough to tear through hide or bone. Our lengthy digestive tract resembles that of the classic herbivore. Most carnivores are anatomically constructed to quickly get rid of the meat they eat before it putrefies, and to eliminate the majority of their dietary cholesterol. We aren't. Our digestion begins in the mouth as the salivary glands secrete an enzyme designed to break down the complex plant cells. Carnivores don't have this enzyme. They secrete an enzyme called uricase that breaks down the uric acid in meat.

THE DANGERS OF MEAT Although designed to subsist on vegetarian foods, man has changed his dietary habits to accept the food of the carnivore, and thus has increased the risks of developing a number of disorders and diseases. Granted, most meats are good sources of high-quality protein. But animal flesh is nearly void of carbohydrates, has little or no fiber, and is a poor source of calcium and vitamin C. It is naturally high in saturated fats and cholesterol, which increase the risk of hardening of the arteries and heart disease. The leading cause of death in America, heart disease, is three times more likely to occur in meat eaters than in vegetarians. Consuming meat doubles our chances for colon and rectal cancer, while tripling them for breast cancer. The high-protein intake of beef eaters places undue stress on the liver and kidneys, two important organs of detoxification. It may deplete our calcium supply, leading to osteoporosis, and the uric acid it contains can settle in the joints, inducing painful gouty arthritis.

In addition, there are unnatural substances in meat and poultry that, when eaten, place undue stress on our systems. These include hormones, antibiotics, tranquilizers, additives, preservatives, and pesticides that are added to the meat in breeding and processing the animals. Such long-term bodily pollution creates a vast overall negative effect on our health, making us susceptible to a host of pathological abnormalities.

Time after time, the public is warned against the nutritional deficiencies of "ill-planned vegetarian diets," or we read that "most nutritionists agree that vegetarian diets can be adequate, if sufficient care is taken in planning them." The fact is that any ill-planned diet should be avoided, no matter what foods are eaten. Sufficient care should be taken in the planning and preparation of all meals—vegetarian and nonvegetarian alike.

ECONOMICS The rising cost of living in general and of meat in particular has forced many people to adopt a vegetarian meal plan. Ounce for ounce, plant foods are more economical than other foods. They supply more fiber and a wider variety of vitamins and minerals. The same amount of protein costs one-fifth as much when obtained from plant sources as from animal sources.

In addition, agribusiness—huge agricultural companies—has dominated the animal food industry; its high technology and centralization have created unemployment and forced many small farmers out of business. Many people choose not to support these companies by not buying meat. The switch to a no- or low-meat vegetarian diet can benefit the individual without disrupting the overall economic structure by tending to support small farmers rather than giant agribusiness conglomerates.

NATURAL RESOURCES The production and processing of animal products demands an enormous amount of land, water, energy, and raw materials. The rapid depletion of these precious, finite resources is of great concern. The grim reality of the fragility of our ecosystem encourages responsible vegetarian lifestyles, which do not involve wasting more resources than they use, as does the meat industry.

FOOD RESOURCES The idea of eating simply so that everyone may eat is supported by the animal-free diet. Our land is capable of supplying food for nearly 14 times as many people when it is used for human food crops as when it is being used to feed livestock, as animals are a grossly inefficient source of nutrition. They need to consume approximately 26 pounds of grain in order to yield 1 pound of flesh. It has been estimated that our current supply of plant foods could nourish more than double the world population if we managed it better. This substantial waste of protein, calories, and other essential nutrients contributes to global imbalances and starvation. Ultimately, our demand for meat must be drastically curtailed if we are to positively affect the worldwide hunger problem.

REVERENCE FOR LIFE Many people are now refusing a dietary style that supports the cruel treatment and wanton slaughter of millions of animals. Since every person who consumes animal products perpetuates the unnecessary and agonizing existence and brutal death of these innocent creatures, these vegetarians actively defy the harsh reality of this inhumane treatment by adhering to plant food diets.

RELIGIOUS BELIEFS There are various contemporary and ancient faiths that advocate abstinence from meat. Some favor spiritual awareness and reincarnation, others emphasize ethical considerations and health benefits. In the East, these faiths include the Hindus and Buddhists; in the West, they include the Seventh Day Adventists.

PERSONAL TASTE Meat consumption is an acquired habit, not an organic necessity. It starts in childhood for most people, backed by the encouragement of generations of misinformed parents. Our natural taste is actually for the full-flavored, wholesome taste of vegetarian cuisine. This is shown by the fact that most people lose their taste for flesh once it is omitted from their diet. Innumerable culinary delights can be concocted from a wide variety of plant foods, including herbs and spices, and these delicious dishes prove that the only limitations that exist are man-made.

A Vegetarian Rotation Diet and Recipes

The recipes in this chapter have benefited from years of research and experimentation. They have been designed to fit easily into a 4-day rotational diet plan in which specific foods such as brown rice, soybeans, or wheat are eaten only once every 4 days. On any one day, a food may be eaten several times in relatively small quantities. (See chapter 11 for a discussion of food rotation.) Additionally, the recipes have been devised according to the principles of proper food combining in order to allow for optimal digestibility, absorption, assimilation, and elimination. Following a diet using these recipes will provide all the protein and fiber that you need, as well as a full spectrum of vitamins and minerals.

The recipes also were designed to dispel the myths that a vegetarian diet must be boring, unappetizing, and nutritionally inadequate. While a macrobiotic diet has been of benefit to many people, too often those who are unfamiliar with vegetarianism consider macrobiotic cuisine, as prepared in many restaurants, to be synonymous with vegetarian cuisine generally. And yet the major cuisines of the world, including those of China, India, the Middle East, and Mexico, are essentially vegetarian, using meat only sparingly, as a spice rather than an entree. Vegetarian cooking can be both tasty and varied.

Being a vegetarian should not be a burden, nor should it alienate you from your friends and family. Of course, at first you may find it necessary to make a certain number of lifestyle changes. You will want to look for a good health food store that is convenient to shop in and provides the products that you need. If some of the ingredients listed in these recipes are unfamiliar to you, see the next chapter for more detailed descriptions. At first you may have to spend a little more time planning and preparing your meals, but with time it will become second nature.

Two important things to remember are flexibility and gentleness. You are learning something new and initially you may well make mistakes. If, for example, you go off of the diet at a party or if you go on a "binge," it will not help to beat yourself up for it. Simply chalk one up to experience and plan on doing better the next time. If you are out with friends at a restaurant that does not serve brown rice or vegetarian meals, don't panic. You will learn to see your way through such situations without feeling embarrassed or making those around you uncomfortable. For instance, you can order the baked potato instead of the rice, and a grilled piece of fish instead of red meat.

The ideal diet involves eating a number of small meals throughout the day. Eating just one large meal can interfere with the proper absorption of nutrients and place a burden on digestion. It can also add surplus calories. Generally, you should eat no more than 3 to 4 ounces of a given food at any one meal. In these quantities, you may eat the same food several times during the day, however. This approach will reduce your overall caloric intake and keep your body functioning with optimal energy. Keep in mind that it is best to meet the body's vitamin, mineral, and protein requirements throughout the day.

If you wish to prepare additional servings of these recipes, increase the amounts of main ingredients (vegetables, fruits, seeds, grains, legumes, flour, etc.) in proportions equal to the existing recipes. Condiments should only be increased by 1/8 teaspoon per additional portion.

First Cycle

DAY 1
BREAKFAST

Warm and Sweet Morning Cereal

1 cup. amaranth
1 1/2 cups fresh pineapple, if possible
if not, 2 1/2 rings canned pineapple

1/2 cup raisins
1 tbsp. honey
pinch cinnamon

In medium saucepan, combine amaranth and 2 cups of water. Lower heat when water begins to boil. Allow to simmer for approximately 25 minutes. While amaranth is cooking, cut pineapple into 1/2 inch pieces. When amaranth is cooked, add pineapple and remaining ingredients. Mix thoroughly. (Serves 2.)

LUNCH

Three-Grain Vegetable Bake

1/2 cup amaranth
1/3 cup basmati rice
2/3 cup couscous
2 carrots
1 1/2 cups or one small bunchwatercress
1/2 stalks celery
1/2 cup pecans

2 tbsp. safflower oil
1/4 cup water
1/4 tsp. basil
1/4 tsp. rosemary
1/2 tsp. fresh mustard
1/2 cup golden raisins

Prepare a medium saucepan for each of the grains (amaranth, basmati rice, and couscous). Place 1 1/4 cups of water in saucepan with amaranth and cook for 25 minutes. Place 1 1/4 cups of water in the saucepan with the rice and cook for approximately 20 minutes. Place couscous in 1 1/4 cups of boiling water, remove from heat, and let stand for 10 minutes. Fluff with fork. Carefully wash carrots and then grate into a small bowl. Rinse watercress and chop. Clean celery stalks and chop. In large mixing bowl, combine all grains and add remaining ingredients. Mix well. Place mixture in baking pan. Bake for 20 minutes in 325-degree oven. (Serves 3.)

DINNER

Italian Vegetable Toss

2 carrots
1 medium zucchini
3 oz. arugula, 1 1/2 bunches
1 cup parsley leaves
2 tbsp. safflower oil

1/3 tsp. dried tarragon
1/3 tsp. dried basil
2 red cabbage leaves
2 tbsp. pine nuts
1 clove garlic, chopped finely

Carefully clean carrots and zucchini. Cut into bite-sized pieces and steam in either bamboo steamer basket or stainless steel steamer. Steam for approximately 8 minutes. Rinse arugula and parsley, pat dry with paper towel and tear into smaller pieces. In separate small bowl, combine oil and herbs. When vegetables are steamed, allow them to cool to room temperature. Transfer them into a large bowl and toss in arugula and parsley. Pour oil mixture into the bowl as well. Place cabbage leaves on each plate and place mixture on top. Top with pine nuts. You may serve this dish with a small filet of fish. (Serves 2.)

DINNER

(2ND OPTION)

Aromatic Indian Sweet Potato Bake

1/2 sweet potato
5 tbsp. amaranth
3 cups basmati rice
1/2 zucchini
1 stalk celery
2 tbsp. safflower oil

1/4 tsp. basil
2/3 tsp. salt
1/2 tsp. curry
1/2 tsp. tarragon
1/2 tsp. cumin

Wash sweet potato and pierce with fork. Place sweet potato in preheated 400-degree oven for 40 minutes or until done. (You can test it by inserting a fork.) In a medium saucepan, place amaranth in 1 1/4 cups of water. Cook for approximately 25 minutes or until done. In another saucepan, prepare rice similarly in 1 1/4 cups of water, and then cook for 20 minutes. While the grains are cooking, carefully wash zucchini and celery. Cut zucchini into 1/2" cubes. Slice celery in 1/4 " pieces. When sweet potato is cooked, allow it to cool so you can handle it. Then scoop the sweet potato out of its skin and place it in a medium-sized mixing bowl with the cooked rice, amaranth and remaining ingredients. Turn the mixture into the baking dish. Bake for 15 minutes in a preheated 375-degree oven. You may serve this dish with a small filet of fish. (Serves 2.)

DAY 2

BREAKFAST

Crunchy Sweet Rice

2/3 cup brown rice
1/2 cup coconut
shredded and unsweetened
1/3 cup cashews
5 small dates

1/2 tsp. cinnamon
2 oz. water
1/4 cup apples, chopped
1/3 cup sunflower seeds

In medium saucepan, cook brown rice in 1 3/4 cups of water. Lower heat when it comes to a boil. Cooking time is about 30 minutes. When rice is cooked, add coconut. Chop cashews and dates finely and add to rice. Add cinnamon. Take half of mixture and puree along with 1/4 cup of water for a few seconds. Then add pureed mixture back to the rest of the rice. Sprinkle sunflower seeds and apples on top. (Serves 1.)

LUNCH

Vegetable Filbertasia

1/2 cup kidney beans
1 cup cauliflower florets
6 spears asparagus
1 1/2 stalks celery
3 medium mushrooms
1/2 zucchini
1/3 cup filberts
1/4 cup water

2 tbs. sunflower oil
1/4 tsp. dried basil
2/3 tsp. dill
1/3 tsp. chili powder
1/4 tsp. celery seed
1 garlic clove chopped
1/2 tsp. salt

Soak beans in large bowl in 2 cups of water overnight. In the morning, rinse beans and replace with 2 cups of fresh water in a medium pot. Cook for 1 3/4 hours to 2 hours until done, adding water to pot as needed. Carefully rinse cauliflower, asparagus, celery, mushrooms, and zucchini. Steam cauliflower and asparagus for 10 minutes. Chop celery, slice mushrooms and zucchini. Chop filberts medium fine. Put filberts in a blender with water, oil, spices, and salt. Place all the vegetables in a serving pan. Top with filbert/kidney bean sauce. Serve at room temperature. (Serves 3.)

DINNER

Nutty Butternut Squash

1 small butternut squash
2 shallots
1/3 cup peanuts
1/4 cup water
1 garlic clove, finely diced

1 tsp. fresh ginger, diced
1/2 tsp. dried basil
1/2 tsp. salt
2 tbsp. sunflower oil
1/2 avocado, sliced

Cut squash in half, remove seeds, and discard them. Place squash in a baking pan with 1/3" water, cut-side down. Bake for 40 minutes at 400 degrees. When squash is cool enough to handle, remove its skin and cut into 1" pieces. Place in medium-sized mixing bowl. Chop shallots medium fine and add to the squash. Place peanuts, water, herbs, salt, and oil in a blender. Mix well. Add this sauce to the squash and the shallots. Place mixture in a greased, covered baking pan at 350 degrees for 20 minutes. When done, place avocado slices on top as garnish. Serve with a small filet of fish if desired (Serves 2.)

DAY 3
BREAKFAST

High-Protein Cinnamon Millet

1 cup millet
1/3 cup almonds
pinch cinnamon

1/4 cup brewer's yeast
1 tsp. vanilla
1 tsp. maple syrup

In medium saucepan, cook millet in 13 oz. of water. When the water comes to a boil, lower heat. Stir occasionally. Cooking time is approximately 30 minutes. In another saucepan, blanch almonds by placing them in scalding water to remove the skins. Chop almonds. Add cinnamon, brewer's yeast, vanilla, and maple syrup. (Serves 1.)

LUNCH

Thick and Spicy Potato Chowder

2 potatoes
4 cups water
1 small tomato
1/2 green pepper
2 carrots
1 cup broccoli florets

1/2 tsp. cumin
1/2 tsp. basil
3 tbsp. sesame oil
1 1/4 tsp. salt
5 scallions, chopped

Peel and quarter potato, and place in 4 cups of water in medium saucepan. Boil for approximately 15 minutes. Place potato in a blender with the water in which it was cooked. Add the seasonings, oil, and salt. Wash the tomatoes, pepper, carrots, and broccoli. Chop into bite-sized pieces. Transfer the potato mixture back into a saucepan. Add the chopped vegetables. Cook over a low heat for an additional 10 to 15 minutes. Top with scallions. (Yields 4 to 5 cups.)

DINNER

Almost Spaghetti Squash Dinner

1 small spaghetti squash
5 scallions
2 small tomato
1/2 green pepper
2 mushrooms

2 tbsp. olive oil
1/4 tsp. dried basil
1/2 tsp. rosemary
1 tsp. fresh garlic minced
1 tsp. salt

Cut squash in half, remove the seeds and discard them. Place the halves in a baking pan with 1/3" water, cut-side down. Bake for 40 minutes at 400 degrees. When the squash is cool enough to handle, remove the pulp or "spaghetti." Carefully wash the scallions, tomato, pepper, onion, and mushrooms. Chop them medium fine. In large skillet, add oil and sauté vegetables along with the seasonings and salt for 5 minutes. Combine all the ingredients in a large bowl. Mix carefully and then transfer to a serving dish. Serve with a small filet of fish if desired (Serves 2.)

DAY 4
BREAKFAST

Banana Barley

3/4 cup barley
2 tbsp. barley malt

1/2 banana, mashed
1/3 cup raisins

In medium saucepan, cook barley in 1 2/3 cups of water for 20 minutes or until done. Add barley malt, mashed banana, and raisins. Mix well. Serve hot. (Serves 2.)

LUNCH

Rainbow Vegetable Salad

1/2 cup soy beans
3 leaves kale
1 cup cauliflower florets
2 carrots
1 yellow squash
1/3 cup Brazil nuts

11/2 tbsp. soy oil
1/3 tsp. garlic, minced
3 tbsp. chives
1/4 tsp. coriander
1/4 tsp. dried tarragon
1/2 tsp. salt

In large bowl, soak beans overnight in 2 cups of water. In the morning, rinse the beans and transfer to a medium soup pot with 2 cups of fresh water. Cook for 2 hours or until done. Carefully rinse kale, cauliflower, and yellow squash. Tear the kale and cut the vegetables into bite-sized pieces. Steam in a bamboo steamer basket or stainless steel steamer for 8 minutes. Chop Brazil nuts finely. Combine all ingredients in a medium-sized mixing bowl. Mix well. Serve hot or cold. (Serves 2.)

DINNER

Brazilian Broccoli Bake

1/2 cup lima beans
1 cup broccoli
3 oz. tofu, small slice
1/2 onion
1 1/2 oz. Brazil nuts
2 tbsp. soy oil

1 clove garlic, minced
1 tsp. coriander
1 tsp. dried parsley
1/2 tsp. salt
1 tsp. mustard

In large mixing bowl, soak lima beans overnight in 2 cups of water. In the morning, rinse the beans and transfer them into a medium soup pot with 2 cups of fresh water. Cook for 1 1/2 hours or until done, adding water to pot as needed. Rinse broccoli and cut into 1/2" florets. Rinse tofu and cut into 1/2" cubes. Peel and slice the onion. Place all ingredients in a large mixing bowl. Add half of the Brazil nuts, the oil, and seasonings. Add the mustard. Mix well. Place in a greased baking dish with lid. Top with remaining Brazil nuts. Bake for 20 minutes in a preheated 350-degree oven. Serve with a small filet of fish if desired. (Serves 2.)

Second Cycle

DAY 1
BREAKFAST

Carob Gruel

1 1/3 cup oatmeal
1 1/2 tbsp. carob powder

pinch nutmeg
1/4 tsp. cinnamon

In medium saucepan, boil 3 cups of cold water. When water begins to boil, add oatmeal and lower heat. Stir frequently. Cooking time is approximately 10 minutes. Add remaining ingredients 1 minute before the oatmeal is fully cooked. Serve hot. (Serves 2.)

Light 'n' Easy Squash Salad

2/3 cup ouscous
3 medium mushrooms
2 carrots
small summer squash
2 tbsp. parsley
1/2 clove garlic, chopped

2 tsp. dried thyme
1/2 tsp. basil
1/2 tsp. salt
6 tbsp. pine nuts
4 cherry tomatoes for garnish

In medium saucepan, combine couscous with 1 1/4 cups boiling water. Remove from heat and let stand for 10 minutes. Fluff with fork. Wash mushrooms, carrots, and squash carefully. Slice mushrooms, carrots, and squash into bite-sized pieces. Steam in a bamboo steamer basket or stainless steel steamer until tender but crunchy. Start with the carrots, steam 5 minutes, then add squash and mushrooms. Rinse parsley and chop finely. Chop garlic. Combine all ingredients in a large salad bowl. Garnish with cherry tomatoes. (Serves 2.)

DINNER

Vegetable Cornucopia Soup with Black-Eyed Peas

1/2 cup black-eyed peas
1/3 cup basmati rice
2/3 cup hijiki, dry
1 1/2 cups watercress
1/2 parsnip
2 carrots
1 stalk celery

1/2 onion, chopped
1 tsp. tamari
2 garlic cloves, finely diced
3 tbsp. safflower oil
1 tsp. coriander
1 bay leaf
1 tsp. salt

In large bowl, soak peas overnight in 3 cups of water. In the morning, rinse well and transfer to a medium soup pot with 4 cups of fresh water. Bring beans to a boil, lower to medium heat, and cover. In medium saucepan, cook rice in 1 1/4 cups of water for 20 minutes. Meanwhile soak hijiki in 1 cup of water and rinse twice. Rinse the watercress and tear into smaller pieces. Clean the parsnips and carrots, and cut into bite-sized pieces. Clean celery and slice in 1/4" pieces. When peas have cooked for 1 1/2 hours, add the cooked rice and remaining ingredients. Cook over a low heat for 25 to 30 minutes or until beans are tender. (Yields 4 servings.)

Tossed Garden Salad

1/2 head red leaf lettuce
1/2 head endive

1/3 red pepper
1/2 cup alfalfa sprouts

Wash lettuce, endive and pepper. Cut into bite-sized pieces and put into a salad bowl. Top with sprouts. (Serves 2.)

DAY 2
BREAKFAST

Tropical Rice Breakfast

2/3 cup brown rice
1/4 cup raisins
1/4 cup sunflower seeds

1/2 banana, mashed
2 oz. fruit juice, optional
1/2 cup coconut

In medium saucepan, cook brown rice in 1 2/3 cups of water. When water comes to a boil, lower heat. Cooking time is approximately 30 minutes. During the last 10 minutes of cooking, add raisins, sunflower seeds, and coconut. When it is completely cooked, add mashed banana. When serving, you may add the fruit juice. (Serves 2.)

LUNCH

Butternut Arugula Salad

1 small butternut squash
3 oz. arugula
1/2 cup alfalfa sprouts
1/4 cup currants

2 tbsp. sunflower oil
1/2 tsp. dried dill
1/2 tsp. dried parsley
1/2 tsp. salt

Cut squash in half and remove and discard seeds. Place squash cut-side down in a baking pan with 1/3" of water. Bake for 40 minutes at 400 degrees. When squash is cool enough to handle, cut into bite-sized pieces. Place in a medium mixing bowl. Rinse arugula carefully to get all the dirt off. Tear off the stems and discard. Then add the arugula to the squash. Add the remaining ingredients. Toss gently so as not to mash the squash. Serve hot or cold. (Serves 2.)

DINNER

Herby Italian Noodles with Rice

1/3 cup brown rice
3 oz. buckwheat noodles
1/2 avocado
4 small marinated artichokes
2 tbsp. sunflower oil
2 tsp. scallions, chopped

1 tsp. parsley, chopped
1 garlic clove, minced
1/2 tsp. dried basil
1/2 tsp. salt
6 black olives, garnish

In medium saucepan, cook brown rice in 1 1/3 cups of water for 35 minutes or until done. Cook noodles according to directions on package. Chop the avocado and artichokes into bite-sized pieces and place in a medium mixing bowl. Add the remaining ingredients. Toss gently. When the rice and noodles are done, place them on plates. Top with the avocado mixture. Serve at room temperature. Serve with a small filet of fish if desired. (Serves 2.)

DAY 3
BREAKFAST

Almond Millet

1 cup millet
1/3 cup dried banana chips
1/3 cup almonds

1/4 cup brewer's yeast
1 tbsp. maple syrup

Cook millet in 13 oz. of water in a medium saucepan for 30 minutes. Add dried banana. Chop almonds. Add them to the millet along with the brewer's yeast and maple syrup. Serve hot. (Serves 2.)

LUNCH

Savory Mushroom Dip

1/3 large potato
5 mushrooms
1/4 onion
2 tsp. sesame seeds
1/3 cup water or broth
3 tbsp. olive oil

1 tsp. salt
1/4 tsp. cayenne
1/4 tsp. cumin
1/4 tsp. coriander
vegetable sticks (celery,
carrots, daikon, etc.)

Peel and wash potato. Slice approximately 1/4" thick and place in a medium saucepan with enough water to cover. Cook until the potatoes are tender when you stick a fork in them. Rinse and slice mushrooms and onion. Sauté in a medium skillet until the onions are a golden brown. When the potatoes are cooked, place them in a blender with all the other ingredients. Puree well into a diplike consistency. Serve with vegetable sticks. (Yield is approx. 5 servings.)

DINNER

Spaghetti Deluxe

1 small onion	1/2 yellow pepper
2 tsp. olive oil	1/3 zucchini
1/4 tsp. dried basil	2 tbsp. tomato paste
1/4 tsp. dried oregano	1/3 cup water
1/4 tsp. cumin	1 garlic clove, minced
2 large tomato	1/2 tsp. salt
6 oz. spaghetti	

Peel and dice onion. Sauté in the oil with the herbs in a 2-quart saucepan along with the tomato paste, water, garlic, and salt. Continue to cook, covered, for 15 minutes on low heat. Cook spaghetti in 1 quart of water in another saucepan for 10 to 12 minutes or until done. Combine with vegetables in a medium mixing bowl. Serve hot with a small filet of fish if desired. (Serves 2.)

DAY 4
BREAKFAST

Chock Full of Protein Drink

1/3 cup Brazil nuts	1 tbsp. carob powder
1/2 cup soy milk	1/2 banana
1/4 cup apple cider	pinch cinnamon

Chop Brazil nuts finely. Combine all of the ingredients in a blender, and blend well smooth and creamy. If you like your drinks sweeter, you may use the whole banana. (Serves 1.)

LUNCH

Hearty Lentil Soup

1/2 cup lentils	1/2 tsp. garlic powder
1 large carrots	1/2 tsp. coriander
1/3 cup corn (may be fresh and	1/2 tsp. dried rosemary
removed from the husk or frozen)	1/2 tsp. dried basil
4 tbsp. fresh chives	3/4 tsp. salt
3 tbsp. soy oil	several parsley sprigs for garnish

Rinse lentils and pick out any pebbles. Cook lentils in medium soup pot with enough water to cover. Bring to a boil and then set on medium heat with the lid on. Cooking time is approximately 1 hour. Scrub carrot and cut into bite-sized pieces. After lentils have cooked for approximately 20 minutes, drop carrots into the pot along with the corn and remaining ingredients. When the mixture has cooked for an additional 30 minutes, take half of the mixture out of the pot and put it into a blender. Puree for 15 seconds and then pour back into the pot. Cook for an additional 10 minutes. Garnish with parsley sprigs. (Yields 4 to 5 cups.)

Nutty Bean Salad

1/2 cup black beans	1 garlic clove, minced
1/3 cup walnuts	1 tsp. tarragon
1 stalk celery	1/2 tsp. dried sage
1 large carrots	1/2 tsp. salt
1 1/2 tbsp. soy oil	

In large bowl, soak black beans overnight in 1 1/4 cups of water. In the morning, rinse the beans and transfer them to a medium saucepan with 2 cups of fresh water. Cook for 1 1/2 hours or until done, adding water to pot as needed. Chop walnuts very finely. Rinse celery and scrub carrots. Cut celery and carrots into bite-sized pieces. Place oil in a wok or skillet and heat. Place all ingredients into wok or skillet and sauté for 5 minutes. Serve at room temperature. (Serves 1.)

DINNER

Hot and Crunchy Veggie Mix

2/3 cup snap green beans	1/2 tsp. parsley
1 cup cauliflower florets	juice of 1/2 lemon
2/3 cup brussels sprouts (about 5)	pinch cayenne
1/3 cup walnuts	2 tbsp. soy oil
1/4 tsp. dried sage	3/4 tsp. salt
1/2 tsp. dill	1/4 cup water

Wash beans and cut into bite-sized pieces. Steam in bamboo steam basket or stainless steel steamer for 10 minutes or until tender. Rinse cauliflower and Brussels sprouts and cut into bite-sized pieces. Steam for 8 minutes. In a blender, place the steamed beans, walnuts, and remaining ingredients. Pour sauce over the cauliflower and Brussels sprouts. You may serve this dish either hot or cold. Serve with small filet of fish if desired. (Serves 2.)

Third Cycle

DAY 1
BREAKFAST

Sweet Cinnamon Couscous

1 1/3 cup couscous	1/2 tbsp. honey
1/4 apple	1/2 tsp. cinnamon
1/3 cup raisins	1/3 cup fruit juice, optional

In medium saucepan, place couscous in 1 2/3 cups of boiling water. Remove from heat. Fluff with fork. Wash and slice apples. Add apple slices and remaining ingredients to couscous. Mix well. Transfer to serving bowls. Add fruit juice if you wish. (Serves 2.)

LUNCH

Milano Bean and Vegetable Soup

1/2 cup mung beans	1 garlic clove, finely diced
1 zucchini	3 tbsp. safflower oil
5 small summer squash	3/4 tsp. salt
1/2 Spanish onion	1/2 tsp. dried basil
1 1/2 carrots	1/4 tsp. dried oregano
2 tbsp.parsley	

Place mung beans in a large bowl with 3 cups of water. Allow beans to soak overnight. In the morning, rinse beans well and transfer into a large soup pot, adding 4 cups of fresh water. Bring beans to a boil and lower to medium heat. Keep the lid on. Scrub zucchini and summer squash. Peel onion and carrots. Chop the vegetables into bite-sized pieces. Rinse parsley and chop finely. After beans have been cooking for approximately 1 hour, add the vegetables and remaining ingredients. Remove half of the mixture and transfer into a blender. Puree for 15 seconds. Return the puree to the rest of the soup to finish cooking for another 30 minutes. (Yields 4 to 5 servings.)

DINNER

Superb Vegetable Rice Salad

1/2 cup amaranth	2 tbsp. safflower oil
1/3 cup basmati rice	juice of 1/2 lemon
1/2 cup watercress	1/2 tsp. salt
2 tbxp. dill	1/4 cup water
2 tbsp. parsley	1/4 tsp. tarragon
1 carrot	

In medium pot, cook amaranth for 25 minutes in 1 1/4 cups of water. In another pot, cook rice in 1 1/4 cups of water for 20 minutes. Rinse watercress, dill, and parsley, and chop medium fine. Scrub carrots well and chop into bite-sized pieces. Place all ingredients in medium bowl and mix well. (Serves 2.)

**DINNER
(2ND OPTION)**

Oriental Zucchini Salad

1/2 cup amaranth	2 carrots
2/3 cup hijiki dried seaweed	1/2 zucchini
1/4 daikon radish	2 tbsp. safflower oil
1/4 tsp. coriander	2/3 tsp. salt
1/2 tsp. cumin	1/4 tsp. garlic
1/3 cup pecan	

In medium saucepan, cook amaranth in 1 1/2 cups of water for 25 minutes. Rinse hijiki and soak three times. Scrub carrots and zucchini. Peel daikon. Cut carrots, zucchini, and daikon into bite-sized pieces and steam in bamboo steamer basket or stainless steel steamer for 8 minutes. In a skillet or wok, sauté the hijiki with safflower oil and herbs for 5 minutes. Combine all ingredients together in medium bowl. Add pecans. Mix well. Serve with small filet of fish if desired. (Serves 2.)

**DAY 2
BREAKFAST**

Fruity Rice Breakfast

1/3 cup brown rice	1 tbsp. fruit conserve
1/2 cup coconut	(no sugar, just fruit)
1/3 cup cashews	2 chopped figs

In medium saucepan, cook brown rice in 1 2/3 cups of water. When water comes to a boil, lower heat. Cooking time is approximately 30 minutes. When cooked, add coconut and cashews. Mix well. Remove from heat. Add conserves and figs. Mix again. Transfer to bowl. (Serves 2.)

LUNCH

Curried Vegetable Rice

1/2 cup split peas
2/3 cup brown rice
1 cup broccoli florets
2 carrots
1/2 zucchini

1/2 onions
3 tbsp. sunflower oil
1/2 tsp. curry powder
3/4 tsp. salt

In medium saucepan, cook split peas in enough water to cover. Bring to a boil then lower heat. In another saucepan, cook rice in 1 2/3 cups of water for 30 minutes. Clean vegetables well and cut into bite-sized pieces. After peas have cooked for 15 minutes, add chopped vegetables, cooked brown rice, and remaining ingredients. Cook for an additional 15 minutes. (Yields 5 servings.)

DINNER

Sunny Squash

1 small butternut squash
3 oz. buckwheat noodles
6 spears asparagus
2 cups watercress

1 tsp. parsley
1 clove garlic, minced
5 tbsp. sunflower oil
3/4 tsp. salt

Cut squash in half. Remove seeds and discard. Place squash in baking pan with 1/3" water, cut-side down. Bake for 40 minutes at 400 degrees. When cool enough to handle, remove the squash from the skin and set aside in a medium-sized bowl. Drop noodles into salted boiling water and cook for 5 minutes. Set aside. Rinse the asparagus. Steam in a bamboo steamer basket or stainless steel steamer. Cut into 2" pieces. Rinse watercress and chop. Add noodles to the squash along with the asparagus, watercress, and remaining ingredients. Mix well, tossing gently. Serve with tossed salad and small filet of fish if desired. (Yields 4 to 5 servings.)

DAY 3
BREAKFAST

Heart-Warming Breakfast

1/3 cup cream of wheat
7 small chopped dates
1/3 cup shredded coconut

1/4 cup brewer's yeast
1/2 tsp. cinnamon

In medium saucepan, cook cream of wheat in 1 1/3 cups of water for 10 minutes or until done. Stir occasionally over medium heat. When cooked, add remaining ingredients. Transfer to bowl. (Serves 1.)

LUNCH

Baked Potato Sesame

1 small potato
3 oz. spaghetti
3 scallions
1 tsp. dried dill
1/4 cup tahini

1/4 cup sesame seeds
1 1/2 tbsp. sesame oil
1/4 tsp. coriander
1/2 tsp. salt
1 garlic clove, minced

Wash potato and pierce with fork. Bake potato for 40 minutes at 400 degrees. When cool enough to handle, cut into 3/4" cubes. Cook spaghetti in a medium saucepan in 1 quart of water for 10 minutes. Rinse scallions and chop medium fine. Mix potato and spaghetti in medium mixing bowl. Add remaining ingredients. Transfer to baking pan and bake for 15 minutes in a preheated 375-degree oven. (Serves 2.)

DINNER

Crunchy Vegetable Bean Salad

1/2 cup adzuki beans
2 tbsp. almonds
5 scallions
1/2 red pepper
1 tsp. parsley
1 small tomato

2 tbsp. sesame oil
1/4 tsp. oregano
1 tsp. salt
1/2 tsp. thyme
1 clove garlic, minced
several leaves of romaine lettuce

In large bowl, soak beans overnight in 2 cups of water. In the morning, rinse beans and place into medium pot with 2 cups of fresh water. Cook for 1 hour or until done, adding water to pot as needed. Blanch almonds by bringing 2 1/2 cups of water in small saucepan to a boil and dropping the almonds into the water. Remove from heat. Let almonds remain in boiling water for 5 minutes and then run cold water into saucepan. Squeeze the skins off and let almonds dry. Sliver the almonds. Rinse scallions, red pepper, parsley, and tomato. Cut into bite-sized pieces. In medium mixing bowl, gently toss beans, almonds, and vegetables. Add remaining ingredients and mix well. Serve cool on a bed of romaine lettuce. (Serves 2.)

DAY 4
BREAKFAST

Creamy Banana Tofu Pudding

1 banana	1 tsp. vanilla
1/3 cup raisins	3 heaping tsp.
3 oz. tofu, small slice	Ener-G Egg Replacer
3/4 cup apple juice	(any powdered egg subsitite)
1/3 cup barley malt	pinch cinnamon
1 tbsp. carob powder	pinch nutmeg

Place all ingredients in blender. Puree until smooth and creamy. Transfer to medium saucepan and cook over medium heat for 5 minutes, stirring frequently. Allow to chill for 45 minutes. (Yields 2 1/2 cups, about 5 servings.)

LUNCH

Mid-Eastern Tempeh

1/3 cup chick-peas	2 tbsp. soy oil
1/4 cup dulse, dry	a garlic clove, minced
2 cup cauliflower florets	1/4 tsp. salt
4 inch square tempeh	1/2 tsp. dried basil
1/2 onion	1/4 cup water
3/4 cup tomato sauce	

In medium bowl, soak chick-peas overnight in 2 cups of water. In the morning, rinse the chick-peas and transfer into medium soup pot with 2 1/2 cups of fresh water. Cook for 1 3/4 to 2 hours or until done. Rinse dulse 2 or 3 times in cold water. Rinse cauliflower and cut into florets. Cut tempeh into 1/2" cubes and put all the ingredients together in a medium mixing bowl. Peel and slice onion and add to mixture. Toss gently. Add remaining ingredients and mix well. Transfer to greased baking pan and bake for 20 minutes in a preheated 350-degree oven. (Serves 2.)

DINNER

Double Bean Delight

1/3 cup lima beans	3 tbsp. water
1/2 cup lentils	1/4 tsp. dried tarragon
6 pieces okra	1/2 tsp. dried sage
3 oz. cauliflower	1/2 tsp. salt
1/2 tbsp. brazil nut butter	1 garlic clove, minced
1 1/2 tbsp. corn oil	

Note: Brazil nut butter is made with a "champion" juicer or a similar grinder In large bowl, soak beans overnight in 2 cups of water. In the morning, rinse and replace with 2 cups of fresh water in medium soup pot. Cook for 1 1/2 hours or until done. In another pot, cook lentils in 1 1/2 cups of water for 25 minutes. Rinse and cut vegetables into bite-sized pieces. Steam in a bamboo steamer basket or stainless steel steamer for 8 minutes or until tender. Transfer all ingredients into a medium mixing bowl and gently toss. Add remaining ingredients and mix well. Transfer to greased baking pan and bake for 15 minutes in a 350-degree oven. (Serves 2.)

Additional Desserts

Multi-Fruit Oatmeal Pudding

1/2 pear	1 banana
2 heaping tsp.	1/4 apple
Ener-G-Egg Replacer	pinch cinnamon
(or any powdered egg substitiute)	3/4 cup pear juice
2/3 cup oatmeal	

Place all ingredients, except for apples, in a blender. Puree. Transfer puree into small saucepan and cook over medium heat for approximately 5 minutes. Wash and cube apples. Add apples to puree and stir frequently. Place in medium mixing bowl or individual dessert dishes and allow to chill in refrigerator for at least 45 minutes. (Yields 4 to 5 servings.)

Tropical Pudding

1 cup pineapple
3/4 cup apple juice
3 tbsp. honey
2 tbsp. Ener-G-Egg Replacer
(or any powdered egg substitiute)

2 tbsp. shredded coconut
pinch nutmeg
1/4 papaya
1/3 cup pecans

Place all ingredients, except for papaya and pecans, in a blender. Puree. Transfer puree into small saucepan and cook over medium heat for approximately 5 minutes. Peel papaya, remove seeds, and cube. Chop pecans. Add both to puree and stir. Place in medium mixing bowl or individual dessert dishes and allow to chill in refrigerator for at least 45 minutes. (Yields approximately 4 servings.)

Mango Strawberry Canton

1/2 small mango
medium strawberries
1 1/2 cups apple juice

2 heaping tbsp. agar-agar
1 tsp. vanilla
7 small dates, chopped

Peel mango and remove pit. Put in blender with 3 of the strawberries. Add apple juice and blend. Transfer to medium saucepan and bring to boil. Lower heat and add agar-agar. Stir and dissolve agar-agar and simmer for 5 minutes. Add vanilla and chopped dates. Transfer to mixing bowl or individual dessert dishes and place in refrigerator until juice begins to gel (about 10 minutes). Drop in remaining strawberries. Chill for 1 hour. (Serves 2 to 4.)

Papaya Brown Rice Pudding

1/3 cup brown rice
1/3 large papaya
1/2 cup shredded coconut
2 small figs

1 1/4 cup pineapple coconut juice
2 heaping tsp.
Ener-G-Egg Replacer
1/2 cup blueberries

In medium saucepan, cook brown rice in about 1 1/4 cups of water for 25 minutes. When cooked, place in blender. Peel papaya and remove seeds. Add to blender along with remaining ingredients, except for blueberries. Puree until creamy and smooth. Transfer to medium saucepan and cook over medium heat for approximately 5 minutes. Stir frequently. Transfer to medium mixing bowl or individual dessert dishes and place in refrigerator to chill for 45 minutes. Serve with blueberries. (Yields 4 servings.)

Blueberry Kiwi Pudding

1 cup millet
1 1/8 cups blueberries
1 smal kiwi
1/2 banana
1/3 cup slivered almonds

3/4 cup apple strawberry juice
2 heaping tsp.
Ener-G-Egg Replacer
1 tsp. lemon juice

Place millet in a small saucepan with approximately 1 1/4 cups of water and cook for 20 minutes. When cooked, put in blender with remaining ingredients, except for almonds. Puree until smooth and creamy. Transfer puree to medium saucepan and heat for 5 minutes over medium heat, stirring frequently. Transfer to medium mixing bowl or individual dessert dishes and allow to chill in refrigerator for 45 minutes. Top with almonds. (Yields 7 to 10 servings.)

Strawberry Tofu Pudding

7 strawberries
2 small slices tofu

3 tbsp. maple syrup
1 tsp. vanilla

Place all ingredients in the blender. Puree until creamy and smooth. Transfer into one medium mixing bowl or individual dessert dishes. Place in refrigerator and allow to chill for 45 minutes. (Serves 2.)

Peach Canton

1 peach
1 1/2 cup apple blackberry juice
2 heaping tbsp. agar-agar

2 tbsp. Barbados molasses
1/2 cup pitted black cherries

Wash and cut peaches into small pieces. Place half of peaches in a blender with juice. Place mixture in medium saucepan and bring to boil. Lower heat and add agar-agar. Stir and dissolve agar, and simmer for 5 minutes. Add molasses. Transfer to medium mixing bowl or individual dessert dishes and place in refrigerator until juice begins to gel (about 10 minutes). Add remaining peaches and cherries. Chill for 1 hour. (Serves 2.)

Peachy Tofu Pudding

1 peach
3 tbsp. barley malt

1 tsp. vanilla
3/4 cup peach juice

Wash and cut peaches. Place all ingredients in blender and puree until smooth. Transfer to medium saucepan and place on medium heat for 5 minutes, stirring frequently. Transfer to medium mixing bowl or individual dessert dishes and allow to chill in refrigerator for 45 minutes. (Yields 4 to 5 servings.)

Blueberry Banana Pudding

1 1/4 cup blueberries
1 banana
1 small slice tofu

1/3 cup apple juice
1 small nectarines, sliced
4 tbsp. almonds

Place blueberries, banana, tofu, and apple juice in blender. Puree until smooth and creamy. Transfer to medium mixing bowl or individual dessert dishes. Top with nectarine slices and almonds. (Serves 2.)

13

Guide to Natural Foods

Whole Grains

Whole grains contain everything needed to nurture themselves, from germ stage to sprout to mature plant. Plant a whole kernel of any grain and, given the right combination of earth, water, and air, it will naturally sprout and grow to maturity. Not so with refined grains. Bury a milled kernel and cultivate it as much as you like; nothing will grow because the kernel is already dead.

Milling the root of whole grains only refines away a wide range of trace minerals and vitamins in the outer layers, resulting in grains that are bulkier and less healthy. Refined grains, robbed of the minerals and vitamins found in the discarded outer layers, strain the body's delicate mechanism of digestion. Nearly all of the B vitamins, vitamins E, unsaturated fatty acids, and quality proteins are found in whole grains, but refining removes most of these nutrients. Even in so-called enriched foods, only a few B vitamins and iron are replaced; the remaining B vitamins, as well as a rich variety of minerals and proteins, are "refined" out.

There are three ways to prepare whole grains for eating: sprouting, soaking, and cooking until tender. All grains can be sprouted in 2 to 3 days, or until the sprout reaches the same length as the original seeds. You can reconstitute some semiprocessed grains, such as bulgur wheat, by soaking them overnight or pouring boiling water over them and allowing them to fluff up.

When you cook grains, first rinse them in a colander or strainer, then pour the grain into a pot of water and swirl it with your hands, removing the hulls and bits of dirt that may float to the surface. Drain the grain through a strainer, dry pan-fry it in a heavy skillet, and add two parts boiling water. Cover the skillet, reduce the heat, and let the grain simmer for about a half-hour (time varies with the grain).

When preparing grains in a pressure cooker, the proportion of water to grain is roughly 2 1/2 parts water for each part of grain. Add grain and water to the cooker and bring them rapidly up to full pressure. When the regulator on the lid makes a juggling sound, the cooker has reached full pressure; reduce the heat to simmer and maintain the same pressure throughout the cooking. Allow the pressure to return to normal before loosening the lid, then open the pot and gently stir the grains, mixing the kernels toward the bottom with those at the top. Let them sit for a few minutes, then mix again.

Most grains at least double in size from their dry to cooked states. This means that 1 cup of cooked grain can feed two or three enthusiastic grain eaters or three to four people eating grain along with other foods. To achieve a sweeter flavor and crunchier texture, try dry-toasting the grain or sautéing it before cooking. To dry-toast, start with a cold skillet, preferably cast iron. To sauté, you must first heat the skillet and then quickly, evenly, coat it with oil. (If the oil smokes, it's too hot.) Whether dry-toasting or sautéing, stir the grain until a few kernels pop and a delicious aroma begins to rise.

BARLEY Barley has much to offer as a solo grain dish. Some of the best barley in the world—consistently high in protein and minerals—comes from the rich soil of the Red River Valley of North Dakota and Minnesota.

Since unhulled barley is almost impossible to cook, practically all barley available in food stores has been "pearled" so as to remove its tenacious hull. The factor to consider here is just how much pearling has taken place; too much results in a whiter product robbed of the nutrients in its outer layer. Look for the darker barley available in most natural food stores.

Allow 30 to 35 minutes to cook simmered barley using 2 1/3 parts liquid (water, stock, etc.) to 1 part grain. The barley can also be browned before adding it to the boiling liquid. Pressure cooking (2 parts water to 1 part grain) takes approximately 20 minutes. If the resulting grain seems too chewy, simply add 1/4 cup more water, cover, and simmer until soft. You might also try cooking barley with other grains, such as brown rice and wheat berries.

Barley can be sprouted but first it has to be hulled (try seed houses and grain suppliers). Harvest the sprout when it's about the same size as the grain. Barley flour can be obtained already milled or ground fresh from the pearled grain. It is often pan-roasted before being used in breads, muffins, and cakes. Recently, researchers have found that barley, eaten daily, is successful in lowering cholesterol levels by 25 percent.

BUCKWHEAT Buckwheat is actually not a true grain but a grass seed related to rhubarb. When raised commercially as a grain crop, buckwheat is unlikely to have been fertilized or sprayed. Fertilization encourages too much leaf growth;

spraying stops the bees from pollinating. The best buy is whole, hulled, unroasted (white) buckwheat grains, known as groats. Roasted (brown) and cut groats are less nutritious, and the roasting can easily be done just before cooking without disturbing the flavor or the B vitamins.

Buckwheat cooks quickly, so it is rarely pressure cooked. Simmer for 15 to 20 minutes in the same saucepan or skillet you first roasted it in, using 2 parts water to 1 part buckwheat. If you prefer a porridgelike consistency, use 3 parts water. Cooked buckwheat can serve as a stuffing for everything from cabbage leaves and collard greens to knishes. Buckwheat flour combined variously with whole wheat, unbleached white, and soy flours is a delight to pancake lovers. Whole grain buckwheat flour is always dark; light-colored buckwheat flour is made from sifted flour rather than from unroasted groats.

A Japanese pasta called soba is now readily available in natural food stores and in Asian markets. It contains anywhere from 30 to 100 percent buckwheat flour. Its subtle flavor and light effect on the stomach should encourage pasta enthusiasts to give it a try. It needs no heavy sauces; try a simple garlic or onion and oil topping.

You can prepare a buckwheat cream for morning cereal from buckwheat flour sautéed in oil in a heavy skillet. Allow it to cool and then return it to the heat, gradually adding water and bringing it to a boil. This mixture is then stirred and simmered about 10 minutes or until it reaches the desired consistency.

Sprout buckwheat from the unhulled groats in half an inch of soil on wet paper toweling and allow it to reach a height of 3 to 4 inches. The sprouts or young grass, called buckwheat lettuce, can then be juiced or chewed. The bioflavonoid rutin, which is reported to speed the coagulation of blood, helping to stop bleeding, is very high in sprouted buckwheat.

CORN Corn, a staple food for thousands of years, has changed from a small shrub with only a few kernels to today's hybrid varieties with 6-foot stalks bearing several ears that contain over 100 kernels apiece. Both white and yellow varieties of dried corn are readily available, but in the American Southwest the blue and varicolored older types of corn are still grown. "Sweet" corn is normally boiled or steamed in water; field corn is likely to be ground into meals and flours. Field corn is allowed to dry out completely, which changes the simple sugars of the grain into starches.

Yellow cornmeal contains about 10 percent protein and is higher in vitamin A than the white variety. The only difference between a meal and a flour from yellow corn is its degree of coarseness. The germ of cornmeal starts deteriorating in a matter of hours, so you should grind your own meal or flour as you use it for cornbreads, muffins, Southern spoon bread, johnnycakes, or whatever. You can fry it in a pan and then cook it with 5 to 6 parts water as a hearty "mush." Adding cornmeal to whole wheat flour in a tempura batter gives it a delicious crunchiness.

Another favorite form of this versatile grain is creamed corn. You can make creamed corn by cutting off the kernels just far enough down to allow the milky, sugary liquid to flow. Pour in enough water or milk to cover, a dash of salt, and cook the mixture gently for a few minutes. Corn flour can also be used in small amounts in whole grain pastas. A variety of Texas Deaf Smith County sweet corn can be sprouted successfully until the sprout is about a half-inch long.

MILLET The many virtues of millet are often overlooked because of its reputation as "the poor person's rice." Being the only grain that forms alkaline, millet is the most easily digestible. It is also an intestinal lubricant. Its amino acid structure is well balanced, providing a low-gluten protein, and it is high in calcium, riboflavin, and lecithin.

Millet is cooked the same way as most grains, with 2 parts water or stock to 1 part grain. Preroasting releases a lovely aroma and adds texture to the cooked grain. Leftover cooked millet is a highly versatile stuffing for anything from hollowed-out zucchini halves to mushroom caps.

Millet meal and millet flour are quality protein additions to any bread recipe. Millet meal also makes a good hot cereal. Sprouted millet makes an excellent base for morning cereal; just harvest the sprout when the shoot is the same size as the grain.

OATS Oats must be hulled before they can be eaten; after hulling they are cracked or rolled into the familiar cereal forms. Rolled oats are shot with steam for a number of seconds and then passed through rollers; thus some nutrients are lost. Rolled oats will cook faster than whole oat groats, but whole oat groats are the most beneficial. Known variously as Irish oatmeal, Scotch oats, or steel-cut oats, whole-oat groats are soaked overnight before being cooked as porridge. (None of these or any other cereals or porridges should ever be prepared in a pressure cooker as they tend to clog the vent on the lid of the cooker.) Whole oats are wonderful in soups. You can add both rolled and whole groats to all sorts of breads and patties.

Oat flour, available at most natural food stores, can be used in equal proportions with whole wheat flour to bake up a tasty batch of muffins. Oat sprouts can be used in soups, salads, and baked goods; just harvest the sprout when it is as long as the groat.

RICE Rice, from a nutritional point of view, means brown rice—whole grain rice which, unlike white rice, has not had its bran and with it much of its nutrition removed. Brown rice is available in short, medium, and long grain varieties, the difference being largely aesthetic. The shorter the grain, the more gluten, which means that short grain rice cooks up stickier and long grain comes out fluffier. There's even a sweet rice grain, the most glutinous of all. Excellent quality long- and medium-grain brown rice comes from southeast Texas and Louisiana; this rice is hulled by a special process that protects the bran layer.

Rice is traditionally simmered, the proportions of water to grain being as follows: short grain—2 1/2 to 1; medium grain—2 to 1; and long grain—1 1/2 to 1. All three varieties take from 25 to 35 minutes to cook fully. Stir regularly to prevent the grains that are on the bottom from scorching.

For pressure cooking, the proportion of water to grain is different: short grain—2 to 1; medium grain—1 1/2 to 1; long grain—1 1/4 to 1. When the rice is cooked, allow the pressure to return slowly to normal. Some of the cooling steam will add moisture to the grain.

Brown rice is a versatile grain aside from its variety of lengths. Rice cream is made commercially by a dry-roasting method, after which the grain is stone ground to a consistency somewhat coarser than rice flour. You can prepare it as a porridge from the whole grain itself, or from prepacked rice-cream powder. Combine the rice with 4 cups of lightly salted boiling water and stir constantly over a low heat to prevent lumping. Rice flour is used extensively in baking, especially by those on gluten-restricted diets. Rice flakes make quick additions to soups or casserole bases when no other leftovers are available.

The flaking process for grains and beans was originally developed to improve animal nutrition. The grains are cooked for 15 to 20 seconds under dry radiant heat and then are dropped onto rollers and flattened into whole grain flakes. Since no wet methods of processing are used, there is only very minimal leaching and modifying of nutrients.

And flaked grains and beans cook in half the usual time. You can add them to breads and casseroles for protein, texture, or taste. In chili, wheat flakes serve to complete the protein of the bean.

A rice-based grain milk called kokoh is available prepacked at natural food outlets. This mixture of roasted and ground rice, sweet rice, soybeans, sesame seeds and oatmeal is good as a morning cereal or tea.

Be careful about your source of brown rice. Commercially produced rice is among the food crops most heavily treated with chemicals.

RYE Rye is mostly known in its flour form, used in bread loaves often flavored with caraway seeds. Especially in its sprouted form, rye is rich in vitamin E, phosphorus, magnesium, and silicon. Like wheat sprouts, rye sprouts sweeten as they lengthen because the natural starches turn to sugar. For salad purposes, use the rye sprout when it's the same size as the grain. Allow it to lengthen up to 1 inch for a sweeter intestinal-cleansing sprout and for cooking. Rye can also be harvested as a grass and chewed for its juice.

The whole rye berry is a good grain, adding chewiness and nutritious value, to combine with rice (use about 1 part rye to 2 parts rice). Rye flakes can be added to soups and stews, or used as a cereal if soaked overnight. Rye flakes, like wheat and oat flakes, make good homemade granolas. For cream of rye, somewhat coarser in texture than rye flour, add 4 parts water to 1 part grain and simmer it over a low heat for about 15 minutes.

TRITICALE Triticale, a highly nutritious grain with a relatively high protein content (approximately 17 percent) and a good balance of amino acids, can be cooked whole in combination with other grains, especially rice (2 parts water to 1 part triticale). Sprouted, it can be used in salads or breads; flaked, in granolas and casseroles. Triticale flour has become a favorite of vegetarians because of its unusually nutty sweetness and high protein content. As a flour it must be mixed with other flours containing higher gluten contents, since its own protein has a low gluten content.

WHOLE WHEAT Today, whole wheat holds a pre-eminent position among grains because of its versatility and high nutritive qualities. Containing anywhere from 6 to 20 percent protein, wheat is also a source of vitamin E and large amounts of nitrates. These nutrients are distributed throughout the three main parts of the wheat kernel or berry. The outer layers of the kernel are known collectively as the bran; there is relatively little protein here, but it is of high quality and rich in the amino acid lysine. The dietary fiber of wheat bran is also the site of about half of the 11 B vitamins found in wheat, as well as the greater portion of the trace minerals zinc, copper, and iodine. Next comes the endosperm, the white starchy central mass of wheat kernel, which contains some 70 percent of the kernel's total protein, as well as its calorie-providing starch. Finally, there is the small germ found at the base of the kernel, which, in addition to containing the same B vitamins and trace minerals as the bran, is the home of vitamin E and the unsaturated fatty acids.

If you use the wheat berry in conjunction with other grains such as rice, you get the entire nutritive value of the grain. Try pan-roasting 1/3 cup of wheat berries with 2/3 cup rice and then simmering them with 2 cups water for 25 to 30 minutes until both grains are tender. You can also eat whole wheat as wheat flakes, cracked wheat, bulgur, couscous, sprouts, and flours (both hard and pastry). The flaking process preserves most of the nutrients of the original form.

Wheat flakes lend themselves especially well to chili dishes, where their addition to the beans provides a completed protein. If added dry to vegetarian chili about 20 minutes before serving, they will break down into tiny pieces to satisfy the appetites of even the most ardent chili con carne aficionados. Cracked wheat (simple coarse-ground wheat) is most often used as a morning cereal cooked with about 3 cups salted water to 1 cup wheat; it is often added cooked to uncooked to breads and muffins.

Bulgur is a variety of whole grain wheat that is parboiled, dried (often in the sun), and then coarsely cracked. This Near and Middle Eastern staple has found its way to America in a distinctive salad called tabouli. Bulgur does not require cooking but is simply reconstituted by spreading the grain an inch deep in a shallow pan and pouring enough boiling water over it to leave about half an inch of standing water. Once the water is absorbed, stir the grain several times with a fork until it's cool. It can then be chilled, combined with greens such as parsley, fresh mint, and watercress, and marinated in a dressing of sesame oil, lemon juice, and tamari.

Couscous is a form of soft, refined durum wheat flour ("semolina") that has been steamed, cracked and dried. It can be prepared for eating by adding 1 cup of couscous to 2 cups of boiling salted water with a teaspoon of butter or margarine if desired, reducing the heat and stirring constantly until most of the moisture is gone. Remove the couscous from the heat and let it stand covered about 15 minutes, fluffing it up several times with a fork.

Wheat also makes an excellent sprout, containing substantially larger amounts of all the vitamins and minerals found in the dormant kernel. The sprout, which sweetens as it lengthens, can be used in desserts.

Whole wheat flour can be made from hard wheat (high protein, high gluten) or soft wheat (lower protein and gluten, high starch), or from spring or winter wheats. Hard wheats are excellent for making bread. The spring wheat contains a higher gluten content than the winter wheat. Soft wheat, either spring or winter, is known as pastry wheat because it yields a fine, starchy flour. Wheat flours are available at natural food stores in many pasta forms—from alphabets to ziti—often combined with other flours such as buckwheat, corn, rice, soy, and Jerusalem artichoke.

Whole grain flours can become rancid. Rancidity occurs when the unsaturated fats in the flour are exposed to the oxygen in the air. The vitamin E in the whole wheat flour acts as a natural preservative, but within 3 months it is exhausted. This problem can best be handled by storing the flour in a cool dry place immediately after milling. There are a number of small natural food companies that mill and distribute their fresh-ground flour. Home grinding machines are now available at many natural food stores.

WHEAT GLUTEN Wheat gluten (kofu, in Japanese cookery) has long been a popular vegetarian source of protein in many places around the world. It is prepared by mixing whole wheat flour and water in a 2 1/2 to 1 ratio and kneading it into a stiff dough. This dough is then covered with cold water and kneaded underwater. As the water clouds up with starch sediment, it is replaced and the procedure is repeated about five or six times until the water remains clear. Then the remaining gluten dough is steamed or cooked in a double boiler for 30 minutes. Kofu may be eaten as is, flavored with soy sauce, or baked in casserole loaves combined with other grains, such as rice and beans.

AMARANTH Amaranth is a native grain. It has been cultivated in the American Southwest for hundreds of years. The plant yields a tiny seed that should be prepared similarly to rice. When cooked, it has a very soft, nutlike consistency.

QUINOA Quinoa (prounced keen-wah), a staple of the Inca Indians, is a delicate, light-textured, high-protein grain that resembles tiny granules of tabouli or couscous. Known as "the mother grain," it is high in complete protein, cooks in 10 to 15 minutes, and approximately triples its volume when cooked, somewhat mitigating its current high price in health food stores.

Beans (Legumes)

The members of the bean family are important, inexpensive sources of protein, minerals and vitamins. Legumes can be cooked whole, flaked like grains, sprouted, ground into flours, even transformed into a variety of "dairy" products.

As a general rule, 1 cup of dry beans will make about 2 1/2 cups of cooked beans, enough for 4 servings. Many beans should be soaked, preferably overnight; these include adzuki beans, black beans, chick-peas (garbanzos), and soybeans. As an alternative to overnight soaking, you can bring the beans (1 cup) and water (3 to 4 cups) to a boil, remove the pot from the stove and cover, let the beans sit for an hour, then cook the beans by simmering after first bringing them to a boil, or by putting them in a pressure cooker.

When using beans for a soup dish, allow five times as much water as beans at the beginning of the cooking process. Don't salt the water until the beans are soft (or after the pressure in the cooker has come down), because the salt will draw the moisture out of the beans.

ADZUKI Adzuki are small red beans that have a special place in Japanese cuisine as well as in traditional Japanese medicine, where they are used as a remedy for kidney ailments (when combined with a small pumpkin called hokkaido). Very high in B vitamins and trace minerals, adzukis should never be pressure-cooked because it makes them bitter.

After overnight soaking, simmer adzukis with a strip of kombu (a kind of kelp) for about 1 to 1 1/2 hours until tender, with 4 to 5 cups of water to each cup of beans. One favorite preparation: add 1 cup each of sautéed onions and celery to the tender beans and then puree them together in a blender. The resulting thick, creamy soup can be thinned with water or bean juice and flavored with a dash of lime juice, tamari, and mild curry.

BLACK BEANS AND TURTLE BEANS Black beans and their close relative, turtle beans, have served as major food sources in the Caribbean, Mexico, and the American Southwest for many years. These beans should not be prepared in a pressure cooker since their skins fall off easily and may clog the valve. A smooth, rich black bean soup, a specialty of Cuba, is made by cooking the soaked beans until tender, adding sautéed garlic, onions, and celery, and then pressing the mixture through a colander (or, more easily, quickly blending it in an electric blender). A small amount of lime juice may be added to lighten the taste.

BLACK-EYED PEAS Black-eyed peas, a Southern favorite, provide a delicious complete protein-balanced meal. Among the quickest-cooking beans, they become tender in 45 minutes to an hour. Eating this bean on New Year's Day is said to bring good luck throughout the year.

CHICK-PEAS (GARBANZOS) Chick-peas, or garbanzos, are so versatile that they have been the subject of entire cookbooks. High in protein, they are also good sources of calcium, iron, potassium, and B vitamins. They can be roasted like peanuts or boiled. After a very thorough roasting, chick-peas can even be ground and used as a coffee substitute. Hummus is a thick paste that combines mashed chick-peas, hulled sesame-seed tahini, garlic, and lemon juice. Bean patés using chick-peas as a base offer many creative opportunities for creating complete proteins by combining different beans. Cooked grains, ground seeds and nuts, raw vegetables, herbs, and miso may all be combined with the cooked beans to produce a sophisticated and appealing paté or paste.

GREAT NORTHERN BEANS AND NAVY BEANS Great northern beans and their small counterpart, navy beans, cook in less than an hour and require no presoaking. They are often used for hearty soups. Cook the beans with 5 to 6 parts water or stock to 1 part dry beans. Firmer vegetables, such as carrots, rutabagas, or turnips should be added one-half hour before the soup is finished; other vegetables, such as onions, celery and peppers, should be added 15 minutes later, either sautéed or raw.

KIDNEY BEANS Kidney beans, standard in all sorts of chilis, will cook in about an hour, after having been soaked overnight. The fragrant brown bean juice produced in cooking the beans makes the addition of tomato virtually unnecessary. Once the beans are tender, try dicing onions, garlic, and red and green peppers; sauté them lightly in sesame oil until the onions are translucent, then add them to the beans. Season them to taste. Rich Mexican chili powder seems to lend more flavor to the beans than does a scorching Indian one. Tamari, a dash of blackstrap molasses, or fresh-grated ginger root can further enhance the beans. For a perfect final texture, add dry wheat flakes to the chili about 20 minutes before serving; this allows time for the flakes to cook and disintegrate, thickening the dish while complementing the protein of the beans.

LENTILS Lentils come in a rainbow of colors, but generally only the green, brown, and red varieties are available in the United States. All are inexpensive and nutritious sources of iron, cellulose, and B vitamins. Lentils require no pre-soaking and disintegrate when cooked, leaving a smooth base to which you can add fresh or sautéed vegetables (including carrots, turnips, onions, and peppers). They sprout well in combination with other seeds and produce large quantities. The flavor of the uncooked sprout is similar to that of fresh ground pepper on salad; when cooked it has a more nutlike taste. The sprouts should be harvested when the shoot is as long as the seed.

MUNG BEANS Mung beans are probably best known in their sprout form, eaten raw or lightly sautéed with other vegetables. They can be cooked as a dry bean, using three times as much water as beans, and then pureed in an electric blender into a smooth soup. The result is rather bland and benefits from the addition of tamari and fresh or dried basil. But as sprouts, mung beans really come into their own. Mung sprouts are rich in vitamins A and C and contain high amounts of calcium, phosphorus, and iron. The hulls are easily digestible and rich in minerals. Mung sprouts can be harvested any time from the second day, when the shoot has just appeared, to the third or fourth day when the shoot is about 4 inches long. Mung beans make a good first choice for beginning sprouters.

PEANUTS Peanuts, though commonly grouped with seeds and nuts, are actually members of the legume family. Their high protein content is well known. In the United States eating peanut butter is virtually a national pastime. Peanut butter can—and should—contain 100 percent peanuts; sugars, colorings, stabilizers, and preservatives are neither necessary nor desirable. A single grinding under pressure extracts enough oil from the nut meal to give the peanuts a creamy texture.

PINTO BEANS Pinto beans are popular in American Southwest dishes and lend themselves especially well to baking. Naturally sweet in flavor, they adapt to many types of seasonings, and once cooked tender, they can be used in casseroles. Pinto flakes cook quickly and reconstitute themselves into tender round beans in about 40 minutes (2 parts water to 1 part dry flakes). Cumin blends nicely with these beans, if used sparingly.

SOYBEANS Soybeans, unquestionably the most nutritious of all the beans, have been the major source of protein in Asian diets for centuries. They are increasingly being viewed as the most realistic source of high-quality, low-cost protein available today on a large enough scale to meet worldwide needs. In addition to high-quality protein, soybeans contain large amounts of B vitamins, minerals, and unsaturated fatty acids in the form of lecithin that help the body emulsify cholesterol. Even the Food and Drug Administration has recognized their value, saying that 25 grams of soy protein a day, as part of a diet low in saturated fat and cholesterol, may reduce the risk of heart disease.

Thanks to their bland flavor after cooking and their high concentration of nutrients, soybeans can be made into an amazingly diverse array of foods. Western technology in recent years has focused on creating a wide range of synthetic soybean foods. There are protein concentrates in the form of soy powder containing from 70 to 90 percent moisture-free protein, isolates (defatted flakes and flours used to make simulated dairy products and frozen deserts), spun protein fibers (isolates dissolved in alkali solutions for use in simulated meat products), and textured vegetable proteins (made from soy flour and used in simulated meat products and infant foods). Most Western cooks also have come across soybeans in the form of full-fat soy flour, soy granules, and defatted soy flour and grits—all of which are available in natural food stores. Full-fat soy flour, which contains about 40 percent protein and 20 percent naturally occurring oils, makes a fine addition to many forms of baked goods. Soy granules contain about 50 percent protein, as do defatted soy flour and soy grits, which are basically byproducts of the extraction of soy oil. Both are used in breakfast cereals, simulated meats, and desserts. Soybeans are also processed into flakes that, unlike raw soybeans, require no presoaking and only about 1 1/2 hours of cooking.

The soybean can be enjoyed in many ways, as tofu (see below), or as a fresh green summer vegetable, simmered or steamed in the pod. Roasted soybeans are now available in many varieties: dry-roasted, oil-roasted, salted, unsalted, and with garlic or barbecue flavors. They contain up to 47 percent protein and can either be eaten as a snack or added to casseroles for texture.

When cooking whole dry soybeans, a pressure cooker can save a great deal of time. Use 2 1/2 to 3 cups of water over a low flame for each cup of dry soybeans. Once the right pressure has been reached, cook until tender—about 90 minutes. Before cooking soybeans by the ordinary simmering method, soak them overnight in 4 cups of water. Bring them to a boil in 4 more cups of liquid and simmer about 3 hours, adding more water whenever necessary.

An interesting soybean preparation called *tempeh* is made from cooked, hulled soybean halves, to which a Rhizipus mold is introduced. The inoculated bean cakes are then fermented overnight, during which time the white mycelium mold partially digests the beans and effectively deactivates the trypsin enzyme, which could inhibit digestion. The soybeans have, by this time, become fragrant cakes bound together by the mold; you can then either deep-fry or bake them into a dish that tastes remarkably like veal or chicken. Tempeh is rich in protein (from 18 to 48 percent) and highly digestible. In addition, like the other fermented soy products and sea vegetables, it is one of the few nonmeat sources of vitamin B_{12}.

Tempeh can be made easily in any kitchen. The tempeh starter (*Rhizopus oligosporus*, mold spores) is available from the Department of Agriculture, complete with an enthusiastic brochure on its use.

A further use of this "queen of the beans" is as a sprout. Significant amounts of vitamin C, not found in the dried bean, are released in the sprouts, which are also rich in vitamins A, E, and the B complex, as well as minerals. The yellow soybean does well for sprouting, and the black variety can also sprout prolifically.

Rinse the sprouts two to three times a day and harvest them when the shoot is from 1/4 to 1 1/2 inches long. As a matter of taste, you may or may not prefer to remove the outer husk before using the sprout. Steaming or boiling the soybean sprouts lightly before eating will destroy the urease and antitrypsin enzymes that interfere with digestion. The sprouts can be ground and used in sandwiches and salad dressings, and they make a fine addition to any sauté of crisp Chinese-style vegetables.

TOFU

Tofu (soy curd or soy cheese) is among the traditional East Asian soy products. Tofu is a remarkable food. It is very inexpensive when purchased at Asian markets or natural food shops and even more so if made at home. Two other related products, tamari soy sauce and miso (fermented soy paste), will be discussed later in this chapter.

You can make your own tofu by grinding soaked soybeans, cooking them with water, pouring the resulting mixture into a pressing sack, and collecting the "milk" underneath by squeezing as much liquid as possible from the sack, leaving the bean fiber behind. The soy milk is then simmered and curdled in a solution containing sea-water brine (called nigari), lemon juice, or vinegar. Any of these three solidifiers will work well, although commercial nigari is most often used for this coagulation process.

After the white soy curds curdle and float in a yellowish whey liquid, they are ladled into a settling box, covered and weighted, and allowed to press into a solid cake. It is then ready for immediate use as is—or for further transformation into a virtually unlimited variety of tofu products. Tofu is high in quality protein and is excellent for creating complete protein, especially when combined with grains. Tofu contains an abundance of lysine, an essential amino acid in which many grains are deficient; on the other hand, grains such as rice are high in the sulfur that contains methionine and cystine, amino acids that are absent in soybeans. These soy and grain proteins complement each other naturally.

Tofu is easy to digest, and low in calories, saturated fats, and cholesterol. When solidified with calcium chloride or calcium sulfate—as in most commercial American tofu—tofu contains more calcium by weight than dairy milk; it's also a good source of other minerals such as iron, phosphorus, and potassium.

Since it's made from soybeans, tofu is free of chemical toxins. Soybeans are an important feed crop for the beef and dairy industries and the spraying is therefore carefully monitored by the Food and Drug Administration.

SPLIT PEAS Split peas, both green and yellow, make a simple soup filled with protein and minerals. They do not require soaking. Start with 1 part dry peas and 5 to 6 cups water and cook about 45 minutes. Once the peas are cooked, the soup will continue to thicken. This leftover paste can be diluted several times in the following days for a quick hot soup. Sautéed onions, tamari, and 1/2 stick of soy margarine complete the soup.

Nuts and Seeds

Nuts and seeds are fine sources of protein, minerals (especially magnesium), some B vitamins, and unsaturated fatty acids. They can be eaten as snack foods or used with other foods to add interesting flavors, textures, and nutritional values.

A general sprouting procedure for seeds and nuts is to soak the dried seeds for about 8 hours (approximately 4 parts water to 1 part seed). Don't throw away the soaking water; use it as a cooking liquid, or water your houseplants with it. Rinse the seeds with cool water and place them in a sprouter.

Keys to successful sprouting include keeping the sprouts moist but never soaked, keeping them moderately warm, rinsing them as often as possible, and giving them enough room so that air can freely circulate around them. Actually, only about 5 minutes a day is needed for growing a successful sprout garden. Use the sprouts as soon as possible. They have a refrigerator life of 7 to 10 days. Sprouts can also be dried easily for use in beverages, nut butter, and spreads. Place the sprouts on cookie sheets for a few hours in a warm room, or keep them in a warm oven until they're dry. Then grind them in a blender, store in a jar and refrigerate.

ALFALFA Many people think of alfalfa as a barnyard grass, which it is. Because its roots penetrate deep underground to seek out the elements it craves, alfalfa is one of the best possible fodders. But the fresh, mineral-laden leaves of this plant are especially nutritious for humans when juiced. Alfalfa seeds purchased at a natural food store may seem expensive, but a few of them go a long way—1/2 teaspoon of dry seeds yields an entire trayful of sprouts. The sprouts have a light sweet taste and are particularly rich in vitamin C, as well as in chlorophyll (when allowed to develop in light). They also have high mineral values, containing phosphorus, chlorine, silicon, aluminum, calcium, magnesium, sulfur, sodium, and potassium. Alfalfa seeds sprout well in combination with other seeds and have a high germination rate. They can also be used when dried.

ALMONDS Almonds will sprout only from the fresh unhulled nut after soaking overnight. They must be kept very moist until their sprouts reach a length of about 1 inch (4 days). They can then be used to make almond milk: a combination of 1 cup of almond sprouts (or merely almonds soaked overnight) blended with 4 times as much water or apple juice. Almonds, which have an exceptionally high mineral content, are delicious raw or roasted with tamari. The raw nut can be sliced, slivered, or chopped, and even can be ground into almond butter.

BRAZIL NUTS Brazil nuts, like other seeds and nuts, have a high fat content. But because they are also high in protein, they are actually not much higher in calories per gram of usable protein than are whole grains. They also offer unusually high amounts of the sulfur-containing amino acids. For this reason, you can serve them to good advantage as a chopped garnish for fresh vegetables, such as brussels sprouts, cauliflower, green peas, and lima beans. These vegetables are all deficient in the sulfur-containing amino acids but high in the amino acid isoleucine lacking in Brazil nuts.

CASHEWS Cashews are also popular nuts that can be added to many dishes. Use them as a layer in a casserole, or simply roast them lightly and toss them in a bowl of steamed snow peas. Cashew butter, from both raw and roasted nuts, is growing in popularity and is well-suited for use in sauces, where it can be diluted with water and miso paste. You can mix it yourself in a nutritious soy "milkshake." Blend 2 cups of plain or sweetened soy milk with1/2 cup of cashew butter; add 2 tablespoons of carob powder, a pinch of salt, and a dash of vanilla extract and nutmeg.

CHIA SEEDS Chia seeds, now available in natural food stores, have long been a staple in Mexican and Native American diets, where they were traditionally used to increase endurance on long hunts and migrations. Although a member of the mint family, chia seeds have a mild flaxlike taste. They can be chewed raw or sprinkled into hot or cold cereals. Since they are in a class of seeds called mucilaginous, which become sticky when soaked in water, their sprouting procedure is slightly different. Sprinkle the seeds over a saucer filled with water and allow to stand overnight. By morning, the seeds will have absorbed all the water and will stick to the saucer. Gently rinse and drain, using a sieve if possible. Then, as with other seeds, rinse twice daily. Also try sprouting the seeds in a flat, covered container lined with damp paper towels. Harvest the chia seeds when the shoot is 1 inch long.

CLOVER The red variety of clover makes a delicious sprout similar in taste to alfalfa. In its sprout form, this forage plant can be an excellent source of chlorophyll. When the primary leaves are about 1 inch in length, spread them out in a nonmetallic tray and dampen them. They should be covered with clear plastic to hold in moisture and placed in a sunny spot for 1 to 2 hours.

CRESS SEEDS Cress seeds are tiny members of the mustard family. They add a zesty taste to salads when used in their sprout form. They are also mucilaginous seeds and so are sprouted in the same way as chia seeds. Harvest the sprouts at about 1 inch long and use them in sandwiches instead of lettuce.

FENUGREEK SEEDS Fenugreek seeds were first used to brew tea by the ancient Greeks. This strong tea is an excellent mouthwash, as well as a tasty and nutritious addition to soy or nut milk. The ground dry seed is one of the components of curry powder. When sprouted, fenugreek can be added to soups, salads, and grain dishes. The sprout should be harvested once it is 1/4 inch long, for it will become very bitter soon afterward.

FILBERTS (HAZELNUTS) Filberts or hazelnuts are tasty nuts that, once chopped, make a delicious garnish for both greens and creamy tofu pudding. These nuts, however, contain an excess amount of calories for the amount of protein they provide.

FLAX (LINSEED) Flax, also known as linseed, is a versatile plant. The fiber of the mature plant is used to make linen and pressed to extract its oil. As a sprout, flax has been used for centuries. At Greek and Roman banquets, flax sprouts were reportedly served between courses for their mild laxative effect. Though flax is sprouted as a mucilaginous seed, its sprouts work well in conjunction with wheat and rye kernels. Harvest when the shoots are about an inch long and serve as a breakfast salad. Taken on an empty stomach, this sprout mixture cleanses and lubricates the colon.

MUSTARD The small seeds of the common black mustard plant will sprout quite readily and are usually available at herb and spice stores. Small amounts of these sprouts add a spicy flavor to salads and sandwiches. Harvest when shoots are about an inch long.

PECANS Pecans are nuts that are cultivated organically in Texas and New Mexico. Though high in potassium and B vitamins, pecans are not good sources of protein. Like filberts, they contain too many calories for the amount of protein they offer. Pecans are delicious as tamari-roasted nuts: dry-roast in a heavy skillet and, when they begin to emit a pleasing fragrance, remove to a plate and sprinkle lightly with tamari.

PIGNOLIAS (PINE NUTS) Pignolias, or pine nuts, have an unusual flavor, but are a poor source of protein. Found in the cones of the small pinon pine, which grows in the American Southwest, these nuts have been used by many Indian tribes as a food staple. Most of the pignolias consumed in the United States, however, come from Portugal. Pan-roasted pine nuts are delicious with green vegetables like peas and beans, and are also tasty in bread stuffings.

PISTACHIO NUTS Pistachio nuts are familiar to many as an Italian ice cream flavor. For snacking purposes, use the naturally grown pistachio rather than the dyed varieties. Like other nuts, pistachios should be consumed only in small quantities, since they are high in calories.

PUMPKIN SEEDS, PEPITAS, AND SQUASH SEEDS Pumpkin seeds, pepitas, and squash seeds are delicious seeds rich in minerals that can be eaten as snacks or ground into a meal for use in baking and cooking. Eastern Europeans, who eat many more pumpkin seeds than do Americans, use them to help prevent prostate disorders. Save the seeds from a pumpkin or squash and sprout them. Harvest when the shoot is just beginning to show (after 3 or 4 days). If allowed to lengthen any further, the sprouts will taste bitter.

RADISH SEEDS Radish seeds, both black and red, make wonderfully tangy sprouts. They sprout easily and work well when combined with alfalfa and clover seeds. They're relatively expensive compared to most sprouting seeds, but you don't need many of these peppery-tasting sprouts to perk up a salad. Harvest these shoots when they're about an inch long.

SESAME SEEDS (BENNE) Sesame seeds, or benne, are popular around the world because of their taste and high nutritive content. Most sesame seeds available in the United States are grown in southern Mexico, where few sprays are used. They are available hulled or unhulled. The unhulled variety is nutritionally superior since most of the mineral value is found in the hull.

Sesame seeds are an excellent source of protein, unsaturated fatty acids, calcium, magnesium, niacin, and vitamins A and E. The protein in sesame seeds effectively complements the protein of legumes, because both contain high amounts of each other's deficient amino acids. Therefore, an especially good addition to a soy milk shake is tahini, or sesame butter.

Used extensively as the whole seed in breads and other baked foods, in grain dishes, and on vegetables, the unhulled seeds can also be toasted and ground into sesame butter, which has a stronger taste and higher mineral content than sesame tahini. Tahini, made from toasted and hulled seeds, is a mild, sweet butter. Tahini is used in the Middle East, where the oil that separates from the butter is used as a cooking oil. Tahini is an excellent base for salad dressing and acts as a perfect thickener for all sorts of sauces. The unhulled seed must be used when sprouting. The sprouts can be used, like the whole seed, in cooked foods or blended into beverages. Harvest when the shoot reaches 1/16 inch in length (usually within 2 days). At this stage the sprouts are sweet, but become bitter with further growth.

SUNFLOWER SEEDS Sunflower seeds are sun-energized, nutritional powerhouses rich in protein (about 30 percent), unsaturated fatty acids, phosphorus, calcium, iron, fluorine, iodine, potassium, magnesium, zinc, several B vitamins, vitamin E, and vitamin D (one of the few vegetable sources of this vitamin). Their high mineral content is the result of the sunflower's extensive root system, which penetrates deep into the subsoil seeking nutrients. Their vitamin D content is partially due to the flower's tendency to follow and face the sun as it moves across the sky.

Sunflowers were cultivated extensively by American Indians as a food crop. In their raw state, sunflower seeds can be enjoyed as snacks or included in everything from breads to salads. The seeds are also available in a toasted, salted nut butter.

Sprouted sunflower seeds should be eaten when barely budded or they will taste very bitter. However, it usually takes 4 to 5 days for the shoot to appear. Unhulled seeds, or special hulled sprouting seeds, are used when sprouting, but the husk should be removed before eating.

WALNUTS Walnuts are a good source of protein and iron. Black walnuts contain about 40 percent more protein than English walnuts (also known as California walnuts in the United States). Walnuts will keep fresh much longer when purchased in the shell. This is true of all nuts. It also brings down the price considerably.

SEAWEEDS Seaweeds rank high as sources for the basic essential minerals, as do green vegetables such as dandelions and watercress. They all contain calcium, magnesium, phosphorus, potassium, iron, iodine, and sodium. Most Westerners dislike the idea of eating seaweed. If they were to sample what they're missing, though, they'd find a new world of taste and high-quality nutrients—especially trace minerals—in the six varieties of sea vegetables available in most natural food stores and food co-ops.

AGAR Agar, or agar-agar (called *kantan* in Japanese, and also known as Ceylonese moss) is a translucent, almost weightless seaweed product found in stick, flake, or powdered form. You can use it like gelatin to thicken fruit juices or purees. Agar also can be used to make aspics and clear molds of fruit juices, fruits, or vegetables. If you tear 1 to 1 1/2 sticks into small pieces and dissolve them in 1 quart of liquid, you will produce a puddinglike consistency. More agar can be used to achieve a jellied texture. When used in stick form, agar should be simmered in liquid for 10 to 15 minutes, to ensure that all the pieces have dissolved. This simmering isn't necessary when using the flaked or powdered varieties.

DULSE Dulse is the only commercial sea vegetable that comes from the Atlantic Ocean (specifically, the Canadian Maritime Provinces). This ready-to-eat seaweed can be chewed in its tough dry state, but a short soaking to rinse it and to remove any small, clinging shells is worthwhile. Dulse can be added to miso soup.

HIJIKI (HIZIKI) Another Japanese seaweed is the jet-black hijiki or hiziki. This stringy, hairlike seaweed contains 57 percent more calcium by weight than dry milk and has high levels of iron as well. Dried hiziki should be soaked in several cups of water for about 20 minutes, then strained in a colander and lightly pressed to squeeze out excess moisture. Once reconstituted, hiziki is best when sautéed together with other vegetables—especially onion and leeks—or cooked with beans and grains.

KOMBU (KELP) Kombu is the Japanese term for several species of brown algae. In English, these are usually referred to collectively as kelp. Kombu is especially rich in iodine, vitamin B_2, and calcium. When using the dried form of kombu, rinse it once and soak for 10 to 15 minutes.

Note that all dried seaweeds increase greatly in size when reconstituted. For example, 1/4 cup of dried hiziki will yield 1 cup when soaked. Save the water in which the seaweeds are soaked and use it as soup stock. Reconstituted kombu strips can be used whole in the cooking water for beans and grains, or can be cut into thin strips or diced for use in soups and salads.

NORI (LAVER) Nori is the most popular Japanese seaweed, also known as dried purple laver. It is sold in the form of paper-thin purplish sheets, with 8 to 10 sheets per package. Laver has been used a food by many peoples. The Japanese and Koreans are the only people to cultivate these plants and dry and press the mature leaves into sheets.

The nori sheets are toasted over a flame until crisp, during which their color changes from black or purple to green. They are then crumbled or slivered and used as a condiment for noodles, grains, beans, and soups. Remarkably rich in protein, nori is also high in vitamins A, B_2, B_{12}, D, and niacin.

WAKAME Wakame is a long seaweed with symmetrical and fluted fronds growing from both sides of an edible midrib. Although generally used fresh in Japan, it is only available dried in the West. It is reconstituted in the same manner as kombu: rinsed once, soaked, and pressed of excess moisture. If the midrib is particularly tough, it can be removed. When used in soups, wakame should be cooked for no more than a few minutes and should therefore be one of the last ingredients added to miso soup. This delicious vegetable is rich in protein and niacin. In its dried state, it contains almost 50 percent more calcium than dry milk.

FERMENTED FOODS: MISO AND TAMARI Miso, a fermented soybean paste, has long been a staple seasoning in the Asian kitchen. It is produced by combining cooked soybeans, salt, and various grains. Barley miso is made with barley and soybeans. Rice miso is made with both hulled and unhulled rice plus soybeans. Soybeans alone are used to make hatcho miso. These cooked and salted combinations are dusted with a fungus mold, koji, which produces the enzymes that start to digest the bean-and-grain mixture.

Tamari is naturally fermented soy sauce. Originally considered excess liquid, it was drained off miso that had finished fermenting. Today it is a product in its own right and is made from a natural fermentation process of whole soybeans, natural sea salt, well water, roasted cracked wheat, and koji spores, all aged for 12 to 18 months. Tamari, like miso, has a range of colors, textures, and aromas as wide and varied as those of wines and cheeses.

Miso and tamari contain between 9 and 18 percent complete protein; the higher the soybean content, the higher the protein. The protein in these products is "predigested": it is already broken down into 17 amino acids, which makes for easy digestion. Also, the digestion-inhibiting enzyme present in raw or poorly cooked soybeans is destroyed by their fermentation. During the microorganic synthesis of miso and tamari, the amounts of the B vitamins riboflavin and niacin increase. In addition, miso and tamari are among the few vegetable sources of vitamin B_{12}, which is actually manufactured by fungi and bacteria in the fermenting mixtures just as it is synthesized in the human intestine.

Miso and tamari are useful in all cuisines, but because of their high salt content—11 percent for the saltiest of hatcho miso and 18 percent for tamari—they should be used sparingly. Miso diluted with water can be used as a base for a sauce made with tahini; a dash of tamari brings out new flavors in familiar grains. Miso also makes a wonderful soup base to which tofu, mushrooms, seaweeds, and many fresh or cooked vegetables can be added.

All of the natural miso and tamari available in the United States today comes from Japan. If a package of miso you purchase has started to expand, you can be assured its contents have not been pasteurized and that the microorganisms are still alive and producing carbon dioxide gas. Get rid of it.

In the future, the United States may begin producing its own fermented soybean foods. A lively market now exists and many people are acquiring the necessary technical know-how. Organic farmers are already producing soybeans, wheat, barley, and rice; the koji starter and engineering skills are always available from Asia. As fermented soy foods play a larger role in American diets, we may start to develop and adapt our own distinctive varieties.

SALT: SOME ALTERNATIVE SOURCES Controversy continues about the virtues and dangers of salt. Some people consume large quantities of salt. Many others attempt to get their salt from the juices of celery, spinach, beets, or carrots. Very little sodium, however, is derived from these supposedly sodium-rich foods. Still other people decide upon, or are prescribed, low-sodium or even "salt-free" diets. People on low-sodium diets have often been suffering from hypertension (high blood pressure) or kidney problems. Overconsumption of salt will lead to hypertension: the salt draws water out of blood cells and vessels, which in turn causes dehydration of the tissues and forces the heart to pump much too strenuously. Overconsumption of salt also clogs the kidneys and creates an excess of water that cannot be properly eliminated from the body.

On the other hand, moderate and intelligent consumption of salt helps the body retain heat by slightly contracting the blood vessels, which is why we tend to consume more salt in cold months. Sodium also helps maintain intestinal muscle tone. You should evaluate your own salt needs according to your physical activity, climate, water intake, and—above all—diet. People in meat-eating cultures seldom need extra salt per se, because they get all they need from the blood and flesh of the animals they eat. Vegetarian or agricultural peoples, however, tend to have a high regard for salt and use it to cook, pickle, and preserve foods.

If you want to eat salt, you should use the natural sun- or kiln-dried variety, which still contains important trace minerals. Refined "table" salt is made fine by high heats and flash-cooling, and then combined with such additives as sodium silico aluminate to keep it "free-flowing." Kosher salt is an exception. It has larger crystals due to its milder processing, and nothing is added to the better brands. Natural salt—rock salt or sea salt—is not free-flowing, but some brands add calcium carbonate, a natural compound, to prevent caking. All salt is or once was sea salt, so differences between salt obtained from inland rock deposits or from the sea are minor and unimportant.

No natural salt contains iodine, which is far too volatile a substance to remain stable for long without numerous additives. But there is an excellent source of iodine from the ocean: sea vegetables, the most common being kelp. These contain a natural, sugar-stabilized iodine—as well as about 4 to 8 percent salt. They are harvested, roasted, ground up, and marketed as salt alternatives.

Another healthful way of adding salt to your diet is to use sesame salt, sold as gomasio. This versatile condiment can be used in place of ordinary salt on cooked greens, grains and raw salads. Gomasio can be purchased in most natural food stores.

Salted umeboshi plums also may be used. These small Japanese plums are known for the high quality and quantity of citric acid they contain. The citric acid in plums allegedly helps neutralize and eliminate some of the excess lactic acid in the body, helping to restore a natural balance. An excess of lactic acid in the body is caused by excessive consumption of sugar. If not converted to body energy, the sugar turns into lactic acid and combines with protein to contribute to ailments like headaches, fatigue, and high blood pressure.

In Japan, these organically grown plums are available in a variety of preser-

vative-free forms—from concentrates to salted plums. In most American natural food stores, only the salted plums are available. These are potent alkaline
sources, excellent to aid indigestion, colds, and fatigue. Umeboshi also have
many culinary uses. Use them to salt the water in which grains will be cooked
or use several in tofu salad dressings instead of tamari or sea salt.

SWEETENERS Carbohydrate sugar is unquestionably essential to life, but try to
get it in as unadulterated a form as possible. Common table sugar has been
processed to 99.9 percent sucrose, devoid of the vitamins and minerals found in
sugar cane or sugar beets. This refined sucrose taxes the body's digestive system
and depletes its core of minerals and enzymes as the sugar is metabolized. For
this reason and others, white sugar has earned a bad reputation and the label,
"empty food."

Carbohydrates include many sugars. The best known is sucrose, or white
table sugar, which breaks down in the body into simpler sugars, glucose and
fructose. There are also starches in whole cereals (together with their own component enzymes, vitamins, minerals, and proteins) that break down uniformly
in the body into simple glucose molecules once they have been cooked, chewed,
and digested. Compared with these refined starches, refined sugars tend to
overstrain the body's digestive system. So, it would seem wiser to get the sugars you need from abundant natural stores in cereals, vegetables, and fruits.
Eaten in moderate amounts, starches are not fattening, contrary to public opinion.

When cooking with natural foods, you should simply replace refined sugars with the richer flavors of naturally occurring sugars. Maple syrup, for example, or honey or fruit juice can substitute for sugar in almost any home recipe.
Maple sugar is expensive and very sweet, so use it in moderation. Use 1/2 cup
of maple syrup instead of 1 cup of sugar and either reduce the other liquids in
the recipe or increase the dry ingredients accordingly. Maple syrup is believed
by some to be a source of the trace mineral zinc. But be sure that the maple
syrup you buy has not been extracted with formaldehyde.

All honeys are basically the fruit sugar fructose, which consists of varying
amounts of dextrose, levulose, maltose, and other simple sugars. The flavor of
honey depends on the source of the bees' nectar. All honey you use should be
unheated and unfiltered so that its natural enzymes and vitamins are still intact.
When cooking with honey in a recipe originally calling for refined sugar, divide
the amount of sugar called for in half and adjust the recipe with less liquid or
more dry ingredients.

In fact, not too much sugar of any kind should be used in cooking or baking, because heat can be destructive to protein in the presence of sugar. This is
especially true when using honey or a refined glucose such as corn syrup. Try
using fruit juices or purees made from soaked dried fruits to sweeten dishes. A
little bit of these natural sugars will go a long way.

Granulated date sugar, available in many natural food stores, is indispensable when your recipe specifically calls for a granulated dry sugar. This sugar has the distinctive flavor of whole dry dates. Another dry sweetener is carob, or St.-Johns bread. This powder comes from the dried pods of the carob tree and can be purchased roasted or unroasted. Use the unroasted variety and toast it yourself for a fresher taste. In addition to its natural sugars, carob is rich in trace minerals and low in fats. Only a small of this strong sweetener is necessary; either mix with the dry ingredients or dissolve in a little water or soy milk before adding to the other liquids. Carob is also available as a syrup. If you are using carob as a substitute for cocoa or chocolate, the equivalent of 1 square of chocolate is 3 tablespoons of carob plus 2 tablespoons of water or soy milk.

From the starches, two grain sweeteners are available: barley malt (also made from other grains and containing the sugar maltose) and a rice syrup called *ame* in Japanese. These grain syrups are produced by combining the cooked grains, rice in this instance, with fresh sprouts from whole oats, barley, or wheat. This combination is allowed to stand for several hours until it has reached the sweet stage, when the liquid is squeezed off through cheesecloth, lightly salted, and cooked to the desired consistency. This thick, pale-amber syrup works well in pastries and sauces. Its semisolid state can be softened by beating it to the consistency of thick honey. It is also sold in health food stores in the West as a chewy taffy.

For those who use dairy products, noninstant dry milk powder is a versatile natural sweetener containing the milk-sugar lactose.

So-called raw sugar, or turbinado, is available in many stores, but is only slightly more nutritious than white sugar. It is 96 percent sucrose, compared with the 99.9 percent sucrose in white sugar. The only refining step to which it has not been subjected is a final acid bath that whitens the sugar and removes the final calcium and magnesium salts. This "pure" sugar was, as a juice from either sugar beets or sugar cane, only 15 percent sucrose. In its final form, all natural goodness has been lost.

Several sweeteners produced in the intermediate stages of sugar refining can be used somewhat more nutritionally than white table sugar. Once the cane or beet juice has been extracted, clarified to a syrup form, and crystallized, it is then spun in a centrifuge where more crystals are separated from the liquid. This remaining liquid is molasses, which is then repeatedly treated and centrifuged to extract more and more crystal until the final "blackstrap" form contains about 35 percent sucrose. Blackstrap molasses also contains iron, calcium, and B vitamins. Another variety of molasses is known as barbados. This milder, dark-brown syrup is extracted from the processes described earlier, resulting in a lighter-tasting product with a higher sucrose content. Sorghum molasses is produced by a similar process, but uses as raw material the cane from the sorghum plant. It has a distinctive, rather cloying, taste and is best used in baking, especially cookies.

UNREFINED OILS For a healthful diet, you should obtain necessary unsaturated fatty acids primarily from unrefined vegetable oils. Like other unrefined foods, these oils still contain all the nutrients present in the grains, beans, or seeds from which they were derived.

Nearly all cooking oils are made by first heating the grains, beans, or seeds; then, to produce "unrefined" oils, they are pressed with a centrifuge and expelled without the use of chemicals or solvents. No further processing occurs, but some firms do filter their "unrefined" oils to remove the remaining particles of the germ. It is better, of course, to purchase unfiltered, unrefined oils with some sediment left in the bottle. Commercial processing also results in the loss of vitamin E, which is found naturally in the oil and is essential for the proper utilization of important unsaturated fatty acids. You therefore benefit very little from refined oils, since they are a poor source of unsaturated fatty acids.

Refined oils also lack the natural odors and flavors that are noticeable in all unrefined oils. The mildest of the unrefined oils are safflower and sunflower. Unrefined sesame oil imparts a unique nutty taste to sautéed foods, while unrefined corn-germ oil gives a buttery taste to baked goods. Everyone has appreciated the full-bodied flavor of unrefined olive oil in salad dressings. Peanut and soybean oil are stronger in flavor and can be better utilized in sautéing, which reduces the intensity of their taste. Unrefined coconut and palm oil are also available in natural food stores; these partially saturated oils are used extensively by Southern cultures for all types of cooking (and in many processed foods).

Another reason for using unrefined oils is that at high temperatures the chemical makeup of an oil is altered and possibly becomes detrimental to health. Many advertisements praise refined oils for their ability to be used at extremely high temperatures, but these high heats are neither necessary nor desirable. Unrefined safflower oil can be used for deep-frying at about 400 degrees, and can withstand higher temperatures than most other oils. Cooking temperatures above this simply aren't necessary. Overheating of unrefined, unfiltered oil causes the germ to scorch and most nutrients to be lost. When substituting unrefined oils for solid fats in recipes, reduce the amounts of other liquids slightly or increase the dry ingredients.

OTHER USEFUL FOODS Bancha tea is high in calcium. It is a coarse, undyed green tea. The leaves, which must have remained on the bush for 3 years, should be roasted in the oven until browned. Bancha twig tea, known as kukicha, consists of the twigs of the tea bush and is generally available. One spare teaspoon of kukicha should be used for each cup of tea, which is prepared by simmering the twigs for about 15 to 20 minutes.

Baking powders are used to make "quick breads" that can usually be put together and baked in less than half an hour and that rise by virtue of the baking powder included. It's best not to use too many quick breads, but they occasionally do lend themselves well to the use of concentrated nutrients such as seeds and nuts, and they can contain a mixture of flours such as whole wheat with fresh ground corn, millet, triticale, and soy flour. Never use sodium bicarbonate in making quick breads. Its action is not only unnecessary but potentially unhealthy, destroying vitamin C and some B vitamins.

Instead, the baking powder you choose should be low-sodium and aluminum-free; aluminum is known to be toxic. Potassium bicarbonate does not destroy vitamin D in the body. Most natural food stores carry this type of low-sodium baking powder, but you can make your own by using 1 part potassium bicarbonate, 2 parts cream of tartar (potassium bitartrate) and 2 parts arrowroot powder. It may be necessary to obtain potassium bicarbonate through a chemical company because it is not generally available at pharmacies.

Nutritional yeast is a natural treasurehouse of proteins, vitamins, and minerals that can be used as a dietary supplement when added to juices or included in cooked dishes. Often called brewer's yeast because at one time it was a byproduct of the brewing industry, nutritional yeast is the tiniest of cultivated plants. The minuscule plants are grown on herbaceous grains and hops under carefully controlled temperature conditions. The yeast plant grows at an astoundingly fast rate. Once it has multiplied many times and matured, it is harvested and dried in a way that preserves all its nutrients. These yeast "flakes" are one of the most economical sources of the B vitamin complexes. In addition to these vitamins, yeast flakes contain minerals such as calcium, phosphorus, iron, sodium, potassium, and many of the amino acids, all of which work in conjunction with the B vitamins.

Many people take several tablespoons of yeast daily. If yeast is to be used in a beverage such as a vegetable juice, the flakes should first be mixed with a small amount of the liquid and stirred into a paste, then added to the rest of the liquid and thoroughly mixed again. A blender will simplify this method of preparation. Yeast flakes also may be added to baked foods such as breads and casseroles or mixed in small amounts with nut butter or bean-paste sandwich spreads.

Thickeners for smooth soups and sauces are usually based on a finely ground starch or flour, the most widely used being whole wheat, rice, and whole wheat pastry. The thickness of a flour-based sauce is determined by the ratio of flour to liquid. One tablespoon of flour to 1 cup liquid yields a thin sauce; up to 3 tablespoons flour to 1 cup liquid, a thick sauce. Cornstarch, corn flour in its finest version, is used in the same way to thicken sauces. Arrowroot powder, or flour made from the arrowroot plant, produces a finer sauce than cornstarch. The arrowroot starch should be dissolved in cold water before being added to hot foods to prevent lumping. Once the arrowroot has been added, simmer the thickened sauce to allow all the flavors to merge.

Kudzu is another high-quality but rather expensive thickening agent. The kudzu plant grows wild in the United States as well as in Japan, where it has long been used in folk medicine, often prescribed for diarrhea and head colds. The crumbly white chunks should first be dissolved in cold water before being added to hot sauces to prevent lumping.

If vinegar is called for in a recipe, never use the white distilled or wine varieties. Use an apple cider vinegar made from whole, unsprayed apples, undiluted and naturally aged. Refined, distilled vinegar has few of the naturally occurring nutrients (such as potassium) and virtually none of the indefinable subtle flavors of slowly aged cider vinegar. Because of the predominance of acetic acid in white distilled and wine vinegars, use them sparingly. Apple cider vinegar, on the other hand, contains a predominance of malic acid, which when wisely used is a constructive acid, naturally involved in the digestive system. Besides its culinary uses for preparing salad dressings and preserving foods, vinegar has long been useful as an antiseptic and blood coagulant. Rice vinegar is also available at natural food stores and in Asian markets. It has a distinctive aroma and taste, so use it with utmost discretion in pickling and salad dressings. Thanks to its natural fermentation, it contains none of the problematical properties of commercial distilled vinegars.

14

Bringing Herbs into Your Daily Life

American interest in herbal medicine has exploded in recent years. We now spend as much as $4 billion annually on products such as ginseng, echinacea, St. John's wort, black cohosh, and ginkgo biloba, to name just a few. Not long ago, we had to seek out an herbalist or visit a health food store to obtain herbal formulas. Today supplements are being manufactured by mainstream drug and vitamin companies, and can be found on store shelves everywhere. The National Institutes of Health has established an Office of Dietary Supplements to maintain a database and fund research into herbals. We read about herbs in our local newspapers and watch reports about them on the television news. It may seem as if herbal medicine is a new field. In actuality, herbs have been used for healing for as far back as we can trace the existence of humans.

A Brief History of Herbalism

In a Neanderthal grave in Iraq some 60,000 years old, scientists found pollens belonging to eight plants, seven of which are still used medicinally by people in that area. *The Chinese Shennong Herbal* lists 365 herbal drugs; it has been historically dated back to 200 B.C., but legend credits it to the Emperor Shennong of around 2700 B.C. Herbalism was not limited to the East. It reached a peak in England in 1653, when Nicholas Culpeper published his *Complete Herbal,* the first and greatest herbal work in the English language.

Yet, soon after that time, the pendulum swung away from the use of herbs, which had become inextricably tangled with magic, myth, and astrology. The Church of Rome objected to these pagan practices and in the 16th century the Swiss physician Paracelsus began to use inorganic cures like mercury and antimony instead of herbals, heralding the near-monopoly of chemical-based medicine that has lasted until today.

The first determined effort in the modern Western world to break this pharmaceutical monopoly came from America in the 18th century. Samuel Thomson, the son of a farmer, lived during a time of great yellow fever epidemics. The accepted medical practice in curing this (and almost any other) ailment was a liberal use of bleeding and mercury, which a healthy patient would be lucky to live through. Thomson instead used herbs and steaming—with great success—but was met with hostility from the orthodox medical establishment, and even imprisoned briefly.

In the 19th century, herbal medicine made a popular comeback. So broad and exaggerated were the claims made for various tinctures, potions, "patent" medicines, and favorite cure-alls like mandrake root, however, that this popularity only contributed to a medical bias against herbal remedies. Modern science's success in synthesizing powerful drugs and the advent of highly rational double-blind testing procedures has confirmed this bias further.

Contemporary Issues and Regulatory Control

The traditional antipathy of the medical orthodoxy, the American Medical Association (AMA), and government bodies like the Food and Drug Administration (FDA) to herbs as medicine or even as nutrition has grounds in several factors. In the age of double-blind testing and standard doses, herbs are difficult to quantify or analyze. Sometimes a single chemical component can be isolated and purified or synthesized. Digitalis, used to treat heart disease, was isolated from the foxglove plant; quinine from the bark of the quinoa tree; salicylic acid (aspirin) from willow bark.

But herbal medicine is by nature an inexact, individualized science. Herbs may work differently on different people. The conditions under which a plant has grown, the time at which it is harvested, or the form that its preparation takes may all modify its effect. And despite successes such as aspirin and quinine, the "scientific" method of isolating, analyzing, and extracting the active ingredient in a plant often doesn't work very well. A chemical that might be isolated as the active component in an herb may in fact be modified by other, less obvious constituents that make it more powerful or moderate its side effects. And sometimes, even with rigorous research, the ways in which a plant affects the body can remain stubbornly mysterious.

A second, no less powerful reason for the particular hostility of the AMA toward herbal remedies is the threat they present to the vastly powerful, multibillion-dollar pharmaceutical industry. Drug sales in the United States, the world's largest pharmaceutical market, reached $86 billion in 1999. Herbal remedies cannot be standardized, packaged, and marketed like drugs. They can usually be grown and prepared by anyone, and cannot be patented. In many cases they cut into the consumption of over-the-counter and prescription medicines. The pharmaceutical companies underwrite the very existence of the AMA.

The problem of regulatory control is a burden to the herbal industry. Because herbs are neither foods nor drugs, they are extremely difficult to define and hence hard to regulate. When the use is medicinal, they can be considered as drugs; when the use is culinary, they can be considered as spices. But it is not always easy to draw the line. The regulations of the Food and Drug Administration (FDA) stipulate that a product that is being sold as a food or a nutritional supplement is limited as to the health benefits that can be claimed to result from its use. In 1998, the FDA proposed that dietary supplements of all types could not imply that they diagnose, treat, prevent, or cure a disease or symptom. In early 2000, it eased some restrictions and allowed supplements to claim to help "common conditions" associated with "passages of life" such as morning sickness and memory loss.

The cost of testing drugs, which tends to be in the millions or tens of millions of dollars, is prohibitive for herb companies, which tend to be relatively small as compared to the huge pharmaceutical conglomerates. This puts herb companies in a bind. Some, aware that the FDA usually takes several years before it will catch up with a company, choose to go ahead without scientific proof of the efficacy of their product.

If the mainstream health industry were to consider the health properties of herbs more seriously, this would not be a problem. Other countries have no such opposition to the complementary use of herbal remedies within an orthodox medical framework. In 1958 Chairman Mao urged that China's traditional sciences of herbal medicine and acupuncture should not be abandoned. China's goal now is to develop medicine that combines both the ancient and the new. For instance, herbal tonics are often used to strengthen a patient's ability to cope with modern chemotherapy. Russia has been committed to research on herbs, carrying out hundreds of studies on Siberian ginseng alone. Even in Britain, the National Institute of Medical Herbalists (created in 1864 as the National Association of Medical Herbalists) is a flourishing—and scientifically respected—body.

In some less industrialized, less wealthy nations, there tends to be a greater acceptance of medicinal herbs. In part, this is simply due to economics. In many countries, if you are poor, your health care will depend largely on medicinal herbs because industrial medicine is only for those who can afford it.

Were conventional health practitioners to include herbal medicine in their training and delivery of health care, a significant improvement could occur almost immediately in the quality of medicine available to patients. In particular, the problem of iatrogenic (doctor-induced) illness would be substantially reduced. The side effects of synthetic drugs are often substantial: The medicines we take frequently make us sicker. In many patient care situations, medicinal herbs could go a long way toward maintaining or restoring health.

Some signs of change are evident. In 1999, the Office of Dietary Supplements at the National Institutes of Health announced awards of approximately $1.5 million per year for 5 years to two universities to study, among other things, green tea extract and soy for inhibition of tumor growth, St. John's wort for depression, and herbal supplements specifically for women.

The Practical Use of Herbs

You don't have to be an herbalist, know complicated formulas, study the chemistry of plants, or learn the Chinese philosophies of herbal medicine to enjoy the benefits that herbs can bring into your life. If you are a novice in the world of herbs, go to a bookstore or library for books in their health and diet sections. Start small, with perhaps five herbs—some good ones to try first might be garlic, rosemary, comfrey, echinacea, and thyme. (Some herbs and their benefits, along with recommendations for the forms and quantities in which they can be taken, are listed below.)

The best way to begin to use herbs is the simplest; incorporate them into your cooking in progressively increasing amounts, or make a tea of one or more herbs. Cookbooks often recommend the kinds of herbs that go well with different foods, but make your own experiments. Just put a few pinches in the stew pot, sprinkle them over a salad, or mix a little with a sandwich spread. Also, start reading the labels on the herbal tea boxes at the supermarket. Pick out a tea you think would taste good. Add an herbal tincture to your shampoo, your skin lotion or massage oil, or your bathtub. Within a short period of time, you will have incorporated a number of different herbs into your life. And you should start feeling better naturally.

Remember, though, not all herbs are equal. How they are grown, harvested, stored, and prepared will effect their potency and usefulness. Fresh and homegrown is always best, because you know the conditions under they have been planted, monitored, fertilized, and cared for. Many nurseries sell not only herb seedlings but also kits that can be used to conveniently grow herbs on the windowsills of city apartments. Investment in a full-spectrum light tube will even allow you to grow herbs on the kitchen counter. If you live in the country and you really know which plants you are looking for, some herbs can be collected wild. Be careful, though; some toxic plants can look very much like useful herbs. It would be best to have someone with an expert knowledge of wild plants in your area along at first. A city dweller should not pick herbs that are just growing in the streets. With people, animals, and traffic circulating around them, such herbs can actually become quite toxic.

When buying herbs form a store, especially in bulk, make sure you use your senses of smell and sight. The herb shouldn't seem dusty nor have a moldy aroma. If it looks more brown than green, then it will definitely have reduced effectiveness. Consumers ought to insist on fresh herbs if they're buying in bulk in herbal stores. The more information you can get about where the herb was grown, how it was cultivated, and when it was harvested, the better. Stay away from potent dried herbs in powder or capsule form. They generally have not been tested for safety or efficacy and are all too often a rip-off. It is almost impossible to determine what the actual ingredients are of a powder inside a capsule; you have no way of telling the age of such a preparation, or even if it is made from the herb it claims to be.

Also, some people may have allergic reactions or other problems with specific herbs. To test those sensitivities, use one herb at a time at first. Try them out, see what they're like, taste them and smell them.

In addition to fresh herbs and dried herbs, there are several other forms in which herbal medicines can be taken. Often the form in which an herbal remedy is prepared is as important in therapeutic terms as which herb is used. *Infusions and decoctions*, two of the simpler forms, are both made with boiling water. Infusions are made by pouring boiling water over dried or fresh herbs, while roots and barks are boiled in water and left to steep as they cool. Distilled or spring water is preferable; the traditional proportion is about 1 ounce of dried herb to 1 pint of water. The pot or cup should be covered to prevent the escape of volatile oils. It should not be made of aluminum, which can enter the preparation in minute amounts.

Tinctures are made by macerating herbs in a mixture of water and alcohol for at least 2 weeks. Water extracts many constituents of plants but oils, gums, and resins are most efficiently extracted in alcohol, which also preserves the preparation. The strength of the alcohol varies. Vodka or brandy can be used to make tinctures at home. Some herb liqueurs, such as chartreuse, were originally a kind of therapeutic remedy in the tradition of the monks who made them, although they no longer have these properties. *Ointments*, which are useful to treat some skin conditions, can be made with herbs and oils.

Herbs and the Immune System

Herbs can play a vital role in our day-to-day lives by stimulating our immune systems. Many people find that their health seems to be sapped by recurring or chronic colds and viruses. Synthetic drugs, far from being a solution, seem merely to encourage new, more resistant strains of bacteria and viruses. People with more serious immune problems, like AIDS and cancer, can help their systems to fight back as much as possible by using herbs to stimulate a healthy immune system.

Dr. Paul Lee, founder of the Platonic Academy in Santa Cruz, California, is one of America's leading authorities on the use of herbs for immune system health and overall well-being. Dr. Lee links herbology, immunology, and molecular biology together in his theory that there is an herbal code in our immune system memory that is carried by our DNA. This immune memory, genetically transmitted from our ancestors, records their own struggle against illness and disease. When the Spanish conquistadors brought smallpox into Mexico, 3.5 million Mexican Indians died; they had no such genetic immunization to ward it off. Few in the world die from smallpox today, because the World Health Organization has effectively eliminated it. But despite all our triumphs in conquering some diseases, it seems that cancer and other immune system diseases have taken their place. Dr. Lee believes that our generation is suffering from a kind of immune system amnesia. We have become detached from the botanical basis of health care and the medicinal herbs that are the natural agents of our immunity.

The body's ancient natural response to herbs is evident to anyone who has grown them. The aroma of specific herbs brings a unique and clear reaction. Anyone with any familiarity with herb gardening would never mistake thyme for oregano or oregano for rosemary, even with their eyes closed. The recent development of aromatherapy is a recognition of the power of our genetic memory of certain herbal substances, which even responds to just the smell of them.

Most humans in the modern world have lost the ancient talent for "intuitive herbalism" that ancient cultures recognized and that animals still possess. Dogs and cats will nibble certain grasses when they feel ill. Sick African chimpanzees methodically seek out the leaves from a bush called aspilia, keep them in their mouths for about 15 seconds, and then swallow them whole. An analysis has shown that the aspilia leaves contain a powerful antibiotic chemical. Humans, however, have largely forgotten how to select herbs we need to keep our immune responses healthy. Certain herbs can augment immunity because we're coded or programmed for them; this needs to be reactivated in our generation because one of the worst health problems that faces Americans today is a collective deterioration of the immune system. If we could restore a botanical emphasis to health care in a widespread way, it would make a great contribution to public health.

Rather than just concentrating on a better immune system, however, look at your system as a whole. As much as possible, consider the elements that contribute to your condition: lifestyle, stress, clinical and subclinical infection, toxins, and anything else that would divert the immune system from functioning properly. Then, with all this in mind, examine the herbs that can help you in these areas.

What to Use for Specific Types of Disorders

Although it is important to try to treat the body as a whole for almost any disorder, some herbs can be suggested as specifics for weakness or disorder in one system or organ:

ANTIBIOTICS: dandelion, garlic, goldenseal, marigold, myrrh, thyme

ARTHRITIC DISORDERS: alfalfa, cayenne and feverfew for pain relief, and sarsaparilla

BLOOD-CLOTTING: cinnamon helps mild, passive hemorrhaging

CIRCULATION/HEART TONICS: barberry, blackberry, and especially hawthorn

CHOLESTEROL REDUCTION: cayenne, ginger, and garlic

CLEANSING AND DETOXIFICATION: barberry, blackberry leaves and fruit, celery, chaparral, goldenseal, rosemary, and seaweeds

COLDS AND FLUS: cayenne, chaparral, echinacea, garlic, goldenseal, osha, and thyme

DIGESTIVE SYSTEM: alfalfa, barberry, celery, chamomile, cinnamon, comfrey, and marigold

DIURETICS: dandelion and celery

IMMUNE ENHANCEMENT: astragalus, echinacea, garlic, ginseng, goldenseal, marigold, pau d'arco, suma, turmeric (especially for allergies), and wild indigo root

LIVER TONICS: dandelion and milk thistleMENOPAUSE: black cohosh, chaste berry, dong quai, licorice, and wild yam

MEN'S HEALTH: saw palmetto

NERVOUS SYSTEM/BRAIN TONICS: avena, chamomile, ginkgo biloba, ginseng, kava kava root, rosemary, valerianPAIN REDUCTION: cayenne and feverfew

RESPIRATORY TRACT: cayenne, garlic, and milk thistle

More information on each herb is contained in the *Glossary of Herbs* below. See later chapters to learn more about herbal remedies for specific diseases, disorders, and conditions.

A Glossary of Herbs

ALFALFA Alfalfa (*medicago sativa*), used as a tea or eaten whole as sprouts in a salad, is rich in a variety of vitamins and minerals, as its roots can reach as far as 30 feet into the ground to gather up essential minerals. Alfalfa is also plentifully stocked with enzymes that can help in the digestive process. Alfalfa is used as a tonic to increase vitality, appetite, and weight—interestingly, it is fed to horses for the same reason. The root of tooth-leaved clover, a close relative of alfalfa (which, in fact, is given the same name—*mu xu*—as alfalfa by the Chinese), has been found to be very successful in curing night blindness. Alfalfa also has a reputation for healing peptic ulcers and is an old folk remedy for arthritic conditions. It may work by cleansing the bowels.

Alfalfa grows wild throughout America and is also cultivated as live stock food and for other commercial purposes. It is a major raw source in the manufacture of chlorophyll. Extracts of alfalfa are used commercially to flavor beverages and food products. It is easy to grow alfalfa sprouts at home for use in salads. Caution should be observed in using alfalfa, however. Some individuals may be allergic to alfalfa. In addition, it is difficult to tell if powdered alfalfa sold in health foods in capsule form is pure or indeed if it is really alfalfa at all.

ASTRAGALUS Astragalus, a Chinese herb, is only now gaining popularity in this country although it has been used for thousands of years in China as the basis of an immune-enhancing therapy called *Fuchang* therapy. The immune system is basic to the Chinese approach to health, which is concerned with bringing the body back into balance. This root is a staple of traditional Chinese medicine and can be found easily at herbal markets. It is best prepared in a decoction, simmering the root for 10 to 15 minutes, then straining while still hot.

AVENA Avena has been a folk remedy for several hundred years as a general nerve tonic for nervous exhaustion and certain kinds of mental disease. It is used in the form of the fresh, undried oat plant—avena sativa—harvested at the milky stage (a seed will give off a drop of milky juice when squeezed). Ayurvedic medicine in India uses avena for opium addiction, as did the eclectic physicians in the United States in the early 1900s. Evidence from studies in Scotland suggests that avena also helps with nicotine addiction, and it may prove effective in treating alcoholism or even heroin addiction. Several companies have now come out with commercial oat extracts.

This extract from the oat plant can be mixed into porridge or baked into cakes or cookies.

BARBERRY Barberry, a common shrub, is of interest primarily because of its bark, although the Japanese barberry's berries were once used to make jellies and relishes. Like goldenseal and yellow dock, barberry bark is yellow because it contains berberine, an antibacterial and antiviral alkyloid. Barberry bark is a tonic to almost every organ in the body. It has excellent bitters, much preferable to those of the marigold, which makes it a good digestive. It stimulates the liver and the gallbladder, aiding not only in digestion but also the cleansing of toxins from the body through the eliminative functions. It is also a tonic to the spleen, which strengthens the immune system. As a laxative, it again plays a role in detoxification. Finally, it increases the circulation.

The bark can be infused into teas or tinctures. To make a tincture, crush about 8 ounces of the bark and add it to a screw-top jar filled with 6 to 8 cups of a clear spirit, such as gin or vodka. Store the tincture in a warm, dark place and shake the jar twice a day to thoroughly mix. After 2 weeks, strain the tincture through a cheesecloth, draining well. Keep in tightly sealed bottles. Instead of alcohol, you could use a sweet cider vinegar.

BLACKBERRY Blackberry leaves are an astringent. Infusion is considered an effective blood cleanser and may be useful for improving the circulation of the blood. Blackberry fruit is useful as a cleansing food to help correct diarrhea. It can also be used as a gargle for throat inflammation or in douching to help with irregular vaginal discharges. A tablespoon or two of dried leaves can be brewed in tea.

CAYENNE Cayenne shares with ginger an ability to help the body metabolize cholesterol. Studies in India have found that it depresses the liver's production of cholesterol and triglycerides, countering the effect of cholesterol-rich foods. It also seems to have a host of other benefits. Chili peppers and other spicy foods act as expectorants in the bronchial passages, benefiting patients with chronic bronchitis and emphysema. Swedish research has indicated that capsaicin—the ingredient that makes a chili hot—desensitizes the lungs to irritants like cigarette smoke. A common cold can be temporarily relieved with a gargle of a little chili sauce in water.

Surprisingly, the capsaicin that stings your mouth in food is also an effective pain suppressant, inhibiting the relay of pain signals to the central nervous system. German researchers discovered years ago that chili peppers seemed to dissolve blood clots. Further research in Thailand has confirmed this finding. After eating hot peppers the blood-clot-dissolving activity increased almost immediately. The effect is short-term, lasting about half an hour, but frequent consumption of chilis in food can prevent clots from building up.

Finally, chili peppers have an effect on the brain; the burning they cause in the mouth provokes the release of endorphins, the body's natural morphine that blocks pain and induces a sensation of pleasure related to "runner's high."

A pinch of finely chopped fresh cayenne peppers added to a curry or chili is perfect for the most benefits. Cayenne is the active ingredient in Tabasco sauce and a few dashes in anything from tomato juice to brown rice adds a healthy jolt.

CELERY Celery has a cleansing diuretic effect, whether it is taken as a tea or as juice. Carrot juice is a good complement to celery. Celery's alkalinity also makes it soothing to the digestive system.

A handful of chopped celery can be added to salads, but it is best when a few stalks are juiced along with carrots or other vegetables. An aromatic tea can be made from steeping a tablespoon of seeds in a cup of boiling water for 3 to 5 minutes.

CHAMOMILE Chamomile is an herb that can be used as a tea or a tincture. Chamomile has a slightly alkalinizing affect on the blood; it helps to stimulate digestion and acts as a nerve tonic. Folk wisdom has aptly given chamomile a reputation as a calming herb. It can be taken at night as a mild sedative. In a bath or as a decoction, chamomile soothes the skin, and it brightens blond hair when added to shampoo. It is antispasmodic when taken internally.

Tea made from a tablespoon of dried leaves should be taken before bedtime to help fall asleep. For swelling or pain in the joints, chamomile oil can be applied. To make the oil, use about 1 ounce of fresh or dried flowers and combine with a half cup of olive oil. Crush the flowers in the oil and let them steep for 24 hours. Strain the flowers out and rub the oil on the affected areas.

CINNAMON Cinnamon is a very effective diarrhea remedy. It can be made into a tea, with just a pinch or two in a cup of hot water. An old-time variant is apple sauce with cinnamon, doubly effective since apple pectin is very soothing to the intestinal tract, as well as delicious.

Cinnamon was also used by the eclectics—a school of 19th century American herbalists devoted to the specific, proven use of herbal remedies—as a first aid remedy to treat mild, passive hemorrhaging, such as blood in the urine or sputum. Many midwives swear by cinnamon for postpartum hemorrhaging. Of course, never attempt to treat any serious bleeding in this way without consulting a doctor first.

COMFREY Comfrey (*symphytum officinale*) is an ancient healing herb. It has a soothing effect on the stomach lining. A British study showed that comfrey activates local hormones called prostaglandins, which protect the stomach lining from inflammation. Comfrey root contains mucilage—a slimy or gelatinous form of sugar that is soothing to digestive tract mucous membranes. Comfrey also contains allantoin, a natural cell healer. It is one of the few plant sources of vitamin B_{12}.

A tablespoon of dried leaves steeped in hot water for 3 to 5 minutes makes a gentle tea. Fresh leaves can be chopped and added to salad.

DANDELION Dandelion is an unlikely healer to most of us who know it as a lawn pest, but in fact the entire dandelion plant is a valuable herbal source. Dandelion is rich in potassium, which makes it an ideal diuretic as it does not leach potassium from the body as diuretics tend to do. Dandelion greens are also very rich in vitamin A, and are an excellent salad ingredient.

Dandelion root has been used for centuries as a laxative, tonic, and diuretic, and in treating liver, gallbladder, and kidney conditions. Its extracts are used in modern pharmaceutical preparations for these properties. Recent Chinese research has shown that the juice of the dandelion fights certain bacteria. It is particularly efficient in treating upper respiratory tract infections, bronchitis, pneumonia, appendicitis, mastitis, and dermatitis. It creates fewer side effects than modern antibiotics, and these disappear as soon as treatment is discontinued.

A handful of tender, fresh leaves can be a delicious addition to a salad. Dandelion juice can be easily extracted by putting a few leaves in the juicer with carrots or other vegetables.

ECHINACEA Echinacea, also known as the purple coneflower, is the most popular herbal immune stimulant in America today. From 1997 to 1998, its market grew 151 percent, with sales of more than $33 million. Echinacea is indigenous to the United States alone, where Native Americans have used it for over 150 years. Nevertheless, echinacea was relegated to the realms of folk medicine until the 1960s, when in-vitro studies focused on its ability to stimulate leukocytes, the infection-fighting white blood cells in our bodies. Echinacea also inhibits hyaluronidase, an enzyme that pathogenic organisms use to break down body tissues to make way for their own spread. Echinacea strengthens the tissues by stimulating the production of hyaluronic acid, the base of the cell membrane in most body tissues. Echinacea helps the body to regenerate new tissue by stimulating fibrocytes.

Echinacea was found to be more effective than cortisone in stopping streptococcus in rats. Echinacea stimulates the adrenal cortex, the area where the corticosteroids—which have a cortisonelike action—are released. Other studies have indicated that echinacea's effect is due to polysaccharides, or sugar molecules, which fool the body into believing that they are pathogens even though they are perfectly benign and nontoxic. Thus, they boost the body's natural immune reaction, giving it a jump start on fighting colds and infections.

There are two kinds of echinacea: echinacea angustifolia and echinacea purpurea. Most research has involved the angustifolia, which seems much more effective. Echinacea should be taken at the first symptoms of cold or flu, every 2 to 3 hours for about 10 days. The root of echinacea can be steeped in boiling water for 15 minutes. The tea should be taken every 2 or 3 hours up to 6 cups a day until symptoms of cold or flu have begun to subside.

FEVERFEW Feverfew (*chrysanthemum parthenium*) is an immune enhancer that lowers inflammation. Its name comes from its ability to reduce fever. Feverfew is good for people with arthritis because of its anti-inflammatory properties.

Attention was first focused on feverfew in England when a miner gave the wife of a medical officer of the National Coal Board a cutting of the plant to cure her migraines. Dr. Stuart Johnson, intrigued by this report, carried out clinical trials in which feverfew completely cured the migraines of 7 out of 10 patients.

The dried or fresh leaves can be steeped in boiling water for a therapeutic tea.

GARLIC Garlic has always had a down-home folk reputation as a restorative; how many grandmothers swear by chicken soup with plenty of garlic for a cold? And this reputation has a history almost as long as written history itself. Jean Carper noted in her best seller, *The Food Pharmacy*, that 22 garlic prescriptions "for such complaints as headache, throat disorders, and physical weakness" were found on an Egyptian medical papyrus dating from around 1500 B.C. The confidence the Egyptians had in garlic is demonstrated by the fact that they reportedly used it to strengthen the workers who built the pyramids. Pliny recommended garlic for 61 maladies in his *Historia Naturalis*; Hippocrates recommended it as a laxative, diuretic, and cure for tumors of the uterus. Garlic has been used to treat high blood pressure for centuries in China and Japan. In first-century India, garlic and onion were thought to prevent heart disease and rheumatism. Garlic even had a reputation as an aphrodisiac in Shakespearean England. It is probable that only the smell of garlic has prevented it form becoming as omnipresent a cure-all as aspirin.

Garlic's distinctive odor is due to its sulfur-containing compounds—the most important being allicin—which also are responsible for many of its therapeutic effects. Allicin is a powerful inhibitor of bacterial growth with an extremely broad spectrum; hundreds of studies have confirmed its effectiveness over as many as 72 separate infectious agents. Not only does garlic directly attack microbes, but it also seems to boost the body's own immune powers. One study found that the immune system's killer cells from people who had consumed large quantities of garlic destroyed half again as many cancer cells in a culture.

Studies also show that garlic lowers cholesterol and thins the blood, lowering the chances of dangerous blood clots. In addition, it is a hypertensive agent. Bulgarian studies have demonstrated that garlic produces dramatic blood-pressure drops in humans. Finally, garlic is an effective decongestant for common colds and can prevent or ease chronic bronchitis.

The best way to get garlic is to grow your own or buy bulbs that are as fresh as possible. Raw garlic is most effective, especially in antibacterial activity, but garlic in cooking retains many of its therapeutic benefits. The garlic sold in health food stores as capsules, pills, and deodorized preparation, however, may have relatively little power. It is the smelly part of garlic that is the most therapeutic. Japanese kyolic paste is one commercial garlic preparation that may approach the value of fresh garlic, but is certainly no better. The best approach is the most simple and natural. If you can't stomach eating garlic cloves raw, cook with it, use it in salad dressings, soups, and garlic bread.

A teaspoon or two of freshly chopped garlic is a healthful addition to all menus. An infusion of 2 cloves of mashed garlic to 1/8 cup of room temperature water can be dripped into each nostril to clear sinuses.

GINGER Ginger is useful for upset stomachs or motion sickness. A double-blind study published in the *Journal of the American Medical Association* compared the effects of ginger and dramamine, a common over-the-counter motion sickness drug, and found that ginger was actually more effective. In addition, ginger had none of the side effects—such as drowsiness—of the commercial drug.

Ginger is an even more effective anticoagulant than garlic or onions. Gingerol, one of its compounds, has a structure very much like that of aspirin, which also thins the blood. Ginger is a folk remedy for menstrual cramps. It reduces blood pressure and cholesterol, stimulates the heart, and has blocked mutations leading to cancer in mice.

Ginger can be taken in capsules, used fresh in cooking, or as a tea. Caution should be taken, especially with powdered ginger, which can burn the esophagus. A slice of fresh ginger should be taken to avoid motion sickness. A few tablespoons of grated fresh or powdered ginger can be used in cooking to add some excitement to your meal.

GINSENG Ginseng is popular herbal product. In 1998, U.S. sales were nearly $100 million. Considered the master herb by the Chinese, Ginseng is probably the most researched herb in the world. It is highly valued in China; in fact, the fist diplomatic liaison between the U.S. and China was a trade agreement for selling ginseng. Ginseng was used as far back as 3100 B.C. in China; around 2597 B.C. it was discussed as a medicine in a scroll. At one time, only the imperial family was allowed to grow or own ginseng.

Wild ginseng, which has been left to grow for 30, 40, or even up to 100 years, is extremely expensive, if it can be obtained at all, and is highly prized. Cultivated ginseng may be uprooted anywhere from the age of 2 to 6 years. Preferably it should be at least 6 years old for optimum pharmacological quality. Interestingly, the soil from which a 6-year-old ginseng root has been pulled is permitted to lie fallow for 10 years to recover its nutrients—an indication of ginseng's ability to pull nutrients into itself. In America, ginseng is grown extensively in the Wisconsin-Michigan area of the Midwest, but most of this crop is exported to Asia.

Ginseng improves physical efficiency and stamina. Experiments with proofreaders found a 12 to 54 percent reduction in misreadings when ginseng was used. It is thought that this results from an improvement of oxygenation of the brain cells. One of the elements found in ginseng, germanium, is a chelator—that is, it can pull heavy metals, such as mercury, lead, or cadmium, out of tissues. Experiments in animals have found that the concentration of mercury in tissue was reduced after the administration of ginseng. Germanium also seems to rid the cells of excess hydrogen; in consequence there is a higher proportion of oxygen, and more efficient energy production.

One of the most fascinating properties of ginseng is its apparent ability to protect the bone marrow against radioactivity. A study presented at a symposium on Ginseng in Seoul, Korea, showed that mice pretreated with ginseng survived intensive x-ray irradiation at a rate some 82.5 percent better than the control group. The damage done to the bone marrow—an important factor because this is where the red blood cells are synthesized—was significantly less in these mice.

Siberian ginseng (*eleutherococcus senticosus*) has been the subject of more than 400 studies in Russia. Discovered as a result of a search for an indigenous substitute for Chinese ginseng, it was found to make mice able to swim half again as far as those without it before becoming exhausted. Another study was done on several thousand carefully monitored telegraph operators, a group in which it was easy to quantify efficiency, for 20 years. Not only was the work efficiency of those who had taken the ginseng greater, but they also had fewer sick days, less cancer, less heart disease, and less diabetes. Back in 1962, Siberian ginseng was added to the official Russian pharmacopoeia. So convinced are the Russians of the therapeutic value of eleutherococcus that it is used by their athletes and cosmonauts.

Ginseng's powers to help the body cope with stress are dramatic and far-ranging. Both panax and Siberian ginseng function as adaptogens. An adaptogen works as a balancing mechanism: it raises low blood pressure but also brings high blood pressure down, for example. An adaptogen has nonspecific properties that enable animals to cope with both physical and mental stress more efficiently, to be more resilient, and to maintain a balance, or homeostasis, under widely varying conditions. As an adaptogen, ginseng helps the body to balance itself under a wide variety of stress factors.

Steep 1 ounce of the macerated root in boiling water for 15 minutes and strain. Also try concocting a tincture of 2 ounces of ginseng with 2 pints of rice wine.

GOLDENSEAL Goldenseal (hydrastis canadensis) has been much misunderstood, and used as a panacea for many ailments. This root is quite powerful, and should be used sparingly and for limited periods of time. The consumer should also be wary, as goldenseal is expensive and may be sold in adulterated preparations.

Goldenseal contains alkyloids, which are strong antiseptic and antiviral compounds. One of these, berberine, has been used to treat malaria when quinine is not available. Berberine gives goldenseal its yellow color. Goldenseal is effective on the mucous membranes of the gastrointestinal tract. It reduces inflammation throughout the body. Goldenseal also indirectly stimulates the immune system by helping to build up the glandular system, rather than directly attacking microbes as its alkyloids do.

Goldenseal also acts as a mild laxative and, as such, detoxifies the system.It is best to chew goldenseal or drink it as a tea with 1/10 to 1/4 of a teaspoon per cup. If it is self-prescribed, begin with a very small amount, slowly increasing to a quarter teaspoon.

An infusion made with 1/4 ounce of goldenseal has been shown to help sinusitis. Also a gargle prepared with a tincture of goldenseal in warm water can soothe a sore throat.

HAWTHORN Hawthorn (*crataegus oxyacanthoides*), the familiar red-berried tree, is used extensively throughout Europe as a heart tonic. In this country digitalis, or foxglove, is used for this purpose, but it is highly toxic. Hawthorn, on the other hand, has none of this toxicity. Hawthorn berries, leaves, and flowers are all excellent for the arterial and peripheral circulation.

Use the leaves to brew a stimulating tea. The berries can be preserved in a tincture and used as needed.

MARIGOLD Marigold, especially the flowerhead, is a very effective herb. The marigold flowerhead is antibacterial, antiviral, and antiseptic. It also enhances the function of the lymphatic system, which in turn aids both the acquired and fixed immune system. The flowerhead is useful in treating superficial wounds.

Most of the benefits of the marigold flowerhead come from its volatile oil. This oil, when extracted, has shown to promote blood clotting and the formation of granulomatous tissue, the first stage of healing in wounds. It also contains salicylic acid, which itself is helpful in reducing the inflammation.

Both the leaves and flowerhead of the marigold contain bitters, which trigger beneficial gastrointestinal responses, boosting the production of hydrochloric acid and enzymes in the stomach. Chefs often use marigold flowers in salads for color, as well as the greens. Do not underestimate the marigold; it is not only beneficial but very gentle. The flowerheads are so light that there is no need to worry about dosage. Sprinkle a few freshly chopped leaves in a mixed green salad.

MILK THISTLE Milk thistle (salybum marianum), a noxious weed to farmers, is effective in treating liver disorders, helping the liver properly process toxins and poisons. Milk thistle contains tyramine, which stimulates mucous secretions. Thus, milk thistle tea can be used to help stimulate congested lungs to discharge their excess fluids and mucous, especially in the winter. Milk thistle is available in tinctures.

MYRRH Myrrh, a resin extracted from the myrrh tree, is packaged in its solid form, looking somewhat like rock candy. Myrrh is used in a number of consumer products because of its antiseptic qualities. For example, it is often an ingredient in natural toothpaste. Myrrh is also antifungal and antiviral. Clinical tests have shown it to fight staphylococcus and *E. coli* bacteria, for which reason it has been used clinically in hospitals in Egypt and India. Myrrh seems most effective in local application, but should not be ruled out for systemic use.

Myrrh is not easily used because of its market preparation. It must first be caramelized—liquified with water over heat—and tends to become a gummy mass when stored in water. The recommended internal dosage is about 1/2 teaspoon. Dissolve a small portion, about an ounce, of the gummy resin in warm water and use as a refreshing mouthwash. Also, sip the liquid as a cure for a stomachache.

OSHA Osha, an herb native to the Rocky Mountain area of the United States, is used extensively in that area for colds, flus, coughs, sore throats, and urinary tract infections.

PAU D'ARCO Pau d'arco (as it is known in Brazil; known as *la pacho* in Argentina), native to South America, has attracted a lot of attention with evidence of its strong antiviral, antitumor, antifungal, and antibacterial action since it was introduced in the U.S. in 1980.

Grind the root into a powder, then fill gelatin capsules. Take 1 capsule twice a day.

PECTIN Pectin is not an herb, but rather a substance found in some plants. The most well-known source of pectin is apples; carrots contain a different variety. Pectin is soluble fiber used commercially to make jello. It is a well-known depressor of cholesterol levels. A more recent discovery is that pectin helps to absorb and remove some toxic metals that can accumulate in tissues, and may increase our ability to withstand irradiation.

Increase your apple consumption for the best quality pectin. Try applesauce or baked apples for variety.

ROSEMARY Rosemary has been gaining publicity recently as an antioxidant, helping to counter the destructive effects of modern industrial toxins and pollutants in the air. Traditionally it has been used as a preservative, especially to keep meats and fats from going rancid. Chemicals extracted from rosemary are used in the modern food industry for this purpose. The folk history of rosemary has been as a brain or memory tonic. This may have something to do with its antioxidant properties. Scientists have found that rosemary promotes menstrual discharge in women and hair growth.

Rosemary oil is used widely in cosmetics such as soaps, creams, and lotions. Infusions of rosemary are used externally for wounds, sores, bruises, eczema, and rheumatism. To use, crush the dried leaves and sprinkle in soups or salads.

SARSAPARILLA ROOT Sarsaparilla root (*smilax ornata*) is an adaptogen (see the entry for ginseng for a definition of adaptogens) that has been around for centuries. It was first introduced to Europe in the Middle Ages as a treatment for syphilis. Although there is no evidence that it can cure syphilis, it may relieve its symptoms. Chemically, sarsaparilla falls into the class of phytosterols. *Phyto* is from the Latin for "plant," and *sterol* is related to the adrenal hormones called steroids, so phytosterols are plant analogues of steroid hormones. Claims have been made that sarsaparilla contains testosterone, the male sex hormone. There is no evidence for this. The related claim that sarsaparilla increases the production of male testosterone, especially in older men, has been suggested by new evidence but not proven. However, sarsaparilla has been touted as a male sex tonic for centuries, all over the world. It is also used as an anti-inflammatory, and it is chemically similar to the clinical steroids used in modern medicine to treat inflammation.

Several major pharmaceutical companies in Germany make a product for psoriasis using sarsaparilla extract. It is also effective in alleviating eczema and other skin diseases, as well as arthritis.

Steep the leaves and berries in hot water for an aromatic tea. The root was once used with wintergreen and sassafras to flavor root beer.

THYME Thyme (*thymus vulgaris*) is mentioned here together with oregano because they are both high in a chemical known as thymol. Thymol is used throughout the pharmaceutical industry; in fact, it is a main ingredient in Listerine. It is a strong antiseptic, effective as an antibacterial, and antifungal. Interestingly, thyme's Latin name is the same as that of the thymus gland, the central organ of the immune system.

Thyme can be used to make a mouthwash, a bath oil, or a deodorant. Oregano and thyme make a wonderful tea that can help against the common cold and mild infections. As a strong tea it is a good wash for minor cuts and scratches. Also use to flavor soups or salads. Crush the dried leaves and sprinkle on foods.

TURMERIC Turmeric, a vivid yellow spice made of ground roots, gives curry powder (and mustard) its classic color. Studies on animals in China and Russia in recent decades have found that turmeric promotes bile secretion, lowers blood pressure, stimulates the appetite, alleviates pain, and reduces inflammation. A recent study in China showed extracts of turmeric to prevent 100 percent of pregnancies in rats. It also seems to have antibiotic properties.

This powdered spice has a subtle taste, but helps support the stronger spices in curries and prepared mustard. Use a teaspoon along with other aromatic spices. Turmeric has been getting a lot of attention lately from evidence of its ability to stabilize mast cells, which line the trachea and intestinal tract and serve as a first line of defense for the immune system. Healthy mast cells have a tight weave that can keep deviant material out of the bloodstream—bacteria, pollen, and protein that has not been properly broken down. Turmeric contains corsitin, a bioflavonoid that can strengthen the mast cells over time.

Many doctors use turmeric for allergies. You might think of the lining of your trachea or sinuses as fabric. Tears or holes in this fabric, or a loose weave, allow things like pollen to enter the bloodstream where they trigger an exaggerated response in the immune system, leading to inflammation and all the symptoms of allergy. Turmeric heals the cracks and tightens the weave, providing greater resistance to allergens. In the same way, food allergies can be lessened by strengthening the mast cell tissue in the intestinal tract.

Although it should not be taken as a panacea, turmeric is very safe and is already used in many foods. It can also be taken in capsule form or made as a tea.

WILD INDIGO ROOT Wild indigo root is not a very popular herb, but it is valuable for its direct antimicrobial activity, helping to fight infections throughout the body and particularly the upper respiratory tract. More important, wild indigo root stimulates the gastrointestinal tract to maintain its levels of hydrochloric acid. This is the first line of defense in the immune system. Without an adequate level of hydrochloric acid in the stomach, microorganisms that enter with the ingestion of food may pass through the stomach and enter the lymphatic or blood systems. Wild indigo root is also a liver tonic, helping to detoxify the body.

The strength of wild indigo root lies somewhere between that of echinacea and goldenseal. A self-prescribed dose should be no more than half a teaspoon in a daily cup of tea, and should not be continued for more than a month.

The root can also be used in prepared ointments to help soothe the inflammation of arthritis. Macerate about 2 ounces of the root and leave for 24 hours in a well-sealed jar filled with 2 cups of olive oil. Shake frequently. Then strain and apply as needed.

PART THREE

Mental Health and Psychological Well-Being

T he first Surgeon General's Report on Mental Health, released in late 1999, reported that 20 percent of the population suffers from some kind of mental illness each year. That means that about 50 million Americans are grappling with severe illnesses such depression, obsessive-compulsive disorder, and schizophrenia, as well as other conditions that do not fall strictly under the rubric of "mental illness" but have a mental component. These include addictions, insomnia, attention deficit disorder, and eating disorders. When you consider that probably an additional 50 million people suffer from intermittent bouts of one or a number of these conditions, then you can see that mental health concerns affect a huge segment of our society.

Yet despite the extent of mental disorders, the American medical establishment has paid little attention to causes, so intent are they on obtaining the relief of the symptoms. Take alcoholism, for instance. There are dozens of studies showing that alcoholics are chronically deficient in certain essential nutrients. Other studies show that when these nutrients are given at optimal levels, the chemical imbalances that precipitate the craving for alcohol are diminished or eliminated, thus biochemically breaking the addictive response.

One would think that the medical establishment would at least attempt to address the ramifications of these studies in the approaches to treatment that are currently favored. But they have not done so. Currently, many tens of billions of dollars are being spent yearly on drug and alcohol treatments, the vast majority of which ignore nutrition-based approaches. Since few of the now-prevalent approaches have been shown to be successful, it is worrisome that nutrition-based approaches continue to be relegated to the margins. We need to look at the fact that when biochemical imbalances are corrected and chemical sensitivities are addressed, the treatments work and with a lack of relapse. This is the kind of cause-and-prevention oriented approach we should be encouraging, for alcoholism and other problems.

Traditional treatments of mental disorders since Sigmund Freud invented his "talking cure" have included psychoanalysis, other psychotherapies, and drugs. While psychotropic drugs can be dramatically effective in some cases of depression, psychosis, and anxiety, some patients are not helped, some require long-term treatment with drugs that have serious side effects, and others become addicted to mood-altering medications.

Orthomolecular psychiatrists are conventionally trained medical doctors with an additional specialization. They seek to identify and treat the root causes of disease. Their objective is to rebalance and rebuild the whole body, not merely to mask or suppress symptoms. They aim to establish equilibrium among the essential nutrients—minerals, vitamins, amino acids—in the body. Frequently, orthomolecular physicians use a high-dosage vitamin regimen, far higher than what the average physician would ever presume would be needed. But it is their experience that only with these very high amounts, these megadoses, do they see the best results. For example, orthomolecular psychiatrists have had striking success in the treatment of schizophrenia, putting the condition into remission by using massive doses of niacin (vitamin B_3), vitamin B_6, and vitamin C. Orthomolecular psychiatrists may use more traditional treatments as well.

15

Depression

Depression is a major health problem that can leave an otherwise healthy person unable to cope with the even the simplest everyday situations. It affects nearly 20 million Americans. This does not include the many individuals who function normally for the most part despite frequently finding themselves in low moods. Two-thirds of those who suffer from true depression are never treated and live their lives in misery without being recognized as sufferers of a mental illness. The American Psychiatric Association estimates that 80 percent of depressed people will recover with appropriate diagnosis and treatment.

Types of Depression

Several types of clinical depression have been identified.

MAJOR DEPRESSION interferes with normal, everyday life. It is characterized by sleep disturbances, agitation, appetite and weight changes, feelings of guilt and worthlessness, and an inability to work and concentrate. Suicidal thoughts may occur. These symptoms may last several months or more.

DYSTHMIA is milder than major depression but it lasts longer. It prevents people from functioning at their full capacity. Some people with dysthmia also have major depressive episodes.

BIPOLAR DISORDER OR MANIC DEPRESSION, which affects about 1 percent of Americans who are depressed, manifests as serious cycles of depression and mania. In the depressed phase, the person may be sluggish, sad, hopeless, and withdrawn. In the manic phase, the person swings to the opposite extreme: hyperactive, energetic, impatient, easily distracted, and too "busy" to sleep.

Most often the changes are gradual, but some people, known as "rapid cyclers," may change moods several times a day. Bipolar disorder is usually chronic and generally begins in the teenage and young adult years.

Causes

BIOCHEMICAL FACTORS For the past 30 years psychiatry has been aware that certain biochemical changes that take place in the brain can both influence and reflect fluctuations in people's moods. A change in the delicate biochemistry of the brain is capable of governing how a person feels at any given moment. A physical deficiency in any of the chemicals responsible for maintaining "good moods" may lead to depression, just as a psychologically stressing factor in a person's life may manifest itself in the body by altering the sensitive chemical balance in the brain, also causing depression or low moods.While   psychiatry has recognized this mind-body connection in general terms for the past three decades, it is only in the last 10 to 15 years that it has actually isolated some of the specific brain chemicals involved. Especially important among these chemicals are substances called neurotransmitters, which are released at nerve endings in the brain and allow messages to be relayed throughout the rest of the brain and the body. Perhaps the most commonly known neurotransmitters are the endorphins. They are responsible for pain relief within the body and are thought to be responsible for the "high" that runners experience after exercise.

Mood swings can be traced to a similar mind-body relationship. Scientists have found that a large number of depressed people have significant deficiencies of the neurotransmitters norepinephrine and serotonin. These neurotransmitters belong to a chemical group called the amines, which are responsible for the control of emotions, sleep, pain, and involuntary bodily functions such as digestion. Almost 90 percent of these amines are found deep in the brain; because of their importance, the normally functioning body has developed a recycling system, called reuptake, by which the nerve cell takes back 85 percent of a neurotransmitter for future use once the chemical reaction has been completed. Only the remaining 15 percent is destroyed by enzymes.

The metabolism of the neurotransmitters is intricate, and deficiencies can occur for many reasons. Dr. Priscilla Slagle, a board-certified orthomolecular psychiatrist who practices in southern California, states that age or genetics may cause one person to use up amines more rapidly than someone else might. She also points out that a defective receiving cell or reuptake mechanism, or a deficiency of the amino acids, vitamins, and minerals that make up amines, may be the culprit here. The nutrient deficiencies involved may result from excessive intake of caffeine, sugar, alcohol, or tobacco. Sugar and coffee can destroy the B vitamins and the minerals magnesium and iron, all of which figure significantly in neurotransmitter formation. Alcohol and tobacco also deplete almost all the B vitamins, vitamin C, zinc, magnesium, manganese, and tyrosine. These nutrients are essential to maintaining a good mood.

STRESS Stress is another factor that can contribute to depression. Most people tend to associate depression with what are called major stressors, such as the loss of a loved one, being fired from a job, or another circumstance which upsets one's life in a significant way. However, even the stress associated with everyday living can directly deplete the vitamins, minerals, and amino acids that are so important in maintaining a good mood. Dr. Slagle explains: "We have found very high levels of the hormone cortisol, which is secreted by the adrenal glands, in severely depressed patients. Indeed, scientists have devised a test that measures the levels of this hormone in the body to determine the degree of depression. When people are depressed and highly stressed, their adrenal glands may secrete higher levels of cortisol, triggering certain enzymes in the body that destroy tyrosine and tryptophan. One would think that under extreme stress the body would compensate for this breakdown by facilitating the survival of these important amino acids. Instead, for whatever reason, these amino acids are used up. I believe that high cortisol levels induce depression in certain people."

SIDE EFFECTS OF MEDICATIONS Dr. Slagle also points out that depression is a common side effect of many prescription medications. The list of medications that can cause depression is quite extensive; it includes antibiotics, antiarthritis pills, antihistamines, blood pressure medication, birth control pills, tranquilizers, and even aspirin. When people are given these medications, they often are not warned that they may experience depression as a side effect. Most orthomolecular psychiatrists believe that drugs for which the *Physician's Desk Reference* (PDR) lists depression as a side effect should include a nutritional program with the prescription in order to replenish the vitamins and amino acids that may be depleted by the medication.

ENVIRONMENTAL FACTORS It is common for depressed people to have a family history of depression. In addition to the genetic factor, such family histories may also be due to common environmental factors, shared experiences in depressed families, and poor eating habits that are passed on from one generation to the next.

Environmental factors may play multiple roles as causes of depression. For example, being raised in a family in which one or more people are depressed may often be associated with poor nutrition. As Dr. William J. Goldwag reminds us, "Just being exposed to depressed people can be an influence, since children learn how to behave by imitation. Also, family members are eating the same food, and if, for instance, the mother is depressed and is cooking for and serving her family, that food is apt to be sparse in nutrients since she is interested in just getting the meal over with and has difficulty finding enough energy to prepare it."

The children of depressed parents may be abused physically or verbally. As a way of handling abuse, a child may withdraw and become depressed and inactive as a defense against harsh treatment from the parent.

Dr. Doris Rapp, a board-certified pediatric allergist and specialist in environmental medicine, adds that mood disorders often lead to battering of family members and intimates: "Husbands batter wives, wives batter husbands, they both batter the children, and boyfriends batter their girlfriends. Mother battering, I might add, is very common. Many of the children I treat beat, kick, bruise, bite, and pinch their mothers. When some individuals have typical allergies and environmental illness, if they have a mood problem, they can become nasty and irritable and angry. All I ask is, 'What did you eat, touch, and smell?'

"To help find the cause I try to discover whether the change in behavior occurs inside or outside, after eating, or after smelling a chemical. It might be a food, dust, mold, pollens, or chemicals, which affect not only the brain as a whole but also discrete areas of the brain. As a result, the allergen or food or chemical exposure may make you tired or, if it affects the frontal lobes, make you behave in an inappropriate way. It could affect the speech center of the brain so that you speak too rapidly or unclearly, or stutter, or don't speak intelligently. It's just potluck as to what area of the brain or body will be affected when you are exposed to something to which you are allergic."

MAGNESIUM DEFICIENCY According to Dr. Lendon Smith, a specialist in nutrition-based therapies and the author of many books on that topic, including *Feed Your Body Right: Understanding Your Individual Body Chemistry for Proper Nutrition Without Guesswork*, craving chocolate is also a sign of depression. It usually means that people need magnesium, because there's magnesium in chocolate. The day before their menstrual periods women often find themselves searching through the cupboards for chocolate. They find a big can of Hershey's and drink it down before feeling better from the magnesium.

"I often had the delightful experience of giving an intravenous mixture of vitamin C, calcium, magnesium, and B vitamins," Dr. Smith says. "Usually it has more magnesium than calcium. Afterward I asked patients whether they would like some chocolate and they told me they didn't need it. It really is connected.

"Women in the sixth month of pregnancy will often send their husbands out for ice cream because the baby is starting to grow fast. The woman has a conscious need for dairy products because she knows they will bring her the calcium she needs, but she also says, 'Don't forget the pickles.' She knows somehow that she needs to acidify that calcium source for the baby. She will not get much out of it and she will suffer from leg cramps."

Dr. Smith explains that once food has been processed, magnesium is one of the first minerals to disappear. "Magnesium is also one of the first minerals to leave the body when there is stress, which accounts for how many women behave a day or so before their periods. They feel stressed because they're losing their magnesium.

"We need to supply magnesium to these people. We can determine who needs it by a blood test and by the sense of smell. If people smell a bottle of pure magnesium salt—magnesium chloride is a good one—and it smells good or if there's no smell, then the person needs it. The blood test we usually use is the 24-chem. screen, the standard blood test.

"Many symptoms of depression, hyperactivity, headaches, loss of weight, and other conditions are related to genetic tendencies. If there is a tendency to be depressed in the family, a magnesium deficiency will allow that tendency to show up. If there's alcoholism, diabetes, or obesity in the family, low magnesium may allow those things to show up in a person. There are reasons for all these things, and nutrition is basic. These patients don't have an antidepressant pill deficiency; they usually have a magnesium deficiency."

The first thing Dr. Smith does when he sees patients is ask what they're eating. "If I find that they're eating a lot of dairy products and that as children they had their tonsils taken out and that they had a lot of Strep throat and ear infections, I know they're allergic to milk and they're looking for calcium. Sure enough, the blood tests will show this. That's the first thing they have to stop. Whatever they love is probably causing the trouble because food sensitivities can cause low blood sugar."

TOBACCO Orthomolecular psychiatrist Dr. Abram Hoffer tells the story of a classic case of a misdiagnosis corrected, enabling one man to start anew after his life had seemingly been ruined. "A high school teacher and principal about 45 years old developed a severe depression. In fact, I believe he was misdiagnosed as a schizophrenic. He exhibited what we call a straightforward, deep-seated, endogenous depression. He was in a mental hospital for about a year or two and was then discharged. He was so depressed that no one could live with him. His wife divorced him and eventually he was living with his aunt, who looked after him as if he were a child. As a last resort, he was referred to me.

"When he came to see me, which was many years ago, I had just started looking into the question of allergies. At that time, I wasn't very familiar with food allergies, but I thought he was a very interesting case and I said to myself, 'He is a classic case of a depression, maybe schizophrenic. He'd be the last person in the world who would respond to this antiallergy approach.' At that time I was using—and I still do—a 4-day water fast. This is a way of determining whether or not these allergies are present. He agreed that he would do the fast, which also involved refraining from any smoking or consuming of alcohol; he had to drink about eight glasses of water a day and nothing else. His aunt said she would help make sure he complied. When he came back to see me 2 weeks later, he and his aunt explained that at the end of the 4-day fast, he was normal. All of the depression was gone.

"This man then began to get tested for food allergies, and he found that not a single food made him sick. But now he began to smoke again. Within a day after he resumed smoking, he was back in his deep depression. The ironic thing was that he had a brother who was a tobacco company executive, who kept sending him free cartons of cigarettes. When we made the connection to his cigarette smoking, he stopped smoking. Thirty days later, after he had been depressed for 4 years and hadn't been able to work, he was back in school teaching. I remember this clearly because the insurance company that was paying his monthly pension was so astounded at this dramatic response that it sent one of its agents to see me, to find out what the magic wand was that I had waved to get this patient off their rolls. This is a classic case of an allergy to tobacco that was causing this man's depression."

Diagnosis

Traditional psychiatrists diagnose depression according to the criteria set forth in the DSM-IV (*Diagnostic and Statistical Manual of Mental Disorders*, 4th edition), which essentially defines major depression as a condition that includes at least five of the following symptoms during the same 2-week period:

1. Depressed mood
2. Markedly diminished interest or pleasure in all or almost all activities
3. Significant weight loss or gain (when not dieting)
4. Insomnia (a constant inability to sleep) or hypersomnia
5. Psychomotor agitation (a hyperanxious state) or retardation
6. Fatigue or loss of energy
7. Feelings of worthlessness or excessive or inappropriate guilt
8. Diminished ability to think or concentrate or indecisiveness
9. Recurrent thoughts of death

While orthomolecular psychiatrists may use this definition as a starting point, they do not confine the diagnosis to these criteria. Orthomolecular psychiatry views depression or any other illness as a unique and individual condition. While there may be certain guidelines, such as those set forth in the DSM-IV, a diagnosis that rigidly adheres to these criteria can arrive at a wrong conclusion either by missing the diagnosis altogether because the person's symptoms are not those normally associated with depression or by falsely diagnosing a person as being depressed simply because he or she has the textbook symptoms.

Often a depressed patient is not aware of the condition, especially when it is complicated by associated physical symptoms. If you suffered from chronic back pain, indigestion, or neck stiffness, would you immediately think that you might be manifesting symptoms of depression? Probably not. You might go to several doctors in search of relief, and there would be a very good chance that none of them would ever consider depression as the root of your problem. Even if someone were to ask whether you were depressed, you might quickly protest if, as Dr. Priscilla Slagle puts it, you "have 'somatized,' that is, put [your] emotional feelings into the body, thereby inducing bodily symptoms."

Sometimes a patient may develop responses to medication that are misinterpreted as purely physical. "For example," Dr. Slagle says, "an acquaintance of mine who lost her daughter through death a year ago became so anxious that her doctor started her on tranquilizers. Although she was on tranquilizers for 6 months, she got worse and worse. When I visited her, it was readily apparent to me that she had severe depression. It was difficult to convince her of this because she could relate only to the anxiety and the insomnia she was having. I started her on a nutrient program, and she improved dramatically in 2 to 3 weeks. Of course, I tapered her off the tranquilizers, because if they are stopped abruptly, one can have withdrawal symptoms which can aggravate the anxiety."

Traditional Treatments

Orthodox treatments for depression range from counseling and psychotherapy to medication and electroshock therapy. However, when a traditional psychiatrist arrives at a diagnosis of depression, more likely than not the next step will be to put the patient on antidepressant medication. Some of the most common of these medications are the selective serotonin reuptake inhibitors (SSRIs) such as Prozac (fluoxetine), Zoloft (sertraline), Paxil (paroxetine), and Luvox (fluvoxamine). They are all designed to increase the concentration of the neurotransmitter serotonin. Other types of antidepressants include the older tricyclics, monoamine oxidase inhibitors, and new inhibitors that act on the brain chemicals norepinephrine and dopamine.

For bipolar disorder, lithium, Depakote (divalproex), and Tegretol (carbamazepine) are used to stabilize moods. If the mania is severe, antipsychotic drugs such as Risperdal (risperidone) may be prescribed. In the depressive phase Wellbutrin (bupropion) and the SSRIs are often used. Some patients receive monoamine oxidase inhibitors or tricyclic antidepressants.

Although the manufacturers claim that there is no evidence of addiction to most of these drugs, they are not without side effects. The *Physician's Desk Reference* (PDR) entry for the monamine oxidase inhibitor Elavil (amitriptyline), for instance, mentions many contraindications, warnings, precautions, and adverse reactions, including severe convulsions and possibly death if this drug is used improperly with other drugs, complications in patients with impaired liver function, hypertension, stroke, disorientation, delusions, hallucinations, excitement, tremors, seizures, blurred vision, dizziness, fatigue, baldness, and elevation and lowering of blood sugar levels.

Because suicidal tendencies are a common characteristic of depression, perhaps one of the most serious problems associated with antidepressants is the potential for drug overdose. The potential for suicide caused by the very medication prescribed to prevent it is further enhanced by the synergistic interaction of antidepressants with alcohol, barbiturates, and other central nervous system depressants. A glance through the PDR indicates that the quantity and magnitude of the dangers associated with Elavil are equally present with the other antidepressants.

Alternative Therapies

DIET AND NUTRITION It is surprising how often diet and nutrition are factors in depression and how effective enhanced or improved nutrition can be in helping someone suffering from depression to improve his or her mood. According to Dr. William J. Goldwag, "Often the quality of the diet suffers in depressed people. If the depression is profound, the individual doesn't even feel like eating. Depressed people who live alone or who are major providers or cooks in the home may not feel like preparing meals or even shopping. They're apt to restrict their nutrition to fast food or anything just to get eating over with." In many cases, weight loss is a symptom of severe depression. In others, there is substantial weight gain.

Dr. Goldwag notes that significant weight loss is likely to bring about "marked deprivation of the essential nutrients, including the amino acids needed to manufacture the proper proteins, as well as a deficiency in many vitamins and minerals. That in itself can aggravate the depression."

Dr. Goldwag suggests straightforward solutions to at least some of the challenges associated with depression: "There are some simple ways to prepare food in advance so that the food has to be prepared less often. I recommend preparing a raw salad once a week. Certain fresh vegetables keep well for quite a while in a refrigerator. There are a whole variety to choose from: carrots, celery, radishes, cauliflower, broccoli, peppers, red cabbage, green onions, snow peas, string beans. They can all be cut up and mixed together. They can be stored in a plastic bag or sealed container. When mealtime comes, a person can take a handful of these vegetables and then perhaps add some other ones that don't keep as well, such as tomatoes and sprouts. You then have a fresh salad that is already prepared with a lot of important nutrients. This is just one way of having food prepared in advance. It's good for people who are depressed and don't have the energy to make a whole meal."

Dr. Goldwag believes that the B-complex vitamins are especially important. "One of the major groups of vitamins to incorporate is the B-complex family. Years and years ago, when people suffered from severe vitamin deficiencies, some of the resultant diseases, such as pellagra, were characterized by accompanying psychotic reactions. That is, the thinking process was the most obvious one to be affected by the vitamin deficiency. Simply providing the proper vitamin, in this case vitamin B_3, or niacin, was the treatment. It cleared up the psychosis.

"There's no doubt that brain function is very dependent on nutrients such niacin and others, because when they're absent there is apt to be some very disturbed thinking. Depression is one of the symptoms that can occur with this.

All of the B complex vitamins are important, but niacin is especially so. As Dr. Goldwag explains, "Niacin is often used in much higher doses than the others to accomplish some of these changes. Niacin is a ubiquitous vitamin. It is being used to improve cholesterol levels, to increase the good cholesterol and reduce the bad. The doses being used are much greater than those used to simply overcome a deficiency."

At the same time, there are plenty of foods that should be avoided. Fast foods can affect mental symptoms by causing blood sugar abnormalities. People who have tendencies toward hypoglycemia, or low blood sugar, should avoid eating too many simple carbohydrates, such as candy bars, which are converted very rapidly to sugar in the blood. As Dr. Goldwag says, "Simple carbohydrate foods temporarily raise the blood sugar, but then they drop it to a very low level several hours later, resulting in depression. This encourages the individual to repeat the cycle of taking sugar or some simple carbohydrate that's converted to sugar in order to feel that high again. This constant seesaw from a high to a low mood can account for many episodes of depression in individuals."

Both alcoholics and chronic dieters often have depressive tendencies. Alcoholics often suffer from symptoms of low mood. Although alcohol may appear at first as a stimulant and mood enhancer, it is in fact a depressant and substantially decreases the ability of the body to extract nutrients from the food we eat. Dieters tend to eat very few B-complex-containing foods, and they often suffer from depression as well.

AMINO ACIDS: TYROSINE AND TRYPTOPHAN A leading authority on the treatment of depression with amino acids and nutritional therapy, Dr. Priscilla Slagle became interested in the treatment of mood disorders as a result of her own depression, which lasted for many years and did not respond to traditional psychoanalysis or psychotherapeutic treatment. Disinclined to use antidepressant medications because of the adverse reactions that so commonly accompany them, Dr. Slagle discovered that "there are natural food substances that will create the same end effects, that is, elevate mood in the same way without causing side effects or toxicity. I started myself on [a program using certain single amino acids to control mood] and achieved very dramatic results. Although I have had tremendous stress over the past 10 years, particularly the past year, I have not had one day of a low mood. This has been a marvelous reprieve, since I have had and therefore understand the pain that low moods can create for many people."

In her book *The Way Up from Down*, Dr. Slagle outlines a safe and easily implemented program of treatment for depression using amino acids and other precursors required for the production of norepinephrine and serotonin. She is careful to emphasize that people should follow the program under the supervision of a physician. For those already on antidepressant medication, it is not advisable to stop abruptly because of the potential for withdrawal symptoms.

Dr. Slagle explains the basis of the program: "It consists of taking an amino acid called tyrosine, which in the presence of certain B-complex vitamins, minerals, and vitamin C will convert into norepinephrine in the brain. This neurotransmitter not only sustains positive moods but also helps our concentration, learning, memory, drive, ambition, motivation, and other equally important qualities. Additionally, it helps to regulate food and sexual appetite functions. Thus it is a very important chemical. The other amino acid used in the program is tryptophan, which forms serotonin in the brain if the requisite cofactors—the B vitamins, minerals, and vitamin C—are present. In addition to sustaining mood, tryptophan has other functions, such as controlling sleep and levels of aggression. People who are quite aggressive, irritable, or angry are often suffering from a marked deficiency in serotonin. Indeed, very low levels of serotonin have been found in the brain of suicide victims at autopsy. ..."With these two amino acids, a good multivitamin-mineral preparation is taken to provide all the nutrients necessary to catalyze or promote the conversion of the amino acids into the neurotransmitters."

Dr. Slagle suggests the following dosages for the two amino acids: about 500 to 3,000 milligrams of tyrosine taken twice daily and about 500 to 2,000 milligrams of tryptophan. Public sale of tryptophan was banned by the Food and Drug Administration in 1990, but the supplement is now available by prescription through most compounding pharmacies. Dr. Slagle recommends that tyrosine be taken first thing in the morning on an empty stomach and then also sometime in the midmorning or midafternoon. Tryptophan, because of its sleep-inducing effects, is taken before bed. Any amino acids used therapeutically must be taken separately from other protein foods, because protein interferes with their utilization. Dr. Slagle also specifies that the amino acids be taken in capsules (tablets can pass through the body undigested) or in the "free form," a preparation in which the amino acids are ready for immediate absorption by the body.

OTHER SUPPLEMENTS Other nutrients that can improve mental and emotional states are listed below:

OMEGA-3 FATTY ACIDS. A study from Harvard Medical School published in the May 1999 *Archives of General Psychiatry* found that omega-3 (fish oil-type) fatty acids may be important mood stabilizers. Thirty people with bipolar disorder received either fish oil or a placebo (olive oil) along with their standard medications for 4 months. Sixty-five percent of those who got the omega-3s improved during this period, compared with only 19 percent of the placebo group. The omega-3s were associated with longer remissions and fewer symptoms.

SAME. S-adenosyl-l-methionine (SAME), available commercially in Europe since 1975, recently became available in the United States. The SAMe molecule is a methionine, an amino acid.

ACETYL-L-CARNITINE. This nutrient crosses the blood-brain barrier and provides the brain with more energy. The energy it provides is a gentle, not jittery, type of energy, and it is especially important for older people, who tend to lose brain cells due to a lack of energy. Between 500 and 1,500 milligrams should be taken on an empty stomach.

LIQUID ZINC. Dr. Alexander Schauss, clinical psychologist, certified eating disorder specialist, and author of *Anorexia & Bulimia*, describes his studies with liquid zinc: "In our eating disorder studies, we used a multidimensional design and evaluated the affective or mood state of our patients for 5 years. One of the first things to improve in patients treated with liquid zinc was the degree of depression that they were experiencing based on psychometric instruments such as the Beck Depression Scale, the Profile of Mood Scales, and other indexes of depression. This suggests that we might consider using zinc as an antidepressant. There is a growing concern among many patients, and even therapists, that antidepressant drugs, such as Prozac, may not be safe, and we are looking at viable alternatives. We have discovered this antidepressive effect and have documented it in patients under blind conditions."

PHOSPHATIDYL SERINE. This nutrient is produced by the body but lessens with age. Taking 200 to 500 milligrams improves the ability of brain cell membranes to receive signals and improves their function. That, in turn, can elevate mood levels, help overcome winter depression, and enhance short-term memory.

HERBS

ST. JOHN'S WORT (*hypericum perforatum*) is an herbal remedy for depression that has become extremely popular in recent years. It contains a number of compounds that have documented biological activity. Studies have shown that it is most effective for mild-moderate depression. Recommended dosage is 300 milligrams three times daily. You'll need to take the herb for about 2 to 3 weeks before you feel any real therapeutic effects. Duke University is now conducting a $4.3 million study of the herb's effectiveness.

Other plants containing chemicals with antidepressant properties include the following:

Pastinaca sativa (parsnip)
Myrciaria dubia (camu-camu)
Malpighia glabra (acerola)
Lactuca sativa (lettuce)
Amaranthus spp. (pigweed)
Portulaca oleracea (purslane)
Nasturtium officinale (berro)
Chenopodium album (lambsquarter)
Cichorium endivia (endive)
Spinacia oleracea (spinach)
Brassica chinensis (Chinese cabbage)
Brassica oleracea (broccoli)
Lycopersicon esculentum (tomato)
Avena sativa (oats)
Raphanus sativus (radish)
Anethum graveolens (dill)
Phaseolus vulgaris (black bean)
Cucurbita foetidissima (buffalo gourd)
Corchorus olitorius (Jew's mallow)

HOMEOPATHY Homeopathic remedies can be quite effective in lifting depression. Dr. Gennaro Locurcioas, a homeopathic physician, says that while money does not create happiness, the king of remedies for treating depression is gold, also known as aurum metallicum. Here he describes this and other remedies for treating depression in women; men can benefit as well.

AURUM METALLICUM. Gold is for a perfectionist woman who has set high goals for herself but is unable to meet them. At first she will become irritable, a state that can last for several months. She feels as if she has lost the love of those around her and that it is her fault. This leads to feelings of frustration, accompanied by a strong sense of guilt, which may push her to suicide in extreme cases. Dr. Locurcioas observes, "At first sight, this woman appears perfect and polished. When we start talking to her, we get the idea that there is an abnormal focus on career and achievement. Being a workaholic just covers up the emptiness inside."

ARSENICUM. This remedy is for depression accompanied by anxiety. The woman is restless day and night. She fears being alone and is constantly calling her friends. She wakes up at night and walks around the room thinking about her fears and anxieties. She is afraid of a poverty-filled future and of death. "Arsenicum is from arsenic," says Dr. Locurcioas. "If we give that to a person, the person dies. But giving homeopathic arsenic to a person is completely safe and better than Xanax."

IGNATIA. This helps depression associated with grief. A woman has lost her child or her mother, or has been disappointed by a romantic relationship. The patient may exhibit physical characteristics such as a tic on the face, numbness, a lump in the throat, and sighing. "According to the homeopathic literature, if the patient says that she gets aggravated when she eats sweets and she improves by traveling, these are signs that ignatia is indicated," notes Dr. Locurcioas.

SEPIA. Sepia is a good example of how homeopathic healing uses substances that relate to a person's symptoms. According to Dr. Locurcioas, "This remedy is made from a black mollusk that emits a black ink. Black is the ink from which the remedy is prepared, and black is the color the depressed woman sees around herself. She sees black in her future. This little sea creature, at some point in its life, will deposit about 300 eggs, which are incredibly big for the size of this little animal, and then it will die. This is the housewife who has had a job and has also had to come home and prepare dinner for the husband and children. For years, she has given the best of her energy to her family and children. Now she is 40, 45, or 50. The children are gone, and she feels as if her mission in life is over. She sees no purpose in her life anymore. She does not hate her husband, but feels indifferent toward him. She does not want to be touched sexually, and cries many times during the day without knowing why. Inside she feels despair and isolation. Physically, she has a dull, inexpressive face, and the muscles of the body have lost their tone. The woman has varicose veins; she is constipated. Sepia is a remedy for the exhausted housewife."

ACUPUNCTURE Acupuncture frees blocked energy, and in so doing naturally lifts depression. Look at what one woman has to say about her experience: "When I was in my 20s, just after finishing college, I would go into a depression whenever I was about to get my period. It came on so suddenly that it was frightening. I went to see a doctor about it and was given a referral to an acupuncturist.

"After I was in treatment for 6 months, my practitioner and I sat down to talk about how I was feeling. I realized then that the depression was gone.

"That was 12 years ago. I've stayed in treatment, although not as regularly as when I first started. It's my primary form of health care. My eating habits and sleeping patterns have become totally regulated. I have been able to lose 40 pounds and maintain my weight without dieting. I also quit smoking without ever trying. I never get sick anymore. I never get colds or flus. In general, I'm much more balanced.

"The whole experience of being brought into harmony keeps me from going to extremes. I don't work too hard, I don't play too hard, I don't rest too hard. I manage to stay pretty much in the center of my life. It's a huge improvement. I often wonder how people live without going through a treatment process like I did."

EXERCISE Physical exercise is another key to lifting depression, especially when accompanied by a nutritious diet, meditation, and vitamin and mineral supplementation. According to Dr. William J. Goldwag, exercise is one of the most profound aids in the treatment of depression: "One of the major errors in the thinking of patients and therapists is the notion that in order to be active, you have to feel better. This is exactly contrary to our approach.

"We recommend that you do first, and then the feeling comes later. In other words, you must do what you have to do regardless of how you feel. This aids in feeling better. You can't wait until you feel good to do something, because in depression that may take days, weeks, months, or even years. You want to accelerate the process."

Dr. Goldwag explains that people who exercise regularly will have days when they just don't feel like doing it. "That's the way depressed people feel about everything. They just don't feel like it. They don't have the energy, the motivation, the stimulation to do even the ordinary things. When it's severe, you may not even have the will or desire to get out of bed in the morning.

"The exercise may consist of very, very simple things, like just getting out and walking, getting up and doing some simple movements, some mild calisthenics, any kind of physical movement that gets the body in action. For some people just getting out of bed and getting dressed is a big accomplishment. That may be the first step.

Exercise has many benefits. Dr. Goldwag adds, "Even doing a little bit of exercise will make you feel more energized later on. Finishing an exercise routine, even one that's fatiguing, after a brief period of rest will give you a feeling of revitalization and of energy and a psychological feeling of accomplishment. It gives a feeling of 'I've done it. It's completed.'"

YOGA AND MEDITATION Dr. Michele Galante, a complementary physician in Suffern, New York, overcame depression in adolescence by learning how to center energy with yoga and meditation: "When I was in my late teens, I went through a period of depression where my energy was low. My whole being was unhappy. My parents and others I loved thought I should try seeing a psychiatrist for a while. I went a few times, but that wasn't satisfying to me. I thought nutrition might help, so I started drinking raw vegetable juices and became a vegetarian. I started eating to detoxify myself and to get myself back to feeling stronger again.

"Then I got into meditation and kundalini yoga. I learned about energy centers and started to learn how inner energy flows through the system. I began to sense blockages and to identify emotions and limiting thoughts that were holding me back. Through practice, I was able to center energy into the emotional center in the chest and abdomen where stabilizing rootedness can occur. That started to awaken inner energies and to strengthen me."

Dr. Galante says that depression is not limited to the mind. "The important thing is to not get too hung up in the head, where we have all these conflicts. Our center is the lower abdomen, where a baby grows in a woman. The Japanese call this the *hara*. In Zen we concentrate the mind and the whole being there. That's the hub of the wheel. The mind can be clearer when you do that, and you don't get hung up living in the realm of thought.

"Set aside 10 to 20 minutes daily to quiet the mind, let tensions drain, open up, and resonate with the environment. Everyone does it in a different way. You can do it with meditation or biofeedback. You can do it with music, yoga, a hobby, it doesn't matter what. Anything that takes you to a creative, quiet place and allows you to recharge. Learn to take the time to express your inner needs.

"I like to ask my patients the question, 'Why do we have a physical body?' My answer is always that we exist as a physical entity to carry around our minds and our hearts, in a sense our spirits, so that we can fulfill ourselves. We can then learn and grow and do what we need to do in life. We are nothing without our emotions. Yet we neglect and suppress our feelings. We don't consider nourishing ourselves in a spiritual way. We need some sort of daily practice."

Dr. Galante adds, "We have a lot of outward pressures. We have rules made by corporations which are fulfilling needs for profits and ruining resources. There is a huge lack of wisdom across the board. The only thing that can make you happy is looking inward. Bring your mind and energies inside. Sometimes, when you start out, all you see is unhappiness and tension. But if you keep at it, sitting down, breathing quietly, not moving, and slowly bringing the mind inside, you will start to feel a sense of peace, relaxation, and buoyancy. That is recharging your battery. That is the most profound thing you can do to bring your energy up."

Patient Story

Depression and anxiety are very difficult. You get up and do the things you feel you have to do. But you don't feel like you are in the flow of life. My conditions were probably not that apparent to the rest of the world, but I experienced them as very uncomfortable, and they took away from my quality of life. I felt stressed much of the time. I had difficulty concentrating. At times I would forget things. Someone would ask me to do something, and I would forget to do it. I knew there wasn't something wrong with my mind. I felt my lack of focus was due more to my being so hyped up and tense.

I felt overwhelmed by ordinary, everyday demands, and I felt exhausted by the end of the day. Many times, after lunch, I would feel really tired, almost like I needed to have a nap. Anxiety and depression seemed to gobble up my energy very quickly. By the end of the day, I was not in the mood for recreational activities. Work wore me out. I would just go home and bug out in front of the boob tube. And I wanted more than that.

Once in a while, I would have a drink and notice a difference; I would be able to focus much better. The reason was that the drink helped me relax. But I didn't want to relax that way. I wanted to find an alternative that would really work for me and help me to feel more joy in my everyday experience.

I went to several physicians, and they prescribed various medications for me. But I couldn't take medicines. They had all kinds of strange side effects, which were just as bad as the anxiety or the depression. The drugs masked my conditions, but underneath they were still there. All they did was make me feel very sleepy much of the time. I would be sitting at a meeting, dozing off, and I couldn't afford to do that. So I took only medications briefly.

I was looking for help when I happened to hear a Gary Null lecture at the Learning Annex. I was very impressed with some of the things I heard about limiting belief systems and how difficult it is to see beyond them. I liked the talk on vegetarianism as well. As a result, I went to see Dolores Perri and was very impressed.

Dolores went over my history and concerns. I really enjoyed talking to Dolores because, unlike most physicians I've encountered, she was very relaxed. I didn't get a sense that we were limited by time; we were done when we were done. Basically, I asked my questions and expressed my concerns. It was a very good experience. After we talked, she recommended certain foods, herbs, and supplements.

I have been following a nutritional routine for about two and a half months now, and I have definitely noticed a very dramatic shift. In particular, my hypoglycemia has disappeared. That's mostly from getting rid of refined sugars and processed foods. I used to feel very restless and nervous if I didn't eat. That's been stabilized, and I feel much calmer now.

My energy level is much, much better with a vegetarian regime, supplements, and herbs. The aloe I've been using is outstanding at perking me up at the beginning of the day.

I feel clearer as well. There are subtle differences in my ability to concentrate. And when I go through the day, I feel much calmer. A couple of days ago, I was late for a meeting through no fault of my own. I had to be late for something I thought was very important. Normally, I would be a complete wreck about it. But because of my new regime, I was calm and centered, and I didn't run up the stairs. I just walked in, explained what had happened, sat down, and joined in.

In the past, I would have been practically shaking from anxiety. This is a real departure, which I attribute largely to my change in diet as well as to my holistic orientation.

I think it's important to know that it's not only a shift in diet that has helped me. I became involved in meditation to clear my mind and help me reach that stillness. I do that in the morning before anything else. In addition, I take a greater interest in the holistic world and participate in seminars. All these different elements help enhance my well-being.—Maria

16

Addiction

The opening shot of the 1990s' film *GirlQuake!* is of a hamburger frying on a grill. In an Arizona diner, a group of overweight American men are smoking, drinking, and chowing down on burgers, hotdogs, fries, coffee, and other junk food. They get their comeuppance when they attempt to rape a bevy of fit, quaintly dressed extraterrestrial Wonder Women, and the biggest food junkie is smothered to death in a gigantic fruit bowl of raw hamburger meat.

One way to look at this scene is as an ironic commentary on addiction: addictions ill fit us for facing life's sometimes unexpected challenges, and one way or another an addiction will kill you if you don't wise up. The scene also serves as a reminder that we can be addicted to other substances besides drugs—such as sugar and caffeine.

The number of Americans using drugs is skyrocketing, though many drug users don't consider themselves addicts. (For example, some people say they take cocaine because it gives them that extra energy to work longer days.) Tens of millions of Americans use drugs. Aside from the two most popular 12-step programs, Alcoholics Anonymous and Narcotics Anonymous, what other approaches to facing and overcoming substance abuse are out there?

There are in fact a number of alternative approaches to beating addiction, including detoxification, eating natural foods, and hypnotherapy or hypnosis. Let's start by talking about detoxification, a process whereby the body is cleansed of the toxins created by the addictive substance.

Detoxification

Dr. Elson Haas is a practicing integrated medical physician and the director of the Preventive Medical Center in San Rafael, California. He is the author of several best-selling books on health and nutrition, including *The Detox Diet*. Dr. Haas describes the best times to detox: "Right now, I'm on day six of my 25th annual spring cleanse, so I've been doing juices and broth. I usually cleanse in spring. That's one of the best times. Seasonal change times are usually more fraught with problems, and a cleanse can help a person. Going into autumn is another good time.

"I live on the West Coast, and even though it's a rainy and lightly cool March day here, back East it's probably colder. Probably a good time out there would be as it warms up into mid-April. Then you can count on a little warmer weather. Because when you do cleansing programs, your body gets a little cooler, so you need to take a little more protection from the cold, and dress warmer. Exercise, keep your body warm and all those things."

Of course, in embarking on a detox program, there are other considerations besides the seasonal. It may be a good idea to begin when you experience congestive problems or are having regular headaches or sluggish intestines. Dr. Haas adds, "Other good times to start are when allergies are kicking up, when blood pressure is getting too high and the cholesterol is rising. Those are times when I, as a physician, would use detoxification as one of my medical treatments. When I see people who have problems of toxicity and congestion, and other things stemming from or related to addictions, I see that detoxification works better therapeutically than almost anything I can do for them. So we have both the time of the year and also the individual time for people when it's appropriate."

Dr. Haas adds, "Anytime you decide to go off any of these substances, you have to get your mind set first. When we are using any of these substances, we are hooked in emotionally. Mentally, we think we need them, and physically, we are slightly dependent on them. This varies with the substance. Nicotine is probably the most addictive, alcohol next, caffeine after that. Sugar is probably the least physically addictive, but emotionally people are really hooked into it."

TYPES OF PROGRAMS Various levels of detoxification can be used. Juice cleanses, dietary changes, drinking more water, getting more exercise and doing steams or saunas all may help in the detoxification process. (See chapter 9.)

Dr. Haas's prescription for the type of detox regimen to follow depends on how advanced the person's level of toxicity is. "If you treat somebody too extremely," he explains, "and she has too much toxicity, then she'll have more symptoms come up and more problems. In any kind of diet change—and the detox diet particularly—there's usually a couple of days of transition during which, as you're starting the diet, you may feel headachy, a cold, irritable. Usually by the third day, you start to click in. It's much like aerobic exercise. The first few minutes are difficult, but as soon as you get into that aerobic state, you think, 'Wow, this feels good. I'm moving forward.'"

Note, however, that people who are pregnant, convalescing from illness, or taking medications, as well as those who have diabetes, hypoglycemia, mental problems, or metabolic imbalances should not undertake any type of cleansing program unsupervised. First they must determine that any proposed supplements or juices are not contraindicated by their medical program. During the program, if the person becomes weak, faint, or dizzy, he or she should have a protein drink made of high-quality soy- or rice-based protein containing anywhere from 20 to 35 grams of protein. Grains such as brown rice, millet, or barley, beans, or a serving of fish may help while cleansing to maintain blood sugar. Eating these foods does not detract from the cleansing program.

Dr. Haas says detox is broadly helpful. "Anybody," he says, "can benefit from a detox program if it is done in the right way at the right time. That's why I wrote *The Detox Diet*, to show people how they can take very simple steps that most anybody can handle. The detox diet provides nutrition for people with fruits and grains and vegetables, which provide many vitamins and minerals. With this diet, you are being nourished while you are detoxing."

Alcohol Addiction

One out of every 13 Americans aged 21 and older has an addiction to alcohol. Alcoholism can affect all aspects of a person's life, including health, career, and relationships. According to the National Institute of Alcohol Abuse and Alcoholism, symptoms of alcoholism include a craving for alcohol, loss of control, increased tolerance, and physical dependency.

Drinking alcohol has serious negative nutritional consequences. "Alcohol doesn't have a lot of nutrients in it," Dr. Haas explains. "People will say wine has a little bit of vitamin C and some nutrients from grapes. Beer has some B vitamins. Yet the levels aren't really that significant. Alcohol also is a diuretic. It causes loss of nutrients through the urine."

Nevertheless, he is not in favor of teetotaling. "When people have a drink here or there and they are eating a healthy diet, it will not cause a problem. In fact, a recent study showed that people who drink wine tend to have a better, more Mediterranean-like diet" and the associated better health, "whereas people who drink beer and other kinds of alcohol tend not to eat as conscientiously."

He adds, "One thing I've seen over the years is that bad habits tend to multiply. People who tend to abuse any substance, whether sugar, alcohol, nicotine, or caffeine, tend to also be less conscientious about how they take care of their bodies. They have other habits which are undermining their health."

Alcohol also irritates the liver, and people who drink more tend to consume more calories. Dr. Haas explains, "Alcohol is a sugar that gets absorbed relatively directly into the body and causes an overstimulation of insulin. Then you are dealing with problems in the whole sugar metabolism. These heavy drinkers then tend to consume less nutrient-rich foods. They get depleted that way. Those are some of the ways that alcohol endangers the body."

What is the best detox program for getting off alcohol? "For alcohol," Dr. Haas advises, "you want a nutrient-rich program. If you have been taking a lot of alcohol, you will definitely need professional guidance and intervention to help get through the period of withdrawal." Dr. Haas finds that the best daily combination of supplements for getting off alcohol is vitamin B, vitamin C, and a combination of calcium and magnesium, which helps alleviate the agitation that accompanies withdrawal. Chromium is another substance that can help in sugar metabolism. He advises a person to take either chromium picolinate or another form of chromium. "You'll need at least 200 micrograms, which is the way they usually come in capsules. Take these a couple times a day to help with processing the sugar."

Another amino acid that can really help is L-glutamine, which affects brain chemistry. "Remember, a lot of the addictions we have are related to the opiate receptors which oversee addiction in the brain. L-glutamine seems to help feed the brain the nourishment it needs. It appears to reduce both sugar cravings and alcohol cravings. It's been used successfully in several alcohol clinics for people with more serious problems. The amount of glutamine that people might use is 500 to 1,000 milligrams, two to three times a day. If you have cravings, you can take more. It's safe. I never see problems with it."

Dr. Haas does suggest that "with any amino acid or any B vitamin, you don't want to use one substance for a long time by itself because you can throw the body off balance a little bit. So if you are using the amino acid or B vitamin for more than a few weeks, you may want to use a whole complex."

Orthomolecular psychiatrist Dr. Abram Hoffer has this advice: "For alcoholism the basic treatment starts with Alcoholics Anonymous. Bill W., the cofounder of Alcoholics Anonymous, first showed that when you added niacin to the treatment of alcoholism you got a major response that you did not see before." Today, there are a large number of very good alcoholism treatment programs in the United States that combine AA's 12-step approach, various social aids, good nutrition, and the right supplements.

Caffeine Addiction

How can detox help you escape the clutches of caffeine addiction? First, let's make it clear how bad for the body caffeine is and how people come to ignore its negative effects. "If you do something for the first time, such as drink alcohol, smoke a cigarette, or have a cup of coffee," Dr. Haas says, "you will be aware of the irritating, stimulating, or sedating effects of the substance." When people start to use any of these substances regularly, however, they tend to overlook those initial effects. They now have an addiction and take the substance not so much to feel the original sensations as to counteract the withdrawal symptoms.

Caffeine is bad for you, particularly over time. In the short term, it raises your blood pressure. It can also make you hyperagitated, increase anxiety, and affect sleep. Over time, because caffeine is a diuretic, it causes the loss of many minerals, such as calcium, magnesium, and potassium, particularly through the urine. The result of these losses is a more permanent increase in blood pressure. Two other long-term effects of caffeine are to weaken bones and to create mineral deficiencies, both of which can lead to a variety of other problems.

In women, Dr. Haas notes, caffeine seems to increase the incidence of all kinds of cystic problems, such as fibrocystic breast tumors and uterine fibroids. Studies on the relationship between caffeine use and cancer have produced conflicting results. However, a number of studies suggest that caffeine does increase the risk of certain types of cancer.

Dr. Haas observes that "most people, when they go off caffeine, will have some secondary effects, usually a tension headache, at least for 24 hours. Sometimes they will feel agitated or fatigued. They are going through a short-term withdrawal. If they have a very large habit, it may last 48 hours, but usually it's only 24 hours." Dr. Haas says that some people can mitigate the withdrawal headache by taking an over-the-counter aspirin, but he thinks it's better to avoid that chemical medication if possible.

Dr. Haas recommends that you begin a detox diet the day before you start getting off caffeine. You can either go cold turkey or try to reduce your intake so that over a week you get down to maybe half a cup a day or less. If you do it gradually in this way, you will have fewer symptoms. According to Dr. Haas, "Many of the withdrawal symptoms happen because of elimination of acid from the foods and chemicals that we're cutting out."

"Doing the detox diet will reduce the withdrawal. I advise that you take additional nutrients, as follows: 2,000 to 10,000 milligrams of vitamin C from calcium ascorbate, 1,200 milligrams calcium and magnesium from citrate, 400 milligrams potassium, 400 milligrams alpha lypoic acid, 200 milligrams ginkgo, 1,500 milligrams of essential fatty acids, a 20 milligram capsule of cayenne pepper, 200 milligrams ginseng, 400 international units (IU) vitamin E, 500 micrograms vitamin B_{12}, and 200 milligrams nonflush niacin.

"Drinking lots of water helps. Also make sure the bowels move. Some people like caffeine because it gets their bowels to move in the morning. It stimulates the intestine's peristaltic activities. For these people caffeine withdrawal may cause constipation. Now not moving your bowels enough can cause more toxins to back up, and you will feel worse. So it's really important to do what you can about this. Even a day or two after you go off caffeine, you might get something from the natural food store such as laxative tea or laxative tablets or find other means of cleansing the bowels."

Sugar Addiction

Many people may debate whether sugar is addictive in the same way nicotine and alcohol are addictive, but it is definitely a hard habit to break. Dr. Haas notes: "When I talk to people about cleaning up sugar because there are so many books out now recommending lowering sugar intake and mentioning the problems with refined sugar, I find that it is an emotional problem above all. People were trained so early on that sugar is a reward. Sugar is sweet. All the love-talk words involve sugar. You're 'sweet on someone,' the person is your 'honey' or 'sweetie.' Sugar is associated with love and reward. So it's hard to break that emotional pattern."

Yet getting rid of sugar improves health. "When women who have problems with their menstrual cycle, who are irregular, who have pain, who have PMS clean that sugar out of their diets, often within a couple of months they are feeling a lot better, as long as they are taking some other nutrients," says Dr. Haas.

Not only does sugar affect behavior and moods, it is responsible for quite a few health problems. As Dr. Haas tells it, "Although some studies have refuted these findings—studies sponsored by the industry, I might add—researchers have found that sugar causes problems in kids in their focus and behavior. I think it causes increases in candida and parasites. It causes weakness in the digestive tract. Clearly, it's a cause of tooth decay. It has some causal relation to obesity, diabetes, and chronic digestion problems, as well as menstrual irregularities. It also hooks into alcohol abuse."

He has seen psychological problems that he believes had strong roots in the patient's sugar intake. "I've had a number of young women patients who came in. They were on medicine for depression and other low moods. When I interviewed them about their diet, which their psychiatrist never did, it turns out they are drinking a quart of Coke or Pepsi or one of those heavily sweetened beverages a day. So they were getting in the neighborhood of 40 to 50 teaspoons of sugar a day. Those intakes are really influencing their moods. The women who I've gotten to pay attention to their diets and get off sugar have been able to reduce their medicines and be more stable without these psychoactive drugs."

He echoes a theme that recurs throughout this book: "I think there's a lot to be said about how lifestyle and these habits affect our health and sanity. One of the key overall views is that when people don't feel well they need to look at their lifestyle first and see if there are factors in the way they are living that may be contributing to their decline. Then they should look at natural remedies. Lastly, I would tell them to turn to medicines, which I still use in my practice because I think that's part of being an integrated doctor. I use any system that I think is going to be of benefit to my patients. Sometimes people do need prescription medicines to help them get out of trouble. If they lived better, however, they wouldn't be getting into that trouble in the first place."

To really eliminate sugar, he encourages people to read labels and work on cleaning up their diet as a whole. He commonly sees people who have some form of yeast infection, or candidiasis. They also have problems with moods, energy, and brain function, secondary to the yeast fermentation process in their intestinal tract, which causes toxins to get into their bodies. A key to recovery for such a person is to eliminate alcohols and sugars to stop feeding the yeast.

"Usually, within 3 or 4 days of cutting out the sugar, the person will feel a change. She doesn't have any symptoms in the way she would from alcohol withdrawal, but for the first couple of days she may feel headachy and moody. This will only last a day or two.

"Again, if you drink more water and you take your extra Bs and other supplements, you'll have a smoother transition. Typically, by the third day and definitely within the week, you'll notice smoother and more balanced energy and better brain function."

Dr. Haas is not against sweets per se. Breaking sugar addiction, he says, "doesn't mean we can never eat anything sweet. Fruits are sweet, and they are some of the purest foods that we have. Most sweet foods are based on extracts from either grains, such as corn syrups, or from other plants that are naturally sweet. Overall, we just want to balance out the diet."

Food Cravings and Addictions

Jerry Dorsman makes the unusual point that food addictions are harder to kick than drug or alcohol addictions. He's a certified addiction counselor from Oakton, Maryland, and the author of *How to Quit Drinking Without AA* and *How to Quit Drugs for Good*.

"Let me begin by saying that in my clinical experience, it is harder to get people to change their diet than to break an addiction to drugs and alcohol," Dorsman says. "I've seen statistics on this recently that show we have a 30 to 40 percent success rate for people breaking addictions to substances; but there is only about a 5 percent success rate for people who are trying to change diet and get away from bad food habits.

"The reason for this, I think, is that we have deeply ingrained addictions to food. Our body has come to expect certain foods in our diets. We have a metabolic expectation. If we don't get those foods, we begin to crave them. If you take a look at it, we've been eating foods since we've been 1 year old, whereas, typically, drugs or alcohol aren't started until we are in our teens or early twenties. So they have had a shorter period of time in which to change the body. I think it's a longer-term, more deeply ingrained pattern that creates the difficulty in changing diet."

To break food addictions, one has to get a handle on cravings. According to Dorsman, "The more balanced we can make our diet, the healthier it becomes. The addiction causes a certain imbalance in the body. The body has to be constantly prepared to metabolize this substance which it's experiencing over and over. This creates a severe imbalance. Our natural response is to balance it. The place to start is dealing with this physical part of cravings. By changing the diet based on the contractive/expansive as well as the acid/alkaline balances, we can really begin to settle our metabolism and find greater peace based on diet alone. In fact, in my opinion, changing diet is the number one stress-reduction technique available.

"A second way to handle cravings is just wait it out. Most cravings, according to scientific studies, last for only about 5 to 10 minutes. Once we know that up front, that particular piece of knowledge can help us beat these cravings. You can think to yourself, 'Hey, I just have a few minutes here to wait this out and manage it.'"

The basic difficulties in resisting cravings—and this applies to any type of addiction, from food to drugs to alcohol—can, in Dorsman's opinion, "be broken into two categories: problems that substance use caused and problems it concealed. The most common problems that substance use causes are the physical problems, because of the biological effects of the drug or alcohol or food on the body, which are very devastating at the cellular level and to the nerve cells. The problems that are concealed are emotional ones. Those are problems which, when a person drank or used drugs or binged on food, tended to go away, because the person could ignore such things as depression, anxiety, and anger. Those emotional difficulties a person ignored when drinking or drugging or bingeing will come back up when the person puts down the addictive substances."

Using Addictions to Battle Depression

If you are taking a substance because you are depressed, your depression may be physiologically induced, perhaps due to some form of brain imbalance. You might have an underactive thyroid, for example, or a blood-sugar imbalance—whether high or low blood sugar. Either of these conditions can be manifested as depression. In order to get away from the chronic feeling of emptiness that frequently accompanies depression, people will start to drink.

One of the reasons people drink is that it takes away the feelings: both the highs and the lows. It gives the drinker a sense of being in a never-never land. The same is true of many drugs. People take drugs because it gives them a euphoria they wouldn't have achieved on their own or that they may have had but could not sustain. So they keep going back to it. Once you get used to that, it's quick and easy to just stick a needle in your arm or put some form of narcotic up your nose. You drink it or ingest it. None of this helps us resolve the underlying conflict, which may be biological, psychological, or a combination of the two.

I have found that the best way to approach this is to get the person into a systematic cleansing program—and there are many—where the person actually breaks all physical addictions, and not just to one thing like sugar, but also every other thing they could be allergic to. That seems to be a major first step. The person's energy comes back. A very big thing about any addiction withdrawal is the lack of energy. So when you substitute for the energy they had been getting from the drug by giving it to the person naturally, through the body's own process of metabolism, the person feels better.

Then you start to rebuild the center of the brain with phosphatidyl serine, 500 milligrams, acetyl L-carnitine, 500 milligrams, phosphatidyl choline, 500 milligrams, and with certain herbs that are known to have an impact like feverfew and green tea. Also flood the body with flavonoids. The person should also juice, juice, juice, taking anywhere from four to six glasses of fresh-made organic vegetable juice a day. Within 6 months to a year, I have seen people who have been totally addicted clear up about 80 percent, stay off, and not come back.

Hypnotherapy

Another health practitioner with experience in dealing with addictions is Michael Ellner, a medical hynotherapist with a private practice at the Chelsea Healing Center and co-author, with Dr. Richard Jamison, of *Quantum Force.*

Ellner begins by explaining that anyone a healer works with is an individual who has his or her own story about why he or she does something. Ellner says, for example, that there are many underlying reasons why a person might use food as the addiction of choice. "Some use food to fill up the empty feeling they have. Other people have social issues with eating. Such a person might eat wisely when at home, but in social situations, just to be part of the crowd, may indulge in food that ordinarily would not be appealing. If the person is very active socially, then suddenly it becomes habitual, almost a license to eat junk food.

"Some people use food as a shield. Very often when a relationship ends, a woman puts on 10 to 15 pounds. It provides a cushion, because people are unlikely to hit on her. The woman gets a little bit of space. Very often when she begins to feel better about herself and is ready to go back into the world, it occurs to the woman that it is time to let go of the extra pounds. I can help the person do that very quickly."

Explaining his treatment for addiction, Ellner uses tobacco addiction to illustrate. "To deal with any addiction, I use one of two ways. For people with combined physical and psychological addictions, in the case of cigarettes, for instance, I work as an adjunct to an acupuncturist. She helps the person resolve the physical addiction, while I am working to help resolve the psychological addiction."

The treatment begins when the addict decides he or she wants a change of behavior. The next step is to develop the self-confidence and self-esteem necessary to move forward, which means stopping the addictive behavior.

"I use hypnotic conditioning to help the person create a shift. The shift would make the desire to be smoke-free much more important to the person than any impulse to smoke. Ordinarily, the impulse to smoke is much stronger. The hypnosis enables the person to make choices rather than responding to preconditioned reflexes."

To some people, the very word "hypnosis" has a stigma attached to it. Ellner comments: "If you ask 50 of the leading experts in the world about what hypnosis is, then you'd probably get 50 different answers. When I use the word 'hypnosis,' I'm talking about a way to help a person change neurological patterns. This is done through imagery, metaphor, and the power of suggestion."

Hypnosis is actually a communication tool. "There are a number of practices that are quite popular and are in fact hypnosis, but the practitioners avoid using the word. An example would be guided meditation. Guided imagery and visualization are also forms of hypnosis. Many meditation practices are forms of self-hypnosis. I myself am working very hard to educate the public to understand the word and to appreciate that hypnosis is one of the most powerful self-help tools available.

Ellner's clients who are dealing with smoking addiction often find relief in just one session, especially if they also have some adjunct sessions with an acupuncturist. "These two systems work very well together to help a person stop smoking very quickly and with little or no withdrawal.

"With food issues, it could take between four and eight sessions. There are a lot of additional areas that have to be worked with that involve building self-esteem, building a better self-image, helping a person gain confidence."

For people with alcohol and drug addictions, Ellner tries to get the person involved in another rehab program and to act as an adjunct. "I will recommend different programs for helping a person stop using drugs and stop drinking. Then the hypnosis would take the edge off. It would give the client a higher quality of motivation."

A substance abuser may find that it's not so difficult to stay off drugs in the rehab environment, but going back home is a different story. When the person goes home, all of the things that contributed to the problem in the first place may still be there. Ellner says he could help the person address this hypnotically in such a way as to "create space and disassociate from those triggers that ordinarily lead back to the addiction."

He mentions some triggers that may start a person drinking. "We live in a country where the founding principle is freedom of speech. Yet the greatest phobia in America is public speaking. You'd be amazed at how many people develop drinking problems because they have a drink or two before they have to speak. It becomes a ritual. Very often, it diminishes the quality of whatever they're saying, but they can't appreciate that. The speaker feels helpless without that drink or two.

"The situational triggers produce anxiety and the anxiety says, 'Hey, I need a drink. Maybe I need a drink and a cigarette.' With the hypnosis, the same stimuli can now create a relaxation response. Instead of anxiety overwhelming the person in that situation, suddenly the person feels calm and peaceful. Suddenly, speaking to the people in front of her is as natural as taking a deep breath. The person is in the same situation, but the triggers don't provoke the same response, don't produce the old unwanted behavior. In that respect, in conjunction with a program and a support system, most people can turn these behaviors around rather quickly and dramatically."

Another adjunct to his counseling is nutrition. "When I am working as an adjunct to the acupuncturist, I have the acupuncturist also do nutritional counseling. If I am not working with her, I would refer the client to a nutritionist. One of the more popular programs I recommend is to join one of Gary Null's study groups, which provides peer support and a firm education about nutritional issues and gives people something to do that is a good use of their time. This is very important in making this kind of change."

Toxic Thinking

Ellner speaks passionately about how thought processes can have a negative impact. "To me, the biggest and most dangerous addiction is toxic thinking. People are very often addicted to negative beliefs, negative opinions about themselves and the world they live in. This addiction really diminishes one's quality of life. Instead of having fun, life is always a drag. Very often, that primary addiction gives rise to all the secondary addictions that people put all their time and energy into. One of the first things I do is make people aware of the nature of toxic thinking. Then I help them do a mental detox and change the way they think.

"As a part of that I use meditation, creative visualization, and other forms of hypnosis. One of the most engaging forms of hypnosis comes about when a person has some kind of creative pursuit, whether it's strumming a guitar and going into an enhanced state of consciousness, or reading a very exciting book, or taking a walk and having contact with nature. All those things are hypnotic experiences. All those things involve moving from one state of consciousness to another. I encourage a person to get very active in everyday life."

Patient Story

I am a recovered alcoholic. It's been about 7 years that I've been off alcohol. At first, I ate a lot of sugar in cakes and things like that. One of the psychological-emotional components of my behavior was that I always had a very difficult time getting started in the morning. The first thing I would think about when I got up was what I was going to eat, which usually included cereal with sugar, a pastry, and sugar-laden coffee. There has been a slow, progressive bettering of my diet, but there has still always been the sugar craving. Sometimes I would be able to get away from it for a week or 2 weeks, but it would always creep back in.

Recently, I completed a 7-day fast and a colonic cleansing and I found that after that cleansing process the craving pretty much disappeared. Also, I wake up in the morning feeling rather alert, and I don't have this compulsion to eat sweets. I think that because I am staying away from sugar, I generally am having better days psychologically.—Bob

17

Anxiety Disorders

N early 20 million Americans suffer from anxiety disorders. Traditional medicine seeks to alleviate anxiety by calming the nervous system.
Unfortunately, as John Douillard, Ayurvedic physician and author of *Body,
Mind and Sport*, explains, "Giving a sedative in this situation will only suppress
symptoms and may deplete the nervous system further, making the situation
chronic." Instead of being depleted, "the nervous system must be built up and
rejuvenated so it can put itself to sleep, stabilize its energy and moods, and stay
that way."

Causes

Anxiety can have many different causes. Psychiatrist Helen Derosis, author of
Women and Anxiety, points to external pressures on people who lead busy lives
and have never learned to plan properly and set priorities: "Practically everyone
I encounter in this country is anxious to some extent. One can be slightly anxious or very anxious, anxious occasionally or continuously. The most devastating type involves being anxious all the time over the little things we have to do
everyday. People worry that somehow things will not turn out right for them."

Dr. Derosis continues, "A woman about 25 years old came to me who was
very bright and educated and was working for a large TV company. She wanted to be a producer, but was only a gofer, though at a very good salary. She was
very upset, disappointed, and angry. She would cry to her husband every night
when he got home. Yet as soon as she realized it wasn't possible to achieve that
goal so quickly and saw that life was not as easy as she thought, she calmed
down.

"Earlier, a doctor or psychiatrist would have treated her with Valium and said her problems were not real, all in her head. Remembering those older treatments, a patient will come in today asking for medication, which is not a solution. Getting over anxiety involves growing. If you can keep growing, you will have problems, but the constant activity of being alive, thinking about what you want to do next, and planning how to achieve it will keep you from being bogged down in anxiety."

How Metabolism Affects Anxiety

From the perspective of orthomolecular psychiatry, practically any nutritional deficiency that affects the mind—and almost all do in one way or another—can cause anxiety as a symptom.

A glucose tolerance test is important in determining whether sugar is being properly metabolized. Anxiety attacks can occur when sugar levels get too low, as in hypoglycemia. Hypoglycemia can also cause a rebound effect when adrenaline is secreted to raise blood sugar levels. This adrenaline rush also causes anxiety. Orthomolecular psychiatrist Dr. Michael Lesser checks out sugar tolerance "rather than getting involved immediately in looking for Oedipal or pre-Oedipal fantasies," because in a recent review of his cases he found that 92 percent of people with neuroses had abnormalities in the glucose tolerance test.

Dietary recommendations based on the results of a glucose tolerance test may help a patient far more effectively, quickly, and safely than either psychotherapy or drug treatment will. The main objective is to create stability so that sugar levels neither drop nor rise too sharply or rapidly. For a person with hypoglycemia, a high-protein diet is recommended by Dr. Lesser because it digests very slowly, sending just a small trickle of sugar into the bloodstream so that the blood sugar is kept stable for a long period of time. Then, when the patient eats frequently, the blood sugar remains stable. "I have these patients eat six or seven times a day, small snacks so as not to put on weight," he reports. "Actually, they can handle more calories than they could if they were eating one, two, or three large meals a day because the body is set up to metabolize the small meals frequently. When you have a large meal, you cannot metabolize all that nutrition, and the body turns a portion of that into fat."

The Role of Digestion

Dr. Walt Stoll, a board-certified family practitioner who combines his traditional Western (allopathic) training with holistic healing practices, has found that anxiety disorders are often linked to an inability to completely break down proteins during the digestive process into their amino acids.

"Just three or four amino acids still hooked together (peptides), if they get through the intestinal lining, can stimulate the immune system to make antibodies against them. Since the body is also made up of peptides hooked together to make proteins these antibodies can attack us. To an antibody, a peptide is a peptide. It frequently doesn't matter whether the peptide came from outside the body or is a part of the body. It is now being found that many of the chronic diseases that are so baffling to the allopathic disease philosophy of conventional Western medicine are related to autoimmune processes.

"In addition, "some of these peptides have been found to be identical to certain brain hormones (endorphins) that are associated with panic attacks, depression, manic depression, schizophrenia, and other conditions. In these cases—with more certain to be discovered—there is no need for the immune system to be involved; the effect is direct. The two first examples to be discovered were peptides from imperfectly digested casein (milk protein) and gluten (wheat protein). Of course, these are the two most commonly eaten foods in our culture."

Dr. Stoll usually sees patients after they have tried a number of different therapies. "These patients come with stacks and stacks of records documenting that nothing seems to have worked in spite of every imaginable test having been done and every imaginable treatment having been tried. Psychoactive drugs have either worked poorly or have even caused the problem to worsen because the side effects exceeded the benefits.

"Since every other conceivable cause has been ruled out by the time I get to see them, I am free to look for the things that have not been evaluated. One of the first things I look for is how well the lining of their intestinal tract protects them from their environment. I frequently find that either they don't have the normal bacterial balance in the colon or that they have gone beyond that stage to having candidiasis. Candida can escape from our control only if the normal bacteria are not under control. If Candida has converted from the yeast form, which is a normal part of the intestinal flora, into the disease-causing fungal form, it further damages the lining so that the leakage of peptides is much greater.

"The greater the amount of peptide leakage, the more likely it is that the brain will interpret these protein particles as being identical to the endorphins it produces during panic attacks, depression, and the like. This leakage is responsible for the increasing sensitivities we see in patients who are sensitive to environmental substances other than foods. In most cases, it is much simpler to correct the leakage than it is to eliminate the substance. But why not do both?"

According to Dr. Stoll, dramatic improvement is often seen once the reason for the leakage is corrected. "The antibodies involved last only for 72 hours. Once the leakage is stopped completely, symptoms lessen substantially in just a few days; even a reduction of the leakage helps. There are many patients today who have had that kind of experience. Not everyone's mental symptoms are caused by poorly digested food playing tricks on the brain. However, in my experience it is the most commonly missed diagnosis and one that is relatively easy to resolve."

Identifying Causes of Anxiety

In Dr. Helen Derosis's plan for reducing anxiety, the first step is to identify one thing that causes anxiety or creates tension, guilt, anger, and so on. One of the main problems in anxiety is that the person cannot discriminate between "distracting and anxiety-producing components" of life.

"For example, one of my patients had a teenage son who was troubling her a great deal. She said her son was coming to the dinner table that summer without any shoes, in his underwear, and with dirty, unkempt hair. She would yell at him, then they would argue, and he would get up and stomp out. Then she'd feel bad because she was kicking him out. In other words, those little details of life. So I asked, 'What is it that bothers you the most?'

"She responded, 'It's his wearing underwear to the dinner table.' Then she added, 'But he does so many things to get me mad.'

"I stopped her and said I wanted only one thing. Then I asked, 'What could you do about that one thing?' This was the second step. Once you have isolated a problem, you have to plan what you are going to do about it.

"I also suggested that she behave in a low-key way, for she had been carrying on just as her son did, and it never got her anywhere. In fact, it made things worse.

"She was able to keep quiet for quite a while and then she thought, 'What if I got him some summer shorts. Maybe he might wear them.'

"So she asked him if he might like them and he said, 'Yes.' She did that, and he wore them all summer. Every once in a while, she would grab them and put them in the washing machine. As a result, their whole relationship changed. But this change involved one of the little details that can make life easy or anxiety-filled."

Diet and Nutritional Remedies

Orthomolecular treatment of anxiety involves approaches that would rarely be thought of in traditional psychiatry. These include metabolic studies, digestive analyses, diet modifications, and stress-reduction techniques.

Dr. Michael Lesser stresses that good nutrition is also important, since junk foods can spur anxiety. Simple, processed carbohydrates such as white sugar and white flour products may give a quick lift to the a person with hypoglycemia, but this is followed by excessive insulin secretion that drives the blood sugar down again, only to be pumped up once again by an adrenaline rush. This episode leaves a person with cold hands, jitters, anxiety, and panic.

Special nutrients can help alleviate this problem, especially chromium—also called the glucose tolerance factor–which helps normalize blood sugar. Zinc and the B vitamins, especially thiamine and vitamin B_1, are also beneficial. Niacin, has also been identified as an antistress factor. It lowers cholesterol and triglyceride levels, which are increased by anxiety, and affects the brain in ways that are similar to the effects of tranquilizers. Dr. Lesser is convinced of the efficacy of this nutritional approach, but emphasizes the need to be patient when looking for results.

It may take months for the condition to begin to clear because "the body has been often run-down for a number of months or years, and you have to gradually repair all the cells in the body. The old cells have to die off and be replaced by new ones that are better nourished. The natural life span of cells varies throughout the body. Some, such as blood cells, live 120 days, so you cannot really expect sudden dramatic improvement unless the condition has come on suddenly and you have caught it early."

According to Dr. Allan Spreen, a specialist in nutrition-based medicine, anxiety disorders respond to treatment with certain natural substances. The advantages of treatment with natural substances can be numerous and substantial: by freeing people from having to take more toxic medication, the holistic approach can spare the patient the medication's side effects as well as the extra expense.

"Some amino acids, when given individually," says Dr. Spreen, "can be very effective in calming down the symptoms of anxiety disorders and panic attacks." For example, tryptophan, which has been banned from public sale as a nutritional supplement, "was used as a sleeping agent until there was a problem with some batches of it being contaminated, which caused a syndrome that was related not to the tryptophan but to the contaminant. Some doctors use tyrosine for depression and anxiety. The 'DL' form of phenylalanine is often used on a short-term basis for depression and can be very effective if given correctly. It can lessen anxiety and depression in people by giving them more of an 'up' mood. Phenylalanine is also an appetite suppressant for many people. If they're given correctly, there seems to be no toxicity associated with amino acids, and they're much cheaper than antidepressants or antianxiety prescription medications."

Another nutritional approach is advocated by Dr. Steven Whiting, author of *The Complete Guide to Optimal Wellness*. He argues, "Once we have addressed the question of whether you are eating the proper foods, then you need to take certain supplements."

For Dr. Whiting, key supplements are calcium and magnesium. "We have been told that the B complex is centrally important. Although this is true, the importance of calcium and magnesium should not be underestimated. Remember, at periods of high stress, calcium and magnesium as well as vitamins

C, vitamin B_1, vitamin B_{12}, and pantothenic acid are consumed by the body at a phenomenal rate. One recent clinical study showed that up to 1,200 milligrams of pantothenic acid can be consumed in a 24-hour period of severe anxiety. With the recommended dietary intake of those nutrients well below that, we can see it is not sufficient for high-stress periods.

"So in addition to these supplements that are commonly given for stress, calcium and magnesium are probably the best weapons we have because of their action on the central nervous system. I would recommend 800 milligrams of calcium and 400 milligrams of magnesium every 4 to 6 hours, as well as at bedtime. By accelerating that, you can create what I designate 'a natural tranquilizer replacement.' While it should be used only for short periods of time, it certainly can be used for 3 to 5 days with no side effects whatsoever."

Dr. Whiting also believes in using vitamin and mineral supplementation to replace tranquilizers. He notes, "A combination which I have used successfully to replace such harmful drugs as Valium and Librium goes as follows: calcium at 600 milligrams, magnesium at 400 milligrams, vitamin B_6 at 200 milligrams, potassium at 1,600 milligrams, and vitamin B_{12} at 500 micrograms every 4 hours under the tongue. This is used every 4 to 6 hours. We have had a phenomenal response with this, in terms of removing people's need for these highly habit-forming drugs."

Herbs

A number of herbs have been found to help reduce anxiety. These include:
piper methysticum (kava kava root)
scutellaria lateriflora (skullcap)
valeriana officinalis (valerian)
eschscholzia (California poppy)
passiflora incarnata (passionflower)
matricaria chamomilla (chamomile)
artemesia vulgaris (mugwort)
See chapter 19, Insomnia, for further discussion.

Stress Reduction

In addition to dietary modifications and nutritional supplements, anxiety may be ameliorated by relaxation techniques, yoga, massage, exercise, and stress management. An orthomolecular psychiatrist will often suggest these approaches before turning to drugs. Drugs, unlike nutrients or stress-reduction techniques, often become addictive. If you suffer from anxiety and then develop an addiction to drugs that were intended to help that problem, you will only have augmented the agony you were trying to eliminate. In addition, the direct side effects that drugs often have may leave you less capable of living a normal, healthy life than you were when you first underwent treatment.

Orthomolecular psychiatry also puts psychotherapy on the back burner. The shortcoming of psychotherapy, according to Dr. Michael Lesser, "is that most people who suffer from anxiety have only a limited capacity to deal with it through insight psychotherapy. There is a real risk and danger that an individual, by concentrating on her pathology—phobias and anxiety—and by delving deep into her childhood and looking for trauma, will become 'fixed' on the idea of her pathology. Rather than becoming more able and competent, she will become fixed in her neurosis and in some cases will become even more anxious as a result of exploring the so-called unconscious. I have seen many cases—I am not saying this occurs in every case; perhaps I am seeing only the failed cases—of individuals who have been in psychotherapy for 4, 6, 8, or even 12 years with no apparent improvement. It seems to me that when a case goes on that long, someone should think about the possibility of using another approach."

18

Eating Disorders

Paul Goodman, a radical social theorist of the 1950s and 1960s, wrote one of the most interesting analyses of *On the Road* by Jack Kerouac. That 1957 novel was about dissatisfied youth, dubbed "beatniks" by the press, who restlessly moved about the United States, dissatisfied with the anti-intellectual culture and conformism of the Eisenhower years. Most critics either decried or fulsomely praised the book, depending on their reaction to its literary and political message. In his review Goodman looked at what the novel's protagonists, who had become role models for disaffected youth, ate for dinner, noting that their favorite foods were hamburgers and French fries. In a time before fast-food restaurants, this was an avant-garde cuisine. Goodman argued, though, that this soft type of food, which does not have to be chewed, symbolically represents a desire to avoid conflict. Not only were the beatniks dropouts who didn't want to get involved in the success-oriented rat race of American society, they didn't even want to commit to masticating their food. For Goodman this indicated a lamentable withdrawal from life's struggles.

Whatever the merits of Goodman's analysis, his basic point—that what people eat says a lot about who they are—is repeatedly illustrated in this chapter as we look at various eating disorders and fad diets.

Food Cravings and Emotional States

Dr. Doreen Virtue, former director of a clinic and inpatient psychiatric unit specializing in eating disorders, has a Ph.D. in counseling psychiatry and is the author of several books on dieting and health, including *Constant Craving from A to Z.*

The first thing to do in approaching the topic of food cravings is to distinguish between a craving and a desire to compensate for nutritional deficiencies. "Most nutritionists would have you believe that nutritional deficiencies are at the heart of all food cravings," she says. "The problem with that approach is that it still leaves many food cravings unexplained. Food cravings tend to be so specific. For example, a person may crave a hard-boiled egg but not a soft-boiled egg. Or a person may want a chocolate candy bar but not chocolate pudding. It sounds bizarre and a little childish, but anyone who has experienced food cravings will understand how intense and specific they can be.

"Another reason why nutrient deficiencies may not be the only possible cause of these cravings is that not everyone satisfies his or her craving for food before the craving passes. Just as mysteriously as the food craving appears, it may vanish. A food craving can change as easily as a person's state of mind." Dr. Virtue has been researching food cravings for 12 years and has found patterns that correlate with people's personalities and emotional issues. Again and again, for instance, she found that someone who craved, say, bread was very different from someone who craved ice cream. It's similar to drug-taking behavior. Someone addicted to marijuana, say, has a very different personality and style than someone addicted to another drug.

Noting this correlation, she says, "I investigated further to look at the correlation between personality, emotional and spiritual issues, and how they are connected to food cravings. I did a great deal of research in university libraries, looking at the psychoactive, that is, mood-altering, chemicals found in different foods. I'm not talking about chemicals such as pesticides. I mean the inherent properties, such as vitamins, minerals, amino acids, and so on, that actually can increase or decrease our blood pressure and trigger the pleasure centers of the brain and other areas, chemicals that really affect our moods and energy.

What I found is that we all tend to act as intuitive pharmacists. We tend to crave foods that will bring us to a state of homeostasis, which means balance or peace of mind. Whenever we are upset, it is normal for us to do something to fix that. If we don't want to take direct action, for instance, by making changes overtly in our lives, a more covert way of dealing with the upset is food cravings, which are cravings for a chemical that will make the body feel at peace."

From this point of view, Dr. Virtue believes that food cravings should be dealt with by trying to understand their underlying emotional sources. Instead of getting angry at yourself for having food cravings, thinking, Oh, I'm so weak. I should have more willpower, it's better and healthier to listen to those cravings, which are a form of intuition. As Dr. Virtue puts it, "Deciphering them is almost like dream interpretation. They can give us guidance in our lives and help us in many ways."

We noted earlier that a food craving is not due to a nutritional deficiency. Nor is it due to physical hunger. Dr. Virtue explains, "Let's think about the difference between emotional hunger and physical hunger. They can feel identical, and actually, this is one of the most important points in managing the appetite: to know the difference between emotional cravings and physical cravings."

She notes several underlying differences. For one thing, emotional hunger comes all of a sudden, out of the blue. As she puts it, "You feel like you are starving. Whereas physical hunger is gradual, at one moment you might just feel a little pang in your stomach, then over the course of the next hour or so it grows into a voracious hunger."

The second difference is that emotional hunger is usually for a very specific food. It has to be rocky road ice cream or it must be a pepperoni pizza. Physical hunger, while it may have preferences, is open to different types of food. It doesn't require an exact type of food to be satisfied.

Third, Dr. Virtue says, "Emotional hunger is always above the neck, whereas physical hunger is based in the stomach. Emotional hunger is a kind of 'mouth hunger' where in your mouth you get a taste for a certain thing. It's a very cerebral type of hunger. It is also very urgent. It has to be satisfied now, whereas physical hunger says, 'I am hungry but I could wait 15 minutes or a half hour if I needed to.'"

The demanding nature of emotional food cravings is due to the urge's misguided attempt to fill an emotional hole: "One of the reasons emotional hunger is urgent is that it really is uncomfortable with the feeling and wants to make that feeling go away. Emotional hunger also is usually paired with some upsetting emotion. And if we stop for a moment when we are experiencing this emotion and ask, 'Could there possibly be something that upset me that I wasn't acknowledging?' as we go into introspection, we usually see that a clerk was rude or a driver cut us off on the road. We are upset, not really hungry."

Physical hunger arises from a real physical need, not from emotional needs. Emotional hunger, since it is not related to actual physical need, has a strong psychic component: "When we do try to satisfy it, we almost go into a trance where we are eating without realizing we are eating. It's as if someone else's hand were holding the fork or the spoon. It can be designated as 'automatic' or 'absentminded' eating. With physical hunger, you are more aware of, more tuned in to what you are eating: you are satisfying it."

This is why many holidays involve overeating and eating foods we normally would not touch: "One reason that, for instance, most people can think of a Thanksgiving when they overate is that a lot of intense emotions take place around that holiday. Maybe you are with your family and someone overdrinks and gets into an argument, or it may be all these emotions in a happy way. So one of the reasons we overeat at Thanksgiving is because of these intense feelings we may not know what to do with. Even after we are stuffed, we keep going. Of course, the food is delicious, but this goes beyond that, because true physical hunger stops when you are full."

SPECIFIC TRIGGER FOODS Usually, if you really look at it, Dr. Virtue notes, there are a few trigger foods that cause a voracious appetite. If you want to find out what your triggers are, you can ask a friend or someone who eats with you, "What kind of food do I seem to binge on?" If you are aware of your own food cravings, you can ask yourself, What's going on and how do I feel?, the same way you would about stress.

Dr. Virtue says, "What I've found is that several factors are involved that correlate the particular trigger food to the emotions. One is the texture. Is the food crunchy or soft or chewy? The next is the actual physical components and the underlying chemical properties that either increase or decrease blood pressure, elevate or lower mood, and create neurochemicals that alter mood. The last thing is the flavor or the taste, whether it's spicy, salty, sugary. All these things have to do with who we are as a personality."

Again, identifying your trigger foods is a way to understand what your underlying fears and other emotions are expressing. "Instead of getting mad at ourselves for craving these things," she counsels, "we need to see our cravings as a blessing in disguise. It's the body's way of talking to us. It's just like when a person puts his or her hand on a hot plate. Then the body talks back and says, 'Get that hand off that heat.' Our appetite is trying to do the same sort of thing and give us a message."

THE FIVE CORE EATING STYLES Food cravings, Dr. Virtue observes, are paired with specific ways of overeating, or what she calls core emotional eating styles: "There are five core emotional eating styles. Although most people center on one style, it is possible to be more than one. Some people are all five, although that is very uncommon."

The first type of overeater is the binge eater. "This is a very black-and-white eating style," Dr. Virtue says. "You are a binge eater or you are not. It's a person who, in response to a certain trigger food, as if she or he had an allergy, goes on an eating binge when she or he tastes this food. Refined white flour and sugar are very common binge foods. Such people actually need to abstain, as if they were alcoholics staying away from alcohol, in order to manage their appetites."

The second type of eater is the mood eater. This person is often very sensitive and intuitive, and overeats in response to strong emotions. Keeping a food journal that lists the foods craved and eaten and the accompanying emotions may help this type of eater to find a better solution.

The third type of overeater is the self-esteem eater. "This is the person who, often because of life events, has low self-esteem and issues about worthiness," Dr. Virtue says.

The fourth type is the stress overeater: "This person will overeat when there is a lot of tension in the air," Dr. Virtue explains. According to Dr. Virtue, a stress eater does really well by exercising, and adding some fun and relaxation into the week. Spending time outdoors is good, as is any kind of spiritual practice. Meditation and yoga are helpful for stress eaters.

The fifth type of overeater is the snowball-effect eater. "This is the kind of person who, just like a snowball rolling down a mountain, will gain speed and momentum in eating after going on a strict diet," Dr. Virtue says. She adds that the person will say, "'I'm not going to eat anything except for three little things at each meal.' This is unrealistic. Every day she begins adding more and more to the diet without realizing what is going on. As her plate gets fuller, her weight goes up, like a snowball."

Dealing with these types of unregulated eating, then, means following the Socratic injunction, "Know yourself." Once you understand which emotions and situations are driving you into these unwanted patterns, you can take steps to satisfy your emotional cravings in less destructive ways.

Insulin Reaction and Overeating

Having examined the emotional basis for overeating, let's look at its biological basis in the body's glucose cycle. Colette Heimowitz has a master's degree in nutrition from Hunter College, is certified in health and nutrition by Pratt University, and has 20 years of clinical experience in weight management.

The number one biological cause of obesity in our sedentary population, she maintains, must be understood in terms of insulin resistance: "In a normal homeostasis, an individual ingests a carbohydrate and it raises the glucose levels in the blood. When someone eats protein or fat, by contrast, this doesn't happen. Once the glucose level rises in the blood, it sparks an insulin response from the pancreas. What the insulin does is take the glucose to the peripheral tissues, either to the fat cells, the liver, or to muscle as storage. When we age, as a result of years of eating refined carbohydrates, maintaining high-sugar diets, and living a sedentary life, the insulin is no longer efficient at taking the glucose to the peripheral tissue.

"One of two things happens. Either the glucose levels remain high or the insulin is constantly being produced—overproduced in a prediabetic state—and fat is constantly being stored. When we are sedentary, the process of burning glucose for energy is not happening. It will even provoke the reaction more."

Among the factors that contribute to insulin resistance, "one, of the utmost importance, is lifestyle, a sedentary lifestyle. Some research was done with retired master athletes. Glucose tolerance tests with insulin levels were studied before putting them on bed rest for only 1 day. The glucose tolerance factors were normal, and the glucose in the blood was normal, because they were still leading an active life, not an elite athlete life, but still one that was active. After one day of bed rest, the glucose tolerance test was repeated and the glucose levels were much higher."

Equally important, Heimowitz says, was a history of eating refined foods, which "the American public is known for—taking the bran out of food, taking the fiber out of food, and replacing the essential fatty acids with hydrogenated fats. This causes a complete stress on the insulin level. The glycemic index of foods [a measurement of the amount of glucose found in the blood as a result of eating a specific food] is much higher, provoking more of an insulin response. The pancreas eventually gets trigger-happy."

There is also a genetic component. It has been shown that people whose parents have a history of diabetes or cardiovascular disease have a weak gene that makes them susceptible to this particular condition. She says, "They especially have to be careful and have an active lifestyle and a low-saturated-fat, higher-protein, lower-carbohydrate diet."

TREATMENT To alter this continuous fat and flabby syndrome, a lower-carbohydrate diet is needed to give the pancreas a rest. Heimowitz recommends eating "low-glycemic-index-type foods, that is, complex whole foods such as fruits and vegetables." She also recommends specific supplements for the insulin-resistant individual.

Alpha lypoic acid is the biological spark plug in converting glucose to energy. She states, "It can lower and stabilize glucose levels and stimulate insulin activity. Some research was done with diabetics being given 600 milligrams daily, and it stabilized their glucose levels without any medication. A nondiabetic or hypoglycemic person could probably use 200 to 300 milligrams a day."

The mineral vanadium, found in vanadyl sulfate, also reduces insulin resistance; 15 to 30 milligrams a day is appropriate.

Chromium is a component of the glucose tolerance factor, a molecule essential for normal insulin function in glucose metabolism. Usually 200 to 1,000 micrograms daily is the range for a beneficial effect.

Heimowitz also emphasizes "essential fatty acids, which are grossly lacking in the American diet and also improve insulin sensitivity and reduce insulin resistance. So supplementing the diet with 3,000 to 6,000 milligrams of the omega-3 fatty acids is appropriate."

Vitamin E is also important. It relieves some of the oxidative stress caused by excessive glucose, which results in free radicals. It will also reduce the risk of cardiovascular disease. Heimowitz adds, "Excessive insulin also causes a lipidation of the triglycerides, and that causes free radical pathology. The excessive insulin also thickens the aortic valve. You are at a higher risk of cardiovascular disease. The vitamin E should be anywhere between 400 and 800 international units (IU) daily."

Zinc also influences carbohydrate metabolism, increases the insulin response, improves glucose tolerance, influences the basal metabolism rate, and supports thyroid function; 50 to 100 milligrams of zinc a day is important.

Magnesium helps maintain tissue sensitivity so that insulin is more effective at taking that glucose to the peripheral tissues. Magnesium helps control glucose metabolism and also decreases sugar cravings; 500 to 1,000 milligrams a day is recommended. "Sometimes," she cautions, "when you go as high as 1,000 milligrams it may cause diarrhea, so the dose should be determined individually. People should start at 500 and work up slowly."

Heimowitz notes that manganese has been shown in studies to be important for insulin activity: "Manganese-deficient rats showed reduced insulin activity and impaired glucose tolerance. This lack also lowered glucose oxidation and the conversion of triglycerides in the rats' adipose tissues. However, the manganese should be dosed in relation to zinc and copper because they will compete at the cell site. So as little as 35 milligrams of manganese is all you need. The proportionate amount of zinc would be 100 milligrams."

She notes further, "If someone has hypotension because of the insulin resistance, the amino acid tyrosine could also help control the hypotension; 1,500 to 3,000 milligrams daily is appropriate. Hawthorn berry, an herb, can also help control hypotension; 240 to 480 milligrams is a good range.

"When there is cardiovascular involvement, with a high risk, especially with low HDL [high-density lipoprotein] and elevated triglycerides in individuals with insulin resistance, coenzyme Q10 is also appropriate. I suggest 100 to 200 milligrams a day."

Lack of exercise also causes blood sugar problems. Thus, exercise is key. Heimowitz recommends that "for exercise, we look at the fitness level of the individual. I wouldn't tell someone who has been a couch potato to go out and exercise an hour a day. The fitness level needs to be increased slowly so the body can adjust to the different mechanisms that are going on.

Why Popular Diets Don't Work

THE HIGH-PROTEIN, LOW-CARBOHYDRATE SCAM The multifaceted approach to combating eating disorders presented so far combines assessing your emotional state, exercising, eating right, and taking supplements. This is in contrast to the faddish, highly touted wonder diets that appear in the media every season. These diets are more often feel-good panders to eaters' worst cravings than scientifically sound practices.

Dr. Joel Furman is a board-certified physician in private practice in Belle Mead, New Jersey, who specializes in preventing and reversing diseases through nutritional methods. He is the author of *Fasting and Eating for Health*.

"High-protein, low-carbohydrate diets have become increasingly popular over the past few years," he notes, "and doctors who promote these diets list a number of reasons why people with weight problems need to get onto this type of diet. One reason they give is that these people's bodies do not metabolize carbohydrates properly, a condition popularly referred to as insulin resistance."

"In fact," Dr. Furman cautions, "such diets, promoted in some of the most heavily promoted, best-selling diet books, are among the most dangerous. Among these books are *Enter the Zone* by Barry Sears, the [Dr. Robert] Atkins books, and *Protein Power* by Michael Eades."

The problem is not the connection between the insulin reaction and bad eating habits but how these books recommend breaking the habits: "All these people who read these books, wanting to lose weight by eating a high-protein, low-carbohydrate diet, remind me of people who want to lose weight by snorting cocaine and smoking cigarettes. In other words, there are lots of ways that may work to help you lose weight, but we are interested in more than just having a person temporarily lose weight. We want a diet that is going to enable us to lose weight and protect our health simultaneously, not something that will end up making us look thin in a coffin or increase our cancer risk."

These diets, he goes on, counsel replacing one bad food, refined carbohydrates, with another, animal fats: "You know, some of these high-protein-diet gurus claim that they have the truth [about the value of eating meat and animal products] and that there's a conspiracy among the 1,500 scientific studies that continue to point to the association between the consumption of meat, eggs, and dairy products and cancer, heart disease, kidney failure, constipation, gallstones, and hemorrhoids, just to name a few. They are overlooking the fact that you must pay a price with your health for eating increased animal proteins as a way to lose weight."

"Of course, there is one good point in what these people say," he adds. "It's true that refined carbohydrates such as pasta, bread, sugar, sweets, candies, bagels, croissants, potato chips, and all the junk food that Americans eat are not doing us any good. This junk now constitutes about 50 percent of the American diet. We know that this food is linked to heart attacks, cancer, obesity, and diabetes. That is absolutely true."

However, the gurus "are taking the fact that these highly refined, low-fiber carbohydrates can cause increased insulin levels, obesity, and insulin resistance, showing that those are dangerous foods and then saying that therefore the diet should be low in carbohydrates and high in animal protein."

"But that's a jump that the nutritional and scientific literature doesn't make. As a matter of fact, there are no data showing that a person on a high-carbohydrate diet rich in unrefined carbohydrates, such as mangoes, cabbage, beans, legumes, and squash, is in any danger. In fact, many studies show that a diet centered on unrefined carbohydrates—vegetables, whole grains, legumes—will not raise blood sugar or insulin levels."

What people don't realize, Dr. Furman continues, is the value of plant protein. "Compare a steak to broccoli, for example. Let's look at the protein comparison for 100 calories of steak and 100 calories of broccoli. Sirloin steak has 5.4 grams of protein for 100 calories, and broccoli has 11.2 grams. In other words, green vegetables are very rich in protein. Beans are very rich in protein.

We can devise a diet that is very low in animal fat or totally vegetarian, but with a good, satisfactory amount of healthy protein.

"People have to realize that there is a big biochemical difference between animal and plant protein. Plant protein lowers cholesterol; animal protein raises cholesterol. Plant protein is a protector against cancer; animal protein is a cancer promoter. Plant protein promotes bone strength; animal protein promotes bone loss. Plant protein has no effect on aging or kidney disease, and animal protein accelerates both of them. In other words, plant protein is packaged along with fiber, phytochemicals, vitamin E, and omega-3 fatty acids. Animal protein is packaged with saturated fat, cholesterol and arachidonic acid."

Therefore, "if you are on a diet such as the Atkins diet or another high-protein diet in order to lose weight, you are paying a price with, for example, the risk of increased cancer."

In Dr. Furman's opinion, after studying the food recommendations of these diets, "I suspect that a person really following one of these high-protein diets that restrict fruit and carotenoid-rich starches—found in foods such as sweet potatoes, corn, and squash—could be more than doubling her risk of colon cancer.

"There are studies that show a clear and dose-responsive relationship between increased cancers of the digestive tract and low fruit consumption. High fruit consumption has a powerful dose-response relationship to reduction of mortality from all causes of death. The only other food that even approaches this powerful effect of reducing cancer is raw vegetable consumption. So I suggest that if you are going to average 60 to 70 percent of your calories from fat and animal products with no fruit, you have to consider that diet exceedingly dangerous."

Dr. Furman describes his own experience of the difference between patients on a plant-protein-rich diet and those on an animal-protein-heavy diet: "Now, I am a physician in practice, so I can watch what happens. In 10 years I may have seen 20,000 patients and treated them with aggressive nutritional interventions that emphasize plant protein. I have a good success rate. I get about 95 percent of my diabetic patients off insulin in two or three months, and this is with a primarily vegetarian diet. Their sugars go down. The long-term effect is that their health improves; their cholesterol drops, and their triglyceride levels drop. It's a diet that is rich in natural foods and unrefined foods."

By contrast, patients who had been trying to control their sugars on high-protein diets did not do as well: "They've gotten some improvement in their glucose responses, but they come in with higher creatinine, and they've hurt their kidneys.

"These are patients who came to me after following the diets recommended by these high-protein proponents. Some came with kidney failure after having damaged their kidneys by eating a high-protein diet. Diabetes itself damages your kidneys enough. You don't have to add to this a diet that accelerates kidney damage." What happens is that the high-protein diet leads to ketosis, a toxic condition in which brain is fed the wrong type of fuel, instead of glucose.

"They used to use ketogenic diets to treat children with seizure disorders when they were unresponsive to medication. Medical studies showed that these diets resulted in very serious metabolic consequences over time. Investigators report that they caused hemolytic anemia, abnormal liver function, renal tubular acidosis, and spontaneous bone fractures. In other words, it's a dangerous way of eating that will age us prematurely and slowly accelerate the calcification of our kidneys and the destruction of the kidneys with time."

Another danger of these diets is that they promote growth. To the uninformed, it might seem that growth-promoting foods are good, but Dr. Furman warns, "If we eat foods that accelerate growth, we speed up aging. Growth is very similar to aging. Laboratory animals that grow the fastest die the youngest. If we feed them foods that maximize growth—especially when they are young—it's almost like we are causing their bodies to age rapidly.

"On a cellular level, the body has to remove wastes and has to repair DNA damage. Eating a diet that activates the cell and activates the DNA and makes the cell replicate and grow is in a sense overworking or overtaxing the body's mechanisms of detoxification and DNA replication. From one perspective, you are prematurely aging the species. With breast cancer, for example, the more slowly a woman grows and the later is her age of puberty, as marked by the first menstrual period, the lower is her chance of developing breast cancer. The object should not be to make our kids weigh 150 pounds by the time they are 12. The object is not to grow as rapidly as possible."

Nutritionists 30 years ago believed it was good to feed kids in a way that maximized growth. But, Dr. Furman suggests, "Now we have learned that the opposite is true. The less we feed an animal, the longer it lives. We want to choose a diet that is rich in nutrients, sure, but low in fats and calories. The only way you can devise a diet that is rich in nutrients and includes an assortment of fibers, phytochemicals, antioxidants, and trace minerals is to eat a large quantity of vegetation in your diet, which has to include green vegetables and things like that. In other words, if we were to analyze the nutrient density of all foods, we would find that vegetables such as salad, broccoli, and string beans would always come out as having the highest nutrient density."

THE BLOOD-TYPE DIET Other popular diets advocate eating according to a person's blood type. These diets have sold many books, and the authors have appeared on all the shows. The authors say, "It's your blood type. You have to eat this for your blood type." I've seen a ton of scientific evidence that could disprove that and show its lack of validity. So why is that approach not being challenged by the American public or the media?

According to Dr. Furman, these diets are popular because they give free rein to people's ingrained bad habits: "I think it reinforces what people want to believe. People are addicted to their rich diets. They are looking to hang on to any reason, however irrational it may be, to not have to change.

"If you talk to smokers, you'll see the same thing. You'll hear how irrational are the reasons they give for why they must still smoke and how they have diminished in their own minds the strong reasons against smoking. The same is true with eating. People want to rationalize why it is okay to do whatever they are addicted to doing.

"The American addiction to such things as junk foods is such that when you stop doing it, you get uncomfortable. The problem is that the American diet is so toxic and so unhealthy that when people try to go off it, when they skip a meal and start eating fruits and vegetables, they feel sick. They get headaches and abdominal cramps. They get shakes and confusion. Then they think that it must be this new diet. It must be that eating healthily is making them sick. They must need this rich animal-fat protein and the junk food. In other words, they don't see that this is a temporary phase that lasts a week or two, when they are withdrawing from caffeine and the rich nitrogenous waste. You might feel a little ill when you change your diet. That slight resistance to change is one basis of people's addiction to harmful foods, and it makes them turn to these quack diets."

Anorexia, Bulimia, and Obesity

Anorexia involves compulsive dieting to the point where the anorectic eats so little that he or she becomes malnourished and may actually starve to death. It is signaled by muscle wasting, loss of menstrual periods in women, body image problems, and an exaggerated fear of becoming fat. Bulimia is characterized by compulsive eating and forced vomiting or the use of laxatives or diuretics to eliminate many of the calories that are consumed during binge episodes. Obesity is seen as an enormous increase in the ratio of fat to muscle, the result of eating to excess, far beyond what the body needs.

Carolyn Costin, author of *The Dieting Daughter* and other books, came to the study of eating disorders through her own experience: "I had anorexia nervosa myself when I was about 16 years old. I had a pretty severe case, was 79 pounds for a few years."

CAUSES In Costin's opinion, a number of seemingly benign factors, such as the emphasis on exercising and dieting in our culture, as well as interpersonal family pressures may cause a person to fall into any of these negative eating practices.

Eating Behaviors

The problem with diets is that they often disappoint their users. "The main thing I say to people about any kind of diet program is, 'Don't do anything to lose weight that you're not prepared to do for the rest of your life, because going on a diet certainly implies that you'll ultimately go off it.'"

So what happens when you go off it? This will lead to disillusionment and weight disorders, such as constantly going on and off trendy diets, unless a person realizes that a healthy lifestyle, not a temporary eating change, is the only answer to maintaining proper weight: "So really, what it always comes down to, always—and everyone ultimately finds this out in the end—is that it's a balanced way of eating and having a lifestyle that is, I think, one that lets you be not just physically healthy but emotionally healthy too."

Another problem is that a healthy desire to exercise can be developed in the wrong way. This, Costin says, is "a little bit like an activity disorder. They can't not do it. There's an addictive component that makes them have to do more and more. Things in their life get put on hold in order to do the activity. They will continue to do it even if they've been injured or are in pain or it's snowing outside. And the way the eating disorders correlate with activity disorders, there are certainly a lot of anorectics and bulimics who also have activity disorder."

In Costin's view, eating disorders are also caused by the way people obsessively codify rules of eating, what she calls "the Thin Commandments." She notes, "Over the years I started to come up with these rules that people with eating disorders have, such as 'If I eat anything, then I have to exercise and burn it off' or 'I have to wear clothes to make myself look thinner. I have to punish myself if I've eaten anything fattening.'"

INTERPERSONAL RELATIONSHIPS

Delving deeper, one finds that eating disorders in women are often rooted in relationships they with their parents, particularly their mothers, though not the type of relationship that's commonly assumed to be at fault. "In the beginning," Costin explains, "anorexia nervosa was often blamed on overcontrolling mothers. But that's way too simplistic." Rather, the problem is the type of role models that mothers sometimes provide for their daughters. Costin asks, "What are little girls learning from these role models about their bodies and about weight and about food?"

Not only those who actually end up with eating disorders but almost all young women and girls are influenced by these role models. Costin says, "When you have statistics that 80 percent of fourth-grade girls report that they're dieting and 10 or 11 percent of those girls report that they're vomiting on these diets, you've got to look at what's happening with their role models."

Costin describes a 6-year-old girl in her waiting room who said she was really excited at having chickenpox. Asked why, she said it meant going to bed without any dinner. "I said, 'Well, what's so good about that?' And she said, 'Because it means I didn't have any calories.' The thing is, she's 6. Her mother was a binge eater seeing me for treatment. But kids are little sponges. And she hears her mother talking about calories are bad and calories are in food, so she just learns that part of being female is trying not to have too many calories."

Fathers also can have a negative influence. "I talk to fathers a lot," Costin comments, "about being conscious about what they say about female bodies when they're reading magazines or watching television or things like that. I talk to them about not just praising their daughters for the way they look, which is a very common thing that fathers do with their little girls. A lot of praise and attention focus on appearance as opposed to internal validation. And also just a lot of paying attention to who their daughter is, doing things with their daughter."

GENETICS

There is mounting evidence that eating disorders have some basis in genetics. Costin states, "It's pretty clear from twin studies that we're going to learn more and more in the next few years about genes that predispose people to inherit this. It's probably going to turn out that there's a biological predisposition. And then maybe a cultural trigger sets it off. Thus, there's a swing back to a more biological basis of these illnesses and not as much of a focus on the big, bad culture. But I think there's no doubt that the culture plays a big role in it, which is why we see over the years an increasing incidence of anorexia and bulimia. But I think it's a combination of someone who has a predisposition and dieting, which is certainly a risk factor. So if more of the population is dieting, more people who have the biological predisposition are exposed to this trigger."

ZINC DEFICIENCY

Some research has shown that anorexia nervosa, bulimia, and obesity may be the result of a zinc deficiency. Dr. Alexander Schauss, a clinical psychologist and eating disorders specialist from Tacoma, Washington, reports that science has long been aware of this connection: "We've known since at least the 1930s that when animals were experimentally placed on diets deficient in zinc, those animals would develop anorexia. Our interest in eating disorders in relationship to zinc has to do with the observation that when humans are placed on zinc-deficient diets, they too develop eating disorders."

"By characterizing three of the most common eating disorders," Dr. Schauss continues, "you can see how vital zinc is. In morbid obesity, when people are significantly overweight in such a way that it could shorten their life span or increase their risk of disease, we know that there is an inverse relationship between the level of obesity and the level of zinc, meaning that the more obese they are, the less zinc they have in the body. We don't know yet whether this is cause or effect, but it is a very important observation because at the other end of the continuum, with anorexia nervosa, self-induced starvation, we also have individuals who are generally always zinc-deficient. We believe there is strong evidence today…that the lower the zinc status is, the more likely it is that the patient will not recover from any treatment plan to resolve the anorexia."

Stress is commonly associated with the onset and continuation of eating disorders and can also be understood in terms of zinc loss, since constant mental stress results in the depletion of this mineral. Women are more prone to stress-related zinc loss than men are and therefore more likely to have eating disorders. Dr. Schauss explains, "The answer may lie in the fact that males have prostate glands and women do not. Zinc is highly concentrated in the prostate in males; it provides a mineral that is essential for the development, motility, viability, and quantity of sperm. If a male is under psychological stress, he can catabolize or seek out stores of zinc in the prostate. Since women don't have a prostate, they will catabolize the zinc from other tissue.

"In women, the richest source of zinc is found in muscle tissue and bone. A common feature of anorexia is muscle wasting and an increased risk of osteoporosis. Anorectics actually catabolize or eat their own tissue as a way of releasing nutrients that they are not getting in the diet. The last muscle, and one that contains only about 1 percent zinc, is the heart muscle. When the body starts to scavenge zinc out of heart muscle tissue, it can interfere with the heart's function, which contributes to bradycardia, tachycardia, arrhythmia, and eventual heart failure. It is particularly dangerous when patients with damaged hearts are in recovery. As they put on weight, they add extra pressure to the heart. That is what killed the singer Karen Carpenter, for example."

NUTRITIONAL TREATMENT Carolyn Costin outlines some of the basic approaches to nutritional therapy. "There are many ways to do nutritional therapy with eating disorder patients," she notes. "One is educational. A dietitian will do some educational sessions. The patients have a lot of myths about food such as 'If I eat anything with sugar, it's going to turn into fat' or 'If I eat anything at night, it's going to turn into fat.' So you send them just to be educated."

Costin also may combine education with therapy. This is needed because "patients' food fears are related to some very deeply rooted psychological stuff. So you combine nutrition therapy and nutrition education."

There are various ways to do this. "For example," Costin explains, "I can send someone to a dietitian, and they get a food plan set up. They get some help, and they go for a few weeks, and then they continue with their therapy, but they don't go back for more nutritional sessions until they're ready to take the next step."

PSYCHOLOGICAL COUNSELING The first step in counseling is to help the person analyze why he or she has this problem. Costin starts off by asking, "Why do you have this disorder? What's good about it? How has it helped you? Let's talk about the advantages of it.' The person needs to understand how the eating disorder has "come to serve a purpose. And that's the whole psychological aspect of it.

"Getting to the emotional aspect is really, really important, and if you don't deal with that, I think you don't really deal with the illness."

SUPPLEMENTS Costin finds supplements helpful in treating eating disorders: "We're using amino acids in some cases with patients instead of medication, and it's working. It's pretty interesting. We use tyrosine and tryptophan and glutamine."

More specifically she recommends "the use of tryptophan, particularly with bulimia nervosa. We use it for people who have trouble sleeping as well. Phenylalanine also, for depression. Tyrosine for depression. For people who are often given medications such as Ritalin, we use a combination of tyrosine, glutamine, and phenylalanine together."

Dr. Schauss adds that liquid zinc may a positive effect in the treatment of eating disorders, as it is directly absorbed into the blood. Powders, tablets, and capsules, which must first be broken down by the stomach and absorbed by the small intestine, do not work as well because many eating disorder patients are unable to digest nutrients properly. Dr. Schauss has found only one brand available in the United States, Zinc Status (supplied by Ethical Nutrients of San Clemente, California), to be effective in clinical trials. Other liquid zincs are not autoclaved (sterile); although they are cheaper, they have not proved effective. Once the patient shows marked improvement, a good zinc supplement will do unless deterioration occurs, in which case the more expensive Zinc Status is needed again.

While results are not usually immediate, taking from several days to weeks, once liquid zinc takes effect, its benefits are long-lasting. According to Dr. Schauss, "In 15 years I worked with hundreds of eating disorder patients. Until I saw this treatment, my colleagues and I felt that the best we could expect in long-term outcome in treating patients with either bulimia or anorexia was maybe a 20 to 30 percent recovery. In our 5-year study, we found that bulimics had a 64.1 percent success rate after recovery on the liquid zinc treatment. In anorexic patients, our 5-year follow-up study found an 85 percent recovery rate. These are extraordinarily high recovery rates for a condition that is considered difficult to treat and insidious."

Another favorable finding is that liquid zinc can lift the depression that is usually associated with eating disorders. Dr. Schauss reports, "In our eating disorder studies, we used a multidimensional design and evaluated the mood state of our patients. One of the first things to improve in patients was the degree of depression that they were experiencing based on psychometric instruments such as the Beck Depression Scale and the Profile of Mood Scales, among other depressive indexes. The fact that we have discovered this antidepressive effect and could document it in patients under blind conditions is of great value."

REFEEDING People recovering from bulimia and anorexia need return to normal eating patterns gradually. Carolyn Costin explains, "In fact, a lot of the deaths that happened early on with anorexia occurred during the refeeding process, because the heart just can't take the volume that you start giving it if you do the refeeding too fast."

In her practice, "We slowly raise the patients' calories. We get lab tests two to three times a week. We take their pulse in the morning and sometimes even during the day and after meals just to make sure their bodies are handling the stress that comes from refeeding. You can't just take someone who's emaciated and say okay, start eating."

COGNITIVE THERAPY Dr. José Yaryura-Tobias, an orthomolecular psychiatrist, also finds that because of the life-threatening severity of a condition such as anorexia nervosa, any nutritional approach must be preceded by a program of cognitive therapy: "Anorexia nervosa, from our perspective, is an obsessive-compulsive disorder that is related to self-image, the way that we perceive ourselves. Basically, anorexia nervosa is the process by which a human being self-starves. Thirty percent of the population who self-starve eventually die.

"In the vast majority of cases, when patients come for a consultation, they are already very emaciated. The chemistry we can measure is very altered. From the biochemical viewpoint, we know that there is a groove related to an area of the brain called the limbic system. This is the hypothalamic area, which regulates sugar, thirst, appetite, and so forth. This information can help us classify some of these patients but does not tell us how to manage and eventually cure the problem. The rest of the problem, we feel, has to do with body-image perception, the way that these patients see their own bodies. They feel too fat. They have different perspectives than the rest of us do.

"How do we treat this condition? Basically, we use a nutritional approach after the patient has undertaken a behavioral program with cognitive therapy. Cognitive therapy is important because the idea is to educate the person about her problems and to discuss with her how many false beliefs she has have about who she is, why she thinks this way, why her body looks the way it does for her, and so forth. So false-belief modification is an important part of treatment."

BREAKING THE CYCLE OF FOOD ADDICTION Dr. Hyla Cass, a holistic psychiatrist who integrates psychotherapy and nutritional medicine, describes her experience as follows: "Some time ago, a psychologist who specializes in eating disorders began to send her clients to me because she had heard that antidepressant medications work for these patients. I had shifted to a more holistic way of looking at things, so I told the psychologist that before I did anything with antidepressants I would try some other things. With certain eating disorders, such as food cravings, the underlying problem is a food allergy. We often crave the very foods to which we are allergic. Typically, it's the very things we want to eat that are the most damaging, that create the symptoms. In fact, it's like an addiction to alcohol: As you abstain from the foods you're addicted to, you begin to have withdrawal symptoms and crave those foods even more.

"In order to break the cycle in cases of food addiction, just as in breaking the cycle with drinking (alcoholics are actually allergic to alcohol), you need to supply the body with the appropriate nutrients. When we correct the deficiencies and restore body balance, the food cravings and allergy symptoms will often be relieved. Rather than having to rely strictly on 'willpower,' it is possible for individuals to break addictive cycles by achieving metabolic balance through avoiding the offending foods and supporting the body with a balanced nutritional program of vitamins, minerals, and amino acids. Often the cravings will then simply go away. It's quite remarkable: With a good vitamin and mineral product, you can often put a stop to the food allergy and its accompanying symptoms.

"I may order a plasma amino acid analysis, a blood test to determine which amino acids—especially among the essential ones which the body cannot synthesize by itself—are low. The amino acid glutamine, in a dose of 500 to 1,000 milligrams, is particularly useful for reducing cravings, including alcohol cravings.

"There are other things to do for food allergies as well," Dr. Cass adds. "Addictions and allergies are often related to magnesium deficiency and can be corrected by supplementation. There are also techniques that can actually eliminate food allergies through the use of acupuncture and acupressure."

"As we can see," Dr. Cass concludes, "there are many ways, other than psychotherapy and medication, to approach what at first seems like a psychological problem."

Dr. Doris Rapp, a pediatric allergist and environmental medicine specialist, gives more details concerning the connection between food cravings and allergies: "In my experience, eating disorders and alcoholism can be related to allergies. Frequently, eating disorders are food addictions. When you have a food sensitivity, there is a certain phase of it that makes you really crave that food. And if you happen to be addicted to wheat or baked goods, for example, you can never get enough of them, with the result that you may become obese. To give another example, men who are addicted to corn may drink a lot of beer and can become alcoholics. They're sensitive to and addicted to the beer, but it's the corn—or sometimes some other component—in the beer that is causing the problem. Sometimes, for those with an allergy to grains, they may feel 'drunk' after eating cereal or certain types of baked goods."

Carolyn Costin, however, disagrees with those who say that eating disorders such as bulimia are an addiction like alcoholism: "It's really, really important that you can be recovered from conditions such as anorexia and bulimia. With alcoholism, you have it and your body responds to alcohol differently. For your whole life you can't have a drink because you are then going to be off the wagon and compulsively drink." This is distinct from eating disorders: "For example, the approach to bulimia shouldn't be, well, okay, if you eat chocolate you binge on it, and therefore you can't eat chocolate. I think that instead we have to learn how to teach you that you can absolutely be in control of this. You have to learn how to have it without bingeing and purging it.

"The bottom line is that the new studies show that people become fully recovered from these illnesses. It takes a long time. The new research shows approximately 5 to 8 years, but the recovery rates are high, much higher than originally was thought. It's like 76 percent full recovery with anorexia nervosa. There's fewer studies on bulimia, but it's pretty good."

Patient Story

Dr. Schauss gives the following account of one patient's recovery:

We were doing blind studies, which means that neither I nor the patients were aware of whether they were receiving a placebo or liquid zinc. One of the women in the study was 47 years old. She was a psychotherapist who had been treating patients with eating disorders for the last 15 years and who herself had bulimia involving about five binge-purge episodes per day for the last 34 years. She could hardly recount a single day in the last 34 years when she did not engage in bulimic activity. We have a protocol in which we give a small amount of liquid zinc, about 5 or 10 ml, which is less than a tablespoon. We ask a person to swirl it around in his or her mouth for a few seconds and to tell us what he or she tastes. Zinc has a strong metallic taste. If the person can't taste the solution, it's evidence of a systemic zinc deficiency. This has to do with a zinc-dependent polypeptide known as gustin that helps us distinguish metallic tastes.

The zinc tasted like water to this woman. Since she couldn't taste anything, she thought that she was receiving a placebo. She followed the protocol, taking about 120 milliliters of the zinc solution spaced out through the day, about 30 or 40 milliliters each time on an empty stomach.

Four days later she called back saying that she couldn't explain why, but she had no desire to binge or purge that day. That was the first day she could recall feeling that way in 34 years. This is very similar to the experience that we have had with hundreds of bulimics we've studied.

We were intrigued about how a simple nutrient such as zinc could cause a major change in the way the brain functions and in the perceptions of the individual. When you've done something for 34 years, whether it's cigarette smoking, nail biting, or engaging in bulimia, you have to wonder how it is possible for that obsessive-compulsive type of behavior to disappear in just 4 or 5 days.

It has now been 5 years since that day, and she has never gone back to bingeing and purging. More important in terms of the study, she received no psychotherapy, nor did she have any contact with me personally. The protocol was given to her by a staff member. So we're quite convinced, in this case and in hundreds of others, that it was the liquid zinc that was effective rather than some tangential treatment.

19

Insomnia

Insomnia is a common problem, affecting one-third of all adults and accompanying many of the disorders discussed elsewhere in this book. People with sleep-onset insomnia have difficulty falling asleep, while those with maintenance insomnia wake frequently throughout the night or very early in the morning.

Causes

Insomnia can be caused by a variety of physical, mental, and behavioral conditions. Among the common causes are pain, anxiety, tension, illness, indigestion, caffeine, and drugs. A major cause of insomnia, especially if it's chronic, is reactive hypoglycemia. This is frequently exacerbated by eating late at night, especially foods with a high glucose level, such as pastries, candy, or even fruit juice. Such foods cause blood-sugar level to go up and then plummet, a fluctuation that can contribute to insomnia. Also, overindulging late at night in highly fatty foods can cause sleeplessness. That's because foods with a lot of fat take four to five times longer to empty from the stomach and be digested than simple or complex carbohydrates do.

Another important cause of insomnia is intake of stimulants. Most of us are aware of the caffeine in coffee, tea, chocolate, and colas. Alcohol, although generally considered a depressant, can have stimulant effects in some cases. In addition to food and drink, certain medications can be culprits in insomnia. Drugs that interfere with the natural sleep cycle include Prozac, the newer drugs related to it, and Xanax.

Exercising in the late evening is another possible bane for the insomnia-prone in that it can overstimulate adrenal levels and excite the musculoskeletal system, resulting in difficulty getting to sleep. Likewise, stress and overstimulating the mind by thinking about unresolved conflicts can be a problem when the goal is sleep.

Conventional Treatment

Many people with insomnia often use over-the-counter or prescription drugs to help them sleep. Benzodiazepines and tricyclic antidepressants are among the medications that may be prescribed by a doctor. Potential side effects include daytime sleepiness, loss of muscle coordination, and addiction.

Herbal Remedies

A variety of herbs can be a real help to those challenged by insomnia. Unlike sleeping pills, herbs won't leave you in a fog in the morning, or feeling like you haven't really slept. Most of these herbs address the underlying cause of the insomnia, a depleted nervous system that cannot settle itself down.

Terry Willard, president of the Canadian Association of Herbal Practitioners, in an article posted on the HealthWorld Online website (www.healthy.net) offers some recommendations:

REISHI MUSHROOM (GANODERMA LUCIDIM). This herb provides daytime calm, decreases anxiety, and adjusts sugar metabolism. It helps to resolve what the Chinese call disturbed *shen qi* (a disturbed mental spirit). It has also been found to boost the immune system, and reduce cholesterol and hypertension. Take three1 gram tablets three times daily.

HOPS (HUMULUS LUPULUS). This age-old sedative can be taken as a tea or combined with other dried herbs in a sleep pillow. To make the tea, mix 1 teaspoon of whole hops into a cup of boiling water. Some people may have an allergic reaction to hops.

VALERIAN (VALERIANA OFFICINALIS). Valerian has been used as a sedative for more than 2,000 years. In Europe it is the most commonly used over-the-counter drug for sleep disorders. Willard recommends that valerian be taken only for short periods or intermittently, when insomnia is at its worst. This is because the herb can become habit-forming, and increased doses may be required if used for a long period. Too much valerian also can make you nauseous. About an hour before going to bed, take a dose of 300 to 400 milligrams of valerian product standardized to 0.5 percent oil.

SKULLCAP (SCUTELLARIA LATERIFLORA). This is a powerful nerve tonic and sedative herb. It can be taken as a tincture of 15 to 40 drops two to three times a day; in combination with reishi, hops, and valerian; or as a tea, using 1 to 3 teaspoons of the root for every cup of water.

PASSIONFLOWER (PASSIFLOR INCARNATA). This is an important relaxant herb. You can find tinctures and extracts in health-food stores. You can make a cup of tea by pouring 1 cup of boiling water over half a teaspoon of dried passionflower. If you're being treated for depression, Willard issues a warning: this herb can reduce the effects of monoamine oxidase inhibitors.

LEMON BALM (MELISSA OFFICINALIS). Lemon balm is used to relax the body and help with sleep. It can be taken as a tea, by steeping 1 to 2 tablespoons in a cup of hot water.

KAVA KAVA (PIPER METHYSTICUM). This powerful anxiolytic (antianxiety agent) and sedative "will probably become one of the most important healing herbs in the next few years," Willard says. Its active compounds, called kavalactones, apparently work directly on the limbic system, which regulates emotional feelings and behavior. A clinical study in Germany found that patients receiving 100 milligrams of kava extract three times daily experienced a significant reduction in anxiety symptoms after only 1 week of treatment. Willard cautions that you should not take this herb if you are depressed, pregnant, nursing, or operating machinery.

CHAMOMILE (MATRICARIA CHAMOMILLA). Chamomile not only relaxes and calms the body, but also strengthens the nervous system. Chamomile tea is a commonly used before-bedtime sedative. You can also take it as a tincture, 10 to 40 drops three times a day; or in capsule form, six 300 to 400 milligram capsules daily.

HERBAL SLEEP PILLOW. Rosemary Gladstar, former director of the California School of Herbal Studies and author of *Herbs for Reducing Stress and Anxiety*, tells how to make an herbal pillow that can be placed next to your head while you sleep: Fill a 4 x 4 inch piece of fabric with dried hops, rose petals, lavender blooms, and chamomile flowers. You might want to put a few drops of lavender oil on top of the pillow as well.

Nutrition and Supplements

Foods with naturally occurring tryptophan in high amounts, such as turkey, eggs, fish, and dairy products, may help you sleep. Other options include calcium citrate and magnesium citrate—1,200 milligrams of each taken any time after dinner; 50 milligrams of the B complex; and 200 milligrams of inositol.

Also, 200 micrograms of chromium in the evening will help stabilize your blood-sugar level. Melatonin, 1 to 3 milligrams before bed, and niacinamide, 70 to 280 milligrams daily, have been found to help some people.

Dr. Robert Atkins points out the efficacy of tryptophan, which has been banned from public sale in the U.S., in the treatment of insomnia: "Tryptophan is very valuable for sleep disorders because serotonin is the sleep chemical. If you take it right when you are ready to go to bed, when your serotonin level is on the upswing anyway, you are really fitting in physiologically with your body's chemical rhythms."

Homeopathy

Homeopathy is based on the principle that "like cures like." Homeopathic remedies are prescribed in minute doses. The homeopathic remedy chosen should correspond to the symptoms described; only one should be used for best results. Sometimes it's a matter of trial and error; if one does not work, try another. Judyth Reichenberg-Ullman and Robert Ullman, naturopathic and homeopathic physicians, describe some of the most commonly used remedies for insomnia in an article posted on HealthWorld Online (www.healthy.net):

ARSNEICUM ALBUM. Recommended for insomnia caused by anxiety, with waking after midnight and restlessness.

NUX VOMICA. Used for insomnia from overuse of stimulants, stress, worries about work. The person usually wakes up in the middle of the night and stays awake.

COFFEA CRUDA. Recommended when you find yourself wide awake at 3:00 in the morning. You feel jubilant and excited, and your mind is racing.

Other Natural Therapies

A gentle neck and head massage for 15 minutes may do the trick in conquering insomnia, and 15 minutes in a warm bath may be helpful as well. Along the lines of positive affirmation, writing in a diary shortly before bedtime can be extraordinarily beneficial. It can be a way of really seeing what you've done that's affirmed your mental, spiritual, and physical health, as well as any deeds you've done that have had positive effects on others. If a person spends some time at the end of each day reflecting on what they've done in the past 24 hours that's been positive, and on plans for the next day, he or she gains a sense of completeness about the day. In a sense, then, diary-writing legitimizes going to bed; it's as if you can now see that you really deserve the good night's sleep you're about to get.

Judyth Reichenberg-Ullman and Robert Ullman also say it's important to prepare for sleep. Choose a time for bed and stick with it. Get ready for bed by unwinding slowly. Your bedroom should be "soothing and comfortable, dim and quiet." Make it a "peaceful sanctuary" used simply as a place for sleeping.

20

Obsessive-Compulsive Disorders

Obsessive-compulsive disorders affect an estimated 6 million Americans. They are characterized by repetitive thinking and the inability to control or put a stop to this thinking process. As orthomolecular psychiatrist Dr. José Yaryura-Tobias explains, these thoughts become urges that are so demanding that it appears to the person who has them that they *must* be carried out. Two of the main compulsions are double-checking and hand washing.

Causes

According to Dr. Yaryura-Tobias, "As to why this condition exists at all, we don't have a sure answer to that question. The behavior may result from a learning process that takes hold during childhood... It may relate to changes in neurotransmitters—the chemical substances in the brain that build bridges between nerve cells so that they can transmit signals from the outside into our system or, in the reverse direction, direct us to act to affect the outside world. The key neurotransmitter that is being studied in this regard is serotonin."

Symptoms

Dr. Yaryura-Tobias talks about some of the peculiar characteristics of obsessive-compulsive behavior: "It usually takes about 7 years or so for a patient to come in for a consultation, which tells us that the condition tends to occur gradually, becoming a part of the patient's behavioral system in a very, very slow manner. It occurs with equal frequency in males and females. Fifty percent of obsessive-compulsive patients manifest their sickness during childhood or adolescence. Later on—primarily after the age of 40—it fades away, and it becomes very rare after age 50.

Conventional Treatment

According to Dr. Robert Atkins, there is some common ground between conventional and alternative medicine. "Both orthodox medicine and complementary medicine, which is the nutrition-based alternative to orthodox medicine, recognize that if a certain neurotransmitter is in short supply, certain syndromes will result. A classic example is that a serotonin-deficient person will often be an obsessive-compulsive. These are the people who can't get out of the house because they've got to make sure the light switches are off or the gas jet isn't on, the people who have to wash their hands 20 times a day, and the people whose desks have to be perfectly neat. These people are serotonin-deficient."

The difference between the conventional and the alternative medical communities lies in how they address the problem. Dr. Atkins describes the conventional approach: "Now there are drugs that block the degradation of serotonin and allow the serotonin level to lift, but those drugs do a lot of other things: They poison a lot of enzyme systems, and that's why so many people got into trouble with Prozac and drugs like that." In addition to Prozac, other drugs used to treat obsessive-compulsive disorders are Anafranil, Luvox, and Paxil.

Alternative Therapies

To treat obsessive-compulsive disorders, Dr. Yaryura-Tobias uses conventional behavioral therapy and an amino-acid approach, along with some other nutrients.

"We basically treat with behavioral therapy. We try to use thought-stopping, exposure (flooding), and response prevention to prevent the brain from repeating the same thought. That is difficult, so we also use cognitive therapy to explain the reasons we think the things we do and try to modify the thoughts."

Behavioral therapy is most effective in dealing with compulsions. Dr. Yaryura-Tobias explains that it's important to expose the patient in some way to his or her fears. "If you have fears of AIDS or of blood, you are exposed to blood or taken to the hospital where there might be patients with AIDS. Or you will read articles on the condition.

"If it is contamination from dirt the patient is afraid of, we teach that person how to touch objects and not to be afraid of them. Then we prevent the patient from washing her hands; in other words, she must remain unclean for a while. I'm talking about patients who, when they are seriously ill, might completely use up one or two bars of soap per day. They might engage in rituals of washing for many hours. They may wash their hands sometimes a hundred or more times a day. Some of these patients will also clean their hands with alcohol or other substances. Sometimes their skin becomes extremely raw. I've seen cases where patients require plastic surgery.

"Overall, the treatment takes about 6 months. With medication there is improvement up to 60 or 70 percent of the time."

People with obsessive-compulsive and anxiety disorders often improve on the amino acid tryptophan. But, as Dr. Robert Atkins explains, "since the FDA [U. S. Food and Drug Administration] ban on tryptophan, pure tryptophan has not been available in the United States, even by prescription. However, some pharmacies will compound capsules of 5-hydroxytryptophan. This compound is an intermediary between tryptophan and 5-hydroxytryptamine, which is serotonin, the neurotransmitter you are trying to build up. The whole idea of supplying a precursor to build up a neurotransmitter that is in short supply is a fruitful approach to treating psychiatric disorders and should, in my opinion, be considered before the use of nonphysiological psychotropic drugs, which have more potential for toxicity."

Dr. Yaryura-Tobias adds, "My colleagues and I were the first to use tryptophan, and with it we were able to reduce and almost eliminate completely the use of drugs for this condition, and we obtained very good results. We were using between 3,000 and 9,000 milligrams per day.

"Then we used vitamin B_6, 100 milligrams, three times a day. Vitamin B_6, pyridoxine phosphate, is a vitamin that is very important for the breakdown of tryptophan into serotonin. The idea behind this was that these patients didn't have enough serotonin in their brains or were very dependent on serotonin or that the normal conversion of tryptophan into serotonin was not occurring.

"When we found by measuring that there was a lack of serotonin, this could be reversed by the administration of L-tryptophan with niacin and vitamin B_6. Some medications also accomplish this result, but with medications we face many types of side effects.

"About 30 percent of patients do not respond to any form of therapy. But it is not a closed chapter for these patients either. An investigation has to be conducted. Now that we have brain imaging, we are able to visualize the brain. We can measure, for instance, the metabolism of sugar in the brain. We find, for instance, that the frontal and temporal lobes and the basal ganglia, which are related to Parkinson's disease, are disrupted. We see the metabolism of the breakdown of sugar and also images of an abnormal brain. The same can be seen with some electrophysiological measurements of brain wave tests and so forth.

"Interestingly, work has been going on using pure behavioral therapy before and after measuring serotonin. With just behavioral therapy, we were able to modify the levels of serotonin in the body. In other words, we may not need medication to change or challenge the presence of a neurotransmitter such as serotonin. Behavioral techniques alone may have an effect."

21

Schizophrenia

Schizophrenia is a group of illnesses of unknown origin that involve disorders of perception and emotion. Schizophrenic illnesses are classified as paranoid or nonparanoid, and they are termed either chronic or acute. According to Dr. Garry Vickar, an orthomolecular psychiatrist, "schizophrenic illnesses as a group are among the most serious biochemical disorders there are; it can be said that schizophrenia is to psychiatry what cancers are to general medicine. The bulk of the lost revenue to society, the bulk of psychiatric expense, and the sheer horror to the families, which is not easily quantifiable, are unfortunately all consequences associated with the diagnosis of schizophrenia."

Symptoms

Among the most disturbing aspects of schizophrenia is the disturbance of thought. Dr. Vickar explains: "These patients may have vague symptoms, go through periods of what German psychiatrists used to call 'stage fright,' and then something happens and they start to believe that their disordered perceptions represent true events. Their strong belief in these disordered perceptions transforms them into delusions, which are simply fixed, false beliefs. Patients will start to believe their delusions and then start to believe their misinterpretation of a perceptual nature. They may hear a voice and believe that the voice is real and represents some real event or real person. They'll act on that.

"The most diabolical part of the illness is the loss of insight, loss of the ability to reality-test. For instance, if you're driving down the street at night and it's dark and hard to see, and you see something at the side of the road, you might slow down to be cautious, thinking that somebody is going to cross the street.

Then you get close enough and see that it's really just shrubs or a mailbox or just part of the normal landscape, and you say, I'm glad I was cautious. If instead, however, you start to distort the original perception and really believe that there's someone who might jump out on the road or that somebody is trying to hurt you and can get in the way of your vehicle, you might take evasive action. In the process, you could have an accident or cause somebody else to have one. You start to distort things without realizing that you are distorting them. That's similar to what happens when the really disastrous part of the illness takes over.

"When you become paranoid and don't know why, you begin to wonder, 'What is it about me that's so bad? Why are people saying bad things about me?' It can become very serious. I had a patient who believed that then-President Reagan was making comments about him—about this individual—and he felt compelled to call the White House and protest to the FBI that he was being hounded by President Reagan. He firmly believed it. When he recovered he didn't believe it, but when he was delusional be firmly believed that the President was, in fact, personally interfering with his life. Such paranoid delusions can become all-consuming and unfortunately very painful."

Early Work in Orthomolecular Psychiatry

Some of the earliest work in orthomolecular psychiatry involved the treatment of schizophrenia. As early as 1952, Drs. Abram Hoffer and Humphrey Osmond, pioneers in the field, conducted a double-blind study on the effects of megadoses of vitamin B_3 (in the form of niacin or niacinamide) on schizophrenic patients. This was the first such double-blind study performed in the field of psychiatry.

They found that schizophrenia is not purely a behavioral or mental disorder but that it also has a basis in biochemical imbalance, particularly a deficiency of niacin. Schizophrenia is among the most difficult psychiatric conditions to treat. But Hoffer and Osmond had good results with the niacin treatment they offered to half a dozen schizophrenics in 1952. One patient—an overactive, delusional, and hallucinating 17-year-old boy—was nearly normal after just 10 days on this treatment and was reported well 10 years later. Encouraged by these results, they then set up a double-blind experiment with 30 schizophrenic patients. Those given niacin treatments did far better than those given only the placebo.

By 1960, they had completed five double-blind controlled experiments, all yielding similar recovery rates. The two-year cure rate was around 75 percent, twice that achieved by placebo. Since then Dr. Hoffer has concluded that early schizophrenics can recover if they receive orthomolecular therapy. A sample study of 27 of those who remained on therapy for 10 years shows that about 60 percent have become well. One example is a woman who burned her house down in response to the voices she heard. After recovering on megavitamin therapy, she started her own business, and now supervises several dozen employees.

Vitamin B₃ Therapy

Dr. Hoffer explains his treatment for the person with schizophrenia: "It's a combination of the best of modern psychiatry, which includes the proper use of tranquilizers, antidepressants, or other drugs, with proper attention to diet and the use of nutrients. The main nutrient is vitamin B_3, which has to be given in large quantities. It's not enough to give the tiny amount present in food. One will have to give many thousands of times as much in the standard dose.

"For the patients I work with, I give 3,000 milligrams per day of either nicotinic acid or nicotinamide, which are both forms of vitamin B_3. I also use vitamin C at the same dose level and sometimes a lot more because vitamin C is a very good water-soluble antioxidant. It is considered the foremost, the most active water-soluble antioxidant present in the human body. That's extremely important.

Dr. Hoffer may use vitamin B_6 as well for some patients. This is combined with an overall nutritional approach that may also include the use of zinc. Zinc and B_6 function together and are extremely important.

"Finally, we use manganese to protect our patients against developing tardive dyskinesia. This is a condition which afflicts chronic schizophrenic patients who are placed upon large quantities of tranquilizers. According to Dr. Richard Kunin, founder and past president of the Orthomolecular Medical Society, when you take tranquilizers for a long period of time you take manganese out of the body, which is the reason patients develop tardive dyskinesia. When you give them back the manganese this condition goes away in most cases."

Dr. Hoffer recommends a diet that is "junk-free." He explains: "I exclude any of the prepared foods that contain additives, including sugar. I also pay attention to patients' allergies, because 50 or 60 percent of all schizophrenics have major food allergies. If these are not detected and eliminated, the patients are not going to get any better."

POTENTIAL SIDE EFFECTS The side effects of this megavitamin therapy are very minor compared with those of traditional treatment. Remember, the aim is to supply optimal amounts of substances normally present in the body and required for good health. As little as 5 milligrams of vitamin B_3 a day is sufficient to prevent the disease pellagra, which only 70 years ago caused hundreds of thousands of people to suffer what was referred to as the four D's: diarrhea, dermatitis, dementia, and death. On the other hand, relatively massive doses of the vitamin can be administered with only minor side effects that disappear as soon as the dose is decreased or the vitamin is temporarily discontinued. The side effects include a tingling or numbness in the extremities and most commonly "flushing," in which parts of the body may become red and sensitive. Dr. Michael Lesser reports that a buffered or time-release form of niacin taken with food and cold liquids has been shown to diminish this problem by helping the stomach handle large doses of niacin. The chemical niacinamide, by contrast, is potentially dangerous in high doses and can cause liver ailments.

Because the B vitamins appear as a complex in nature, a large dose of one of them over time can cause a deficiency to develop in the other members of the complex. Accordingly, during a megavitamin program involving the augmentation of a specific B vitamin such as niacin, the other B vitamins should also be increased in the form of a B-complex supplement.

Other Alternative Approaches

Dr. Garry Vickar emphasizes the holistic foundation of the treatment approach he prefers. "I think in any chronic illness, such as schizophrenia, you have to maximize the person's whole functioning. You want to make them as healthy as possible. You don't want to have an imbalance where your left arm is really maximally in shape because you're a pitcher, but the rest of you is flab. You have to have the whole organism as healthy as possible…

"With the schizophrenic patient I use niacinamide or niacin (more frequently niacinamide because most patients won't tolerate niacin). I tend to use much of what Abram Hoffer has come up with. I look for a minimum of 3,000 milligrams of niacinamide a day with an equal amount of vitamin C. I recommend a B complex with 50 to 150 milligrams of the entire B-complex, mineral balance, depending upon zinc and copper levels. We try to titrate a dose until we reach a level of improvement with the least amount of medicine and the amount of vitamin and mineral supplements that the patient can tolerate."

Dr. Vickar continues, expressing the broad philosophy of his treatment of people with schizophrenia: "I have patients who have been diagnosed as having schizophrenia, and while I don't argue with the diagnosis, it hasn't captured the whole essence of what is going on with that patient. I prefer to see it as an incomplete diagnosis, rather than as a misdiagnosis. Very often the goal, in the schizophrenic diagnosis, is just to subdue behavior. When people are in such states of distress that their behavior is inappropriate, or agitated, or out of control, the goal is primarily to treat that behavior. I think that there is more we can do. We have to try to understand why the patient is doing what he or she is doing—not necessarily psychologically, but in some way biochemically.

"We don't know what the ultimate causes of schizophrenia are. Each new drug that comes along throws the current theory into such disarray that it doesn't apply anymore, because the new drug doesn't work the way that those preceding it did. So I don't think that anybody knows the causes, but there is one thing that we are sure of: We can make a big difference in how a schizophrenic is doing by applying two basic principles, as Dr. Hoffer has indicated: good, sound nutrition and vitamin supplements.

"These are not synonymous. Nutrition has to be the floor upon which the treatment is built. Then, after that, you have to start looking at other factors— whether it be smoking, coexisting alcohol-related problems, dietary disturbances, or absorption difficulties. Also, the patient may not be doing well because what they have been given is, in fact, creating more problems. So we have to be sensitive to such reactions to treatment and continue to modify the treatment all the way along. And again, the approach I find to be most useful is that schizophrenia is not so much a missed diagnosis as it is an incomplete one."

Dr. Philip Hodes, who has spent more than three decades researching, writing, and speaking about holistic health, detoxification, and orthomolecular medicine, describes some additional approaches to the treatment of schizophrenia.

"Today we live in a state of environmental pollution. There are over 90,000 chemicals in the external environment that we ingest through what we eat, drink, and breathe. Contaminants are in the soil, water, air, and food supply. The particles which are toxic penetrate and leak through the blood-brain barrier over time and get into the brain. This process also happens with several of the heavy toxic metals, such as lead, cadmium, copper, iron, arsenic, mercury, and aluminum. These chemicals and heavy metals, by affecting brain chemistry, affect the mind and behavior, so they must be removed. They need to be chelated out.

"Dr. Hal Huggins has shown that the silver mercury dental amalgams are very harmful; when you chew, the mercury is released, causing immune suppression and brain poisoning. Many of the people who have developed so-called 'mental illnesses' are suffering from things like mercury, lead, copper, iron, and aluminum poisonings. These toxic metals affect one's thinking and behavior.

"The orthomolecular approach to schizophrenics is to detoxify them, change their diets, and remove foods that are chemically treated, or that contain a lot of sugar and refined carbohydrates, or that have been laced with pesticides. Then these patients are placed on the optimal doses of nutrients for their individual bodies. The nutrients used include vitamin B complex—especially thiamine, niacin, pyridoxine (B_6), and B_{12}.

"The basic constituents of the human body are proteins, amino acids (the building blocks of proteins), carbohydrates, fats, vitamins, minerals, oxygen, enzymes, nucleic acids, water, and electromagnetic and biomagnetic energy forms. If any of these are unbalanced or deficient, and there are nutritional deficiencies, different conditions and diseases can arise. Our diet is not really a healthy diet: the soil our food is grown in has been overworked; there have been artificial fertilizers added; and the foods are refined, processed, and sprayed with all kinds of chemicals and inundated with all kinds of food coloring and dyes.

"When we eat these foods we become both malnourished and toxic. In answer to those who say, 'Oh, you don't need vitamins. Just eat a well-balanced diet,' I say you can't get a well-balanced diet and you do need extra nutrients to help stave off the deleterious effects of all the chemical pollutants in the environment. With orthomolecular therapy," Dr. Hodes concludes, "many people feel a lot better when they get more nutrients than their diet gives them."

A Final Note

If schizophrenic patients are treated with traditional medicine, they most likely are put on tranquilizers to make them more subdued and manageable. Perhaps psychotherapy sessions complement the drug therapy. Nutrient deficiencies or malabsorption and allergies to common foods—notably wheat in the case of schizophrenia—are almost certainly disregarded. In an attempt to mask the symptoms of the disorder, the traditional physician or psychiatrist is likely to overmedicate the patient, leaving the patient calmer but virtually nonfunctional while completely ignoring the actual cause of the problem.

The orthomolecular psychiatrist, by directly addressing nutritional deficiencies and imbalances from the start, might find a simple biochemical cause for what a traditional psychiatrist would deem a complex and perplexing problem. Mental illness can indeed result from nutritional deficiency, but certainly, as Dr. Michael Lesser points out, "no one has ever claimed that mental illness is caused by a deficiency in Thorazine." Moreover, even if no nutritional cause for the malady is found, such patients can only be made better off by improving their nutrient intake and absorption. Failure to do this can lead to further complications of the mental illness.

Dr. José Yaryura-Tobias points out that some of the more severe cases of schizophrenia—those in which the patient manifests paranoid delusions—are very difficult to treat. While some patients may respond to the administration of certain vitamins or amino acids or to a correction of certain biochemical imbalances, others may not. However, he says, recent studies have indicated that patients who are given Haldol (haloperidol), an antipsychotic drug, appear to have better results when the drug is given in conjunction with vitamin C, which is an important coenzyme in some of the sophisticated functions of the brain. This is an example of how orthomolecular psychiatry can function as an adjunct to conventional treatment.

22

Childhood Disorders

ental health "experts" now tell us that as many as 9 million American children and adolescents may suffer from serious behavioral and emotional disturbances. Some 2 million elementary school children are believed to have attention deficit hyperactivity disorder (ADHD). During the past two decades there has been a significant increase in the number of youngsters who are diagnosed with mental disorders and who, as a consequence, are put on drugs to treat their "disease." These are not just teenagers or even older juveniles: According to a study published in early 2000, the number of children between the ages of 2 and 4 years of age taking medications such as Ritalin nearly tripled during the 1990s.

To what is this alarming situation attributable? Are our kids really more troubled than they were 10 years ago? And if they are, how can drug therapy be the best way to treat them?

Attention-Deficit Hyperactivity Disorder

The following example will address the first two of these questions, namely, how the treatment of childhood mental disorders came to be a major area of modern-day psychiatry. Later we will contrast the traditional approach to these disorders with that of orthomolecular psychiatrists and other health care practitioners in order to provide insights into the many different alternatives to drug therapy available in the treatment of children with behavioral, emotional, and mental problems.

Bobby is 6 years old and has just started the first grade. He is precocious and has been reading and writing for at least a year. He is an only child, has been somewhat spoiled at home, and is used to being the center of attention. He is extremely active and often plays from morning until night. Sometimes his activity gets on his mother's nerves, but on the whole, she and everyone else who knows Bobby find him to be a normal, healthy child who is usually well mannered and considerate.

From the very start, Bobby hits it off poorly with his first-grade teacher. Because he is used to being active, he usually starts to fidget 15 minutes into the class. Often when the teacher asks a question, Bobby blurts out the answer without being called on. The teacher, Ms. Thomas, has admonished him a number of times, and he does try to control himself. Since he already knows what Ms. Thomas is teaching and is not called upon to answer questions, Bobby often becomes bored and restless. He is apt to become absorbed by things going on outside the classroom window to the point where he often does not hear what Ms. Thomas is saying.

Bobby's teacher finds him to be a disruptive influence and believes that he is hyperactive. She sends him to the school psychologist with a report stating that she suspects that Bobby is suffering from what is technically called attention deficit hyperactivity disorder. A copy of the report is sent to Bobby's parents, who immediately become alarmed that something may be wrong with their son. The psychologist examines Bobby, notices nothing out of the ordinary, and sends him back to class with a note to both the teacher and Bobby's parents telling them about his conclusions and asking them to keep an eye on Bobby so that they can alert him if anything new occurs.

A month or so later the teacher files another report. This time, after the psychologist again examines Bobby and fails to notice any aberrant behavior, Bobby's parents are advised that he should be seen by a psychiatrist. After reading the teacher's report and examining Bobby, the psychiatrist concludes that Bobby is in fact suffering from attention-deficit hyperactivity disorder and prescribes Ritalin (methylphenidate).Bobby's parents are somewhat bewildered by this and ask the doctor what the drug is and whether it is really necessary. The doctor explains that while he has not noticed any particular signs of the disorder, symptoms are not necessarily present when the child is having a one-on-one exchange or is in a new setting, such as his office. "Typically," the doctor says, "symptoms worsen in situations requiring sustained attention, such as listening to a teacher in a classroom or doing class assignments." This is why Ms. Thomas has been in the best position to notice and report the disease. The doctor tells the parents that he suspects that Bobby is suffering from a chemical imbalance in his brain which, if uncorrected, could start to affect his performance at school and that bad grades could ruin the rest of Bobby's life. He adds that although scientists do not yet know how it works, Ritalin seems to stabilize children who have this disorder.

At first Bobby's parents are so confused by the diagnosis, and so alarmed that their child is so ill as to require medication for an indefinite period of time, that they simply go along with it. However, shortly after Bobby starts taking the medication, his parents notice that he has become very nervous and complains that he cannot sleep at night. He also shows a marked decrease in appetite and begins to lose weight. They decide to look into the drug more fully and discover that Ritalin is a potentially addictive appetite-suppressing drug of the amphetamine family with numerous side effects, including those already experienced by Bobby: insomnia, loss of appetite, weight loss, and nervousness. When they discuss this with the psychiatrist, he tells them that the side effects are minimal compared with the damage that the boy could sustain if he stopped taking it and that furthermore, Ms. Thomas does not want him back in her class unless she is assured that he is taking the medication.

This example is hypothetical, but it is by no means exaggerated. Every year children like Bobby are diagnosed with nebulously defined "mental disorders" and receive treatment with Ritalin or other even more potent drugs such as Haldol and Thorazine. Since the "diseases" for which these drugs are prescribed first came into vogue in the 1960s, literally millions of American children, about three-quarters of whom are boys, have been labeled and given drugs to tone down their conduct and make it more acceptable to those with whom their energy and activity may collide. While some of these drugs have been studied for use in older children, they have not been tested for use in younger ones. And they have many potential side effects.

In March 2000, in response to published reports about the staggering growth in drug prescriptions for children, the U.S. government announced that the FDA would begin developing research protocols necessary to provide dosage information and labeling for psychiatric drugs in children. In addition, it was announced that the National Institute of Mental Health would begin researching ADHD and Ritalin use in preschoolers. Let's take a look back to see our society has come to this predicament.

Historical Perspective

During the 1960s and 1970s many childhood "disorders" were lumped together under the rubric of minimal brain dysfunction (MBD). The history of MBD and how it suddenly became a childhood disorder provides us with an opportunity to more clearly see into the nature and purpose of much of psychiatric diagnosis and treatment.

The term "minimal brain dysfunction" has been around in medical literature since the 1920s. In its original sense, the term was used to describe learning and behavioral problems that result from identifiable damage to the brain, such as those which sometimes occur at birth or through head injuries. The key was that actual physical brain damage existed that was impairing the child's or adult's ability to do certain things according to fairly objective standards. In 1963, however, all of this changed following a conference held by the U.S. Public Health Service and the National Easter Seal Society for Crippled Children and Adults. A report issued after the conference essentially claimed that the cause of the MBD was organic (of a physical origin within the body) and redefined the term so broadly as to include almost any imaginable form of behavior. According to the head of the Public Health Service at that time, Dr. Richard Maseland [quoting from Richard Hughes and Robert Brewin, *The Tranquilizing of America*], the intent was to single out "that group of children whose dysfunction does not produce gross motor or sensory deficit or generalized impairment of intellect, but who exhibit limited alterations of behavior or intellectual functioning."

The new definition of MBD was drafted by a special task force led by a psychologist at the University of Arkansas Medical School. It included a list of 99 criteria so vague and all-encompassing that the definition would have been laughable had it not become the basis for the psychiatric labeling and medicating of millions of American children. In *The Tranquilizing of America*, Brewin and Hughes further explain:

"It would be difficult to write a more all-inclusive definition for this new disorder subsequently used to label millions of children, but the task force didn't stop there, offering 99 symptoms to help doctors and teachers spot these otherwise normal children. The symptoms include hyperkinesis (too active) and hypokinesis (not active enough); hyperactivity and hypoactivity (activity opposites of a milder nature); 'rage reactions and tantrums' and being 'sweet and even tempered, cooperative and friendly'; 'easy acceptance of others alternating with withdrawal and shyness'; being 'overly gullible and easily led' and being 'socially bold and aggressive'; being 'very sensitive to others' and having 'excessive need to touch, cling and hold on to others'; and 'sleeping abnormally lightly or abnormally deeply....'

"It's unlikely that any child, no matter how normal or healthy, could escape classification under such a hodgepodge of 'signs' pointing to an MBD child in need of treatment."

According to Brewin and Hughes, notwithstanding this basically meaningless cornucopia of definitions, the concept of MBD was enthusiastically welcomed by the psychiatric community, governmental health agencies, educators, and pharmaceutical companies.

How Children are Classified

While the term "MBD" is no longer used in the psychiatric jargon, the concept has by no means been abandoned, nor has the use of amphetamines in its treatment. The DSM-IV (*Diagnostic and Statistical Manual of Mental Disorders*—the official diagnostic guide for psychiatrists) has an entire section devoted to "Disorders Usually First Diagnosed in Infancy, Childhood, or Adolescence." This class includes developmental disorders such as "Mental Retardation," and "Pervasive Developmental Disorders" (including autistic disorder, among others), as well as the "Attention-Deficit and Disruptive Behavior Disorders," such as attention deficit hyperactivity disorder not otherwise specified, conduct disorder, and oppositional defiant disorder.

Nowhere is the DSM-IV more vague or subjective than in the sections concerning and defining childhood disorders. While some of the developmental disorders do contain somewhat more objective criteria, the diagnoses of the "behavior" disorders are very subjective and the symptoms are so wide-ranging that many healthy children could easily fall within their ambit.

The determination of what constitutes normal behavior and what does not is often made by people who have an interest in labeling such things as restlessness and blurting out answers to questions as pathological. In other words, implicit in many DSM definitions is a belief that certain behavior should be controlled and suppressed simply because those in a position of authority may find it troublesome. Even a cursory examination of these definitions reveals that they are primarily directed at a child's behavior at school. Ultimately, then, it is in the school rather than the doctor's office that learning and mental disabilities are first diagnosed.

This is not to say that children do not suffer from emotional and behavior problems that can dramatically affect the quality of their lives. Many doctors treating children for these problems report that such children are often aware of not acting like everyone else and are disturbed and upset by this realization. Few would deny the importance to these children, and to society as a whole, of diagnosis and treatment aimed at getting at the root of their problems and designed to help them live a happy and fulfilling life. However, the treatment of legitimately ill children with safe, caring, and effective therapies is not what we have been talking about here.

Ritalin

Dr. Peter Breggin is a world-renowned psychiatrist and director of the International Center for the Study of Psychiatry. He has authored many books in the field of psychiatry and is considered quite a maverick within the conventional psychiatric community. He shares his thoughts on Ritalin.

"We used to beat our kids and think it was okay. It is no longer considered okay to whip the daylights out of a child. But now we have even more bizarre and potentially more destructive forms of child abuse, such as giving a child toxic substances while that child's brain is growing. This is the basis for how these drugs become addictive. I have cited the data on Ritalin causing psychosis in children. We have animal studies that show when you give amphetamines to animals in the same dose you give to kids and only for a few times, brain cell loss and permanent changes occur.

"There are also new studies showing if you take Ritalin as a child you are more likely to abuse cocaine as a young adult. Ritalin is a schedule 2 drug according to the DEA, meaning it is in the same class of drugs as amphetamines, methamphetamines, cocaine and morphine. Schedule 2 drugs means they have even more addictive potential than Valium and Xanax. It's astonishing that we are willing to do this to our kids.

"In animal studies these drugs suppress spontaneity and autonomy, all searching, exploring and socializing behavior. Because of their effect on the basal ganglia they enforce compulsive behavior. So a monkey that was previously desperate to get out of its cage and play with its neighbor will instead sit quietly behind the bars and pick at its own skin in a compulsive way instead of grooming another monkey.

"That's what we are doing to our kids—making good caged animals. Millions of our children are being suppressed with psychiatric drugs instead of having their needs met. Their needs are for everything from nutrition to inspiring education, consistent discipline at home and unconditional love. They are having their needs unmet when we drug them into submission. It is an abomination. Control is now no longer even a strong enough word. When you are damaging a child's brain in the name of making them sit still in class you have gone beyond social control into brutal suppression."

Dr. John Breeding, a psychologist from Texas and author of *The Wildest Colts Make the Best Horses: The Truth About Ritalin, ADHD and Other Disruptive Behavior Disorders*, tells us more. "The *Physicians Desk Reference*, commonly known as the PDR, is the text that is provided for doctors in which the manufacturers are required to list all the potential effects of drugs.... Among the potential side effects listed for Ritalin are loss of appetite, abdominal pain, weight loss, insomnia, and altered heart rate. And those are just the physical effects....Emotionally we are dealing with things like a basic message to the child that they are defective and that they need drugs in order to cope."

Alternative Approaches to Childhood Disorders

There are a number of alternative approaches to childhood disorders that people should explore before letting a doctor put a child on drugs.

FOOD AND ENVIRONMENTAL ALLERGIES One physician who has had considerable success in the treatment of children with emotional and behavior problems is Dr. Doris Rapp, author of *Is This Your Child?*, *Is This Your Child's World?* and the companion video *Environmentally Sick Schools*. Dr. Rapp practices a branch of medicine called environmental medicine, which looks at the role that the environment plays in people's overall health and well-being. In particular, doctors such as Dr. Rapp are concerned with so-called environmental allergies.

Dr. Rapp explains that most emotional and learning disorders can be caused by allergies in both children and adults. Children can become moody, depressed, suicidal, hyperactive, agitated, or panicky—all for no apparent reason. They may suddenly cry, spit, or kick or hurt others or themselves. Dr. Rapp has "observed that almost any emotional expression imaginable can occur as a result of an adverse reaction or sensitivity to substances in the environment. It sometimes happens in relation to ingesting certain foods or being exposed to certain chemical odors (such as tobacco or perfume), lawn herbicides, chemicals, or pollens and molds. Any of these can cause problems in some individuals at certain times."

Dr. Rapp offered the following observation during a radio interview: "In my office I have seen and documented many patients, young children, who have acted in a very bizarre manner when they have been exposed to something that is unusual. For example, I had one little girl, about 5 or 6 years of age, who became very depressed and wished she was dead on days when it was damp and moldy. When she came into our office and we skin tested her for molds, she became very depressed, pulled her hair over her face, and became untouchable. When her mother walked toward her, she would pull away and scream; she wouldn't let anybody touch her. Then, when we gave her the correct dilution of mold allergy extract, on her own, she walked over to her mother, sat in her lap, gave her a hug and a kiss, and said, 'Mommy, I love you.'

"I had another little boy, about 9 years old, who never smiled. His mother brought in pictures of him at Easter, Christmas, at birthday parties and things like that, and he always looked very dour; he just didn't look happy at all. When we placed him on a diet that merely excluded highly allergenic foods, his mother said that she was really amazed because at the end of 1 week, he was smiling and happy for the first time in his life. When I talked to him, he said that he felt much better on the diet; he said that he didn't want to take Mikey's knife and put it right here, and he showed me where he thought his heart was. He was going to put a friend's knife right into his chest."

WHEN TO SUSPECT ALLERGIES

Dr. Rapp offers some guidelines about when to suspect that allergies may be causing behavioral or emotional problems. "If your parents had hay fever and asthma or any of your children have these conditions, and you have one child who is having behavior and personality problems, you might consider the fact that the dust or the milk that is causing the asthma in one child may be causing bed-wetting or hyperactivity or aggression in the other. If a patient has an allergic history or typical allergies such as asthma or hives, this particular patient may also be having brain allergies—allergic reactions within the brain—that may be affecting his or her behavior or emotions."

Dr. Rapp also states that children or adults who suffer from allergies often have a characteristic look. They frequently have bags or dark circles under their eyes, and many have bright red cheeks and earlobes when they are reacting. Many children with allergic reactions affecting the brain tend to wiggle their legs, fidget constantly, and have trouble remaining seated. Dr. Rapp has also noticed that very often the handwriting and drawings of children will vary significantly when they are reacting. She explains: "The child who is exuberant and all over the place writes in a very large manner. However, the writing may be upside down or backward or in mirror image. But the child who is depressed and goes into the corner frequently writes in extremely small letters. The writing will be as small as it can be, or the child will just write his or her name as a dot. Then, when you treat the child with the correct dilution of the stock allergy extract, he or she can write, and can act in a normal manner.

"I recently saw one 8 year old, for example, who becomes depressed and suicidal each year during the tree pollen season. Last year when she came in, she drew pictures that were very unhappy with sad faces. Then, after we treated her for tree pollen, she drew a smiling face of a youngster who was very happy."

Dr. Rapp describes a 9-year-old boy who became very vulgar whenever he ate certain foods or was exposed to molds. His mother found that he was particularly offensive when he went to a particular school. Dr. Rapp explains: "We went to the school with an air pump, collected samples, and then bubbled this air through a saline solution. We took the youngster, who was sensible and normal at the time, and made him vulgar simply by placing a drop of his school air allergy extract under his tongue. He became vulgar in both his speech and his actions. In addition, he jumped on the furniture and scribbled on walls. He threatened to pee on his mother's leg and do very strange things. When we gave him the correct dilution of the school air, he came right back to normal."

Dr. William Philpott, a leader in the field of environmental medicine and author of *Brain Allergies: The Psychonutrient Connection*, provides other examples of how allergic reactions can affect children:

A 12-year-old boy diagnosed as hyperkinetic had the following symptoms on testing for spinach: he became overtalkative and physically violent, had excessive saliva, was very hot, developed a severe stomachache, and cried for a long time. Watermelon made him irritable and depressed, cantaloupe made him aggressively tease other patients. Once he avoided the incriminating substances in his diet, his hyperkinesis symptoms diminished dramatically. A 4-year-old boy diagnosed as hyperkinetic had a variety of reactions. String beans made him hyperactive, and he wanted to fight with everyone. Celery gave him a severe stomachache, after which he cried and became grouchy. Strawberries made him angry and hyperactive and caused a great deal of coughing. Unrefined cane sugar caused him to be irritable, after which he coughed and developed a stuffy nose. A 12-year-old boy became listless and depressed, and cried when tested for bananas. Then he became aggressive and picked up a stick as if to hit another patient. When he ate oranges, he sang at first but then became very tired, impatient, and eventually wild and aggressive. Rice caused him to experience a sensation of heat, followed by rebellious hyperactivity.

As can be seen from these examples, it is not necessarily unhealthy or "junk" foods that are the worst offenders. Virtually any food can cause problems in a given individual. In fact, one of the major characteristics of allergy is that it is an individualized reaction to substances that ordinarily are well tolerated by other people.

Dr. Theron Randolph, considered by many the founder of environmental medicine (also called clinical ecology), estimates that as many as 60 to 70 percent of symptoms commonly diagnosed as mental are actually caused by allergic-type reactions. Many emotionally disturbed people, especially those with psychoses, develop major symptoms when exposed to foods and chemicals that they frequently consume. Wheat, corn, milk, tobacco, and petrochemical hydrocarbons are some of the more common substances that trigger these allergic responses.

ELIMINATION DIET

There are a few tools that environmental medical specialists use in treating children with allergy-related behavioral problems. The first is an elimination diet, which usually is recommended after the first visit with the physician. In certain severe cases the diet may take the form of a total fast, but usually it eliminates only the specific foods the doctor suspects are a problem for the particular patient. The targeted foods are those that are common allergens (substances that provoke allergies in many people), such as chocolate, dairy products, wheat, and cane and beet sugars, as well as foods that the patient has a tendency to abuse. Environmental medical specialists have found that people are often especially allergic to the foods that they eat most often. Sometimes the frequent consumption can even lead to a sort of addictive-allergic reaction where a person craves the very food that is making him ill.

As food residues can remain in the body up to 4 or 5 days, the object of the elimination diet is to clear the body completely of foods that may be causing problems. If allergy is at the root of the problem and the correct foods have been eliminated, the symptoms will clear at the end of the 5-day period. Dr. Philpott gives an example of how this can work:

"Henry, 17 years old, had been mentally ill for 3 years. Prior use of tranquilizers, psychotherapy, and electric shock had not succeeded in helping him appreciably. He believed that people were out to kill him, and he often had to be placed under restraint because of his attacks on innocent children and adults. He was placed on a fast from all foods and given spring water only. He remained mentally ill until the fourth day, at which time his symptoms cleared; he was released from his restraints. He telephoned his parents, saying, 'I love you. Please come and see me.' On the fifth day of the fast he was fed a meal of wheat only. Within an hour, he began to feel strange and unreal; within an hour and a half, he thought people were going to kill him. He telephoned his parents again, saying, 'I hate you. You caused my illness. I don't want to ever see you again.' Further testing confirmed the fact that when specific foods were withheld, his symptoms cleared, and when he was given wheat, the same paranoid reaction occurred consistently."

The body is particularly susceptible to allergens, particularly after the elimination diet. A small drop of an extract of the substance placed under the patient's tongue can reduplicate symptoms, sometimes very dramatically. This procedure of testing for allergies by placing a drop of extract under the tongue or injecting it subcutaneously is called *provocative testing*, and it is one of the major diagnostic techniques used by environmental medical specialists.

Once the allergies are determined, a technique known as *neutralization dose therapy* is often used to eliminate the symptoms. In this procedure the physician uses increasingly diluted extracts of the particular substance until a dilution is found that reverses the patient's symptoms. This is the neutralizing dose. If you find this confusing don't worry. It is paradoxical, and science cannot explain how a diluted substance can have a more potent effect in relieving symptoms than a stronger solution of the same substance. Because neutralization therapy often is based on very weak dilutions of things such as wheat, milk, and corn, it is an extremely safe and nontoxic form of treatment providing a food doesn't cause a life-threatening medical emergency. It is particularly useful for people who have a moderate allergic reaction whenever they eat a particular food.

FOUR-DAY ROTATIONAL DIET

Another treatment commonly used by environmental medical specialists is the 4-day rotational diet. It is especially useful for patients who are not allergic per se to a given food but become "sensitized" to it when they abuse it or eat it frequently. In this diet almost all foods are rotated so that they are not eaten more than once every 4 days. This way the patient not only avoids the food to which he or she may be sensitive but also decreases the possibility of becoming sensitive to other foods that might have been overconsumed to compensate for the decreased consumption of the "abused" food. (See chapter 11 for more on the 4-day rotational diet.)

AMINO ACIDS, HERBS, AND OTHER NUTRIENTS Dr. Ray Wunderlich, who practices preventive medicine in St. Petersburg, Florida, and is the author of many books, explains his approach to treating children with learning disorders or behavior problems: "We try not to give them Ritalin or amphetamines when they have hyperactivity or attention deficit disorders. Instead we look at their basic quality of life and their lifestyle. Are they troubled by any infections? Do they have allergies? Do they have nutritional deficiencies? Do they have chemical toxicities? Is there some kind of nutritional disorder that is underlying the problem?

"We are directly opposed to the conventional approach, which relies primarily on just treating the symptom by the use of medication. We've determined that very rarely is it necessary to use prescription drugs for these children. The drugs may be needed on a temporary basis while you're testing the patient or while the family is discovering how to reform the diet, for example, or deciding which vitamin and mineral supplements to use. However, in the vast majority of cases—90 percent, I would say—we were able to manage the problem, whether behavioral or academic, without the use of drugs."

Dr. Wunderlich begins by looking at amino acids. "We assess the child's-amino acid pattern through a plasma amino acid test or a 24-hour urine test to spot the amino acid deficiencies and imbalances. We often find that the essential amino acids are not being received by the child. It could be because the diet is so poor, or it could be that the child's digestion and absorption are inadequate, so that the child, while eating well, isn't achieving the amino-acid levels that he needs. We address that issue with supplements to correct either the inadequate input of food or the digestive, malabsorption problem.

"We use herbs in the detoxification process initially. Many of these children are toxic—their bodies react adversely to other elements to which they're exposed. Sometimes, if you give these children vitamins for example, they are unable to take them. The same applies to adults. And when you see that, you know that there is a high level of toxicity in the body and you have to go to some kind of detoxification process. Herbs are very safe and a very convenient way to do that. You get a good response and the family often will see the difference in the child and will then listen more openly to the nutritional message." Detoxification should be done under professional supervision, Dr. Wunderlich adds.

Among the herbs used by Dr. Wunderlich are red clover, goldenseal, black walnut, and acansosyanicide, which comes from blueberries and from pine bark. Dr. Wunderlich explains that these herbs "strengthen the blood/brain barrier and that enables us to protect the child whose brain is more or less on fire—hyper-reactive because of reactions to foods, indigenous chemicals or exogenous toxins. These herbs have been a great help in protecting the brain until we can get the diet changed or the environment cleared up so that it isn't suffering such a toxic assault.

"As far as amino acids are concerned, in some children you have to use just a general, across-the-board supplement including all 8 or 10 of the essential amino acids. In others, we use tryacine, cellalonine, tryptophan, cysteine—particularly the sulphur bearing amino acids—glutamic acids and, of course, the branch-chain of amino acids, particularly in individuals who have an absorption problem.

"Typically we see the most dramatic improvement in the child's use of his or her intellectual ability. It's like putting an engine into gear. The child is better able to listen in class, respond in a communicative way, participate in a dialogue, handle visual tasks—this is enormously important because auditory/visual functioning are linked in learning, and control of eye movement in focusing is a big factor in how well one learns. In many cases, the special lenses which optometrists sometimes prescribe for children with learning difficulties can be discarded several months after these nutrients have been added."

ADD AND NUTRITION Marsha Zimmerman, a certified nutritionist and author of *The ADD Nutrition Solution: A Drug-Free 30-Day Plan*, says that in many cases problems like ADD may be linked to malnutrition during pregnancy. In fact, she says, it may even be malnutrition before conception.

"We are not really preparing very well for conception and neither young women nor men are properly nourished when they conceive children. The women in many cases had a very poor prenatal history. Either they had not been able to keep food down or they didn't have adequate dietary counseling, and the child is totally dependent of course on mother's nutrition during pregnancy.

"The brain develops very early. In fact, between 18 and 21 days the neural fold is developing in the young embryo, and of course the neural fold is what later becomes the brain, spinal cord, heart and all the peripheral nerves. We know of course about the impact of folic acid at that time, but now we are beginning to get insights into the role of fatty acids at that particular time. The brain is uniquely dependent on the correct fatty acids. In particular there is one called DHA or docosahexaenoic acid that the developing embryo needs in very large quantities. The only source of course is the mother. A lot of women are deficient in these fatty acids."

During pregnancy, Zimmerman emphasizes a diet of whole grains and fish. Fatty fish are extremely important, as they are rich in omega-3 fatty acids that are needed for healthy development. Women who don't like or want to eat fish can get these essential fatty acids in a dietary supplement. "Most of the pregnant women that I'm counseling go on a program where they are using DHA in supplement form just to ensure they get adequate levels," Zimmerman says.

Zimmerman explains that ADD is different from ADHD. Attention Deficit Disorder involves attention and behavior but without the hyperactivity. "This is the child who is daydreaming, can't complete tasks, has many things going on at the same time but never finishes anything, has trouble following through with instructions." Children with ADD may have difficulty understanding what time of day it is. "They get confused as to where they are within the day, they forget things, they will complete tasks, or partly complete tasks, and then leave their work at home when they go back to school, and so forth."

A child with ADD can be treated nutritionally, Zimmerman says. Her ADD nutrition solution is a drug-free 30 day plan that fundamentally alters the way children eat. Take carbohydrates, for example. Research has shown that carbohydrates tend to raise serotonin levels in the brain, and serotonin is a neurotransmitter that's calming and tends to put children to sleep. But look at how we traditionally feed our kids: "We give them a high carbohydrate breakfast and a high carbohydrate lunch, and they go off to school and we wonder why they can't concentrate. On the other hand," Zimmerman says, "protein foods provide the necessary amino acids that are precursors of attention grabbing neurotransmitters, namely norepinephrine and dopamine. Just changing the schedule of how you feed children has a big impact on how they will be able to function in school."

In addition to the timing of carbohydrate and protein consumption, food additives play a role in children's behavior. "A child can eat 500 different additives in a day based on the foods that we normally select off the grocery store shelves," Zimmerman says. "We are constantly hitting the brain with things that are going to change the way it functions. We have to get those additives out of the diet. How in the world to you do that? Well, you stay out of the middle of the grocery store. Yet I see parents mindlessly shopping in the store all of the time and just grabbing things off the shelves that either the child wants because they have seen it on television, or because it's easy, it's something that kids like. So we have to reeducate kids taste buds."

In addition, Zimmerman says, we want to replace some of the nutrients that have been lagging because of poor diet. Fatty acids such as DHA, vitamins, zinc and magnesium are especially important.

ADDITIONAL THOUGHTS ON ADHD Dr. John Breeding has some additional advice for parents when a school teacher or counselor brings up the subject of ADHD. "One of the first recommendations I make is to walk through your fear. You need to walk through and realize that you are going to be an activist for your child. Especially if it is a spirited child or a child that doesn't quite fit or cooperate right with the expectations. In other words they are going to be a little hard to deal with over the years, they ask questions, they talk back, maybe they are not well organized, whatever, they draw attention to themselves. The first step is to walk through your fear, realize that the authorities may be walking you down the proverbial garden path.

"The other thing is parents are under a lot of pressure. They are given information, they are given information sheets, and they are given references that all say this is biologically based, that that is what the professionals say. There is a lot of guilt and a lot of pressure."

Dr. Breeding says that parents should not be pressured into making snap decisions about their children. "The key here is not to trust the thinking of anyone who is coming at you from a sense of urgency and pressure about your child. You are in there for the long haul.... Slow down, think about it, be involved, but don't react out of urgency and pressure."

Dr. Breeding shares some other thoughts about ADHD and behavior concerns in children:

"I'm discovering that a lot of elementary schools don't even do recess regularly anymore, or they take it away as a punishment, and this is exactly upside down from what needs to happen with these energetic children. There is also what goes in the child's mouth. Rather than adding toxic drugs, let's look at what is already going in there and seeing if we can help. Maybe there is sensitivity to sugar or some of these food additives and preservatives. A basic common sense approach to more wholesome nutrition can really help.

"The last piece of good information is that large numbers of children in our society are overstimulated, averaging 5 1/2 half hours a day of TV and video versus an average 30 something minutes per week of conversation with their parents. It's a weird statistic. Five-and-a-half hours a day of video and TV results in central nervous system acceleration. That carries over then to tasks that are less stimulating and there is a withdrawal that has to go with that. There is a lot in terms of what parents can do to create an environment that is more conducive to good functioning of the child."

Autism

Autism is a childhood behavioral and neurological disorder. No one understands it but it is a real tragedy for the parents who struggle with it. The incidence has been increasing dramatically worldwide. No one is sure why but there are a lot of ideas out there.

Dr. Jay Lombard is chief of neurology at Westchester Square Medical Center in New York and assistant professor of neurology at Cornell University Medical Center. He has authored a book called *The Brain Wellness Plan*.

"Autism is a very tough disease as any clinician who treats it knows," says Dr. Lombard. "It is common when you incorporate the different manifestations of the disease. The incidence is much higher than previously thought and appears to be increasing."

DEFINITION Autism is a developmental disability that typically appears during the first 3 years of life. Three-quarters of those with autism are male. As defined by the Autism Society of America, "Autism interferes with the normal development of the brain in the areas of reasoning, social interaction, and communication skills." People with autism vary widely in their abilities and behaviors, but may "have deficiencies in verbal and nonverbal communication, social interactions, and leisure or play activities." Other characteristics associated with autism may include repetitive body movements such as hand-flapping, difficulty with changes in environment or routines, and unusual responses to sensory experiences (sights, sounds, textures, etc.).

Making a diagnosis of autism is difficult and confusing. It is based primarily observations of a child's behavior. In the *Diagnostic and Statistical Manual* (DSM-IV), four autism-related disorders are classified under the heading Pervasive Developmental Disorders (PDD). A diagnosis of *autistic disorder* is made when the child displays a certain number symptoms as listed in the manual. When children display similar but fewer symptoms, the may receive a diagnosis of *PDD-NOS* (Pervasive Developmental Disorder, not otherwise specified). *Asperger's syndrome* and *Rett's syndrome*, the remaining disorders, are diagnosed on the basis of observing other specified characteristics.

POSSIBLE CAUSES AND TREATMENT STRATEGIES The causes of autism are not known. Currently, researchers are focusing on neurological and biochemical factors. Psychological causes of autism have been investigated and ruled out.

NEUROTRANSMITTER ABNORMALITIES

"One concept is that there are neurotransmitter abnormalities, in particular serotonin, which is derived from the amino acid tryptophan," Dr. Lombard says. "The patients have too much serotonin circulating but it is not performing its duties. So symptoms like anxiety and sleep disorders are common. One of the strategies is to enhance the beneficial effects of serotonin either nutritionally or pharmaceutically. One of the nutritional compounds that increase brain serotonin levels is L-tryptophan, a precursor to serotonin. The herb St. John's wort acts as a serotonin enhancer in the brain. A new compound is the modification of the amino acid SamE which is s-adenosyl methionine, shown to increase brain serotonin levels."

IMMUNE SYSTEM

Dr. Lombard continues, "The immune system is overactivated in many autistic children, meaning they have chronic ear infections or chronic bowel problems. There is some questionable association with immunization with autism although that is certainly not resolved yet.

"Candidiasis or excessive yeast involvement is something we consider in autism. Reducing yeast is very effective in managing some of the symptoms. We administer probiotics like acidophilus which helps increase the natural intestinal bacteria in the gut and reduce the amount of yeast in the gut."

MITOCHONDRIAL FUNCTION

Dr. Rafael Kellman is the founder of the Center of Progressive Medicine, a holistic medical center in New York that integrates alternative and conventional therapies. He also is an internal medicine physician at the Albert Einstein

College of Medicine. He has looked at the mitochondria as a possible cause of autism.

Dr. Kellman says, "There are a number of causes of autism. There are numerous assaults on children today that include antibiotics and vaccinations. The common denominator is damage to the mitochondria. The mitochondria is the part of the cell that produces energy. When we give children random immunizations or frequent antibiotics it not only kills bacteria but it also kills the mitochondria. Mitochondria is part of our own cells that is responsible for producing energy, also called ATP [adenosine triphosphate]."

Dr. Lombard is also looking at the mitochondria. "This is a common theme in neurological diseases," he says. "Some research I'm working on now looks at the mitochondria. It looks like autistic children are not making enough brain ATP, which is a function of the mitochondria."

NUTRITION AND SECRETIN

There has been a lot of talk about nutritional imbalances and autism. Dr. Kellman has looked at this closely and uncovered certain nutritional interventions that have helped these children. He describes his theory.

"Secretin is a gastrointestinal hormone that the gut releases and is sent to the pancreas. If you use this hormone on children with autism you see a significant, positive result. There is significant improvement in many of their physiological parameters. The question is, why would a hormone that works in the gut affect what we thought was a brain disease, a neurological disease? There is a lot of speculation but I believe it marks a whole new way of thinking about autism, and probably many other diseases as well. In the past we thought the gut was just a blind, stupid tube, but the gut is really a brain itself. We are beginning to see that the mind is not localized only in the central nervous system (what we think is the brain) but rather the mind is interwoven into other parts of the body as well. An imbalance in the gut from antibiotics, poor diet, refined carbohydrates, etc., causes not only gastrointestinal disturbances like diarrhea, constipation, bloating, [and] pain, but it also causes some imbalance in the mind, in the brain that is found in the gut. That imbalance can cause all kinds of physiological and neurological problems because it is affecting the brain in the gut, and possibly the connections between the brain in the gut and the brain in the central nervous system.

"Now we can better understand when people use the metaphor 'gut feelings' or 'I feel it in my gut.' We are beginning to see that if you disturb the brain in the gut you are not only disturbing gastrointestinal function but also actually creating autistic children."

Let's review this concept again. Food goes from the intestine into the bloodstream and the nutrients get into the bloodstream. The immune system plays a role in all this. It is complex and Dr. Kellman breaks it down into an understandable form.

"Numerous hormones and enzymes are involved with the digestion of food. If the digestion is not adequate, the ecosystem of the gut, meaning the different microbes that are found in the gut, becomes unbalanced. Deficiencies in hormones or enzymes, or an overgrowth of yeast like candida or other unfriendly bacteria, can create havoc in the gastrointestinal system. Then toxins can be absorbed through the gastrointestinal tract into the bloodstream. This can cause problems within the body and also activate the immune system. Most of the immune system, about 70 percent, is harbored in the gastrointestinal tract. If the gastrointestinal tract is not functioning properly due to dietary problems, antibiotics, or even stress, that creates a secondary problem in the immune system. It would also create a problem in the brain because there are messages being sent from the gut from those food particles that are being digested.

"A number of neurotransmitters and neuropeptides found in the gut are activated by digestive food particles. If there is a problem with that digestion, then the messages that are sent from food to the cells in the gut and to the neurons in the gut break down. Numerous toxins in the body caused by an immune imbalance that can cause a host of medical disorders. Toxins can cause central nervous system dysfunction, allergies, asthma, and a whole variety of autoimmune diseases. The brain in the gut is not going to send proper messages to the higher brain, the organ found in the cranium in the central nervous system. Results of this improper communication are numerous—headaches, chronic fatigue, depression, anxiety, attention deficit disorder, and autism. I believe autism comes from this primary pathology. That is why you see many autistic children with seizure disorders and hyperactivity. What is the common denominator behind all of this? There is something wrong with the nervous system of the gut and the central nervous system."

Dr. Kellman goes on to explain how to correct the imbalance he sees. "The first thing is the use of the hormone secretin. It is a natural hormone found within the body and not foreign to the body. When we inject secretin into these children with autism the results are really quite phenomenal. We have now treated well over 25 children and I would say about 80 percent of these children have significant changes. For example, children who have made no eye contact in the past are now making eye contact. One child who was never able to go to the bathroom by himself and flush the toilet now can. Some children are now hugging their parents or hugging and kissing their siblings, [children] who were never able to do that before. They are sleeping better. We are doing something to the gut and seeing profound psychological and neurological changes. I would say 90 percent of these children have obvious gastrointestinal disturbances and many of these problems are getting better as well. We have seen absolutely no side effects from it.

"However, this has to be cojoined with a comprehensive approach to improving gastrointestinal function, improving the ecosystem found within the gut by changing the diet, removing foods that create havoc within the gut, changing the whole approach to food, diet and life in general. Some of these children need up to 6 to 8 digestive hormone pills and nutra-supplements. Unfortunately the lay audience takes their advice from the press or popular health food magazines, and they say, 'we'll just take digestive enzymes in 1 to 2 tablets.' These children need a lot more digestive enzymes perhaps than I do or you do. Everyone has to be evaluated individually. Some of these children need extremely high doses of digestive enzymes. Some of them need high doses of hydrochloric acid or zinc. They have an increased need, they are not absorbing their nutrients properly and their whole 'metabolic machinery' is vastly different from the average person."

Part of Dr. Kellman's program involves detoxification. With this program he can unload the toxins and support the liver to do a better job of detoxifying the body. "When the gut is imbalanced, numerous toxins are secreted into the bloodstream. They overload the liver and central nervous system and any type of neurological or psychiatric disease can occur. Most doctors dismiss these people as crazy because they don't fit into their medical categories. The detoxification program also involves a number of nutrients that help the liver enzymes so the liver can better detoxify. Each person has a unique biochemical need and therefore the detoxification program has to be tailored to each specific person. Luckily the testing is available to them but of course is not known to most conventional medical doctors."

MEGADOSE VITAMIN THERAPY

Dr. Bernard Rimland, a research psychologist, has done extensive work in childhood disorders. While recognizing the role that load allergies can play in many of these disorders, Dr. Rimland has also explored the role that vitamins in "megadoses" can play in such conditions as autism and hyperactivity. Dr. Rimland focused his research particularly on autism, a condition that manifests before the age of 3.

Dr. Rimland's research, which has been confirmed by researchers in France and around the world, indicates that children with autism have deficiencies in certain nutrients, in particular vitamin B_6. For some unexplained reason, these children require these nutrients in much larger amounts—up to 50 milligrams a day more—than typically developing children, who require only 10 to 15 milligrams daily. To maximize the effectiveness of this B_6 supplementation program, magnesium is also given. It is a very important mineral here because it can dramatically enhance the effectiveness of B_6. In addition, Dr. Rimland gives the rest of the B-complex, zinc, and other complementary minerals. "If that is done," he explains, "the individual's body has the maximum chance of using the vitamin effectively when it is given in large amounts to correct the metabolic error it is prescribed to correct."

Dr. Rimland's studies indicate that between 30 and 50 percent of children treated with vitamin B_6 and other nutrients show significant improvement.

Not only do they improve behaviorally, his studies have shown that their objective tests improve as well. Urine tests run on children with autism indicate that they have much higher concentrations of a phenol called homovanillic acid (HVA). When given vitamin B_6, their HVA levels often normalize along with their behavior. Additionally, certain abnormal brain waves tend to normalize after the treatment. "So," says Dr. Rimland, "the B_6 and magnesium treatment has been shown to improve autism behaviorally, electrophysiologically, and biochemically."

Another study showed that vitamin B_6 is at least as effective as Ritalin in ameliorating hyperactivity in children. The B_6 was found to be safer and cheaper, and its beneficial effects lasted longer. Even though this was a well-documented, carefully controlled double-blind study published in a reputable medical journal (*Biological Psychiatry*) it could not shake most medical professionals from their bias against nutritional approaches to mental and behavioral disorders. "Pediatricians, psychiatrists, and other physicians," observes Dr. Rimland, "continue to give kids Ritalin instead of B_6 to control their hyperactivity."

PART FOUR
Musculoskeletal Fitness

13

Pain Management

A Gallup survey released in 2000 revealed that nearly 90 percent of American adults experience pain at least once a month. Every day millions of people wake up knowing they are going to contend with pain, whether it be from back pain, arthritis, muscle injury, or a host of other conditions. Many believe that they just have to live with the pain. Unfortunately they do not realize that there are varied ways of treating pain naturally.

In this country we need a different approach to acute and chronic pain. We need to go from treating just the symptoms to treating the sufferer holistically. Getting the proper nutrition through sensible eating and ingesting natural supplements, including minerals and herbs, are key ways of treating pain. Other methods such as chiropractic, shiatsu, acupuncture, and the Trager and Alexander techniques also have a part to play. In this chapter, we survey a broad range of healing strategies that can be used by anyone suffering from chronic or occasional pain.

Dr. Art Brownstein, author of *Healing Back Pain Naturally*, is a clinical instructor of medicine at the University of Hawaii who also teaches yoga. He was a back pain patient himself for 20 years. Like many of the 50 million Americans who have chronic back pain, he ended up on an operating table in a futile attempt to relieve his suffering. He describes his experience and how it bolstered his views on alternative healing:

"I've got two vertebrae that are only half way there, and I was getting worse after the surgery to the point where I couldn't work for 3 years as a physician. I got hooked on the narcotic pain pills, and I was depressed and suicidal. At the end of the 3 year period I was offered another operation, at which point I remembered my professors in medical school saying 'physician heal thyself.' To make a long story short, I ended up traveling around the world several times during the next 3 to 7 year period and discovered some very simple, ancient mind-body healing techniques, including yoga, which allowed me not only to heal my own back pain naturally, but also to help thousands of others."

Dr. Brownstein's back pain protocol emphasizes the importance of the muscles in supporting the health of the back. "When people have back pain they automatically assume, because it is so painful, that there must be a problem with the discs or the bones. And that is what conventional medicine focuses on with its diagnostic tests such as MRIs and x-rays. Muscles don't show up on MRIs or x-rays so in performing these tests, physicians are simply bypassing the most important system."

Often, Dr. Brownstein says, the back problem relates to the condition of the muscles. "If you look at other cultures that have very little furniture and very low-tech kind of societies, they have virtually no back pain. We spend so much time sitting down, sitting at our jobs, sitting while we are driving, that these muscles in our back just don't get used....We have to really tone our muscles in our backs and stretch them....Yoga is an effective strategy for this."

Stress management is also part of his program. When people are under mental stress, the nerves are overstimulated. This can cause the muscles, including those of the back, to tighten and contract. If you have pain in your back, it will get worse. "If you don't have pain," Dr. Brownstein says, "you are an accident waiting to happen. Just bending forward and picking a paperclip off the floor can send your back into tremendous spasms." Among the stress management techniques Dr. Brownstein uses are breathing, relaxation, meditation, and visualization.

Diet is also part of Dr. Brownstein's program. He explains, "I've discovered a very strong connection between what you put in your body, and not only every cell and tissue of your body but particularly your back."

Take coffee, for example. "I had a patient who had been to the top specialists all over the country—the Mayo Clinic, John Hopkins, Harvard," Dr. Brownstein says. "[T]hey all were recommending surgery for him. I asked him about his diet and he was drinking 8 to 10 cups of coffee a day. I asked him if he would be willing to quit it and reluctantly he agreed. Of course he had the caffeine withdrawal headaches but after 2 to 3 days he got over that. Within 3 weeks his back pain was totally cleared up. So it can be something that simple."

Diet

As Dr. Brownstein's example shows, one of the most important ways to combat back and other types of pain is by guiding your diet to avoid abrasive foods and concentrate on those that build up the body's biochemistry. You should eat in the same way you should drive—defensively.

It seems that people are really taking a new look at diet, especially people who used to think that relief from aches and pains could come only from a jar or bottle or from even more drastic remedies like surgery. Not in every case, but in many cases, we're finding that diet can be the most powerful medicine.

One physician who has been looking is Dr. Neal Barnard, author *of Food That Fights Pain* and president of the Physicians' Committee for Responsible Medicine, a nationwide group that promotes preventive medicine and address-es controversies in modern medicine.

As he sees it, there are four ways in which pain is manifested in the usual course of an illness. He uses arthritis as an example. First, there is some type of injury. Second, there is inflammation with redness, swelling, and stiffness. Third, there is irritation of the nerves that transmit the pain signals to the brain. Fourth, the brain receives the signals.

Dr. Barnard explains that there are three steps that must be taken in using diet to help with health problems. First, it is necessary to look for possible trig-ger foods. These are foods that commonly set off pain: dairy products, wheat or citrus for some people, tomatoes, meat, and eggs. "We want to do a little detec-tive work and see which one is a trigger for an individual, because the triggers may be different for each person," Dr. Barnard counsels.

The second step is to find out which foods are safe to eat. "We focus on the pain-safe foods, which is fairly simple to do."

The third step, which Dr. Barnard believes is especially necessary for women, is to use foods to balance hormones, especially if the pain is associated with menstrual or breast pain. Because low-fat, vegetarian diets reduce hor-mone swings and stop the overly aggressive thickening of the uterine lining that is often aggravated by a bad diet, they can dramatically reduce pain.

Dr. Barnard summarizes: "If we put these all together, what we are going to do is tailor the diet intervention to the individual's condition. Getting away from the animal products is certainly very important if you want to open up the arteries again, but if you have migraines or arthritis, we want to look at the specific food triggers. Sometimes that can be a food that would otherwise be quite healthy, such as a tomato or a grapefruit. If you are sensitive to them, you should learn that."

The most striking thing in Dr. Barnard's plan is that a patient doesn't have to be resigned to making a difficult diet change for a long period of time. Positive results often occur quite quickly. If a person has arthritis, for example, it may take as little as 10 days on a new diet to see a difference.

FOODS THAT WEAKEN RESISTANCE TO PAIN In contrast to normally innocuous foods such as strawberries, which may trigger a pain reaction in certain people, some foods may weaken the body's ability to resist pain. Coffee is one of those foods.

Dr. Barnard mentions sugar as another substance that lowers a person's pain tolerance. "Sugar never gets good press, and I'm sorry I have to add to the list of its problems. In a research study, people have taken volunteers and put a little metal clip on the web of skin between the fingers. Then this clip is hooked up to an electrical generator. The participants are given a little bit of electrical energy, which is gradually increased, and asked when they can feel it and when it becomes intolerable. Those numbers are written down. Then they are given sugar and the progression is repeated. These studies find that after ingesting the sugar, they feel the pain sooner and it becomes intolerable sooner.

"The same is true with people with diabetes. If you have adult-onset diabetes, when you have high blood sugar, you are more likely to feel pain more acutely. You are more likely to feel it sooner and find it intolerable at lower levels. Something about sugar changes brain chemistry so that pain is more intense.

"I've been so struck by the fact that people would start their breakfast with a cup of coffee, which reduces pain, then add a little sugar, which will increase pain sensitivity. It goes on for the rest of the day, where we are mixing up foods that cause and reduce pain."

PAIN-SAFE FOODS Pain-safe foods include rice—any kind of rice, but especially brown rice—and cooked green vegetables such as broccoli, Swiss chard, and spinach. If you get an upset stomach from broccoli, cook it a little longer; this knocks out some of the vitamins, but the proteins in the broccoli are what cause stomach irritation in some people. Also, cooked orange vegetables such as sweet potatoes and carrots are pain-safe. Cooked yellow vegetables such as squash are also good. For fruits, pick the noncitrus ones, especially dried or cooked.

PAIN-REDUCING FOODS Dr. Barnard has also found that some overlooked foods are especially good for dealing with pain. "One of the things that we like to use is hot peppers, jalapeno peppers. The zing in the jalapeno is from a chemical called capsaicin. This doesn't just make your mouth hot, it actually changes what happens in the nerves. It stops the nerves from being able to conduct pain. Pharmaceutical manufacturers have taken this capsaicin straight out of the pepper and mixed it into a cream, which is applied externally. Two brands of capsaicin cream in the United States are Capsin and Zostrix.

"Capsaicin can be useful if you have superficial pain, such as the pain of shingles, which can be just miserable, or if you have mastectomy pain. At first when you put on the capsaicin, it tingles and may even burn a little just as a hot pepper would. Do it day after day, and gradually the pain will diminish. You will still feel touch and pressure, but you won't feel pain. Give it a couple of weeks to work."

Herbal Remedies

Herbs eliminate pain by dealing with the underlying causes. There are different types of pain. Some are inflammatory, hot, and pounding. Some are due to toxins in the body that need to be cleansed. Proper herbal treatment can help the body do away with both the pain and the causes of the pain.

For women, herbalist Letha Hadady offers the following recommendations: "We must approach the pain of PMS (premenstrual syndrome) from both the emotional and physical sides. Emotionally, there are two types of PMS. One is the angry type. Aloe root is recommended for this. It cleans the system and cleanses the liver. It may taste a little bitter, but it is easy to take when added to a little apple juice. A stronger gall bladder and liver cleanser that lessens the impact of 'angry' menstrual pains is the Chinese preparation *lung tanxieganwan*. Twenty percent ginseng, it aids digestion and reduces anger. It also calms and quiets headaches and other pains.

"The second type of PMS is weepy. It comes from sadness and excess phlegm brought on by eating foods that are too rich, sweet, and oily or by drinking too much milk. Eating radishes, parsley, or barley soup will cut down on the phlegm. A remedy for this type of pain is homeopathic pulsatilla."

To treat both types of menstrual pain, warming herbs such as cinnamon and myrrh are invaluable. Capsules or drops taken in tea will increase blood circulation and clean the uterus, inducing a more complete period that does not start too early, stay too long, or finish early only to begin prematurely. A warming and cooling remedy for the pain is as follows:

1/2 cup of aloe vera gel

10 drops or one capsule of myrrh

Apple juice This combines the cleaning action of myrrh with the cooling of aloe.

Vitamins, Minerals, and Other Supplements

Most people know that minerals are essential for building up the body, maintaining the body's fluid balance, and helping with many chemical reactions. Let us look specifically at how minerals and vitamins have proved effective in treating pain.

Dr. Luke Bucci, the author of *Pain Free: The Definitive Guide to Healing Arthritis*, states that for handling spinal problems, carpal tunnel syndrome, or arthritis, an antidepressant may be helpful. Carpal tunnel syndrome occurs when repetitive tasks cause the tendons in the wrist to become inflamed; this squeezes the nerves, which then tingle and go numb. About one-third of cases can be cured by the administration of vitamin B_6 (100 mg/day) to which can be added vitamin B_2 (50 mg/day). To deal with the pain of the condition, one should take St. John's wort (Hypericum perforatum). This substance has a molecule that works like a pharmaceutical drug without any of the drawbacks or side effects.

Magnesium salts are also useful for those with pain from torso or joint aches. Many people are already deficient in magnesium. This calmative mineral is obtained from nuts and seeds that are raw and not roasted. Nuts are also beneficial in that they contain essential oils, including the omega-3 fatty acids, which also have mild anti-inflammatory properties that help reduce pain. For torso and joint problems, intake of magnesium citrate salts should be 400 milligrams per day, divided into doses of 100 to 200 milligrams.

Sound sleep is an essential part of good health. For people who have trouble sleeping due to headaches or other pains, there are a number of useful supplements. Valerian, hops (the same element found in beer), skullcap, or passionflower can be used. These supplements, which can be mixed, should be taken a half hour before going to sleep, in either capsule (one or two) or tincture form. You might also try taking 1 milligram of melatonin before sleep.

For the pain arising from PMS, GLA (gamma-linolenic acid) is valuable. It can be obtained from evening primrose oil, black currant seed oil, or borage oil. The sufferer should take three to six pills per day. As an adjunct to GLA, vitamin E is helpful. Also to be taken is vitamin B_6 (100 mg/day) and magnesium, which smoothes muscle contractions.

Here as with all vitamin therapy, the patient must follow through, taking the supplements consistently for two or three months, to be assured of the effects.

The pain of sciatica, a pinched nerve running down the leg, can be reduced by reducing the inflammation at the nerve root. Here one should try a proteolytic enzyme such as bromelain, papain, trypsin, or chymotrypsin to support the body's natural healing properties.

General musculoskeletal pain can be relieved by a number of substances. L-carnitine allows the body to burn fats and soak up excess lactate, which may be causing pain. Also helpful with muscle aches are the methyl donors, such as DMG (dimethyl glycine) and TMG (trimethyl glycerin), taken in doses of 100 milligrams per day.

To reduce the soreness after exercise, one should take vitamin E (400 to 800 IU/day), which prevents the leakage of enzymes from the muscles.

A final way to approach pain is to modify the way the brain perceives it. DL-phenylalanine (DLPA), which is a synthetic amino acid, slows down endorphins, making the ones you have work better. Taken in a dosage of 500 milligrams three times a day, it reduces chronic pain while getting the sufferer off analgesics.

Chiropractic

Chiropractic treatment involves the manual manipulation of vertebrae that become misaligned, causing nerve pressure and energy blocks to various organs. This manipulation is called an adjustment. It involves the chiropractor's gentle application of direct pressure to the spine and joints. The chiropractor may squeeze or twist the torso, pull or twist the limbs, or wrench the head or back. What the chiropractor is doing is readjusting the spinal column to restore the normal vertebral relationship. This eliminates the body's energy blocks and keeps life-sustaining energy flowing freely to the vital organs.

Chiropractic is effective in dealing with pain and as a preventive treatment because it relieves nerve pressure. The buildup of this pressure is cumulative in its erosion of the health and integrity of specific body organs or regions. If one vertebra is out of relationship to the one next to it, a state of disrelationship is said to exist. This disrelationship throws off that vertebra's environment, that is, the blood supply and detoxifying lymphatic drainage surrounding it. When this occurs, a congestion of blood, toxins, and energy creates pressure that upsets both local and systemic homeostasis, or balance.

Tissues all need normal nerve functioning in order to transport required nutrients to the cells. Insofar as the vertebrae are misaligned, the blood becomes congested and slow in its delivery, creating the absence of this nutrient supply. The cell's normal activity is thereby hindered, and it becomes irritated. Moreover, once the cell's metabolic processing is interfered with, its waste-removing lymphatic servicing to that area is diminished. This leads to toxic buildup that causes further irritation and inflammation. The chiropractor is concerned with alleviating all these problems.

Acupuncture

Acupuncture sees pain as being derived from blocked energy or *qi (chi)*. In treating this blockage, the practitioner has to determine whether it stems from an overabundance or a deficiency in energy, so that treatment can be adjusted depending on whether it is necessary to strengthen or decrease *qi*.

The acupuncturist first records the patient's medical history in the manner of a conventional doctor. Then, with the patient lying down or seated, depending on the area to be treated, fine-gauge, stainless steel needles are inserted into significant points and meridians to exert different physiological effects on the body and induce both relaxation and energization. The patient will remain in this position for 20 to 30 minutes, though an appointment with an acupuncturist may last up to an hour, since part of the time will be spent consulting about the employment of other traditional and herbal treatments that might be recommended. Bodywork and massage may also be included in the session.

Dr. Christopher Trahan notes that the treatment will have analgesic and anesthetic effects, block pain, and accelerate recovery from motor nerve injury. Moreover, it enhances the immune system, which has a sedative effect; helps with muscular spasms or neurological problems; has a homeostatic effect in that it helps balance blood pressure; and has positive psychological effects, acting directly on brain chemistry.

Many patients with chronic low back pain find that acupuncture will not only help break the pain cycle, but also allow them to reduce pain medications and participate more vigorously in physical therapy. Dr. Emily Kane, a naturopath who practices in Juneau, Alaska, says in an article on the website of the American Association of Naturopathic Physicians (www.naturopathic.org) that experiments have shown that acupuncture stimulates the nervous system to release endorphins as well as other chemical pain relievers in the body. Some people get immediate relief from low back pain after the first acupuncture session, but she recommends having six or eight sessions within a short period of time before assessing whether or not it is working for you.

Bodywork

SHIATSU Shiatsu is based on the principle that a vital energy, called *qi (chi)*, flows through the body. The primary cause of pain is an imbalance of this energy. The goal of the healer is to balance the client's energy so that pain and discomfort do not manifest or, if they do appear, will be relieved.

As bodywork practitioner Thomas Claire explains, thumbs, fingers, palms, forearms, elbows, and even knees are used to apply pressure to specified points in the body to modulate the flow of energy. During a shiatsu treatment, the client lies on the floor on a comfortable padded surface, such as a futon, fully clothed or undressed to her or his level of comfort. What the client feels is pressure, which can be gentle or deeper at the places where the practitioner is working. As the pressure continues, the patient generally feels relaxed and energized at the same time.

Shiatsu is good for treating a variety of different pains. It is especially beneficial in combating chronic pain in the back, neck, or shoulders, but it has also proved effective in treating whiplash, herniated discs, and problems affecting the nervous system, such as Bell's palsy.

A shiatsu healer concentrates on certain pressure points that have metaphoric names that tell us something about what they do or how they are to be worked with.

The first point of interest is on the ankle and called Spleen 6. It is at the meeting of three yin meridians and is the most powerful point for tonifying the feminine energy in the body. It can be located by placing the little finger on the border of the inside ankle and counting up four fingers. At the very top of these fingers, and at the center, is Spleen 6. To modulate the energy, you can put pressure on this point with your thumb, pushing three times in succession for 7 to 10 seconds each time. This pressure will stimulate the feminine energy, helping a woman control PMS and irregular cycles. Moreover, since all people have feminine and masculine sides, use of this point can also be beneficial to men and can help with sexual problems such as impotence.

The corresponding point for male tonification is called Stomach 36. To locate this point, find the indentation just outside the kneecap. Put one finger at this indentation and go down four fingers. There you'll find Stomach 36, which is also known as Leg 3 Mile. This second name is given since, it is said, if you have a strong Stomach 36, you will have enough stamina to walk three miles with no trouble. Manipulation of this point can lead to a tonification of masculine energy as well as the whole body. For women, this point can be used to ease childbirth and labor pains.

A third important point, located at the middle of the web of the hand, is Large Intestine 4, also called Meeting Mountains. The latter name is derived from the "mountain of flesh" found jutting up between the thumb and index finger when you close your hand. To locate this point, find the highest point on that protruding flesh and then open your hand. This point should be pressed three times running for 7 to 10 seconds to tonify the upper body. Pressing this point can also help with nausea, vomiting, colds, and constipation.

Pericardium 6, or the Inner Gate, is found on the forearm. If you flex your hand, you'll find two tendons that pop up on the inside of your wrist. Go up these tendons and press. This point is particularly good for controlling nausea, such as that from morning sickness or motion sickness.

Another valuable point is found right in the middle of the palm. Pressing it can relieve tension such as that arising from a stressful work environment or relationship.

Runny nose, allergy, colds, and sinus infections can be treated by putting pressure on the point called Welcome Smell, so named since nearly any smell is welcome to a person whose nasal passages have been blocked. To approach this point, take the index finger and bring it in at a 45-degree angle to the crease under the nose. This pressure can be applied on either side of the nose, although it is not recommended that both sides be touched simultaneously because this might interfere with breathing.

In fact, all these pressures can be applied to either side of the body, since the meridians are bilateral and bring the same energies to each side of the body.

TRAGER TECHNIQUE The Trager technique is a way of working with the mind and body simultaneously. According to the philosophy behind this technique, pain comes from the accumulated action of the patient frequently tightening his or her movements and posture. To correct it, the practitioner uses gentle motions to increase the patient's pleasure in the quality of the tissues and decrease the restriction and the sense of holding. The practice works by reaching into the functional subconscious with particular qualities of movement, posture, and sensation. Gentleness is emphasized so that no message will be sent to the body alerting it that pain is on the way or causing the patient to tighten up. The movement reaches into the central nervous system with a motion at once pleasurable, lengthening, softening, and opening, conveying this sensation to the tissues and joints. The movements can be very small and internal or can be done at the periphery of the body in the limbs. In the latter case, the limbs are used as handles to reach the core.

Roger Tolle, a Trager practitioner, says that some clients will feel results immediately as the touching allows them to release pain. In other cases, it takes a repetition of the information into the body and mind, which will gradually allow the client to relearn how to go about daily activity with a different quality of motion.

The Trager method works particularly well against pain in the temporo-mandibular joint (TMJ), neck, back, pelvis, and carpal tunnel.

ALEXANDER TECHNIQUE Jane Kosminsky, an Alexander technique teacher, describes this modality: "The Alexander technique is an educational tool that teaches us first how to balance our heads well at the top of the spine. It teaches the correct use and relationship of the head to the spine and the spine to the limbs. We deal with the problems of the lower back, the arm or the leg by focusing first on the balance of the head and its relationship to the spine."

Actual exercise is not part of the Alexander program. "In Alexander we don't do exercise, we don't try to fix ourselves," Kosminsky says. "We notice what we are doing and then we make the decision to say no to a habit that is not good for us. For example, we note excessive tension, crunching in the spine, pulling in the shoulders, and then we use the technique of visualization to effect change."

ROLFING According to the practitioners of Rolfing, pain is due to chronic short-enings in the tissue. Correction of this pain can be accomplished through soft tissue manipulation. This manipulation acts to create order in the body so the client stands tall and free of restriction.

David Frome, a physical therapist, states that Rolfing is done in a 10-session series designed to address all the shortenings in the structure systematically. Each session works in a different area. In the first hour, for instance, concentration is on the trunk, shoulders, and hips. In the second hour, work is done on the back and lower leg. Going through the complete series allows the therapist to work through all the body's shortenings. During a session, a patient may experience a tingling sensation and a sense of release. The patient should strive to draw the deepest possible breath to aid in treatment.

The major goal of the treatment is not pain relief per se, but it has been found to help with TMJ pain, frozen shoulder, tennis elbow, carpal tunnel syndrome, chronic hip problems, sciatica, cervical neuropathies, and knee, foot, and ankle problems.

CRANIOSACRAL THERAPY The sacral region is at the bottom of the spine. Between it and the head there should be a balanced rhythmic motion maintained for the health of the organism. When pain arises, it may be due to a restriction that disturbs the harmony between these two regions or between them and the rest of the body.

In craniosacral therapy, the practitioner places his or her hands on the client's body in such a way as to try to bring the cranium (skull) and sacrum back into alignment, reestablishing a natural rhythm. Charles A. Kaplan, the founder and director of the Center for Pain Management, points out that this hands-on technique usually centers on touching the head or lower back but can be done anywhere, such as on the fingers or toes. Some patients will go through a first treatment and not feel anything, but most will leave the treatment table feeling very relaxed and stress-free.

Craniosacral therapy is recommended for dealing with muscular and skeletal pain, headaches, pains in the back and neck, sports injuries, sciatica, and nerve pain. It can also be beneficial to those recovering from pneumonia or bronchitis, helping by loosening the ribcage. Craniosacral therapy is a tremendous stress reducer.

Magnet Therapy

With an ancestry as old as that of acupuncture and shiatsu, magnet therapy also acts to influence the body's energy. Dr. Jim Joseph mentions that the healing power of magnets was known in China over 4,000 years ago. Such ancient fathers of medicine as Galen and Aristotle discussed magnets, as did Paracelsus, one of the founders of chemistry. The value of magnet therapy was a tenet of Mesmer and others in the 19th century and is still being developed and practiced today.

Down through history, magnets have been used to deal with the causes of various ailments. As Dr. Joseph remarks, "Pain is a messenger. We don't want to kill the messenger but find the cause."

Pain in the body can be caused by positive energy being drawn to the site of injury. To bring about this transfer, the brain sends out a negative signal. Using the negative side of a magnet can augment and assist that reaction. Furthermore, around an injury there will be an acidic buildup. The negative side of the magnet is an alkalizing force that can help alleviate the pain accompanying this acidity.

A second source of pain arises when a person is overworked or suffering from undue stress, causing that person's cells to be overly positively charged. Putting a negative magnet on a weakened area will repolarize the cells, restoring the balance between positive and negative charge.

The distortion of the cells' polarity and resultant pain may also be caused by our technological environment. We are swamped with positive electromagnetic pulses coming from televisions, radios, electric clocks, and all the other electrical devices around us. The pulses of their fields are not congruent with the one found in our body and can throw us into disharmony and disease.

Magnets can be obtained in a plastiform case that can be molded and shaped for a particular area. They last indefinitely and are low priced. A medium-sized magnet may cost $20. Healing magnets are color-coded with the negative pole green and the positive red. The positive side of the magnet is active and sun-oriented; the negative side is relaxing and earth-oriented. All the treatments discussed here utilize the negative pole. One must be careful with the positive pole, since positive magnetism causes growth in any biological system, even cancer. Treatment should last from 20 minutes to overnight. The magnet's power should be from 1,000 to 6,000 gauss.

A magnet can be wrapped with Velcro on the area to be covered. Special wraps in which the magnets are inlaid in Velcro are available. These wraps can be placed on most parts of the body, though they should not be used on the eyes. Negative magnetism attracts fluids and gases, and a negative magnet placed near the eye would draw out its fluids. If work is to be done on the eyes, the magnet can be placed off to the side. From this position, magnetism can be exerted on cataracts to reduce oxidation and free radical development. The magnet's value in reducing oxidation is due to the fact that oxygen is paramagnetic. When you breathe, you are pulling negative energy from the earth into your body.

At night, it is useful to lie on a magnetic bed pad and put magnets behind the head, where they will bathe the pineal gland in energy. This will induce a restful night's sleep. By using a magnet, one can feel rested even after sleeping fewer hours than one normally does. The magnet has also been known to increase sexual abilities.

The magnet can help with shoulder pain, pain in the rotator cuff, and aches in the lumbar region of the back. Magnets can be attached to the head or neck to deal with hypothyroidism, depression, migraine headaches, and problems with the vestibular system. For depression, the magnet should be placed near the occipital lobe.

The Mind-Body Connection

Some therapists, like Dr. Art Brownstein mentioned at the beginning of this chapter, recommend a more eclectic approach, one that looks for and relies on the often-overlooked synergies that flow between the mind and the body. Dr. Ron Dushkin brings up a number of points to consider in dealing with pain. He notes first the importance of relaxation, which will quiet and calm the nervous system. Remember that when we feel pain, we also are feeling a layer of stress on top of that pain. If the layer of stress is relieved, the pain will diminish significantly.

Human touch can also play a part in relieving pain. As babies we like to be touched and as adults we still find this important.

A third overlooked factor in healing is humor. The writer Norman Cousins tells the story of how he was hospitalized with a critical health problem. As he saw it, a lot of his physical deterioration was due to stress and negative thoughts from that stress. He reasoned that if we can create disease with stress, then by alleviating stress through means such as humor, we can cure disease. He had a movie projector brought into his hospital room and began showing Marx

Brothers films and other comedies. Soon his room became a place of congregation for other patients who wanted to enjoy the shows. It got rather chaotic because so many people were coming into his room and laughing. You're not supposed to laugh in a hospital. Some people were scandalized. Cousins said that the doctors would give him blood tests before and after he had been laughing at a humorous film and would find an improvement after the film. He also had less pain after laughing.

Guided imagery is also an element of the mind-body connection. With this technique, a sufferer places a hand over the injured area and invites the other cells in the body to go to the aid of the damaged area. After all, the body's cells always work together, and this is one way to encourage their interplay.

All the methods mentioned as part of the mind-body connection get the patient to take charge of personal recovery. Many people are strong in many areas of life—pursuing a career, forming good relationships, playing sports—but when it comes to their own health, they turn over all control to a doctor. To really escape pain, the patient must play a big role in the recovery process.

24

Arthritis

More than 40 million Americans suffer from some form of arthritis. Some 250,000 children have the disease, and its prevalence is rapidly increasing. We know the kind of discomfort this can mean: swollen joints and excruciating pain. It can be so bad it prevents a person from having a quality life.

With so many millions suffering from arthritis, maybe we should be thinking of something by way of treatment other than simply dulling the pain with drugs or performing dangerous and expensive operations. As you will see in reading this chapter, alternative practitioners have been thinking this way for years with quite astounding results.

There are signs that alternative therapies are starting to gain some of the recognition they so rightly deserve. A report published in March 2000 in the *Journal of the American Medical Association* concluded that two popular nutritional supplements, glucosamine and chondroitin compounds, are safe and "have some efficacy in treating osteoarthritis symptoms."

The Arthritis Industry

More than 15 years ago, *The New York Times* ran an article on arthritis in its Sunday business section. The title, "Arthritis: Building an Industry on Pain," together with its placement in the business section (as opposed to the health, lifestyle, or human interest section), gave the article a uniquely realistic point of view. For many people, arthritis is not a health issue per se but a very lucrative growth industry. Although the article is an old one, this view remains prevalent. Using the example of Ann, a fairly typical arthritis sufferer, the article reveals how the symptomatic approach to arthritis that is typical of traditional medicine offers little in the way of health benefits while providing tremendous profit-making opportunities for those involved in the arthritis industry.

Ann began to suffer from arthritis at age 28. She was walking downstairs when her knees suddenly gave out, followed by a sharp burning pain. Ann's doctors diagnosed her as having rheumatoid arthritis and started her on an arduous and expensive journey through the maze of treatments used to battle arthritis in the United States. According to the *Times*, Ann spent more than $200 a year on medication (this is probably a very conservative estimate compared with the amount most arthritis sufferers spent on antiarthritics during that period, and of course, medical costs have increased since the article was written in 1985).

This included a daily dosage of 8 to 10 Ecotrin (aspirin) tablets, a prescription pain reliever, and 5 milligrams of the steroid prednisone. She visited the doctor at least once a month at $20 to $50 a visit. Even with all this medication and regular medical attention, Ann was physically incapacitated. She found it necessary to acquire a number of new arthritic devices designed to replace her ever-decreasing mobility: $35 for a walker, $25 for a set of canes, $15 for a reacher to get objects from shelves or retrieve them from the floor, and $130 for a padded bathtub seat. Ann also had four joints replaced at a cost of $15,000 per joint. "And so," the article concluded, "Ann is one of the nearly 40 million consumers of the arthritis industry. It may sound odd to label arthritis as an industry, but in fact any disease—cancer, diabetes, AIDS—is not only an affliction, it is an employer. For thousands of people and scores of companies, battling arthritis is a livelihood."

The *Times* estimated that arthritis costs this nation $8 billion to $10 billion annually in medical bills and adds to those figures another $7 billion in lost wages and taxes resulting from absenteeism.

Arthritis medications are one of the pharmaceutical industry's biggest and most lucrative products. Additionally, according to the *Times*:

"Drug company estimates suggest that arthritis relief accounts for anywhere from one-third to one-half of the $900 million in annual aspirin sales.
"Some arthritis sufferers gulp down as many as 10,000 aspirin tablets a year, 30 a day. The extra-big bottles, with as many as 1,000 tablets, are earmarked for arthritis sufferers.

"It is hard to pinpoint how much drug-makers earn from arthritis because antiarthritis products also are taken for headaches, trick knees, and the many other guises of pain. But when one considers all the drugs that find use in fighting arthritis, the market bulges to something close to $3 billion in retail sales, according to analysts. Over-the-counter sales make up more than half of that total, but the swiftest growth comes from prescription drugs."

The arthritis industry remains extremely lucrative today. According to the Arthritis Foundation, the estimated annual cost of arthritis to the economy is some $72 billion in medical care and a whopping $77 billion in indirect costs such as lost wages. Additionally, according to the foundation, individuals with rheumatic disease average eight doctor visits per year, twice the average number for persons with other conditions.

The arthritis establishment, which includes the pharmaceutical companies, special-interest organizations such as the Arthritis Foundation, and specialized medical personnel such as rheumatologists, physical therapists, and surgeons, has consistently maintained that arthritis is an incurable disease. Therapeutically, this translates into the possible need for physical therapy, ad hoc surgical intervention to replace joints, and a lifetime of medication that, even if it is effective at relieving pain, does nothing to address the cause or arrest the progression of the disease. Economically, addressing arthritis as an incurable disease is a prescription for steady long-term profits.

What Is Arthritis?

The word "arthritis" means pain and swelling of the joints. A joint is the place where two bones meet. Cartilage covers the end of each bone and prevents the bones from rubbing together. The joint capsule surrounds the joint and protects it. Special membranes surround the joint and cover it with a fluid that lubricates it. Muscles and ligaments around the joint provide support and make it move. When all these parts are working right, the joint moves smoothly and easily, but when something is wrong with the joint, arthritis may develop.

There are many types of arthritis. Some of the most common are described below.

Osteoarthritis

Osteoarthritis, also known as degenerative joint disease, is the most common form of chronic arthritis. It is estimated to affect more than 20 million Americans. In osteoarthritis, the cartilage is worn away so that the bones rub against each other. When the cartilage breaks down, the joint may lose its shape. The ends of the bone may thicken and form spurs

Adds Dr. Jason Theodosakis, whose treatment program is profiled later in this chapter: "At a biochemical level, the breakdown of cartilage is happening more rapidly than the buildup of cartilage. That brings up an important point. Cartilage on the end of the bones is not like a pencil eraser, which, once it is rubbed off, is gone. It is constantly breaking down and being replaced."

Osteoarthritis most often affects middle-aged and older people. Many people consider it a part of the aging process. The joints of the fingers, neck, low back, and legs are usually involved. Symptoms include joint pain, tenderness, stiffness, loss of function, and restricted mobility. Diagnosis is made by physical examination, x-rays, and ruling out other types of arthritis.

Rheumatoid Arthritis

Rheumatoid arthritis, one of the most destructive forms of arthritis, is a severe inflammatory condition that affects the joints as well as other body organs. It is an autoimmune disease in which the body attacks its own tissue. More than 60 percent of the 2 million Americans with rheumatoid arthritis are middle-aged women. Symptoms include pain and swelling in many joints, morning stiffness, afternoon fatigue, and low-grade fevers. Significant joint deformity and disability may occur.

Rheumatoid arthritis can be difficult to diagnose. It often begins gradually and may resemble other types of arthritis. The condition is unpredictable, marked by episodes of remission and exacerbation.

Gout

Gout is a form of inflammatory arthritis caused by excess uric acid in the body. This excess can result from overproduction by the body itself, decreased elimination by the kidneys, or increased consumption of foods containing purines, which are metabolized into uric acid. Foods that are particularly high in purines include meats and seafood. Alcohol also increases uric acid levels. Acid crystals, which build up and congregate in the joints, are identified as invaders by the body's white blood cells. The cells attack the joints, creating painful episodes of inflammation.

Acute gouty arthritis is a sudden affliction that may last a few days to a few weeks and then disappear temporarily. Usually just one or a few joints are affected. In most cases, the big toe is the initial target. Often a person is awakened from sleep with intense pain. Gout tends to run in families, and commonly affects overweight men in middle age. Gout also may result from blood disorders or cancers, or from the use of certain drugs. The symptoms of gout may appear following periods of excessive eating or drinking, or physical or mental stress.

Causes of Arthritis

A host of factors are triggers for people who are genetically susceptible to arthritis. All in all, arthritis seems to be an accumulation of deficits of which we are unaware. This is Dr. Ray Wunderlich's opinion: "We talk about inadequate repairs, inadequate defenses for our body. As we go along with inadequate food, digestion, metabolism, and porosity of gut, we develop increasing levels of immune disturbance, and the joints are a major place where this manifests. That may be because of their movement or because of the tremendous amount of connective tissue around them."

Connective tissue disorders are very common in our society. Connective tissue needs high amounts of vitamin C, glucosamine, and appropriate minerals such as silica, magnesium, zinc, and pantothenic acid. "Without these," says Dr. Wunderlich, "there will be a decline of the connective tissue, which is the glue that keeps our bodies together. As the body sails along through space in our journey through life, we get bombarded with more and more toxins. Rachel Carson was right. It's a toxic planet, and it's not getting any better."

At this point, I want to underline how central environmental stress is to arthritis, as it is to so many other illnesses. There has been an intellectual blind spot on our medical, health, and legislative screens. We look out there and we see herbicides, pesticides, genetically engineered foods, pollution in our water—so much new pollution that government regulators cannot even abide by the old standards, and so they keep raising the allowable amount of toxins in the body.

Once, for example, they said we had to maintain zero tolerance of PCPs. Then they found that many people had 2 parts per million of PCPs in their bodies, and so they just raised the standards and said that was allowable. But then they discovered that people had more that that in their bodies, and so they said 5 parts per million were allowable. Then it went to 10 parts. And people were saying, "Gee whiz, why don't you clean up the environment and stop raising the body's tolerance levels because there are no studies showing that we can actually tolerate this stuff?" There are 100,000 man-made chemicals, and there is no way to understand what's going to happen when they are synergistically mixed in our diet, air, and water.

We always have this risk-benefit ratio in government studies, where the risk is always to the consumer and the benefit is always to the manufacturer. It's never reversed.

Traditional Diagnosis and Treatment

Typically, arthritis is diagnosed on the basis of a patient's symptoms, which most commonly include pain or swelling in the joint areas or some limitation of movement. Some diagnostic tests and x-rays may show abnormalities in the joints, but often these tests are not accurate. Thus, the patient's symptoms are the central factor in determining the diagnosis.

Because medical students have been taught that there is no cure for arthritis, as doctors they do not look for the cause of the disease but instead focus on alleviating the symptoms. This approach can be very dangerous because many of the drugs used to counteract pain and swelling can have serious side effects. Even aspirin, which is ordinarily considered one of the least toxic medications and normally constitutes the first line of attack in the traditional treatment of arthritis, is not without side effects. In the treatment of arthritis, aspirin is given in large doses on a constant basis. Consequently, arthritis patients have consistently high levels of aspirin in their systems; this can result in dizziness, ringing in the ears, intestinal tract bleeding, and kidney damage.

When aspirin does not work or when an arthritis sufferer develops adverse reactions to it, other medications called nonsteroidal anti-inflammatory drugs (NSAIDs), such as the widely advertised Motrin, are used to control inflammation. Since these drugs are nonsteroidal (i.e., do not contain cortisone), they are less toxic than are some medications commonly used to combat inflammation, but they nevertheless have side effects.

NSAIDs came onto the market as effective alternatives to aspirin, which had caused internal bleeding in many long-term users. Ironically, while the NSAIDs are less effective than aspirin as anti-inflammatories, they also have side effects that include gastrointestinal bleeding and peptic ulcers. Other side effects include dizziness, nervousness, nausea, vomiting, and ringing in the ears. If these drugs are unsuccessful, doctors often prescribe cortisone-derived drugs such as prednisone. These drugs are notorious for their severe toxicity. They interfere with the immune system, leaving the patient defenseless against infection and other diseases. Cortisone-type drugs also interfere with the body's healing ability, and it is not uncommon for a person taking these drugs to have bone fractures or wounds that do not heal for long periods.

Some rheumatologists (doctors who treat arthritis patients) use gold injections. This method of treatment was abandoned years ago because it was considered too dangerous, but today gold treatments are finding their way back into medical practice. Another technique finding acceptance among arthritis doctors is the use of chemotherapy drugs. The theory behind this drastic measure is that when a patient's immune system is knocked out, the patient's body is no longer able to form the antibodies that may be causing the inflammation in his or her joints. Other techniques include radiation therapy in the area of the inflammation, again with the intent of destroying the patient's immune response, and plasmaphersis, a procedure by which a patient's blood is drained, filtered to remove antibodies, and then reinjected into the patient.

While the traditional medical approach to arthritis is undeniably becoming more sophisticated, it also appears to be missing the mark. Not only do these treatments fail to get at the cause of the disease, they are becoming more expensive, invasive, and toxic and lead to the inevitable question, Do the ends justify the means? When traditional medicine begins to turn to anticancer therapies to treat arthritis—therapies that often are cancer-causing themselves and result in side effects ranging from nausea, hair and weight loss, to depletion of the immune system—this question becomes even more pressing.

Dr. Warren Levin of Physicians for Complementary Medicine recalls that a couple of years ago the American Medical Association (AMA) put out a series of videotapes to teach physicians how to take care of and diagnose rheumatoid arthritis. The lecturer on the tape was adamant that nutrition has nothing to do with arthritis: "His whole face filled the screen, and he said, 'Nutrition has no place in the treatment of arthritis. We can use drugs.' That is the AMA way. They have not come to Physicians for Complementary Medicine to see what success we have with our methods and how the vast majority of our patients dramatically improve without the use of the toxic drugs that characterize American medicine's treatment of arthritis."

Alternative Treatments

"The way I treat arthritis is probably quite different from the approach of most physicians," says Dr. Peter D'Adano, a naturopathic physician. "As a naturopath, I was taught that we should not always think about treating a disease but about treating a person. Arthritis is a very good example of a disease that is highly individualized. Not only are there different types of arthritis, but people get it and express it in different manners."

It's a good idea to try to listen to the body and realize that it has an intelligence. In other words, if you are following a certain lifestyle and your problems are the result of that lifestyle, a change in lifestyle may change the illness.

People say that as the body gets older, the most natural thing in the world is for it to get decrepit. But give the body credit for the intelligence it has. When the body tells you something, if you listen and follow what it says, you will improve.

DIET AND NUTRITION Dr. Peter Agho of the Healing Center says, "I do diet. Not just for arthritis. The thing about the whole diet is this. Change the diet, and the arthritis—along with obesity, high blood pressure, and other problems—will get better. The diet should include fresh fruit, including fresh fruit juice, and vegetables. You should eliminate animal fats and cut high-fat foods."

Dr. Howard Robins outlines his treatment: "We use a complete vegetarian diet, including a lot of green, leafy vegetables. These are important because of all the phytochemicals and phytoestrogens that help in all the chemical processes that are necessary to getting well again. We give them juices, six to eight fresh green juices a day—the best way to take in these chemicals."

Dr. Luke Bucci, author of *Pain Free: The Definitive Guide to Healing Arthritis*, notes that part of the reason people get arthritis is the lack of essential nutrients in a highly processed, refined diet. Sure, you get plenty of calories, protein, and fat—usually the wrong kind of fat. What you do not get is just as important—the minerals: magnesium, zinc, copper, manganese, boron. Many people are not aware of boron as a nutrient, but boron may turn out to be essential to our joints' health. These are what you do not get with the current, typical American diet. We lack the substances that enable the joints to repair themselves from the damage they sustain. That is why you want to start eating a whole-food diet that is rich in organic vegetables, fruits, and nuts.

Dr. Rich Ribner tells this story: "Recently, a woman came to the clinic with a terrible case of arthritis. She was in terrible pain and had been taking anti-inflammatory medication and tranquilizers. She was miserable. She said she thought about killing herself. I said, 'Stop this nonsense. I'm going to ask you to do something. You may not even want to do it.' She said, 'Anything.' I said, 'Between now and next week, I want you to drink six to eight glasses of water a day, but it has to be distilled or spring water. And eat nothing but brown rice, just brown rice.' 'But, but...' she began. 'Wait,' I said, 'You were talking about killing yourself. So listen, I'll add a few green vegetables to that.'

"You have to make sure there is a cleansing. Make sure they drink the water. Have a bowel movement daily.

"Well, this woman was so desperate that she stayed on the diet 1 week. When she came back, there was marked improvement. She still had a long way to go, but there was a change."

SUPPLEMENTS Vitamins, minerals, and nutritive substances can play important roles in the treatment and prevention of arthritis. There is some evidence that the essential fatty acids furnished by substances such as cod liver oil, linoleic acid, and marine lipids, by replacing missing fatty substances in the synovial fluid, can be important in treating arthritis. The synovial fluid consists primarily of mucin with some albumin, fat, epithelium, and leukocytes. When the joint surfaces become irritated and undergo degeneration, some of the fat from the joint itself is lost. This fat acts as a lubricant and keeps the joint surfaces apart so that the cartilage-covered bone ends are protected and can move smoothly. When a person takes extra cod liver oil or other essential fatty acids, the oil goes to the joints and provides more lubrication.

Vitamin A, which is found in large quantities in cod liver oil, is also important for the maintenance of the mucous membranes of the body, which manufacture mucus to cleanse the body of infectious bacteria and toxins. Without adequate supplies of vitamin A, infection and accumulation of toxic materials can set in around the joints. Furthermore, a vitamin A deficiency can lead to insufficient production of synovial fluid; when this occurs, the joints lack proper lubrication, the cartilage becomes subject to drying and cracking, and movement becomes difficult and painful.

Because lubrication is vital to the smooth functioning of the joints, vitamin E, whose primary role is to protect against the destruction of the essential fatty acids by oxidation, is also an important antiarthritic nutrient. Both vitamins E and C, which generally act as free radical scavengers within the body, can be especially important in the treatment as they can "clinch" the free radicals present at the site of inflamed or irritated joints, thereby decreasing pain, swelling, and inflammation.

Many symptoms of arthritis are alleviated by establishing a proper balance of calcium and phosphorus in the body, since these are the two minerals most responsible for bone formation and healing. This can be one of the most confusing aspects of arthritis, because x-rays of arthritic joints often show excessive calcification. Afraid of further calcification, patients mistakenly believe that they must avoid calcium-rich foods. Actually, the calcification is due not to an excess of calcium but to malabsorption of existing supplies caused by an imbalance in the ratio of calcium to phosphorus. This imbalance is caused by two major factors: (1) excessive consumption of foods containing high levels of phosphorus such as meat, dairy products, and soft drinks and (2) the process of joint degeneration, which releases high levels of phosphates. This excess phosphorus at the joint site binds with calcium and results in calcification. Taking extra calcium orally does not contribute to this localized calcification. Rather, by increasing calcium levels in the blood, it draws the excess phosphorus away from the joints to bind with the blood calcium so that both are eliminated; this in turn inhibits calcification around the joints.

It should be noted here that soft drinks are the number one source of phosphorus in the American diet today. These drinks contain more phosphorus than most other foods or beverages, and the typical American consumes nearly 500 gallons of them a year. According to Dr. David Steenblock, excess phosphorus is one of the major contributing factors to the development of osteoarthritis. He says, "We see this clinically in many people, who come with osteoarthritis in their early 40s who are large consumers of soft drinks, who also consume excess quantities of meats and other high-phosphorus foods, and who do not eat enough of the green, leafy vegetables which contain calcium." The other problem associated with soft drinks is that most of them contain citric acids, which bind calcium and cause it to be excreted. "So," says Dr. Steenblock, "not only is there extra phosphorus in the soft drinks, they contain the material that takes calcium out of the body. If you want to develop osteoarthritis, that's a very good way of doing it."

Other useful supplements include glucosamine and chondroitin. According to Dr. Luke Bucci, these substances act to "convince" your joint tissues to repair the damage caused by arthritis.

Several studies have shown that a small supplemental dose of boron, about 3 to 6 milligrams a day, can reverse the symptoms of osteoarthritis. Magnesium also is helpful.

AVOIDING CERTAIN FOODS AND CHEMICALS Arthritis may be caused or exacerbated by allergies to foods and chemicals. Dr. Warren Levin says that removing offending substances from the patient's environment can produce dramatic changes.

Some doctors believe that arthritis is caused by the foods a person eats most often. Dr. Morton Teich stresses that the food the patient wants the most may be the problem. Studies have shown that milk, for example, can cause severe allergies and arthritis.

Dr. Teich also warns us about the glycoproteins in milk, wheat, corn, and cinnamon, as well as inhalants such as dust, mold, and pollen. Chemicals and food additives are also potential contributors to allergies and arthritis.

HERBS Letha Hadady, an herbalist, tries to eliminate the toxins that result from poor digestion and poor circulation. She shares some of her herbal remedies for total health.

In dealing with arthritis, one thing you must have every day is alfalfa. You could chew 10 tablets a day with a little water to eliminate much of the uric acid that can build up to create joint pain. Rhubarb also eliminates acid. It is a laxative, but it also breaks apart the painful crystals that form around your joints.

Dandelion greens are full of vitamins and minerals. Dandelions break down pain-giving acid, too.

Star fruit is a sweet, delicious fruit you can find in the grocery store or at the vegetable stand. Juice it. Add a cup and a half of cold water. Taken three times a day, it can eliminate inflammatory joint pain, bleeding hemorrhoids, and burning urine. It is cooling and cleansing.

It is important to realize that everyone's arthritic pain is not the same. Do you wake up in the morning with your joints feeling stiff and sore? Do they feel better after you move them around and after you exercise? If so, you need to take warming, tonic herbs that build vitality, increase circulation, and warm joints. Add a pinch of turmeric to your stews. Turmeric and cinnamon are a good combination for achy shoulders. If you have rheumatism that gets worse in cold weather, add a quarter of a teaspoon of turmeric and cinnamon to a little water and drink it as a tea.

Asafetida is a spice that is available in Indian stores. A little asafetida added to cooking beans or other hard-to-digest foods will help cleanse the body and warm the joints.

Also useful is the resin myrrh; a few drops added to your tea will make your joints feel warm and your blood move, thus improving the circulation.

Hadady says that Asian medicine uses many herbs that can be added in cooking. For example, *tang kuei* increases circulation and warms joints. Another classic Chinese remedy, one that Chinese doctors have used for generations, is *du huo jisheng wan*. Hadady's favorite—*guan jie yan wan*—is translated as "walk as smoothly as a tiger." Other Asian remedies include raw Tienchi ginseng, Efficacious Corydalis, *tien ma*, Three Snakes Formula, Mobility 3, Clematis 19, *du zhong, leigong ten pian,* and *rinchen dragjor-rilnag chenmo.*

CHIROPRACTIC Many arthritis sufferers interviewed for this chapter said that of all the things they tried to eliminate the pain, going to a chiropractor helped the most.

Dr. Mitchell Proffman, a chiropractor at the Healing Center, showed me two x-rays. The first showed bones that were nice and clean and square in shape; the second showed degeneration of the bones.

He showed what arthritis looks like in the human body: thinned disks and a little lip or spur, the body's defense mechanism to heal or shore up the area so that it does not totally disintegrate. He said a person might have a pinched nerve somewhere in the body, in the neck, for example. He administers a gentle push with his hand, which is not painful, to move the bone back into position. The nerve energy comes through, and the joint can start to heal.

RECONSTRUCTIVE THERAPY The noted physician Dr. Arnold Blank has used reconstructive therapy to treat arthritis. Reconstructive therapy, created in the 1920s by the osteopathic physicians Gedney and Schumann, works by stimulating the body's ability to heal itself. The doctors found that by injecting substances that caused a slight irritation to these tissues, they could help the blood vessels grow into the region, thus bringing more oxygen, vitamins, and minerals, as well as fibroblast growth factor, into the cartilage, promoting tissue growth.

Dr. Blank introduced me to one of his patients: "George has had an injury to his shoulder due to chronic overuse. I have been injecting into the ligaments in and around his shoulder joint. This therapy works best when the patients are in an optimal nutritional state. Vitamin and mineral levels are important in our healing response and ability. The injection consists of a variety of different liquids. Primary liquids I use are calcium, lidocaine, and saline. They take a moment and really aren't painful. The majority of patients feel improvement after the first three or four treatments, developing some strength and feeling less pain, even increasing the range of movement.

"The nutrients we may use, natural ones, include substances that have an anti-inflammatory effect, such as vitamin C, shark cartilage, sea cucumber, glutathione, and glucosamine sulfate. All these substances are used once reconstructive therapy has begun because the new blood vessels going to the tissues will enhance healing. These nutrients may not work well when there are no blood vessels going into the area, and so they should be administered after the therapy has begun its work."

Another patient recounts his experience: "I injured my back and didn't realize it until I started getting aches in the back of my leg. I had heard about reconstructive therapy, so I started on my back, had so many treatments, then I went to the hip, knee, and shoulder. They all feel great at present."

ACUPUNCTURE Acupuncture has been used by countless people throughout the world to help alleviate the pain and suffering of arthritis. Dr. Yuan Yang of the Healing Center explains briefly how this works. "We put the needle around the joint to create circulation, taking the pain away. There may be cold, blocked blood and low energy, so I apply the needle for smooth blood flow. Moving blocked energy takes the pain out."

PHYSICAL THERAPY Shmuel Tatz works at Medical Arts at Carnegie Hall with an exercise physiologist, doing mostly hands-on treatment. He typically works with people who have arthritic problems from overuse syndromes or accidents. He works directly on the joints. For example, for a pianist who has problems with the hands, he will try to move the bones, separating the joints to make more space.

As Tatz explains, "Today in physical therapy we use many modalities. One of these is magnetic pulse therapy. We know of the positive effects of magnetism on the body. Scientists have developed a machine with different programs so that we can adjust for every different situation.

"We put electrodes on the body, for example, on the hip joint. Here it stays for 15 to 20 minutes. Usually patients report a very mild relaxing sensation, and the pain decreases.

"Many people with pain from osteoarthritis are afraid to be touched. People with a swollen knee, for instance, can do reflex therapy. For the knee we touch an acupuncture point on the ear, which gives relief."

Once this manipulation has had an effect, they start to exercise the knee by putting the legs in slings, relieving the pressure on the joint and making it easier for the patient to move the body. Trying to open the joint and make more space around the bones allows for better circulation. Movement is very important for people with arthritis.

One patient, Lori, speaks about her improvement:

"Here at Medical Arts I was able to receive physical therapy, which has enabled me to avoid surgery and has greatly improved the quality of my life. I'm still dancing."

YOGA Molly McBride, a yoga instructor, believes you do not have to stop working on your health simply because you may have some physical limitations. Even by working with something as simple as a chair, it is easy to stay fit and help yourself with the problems of arthritis.

The basis of yoga is breath and breathing practices, she says, which help circulation and also help flush the body out by collecting toxins so that they can be exhaled. Breath is the foundation of all the yoga stretches.

"We start with just taking a simple breath; the basic beginning exercise is a three-part breath. Let the air fill the abdomen, then the ribcage, then the upper chest. Exhale, letting the breath exit the upper chest, then the ribcage, and then abdomen. Inhale, exhale."

It is important to take time every day to do these breathing exercises. A really good time to do them is first thing in the morning, when your stomach is empty; if you have eaten, wait a few hours before you start. These breathing exercises can be combined with some simple joint lubrication exercises. To regenerate the body and increase the flow of oxygen through the system, to help release all the toxins that build up in the muscles and the protective cartilage around the joints, try simple yoga exercises.

Specific Treatment Approaches

In the following pages, we discuss some specific alternative approaches to treating arthritis. Although there are many other approaches, these have had a consistently high success rate, are not toxic or expensive, and in some cases may get to the cause of the disease rather than merely masking its symptoms.

TREATMENT FOR GOUT Traditional medicine treats gout symptoms with drugs to relieve pain and decrease uric acid levels in the body. These drugs include colchicine, corticosteroids, analgesics, uricosuric agents, and allopurinol. They may be beneficial but they do have side effects. More important, they're reactive, not proactive.

An article on www.healthwell.com from Integrative Medicine Communications provides a good summary of the alternative and complementary ways to prevent and treat this painful condition. First, it's important to maintain a healthy weight, drink adequate amounts of water, avoid alcohol, and eliminate or limit foods that contain purines. Beef, goose, organ meats, muscles, herring, mackerel, and yeast contain high amounts of purine, Moderate amounts of purine are found in other meats and fish, as well as spinach, asparagus, lentils, mushroom, and dried peas.

Helpful nutrients include berries, vitamin C, and folic acid. Cherries, hawthorn berries, and blueberries all contain anthocyanins, a class of natural dyes that have been found to reduce inflammation and enhance the quality of collagen. They also act as antioxidants. According to Dr. Muraleedharan Nair from Michigan State University in a 1999 article in *Newsweek*, the anthocyanins in tart cherries are 10 times more effective than aspirin in reducing inflammation. As an added benefit, they don't irritate the stomach like aspirin does. Half a pound of cherries per day for 2 weeks has been found to lower uric acid levels and prevent episodes of gout. Also beneficial is cherry juice, 8 to 16 ounces daily.

Eight grams of vitamin C daily have been found to reduce uric acid levels in the blood. Caution must be noted, however, as gout symptoms will get worse in some people with this amount of vitamin C. In terms of folic acid, 10 to 75 milligrams daily are recommended.

A good herbal remedy for gout is bromelain, 125 to 250 milligrams three times a day during an attack. Also recommended is Devil's claw, which can be taken in the following dosages: 1 to 2 grams three times daily of dried powdered root, 4 to 5 milliliters three times daily of tincture, or 400 milligrams three times daily of dry solid extract. Both of these herbs act as anti-inflammatories.

Among the homeopathic remedies used for gout are the following;

ACONITE, recommended for burning pain, anxiety, and restlessness that comes on suddenly.

BELLADONNA, recommended for intense, throbbing pain that increases with motion and decreases with pressure.

BRYONNIA, indicated for pain exacerbated by motion and decreased by pressure and heat.

COLCHICUM, suggested for pain that increases with motion and weather changes.

LEDUM, for swollen, mottled joints that respond better to cold than heat.

In addition, hot and cold compresses, and bed rest may help.

DR. JASON THEODOSAKIS: MAXIMIZING THE ARTHRITIS CURE Dr. Theodosakis is the author of *The Arthritis Cure* and *Maximizing the Arthritis Cure*, and a board-certified physician trained in exercise physiology and sports medicine. He is a lecturer on preventive medicine, a clinical professor at the University of Arizona College of Medicine, and the director of its Preventative Medicine Residency Training Program.

He describes his arthritis program: "I've come up with my arthritis program out of necessity, both to treat patients and for personal use. I see a lot of patients mainly with osteoarthritis but also with the other types of arthritis.

"My program is an integrated, comprehensive approach to creating a situation that optimizes the buildup of cartilage. I will basically use anything—diet, exercise, even medicine when it's called for. We hit it from all angles, including the psychological aspects.

He notes that his program addresses the causes of arthritis: "I believe that the hallmark of good medicine is not to just treat but to get an accurate diagnosis of where the problem originates and then try to reverse the reversible conditions whenever possible, in line with the knowledge of how the arthritis originated. If you have gout, for instance, with these crystals in your joint, you wouldn't want to just go through the standard treatment protocols for osteoarthritis, such as taking anti-inflammatory pills, because that won't eliminate the crystals."

Nonsteroidal anti-inflammatory drugs (NSAIDs), he remarks, are part of a $37 billion worldwide market that involves such huge corporations as Whitehall-Robins, which makes Advil and Motrin; other NSAIDs are Aleve, which is naproxen sodium, and aspirin. According to Dr. Theodosakis, these drugs may cause serious problems such as bleeding ulcers, kidney dysfunction, and adverse drug interactions. "At a rheumatology conference I was at, it came out that none of these anti-inflammatories have been studied long term," he says. "Studies have suggested that they may even worsen the condition."

Dr. Theodosakis's program can be broken down into the following components: diagnosis, supplementation with glucosamine and chondroitin, a change in biomechanics, exercise, and medical approaches.

DIAGNOSIS

"The very first step is getting an accurate diagnosis and working with the physician," he explains. "Be up front with your doctor. In my book, I lay out what you should be telling your doctor and what your doctor should be asking you, the tests you should getting for a diagnosis, and so on. Even if you are in a managed-care setting where you get only 5 or 10 minutes with your doctor, you have to know what information to get to use that time optimally. Getting an accurate diagnosis so you'll know what you are treating is step one."

SUPPLEMENTS: GLUCOSAMINE AND CHONDROITIN

Glucosamine and chondroitin are natural supplements from seashells and cow's cartilage, respectively. When taken orally, they improve the balance between breakdown and buildup of cartilage. Several recent studies support their use. "These supplements are part of a treatment," Dr. Theodosakis cautions. "Alone, these supplements are not the answer; they need to be part of a complete program.

Dr. Theodosakis has a web site listing the studies on glucosamine and chondroitin (www.drtheo.com). Further, he states, "I also set up a national reporting center for drug side effects related to glucosamine and chondroitin to see if any negative effects have been noted. So far, although millions of people are using these supplements, I'm not aware of any side effects. And I would be the first person to be aware of them if they were occurring."

The one problem with these supplements is that there are about 100 different brands on the market. In Dr. Theodosakis's opinion, "maybe as many as 30 percent do not meet the label claims. In other words, you are not getting what the bottle says. This is a very big concern of mine."

BIOMECHANICS

Biomechanics refers to the way the body absorbs shock from everyday movement. "You have different forces on your joint," he says, "and if you learn to dissipate these forces throughout your body, there is likely to be less damage to your cartilage. People can learn to improve their biomechanics. They certainly do in the sports arena, which you will see if you look at athletes as well as performers in such disciplines as ballet. They have wonderful biomechanics and can absorb and dissipate tremendous shock. So my patients are taught how to alter their biomechanics."

EXERCISE

Exercise is absolutely necessary for arthritis sufferers, but the wrong kind of exercise can worsen the condition. You need a specific program for whatever ails you, Dr. Theodosakis says. If you have a hip problem, for example, you will need to do the appropriate exercises for that.

DIET

Another component of Dr. Theodosakis program is diet. He remarks, "The fasting in order to detoxify the body, the juicing, the vegetarian diet are all things I agree with 100 percent.

"Diet has a tremendous impact on arthritis for several reasons. One is weight control. A major risk factor for getting arthritis is being overweight. For example, women in the highest fifth of weight are eight times more likely to get arthritis of the knee than are women in the lowest fifth. Another factor is that different foods will either aggravate or alleviate arthritis. Some of the fish oils, omega-3 fatty acids, can help, while certain components of meat, such as arachidonic acid, can worsen the condition. You also need to eat a wide variety of fruits and vegetables, making sure you get a wide variety of nutrients and also taking supplements. With these nutritional elements, we are making sure your body has the optimal environment to win this cartilage battle."

MEDICAL APPROACHES

Dr. Theodosakis also incorporates medical approaches into his program. This may, include prescription drugs, surgery, and treatment for depression associated with arthritis.

RESULTS

Dr. Theodosakis describes what he calls "one of my most remarkable cases," that of one of his nurses. "She is about 40 years old. She had terrible arthritis, to the point where she was going to have her knee cartilage scraped off, she had so many crystals in it. She used my program for about 4 months and saw tremendous improvement. She was taking the supplements at that time, then she stopped taking the supplements—that was about 2 years ago. Now she's become a runner; she did a half marathon. But she would have been crippled if she had had the surgery.

"I have had a number of patients who were scheduled for joint replacement therapy and after going through this program were able to avoid the surgery. Many are pain-free. It won't reverse the bony changes that occurred in the joint, but it gives them the opportunity to exercise and do some of the things they want to do."

DR. ROBERT LIEFMAN: HOLISTIC BALANCED TREATMENT Holistic balanced treatment (HBT) is derived from the work of the physician Dr. Robert Liefman (1920–1973). Dr. Liefman first used this treatment in 1961, after 20 years of research. Since that time more than 30,000 arthritis sufferers have received the treatment, and many of them are living pain-free, normal lives.

HBT is based on the results of Dr. Liefman's research, which showed that many arthritis sufferers, especially those with rheumatoid arthritis, have specific hormonal imbalances. Within the body there are naturally occurring hormones called glucocorticoids whose role is to reduce inflammation and raise the level of simple sugars in the blood. One of the ways these hormones raise blood sugar levels is by converting nonglucose molecules such as protein into glucose. If unchecked, these glucocorticoids can be responsible for the collagen breakdown of cartilage in joints, which may be a contributing factor in the development of arthritis. The glucocorticoids are balanced within the body by other hormones, such as testosterone and the feminizing hormones, which include estradiol; these hormones induce tissue building and hence balance the tissue-wasting effects of the glucocorticoids. If the body is not regulating these hormones, there are therapies to correct these imbalances. Dr. Liefman developed formulas consisting of varying amounts of three basic ingredients: (1) prednisone, an anti-inflammatory steroid, (2) estradiol, an estrogenic hormone, and (3) testosterone.

According to the proponents of HBT, the anti-inflammatory property of the steroid prednisone and the healing properties of sex hormones can be used to treat arthritic conditions with minimal side effects because of the balancing action between the different components. The anabolic, or building, quality of the sex hormones acts to control the catabolic, or destructive, effects of the steroidal drug therapy (these effects include infection, decreased immunity, improper healing, suppression of pituitary and adrenal function, and fluid retention). The feminizing and androgenic activities of sex hormones are kept in check both by the catabolic nature of the glucocorticoids and by careful adjustment of the concentration of the sex hormones in accordance with the specific requirements of the individual patient during treatment.

THE SUCCESS OF HBT

In contrast to the symptom-suppressing approach taken by the traditional medical establishment, HBT is designed to address the causes of arthritis. It does this first by restoring a positive protein-building balance within the body through the administration of the trihormonal formulas, which works to stop pain and inflammation. Second, according to Dr. Henry Rothblatt, "HBT is never administered without considering the particular need of the individual patient. The medication is adjusted for every patient so that the proper tissue-building and healing response can be obtained. Respect for the uniqueness and the unique need of the individual patient is one of the essential principles of the holistic approach to medicine."

Dr. Liefman developed four basic formulas to account for the different requirements of each individual using HBT: (1) White Cap, which contains prednisone, testosterone, and estradiol, (2) Black Cap, which has only prednisone and estradiol, (3) Red Cap, which contains prednisone and testosterone, and (4) Green Cap, which contains only prednisone and is used only to allow women to shed the endometrium proliferation caused by the intake of the estrogen-containing preparations. In turn, the proportions of these different compounds may vary from individual to individual and may be altered for the same person during the course of treatment.

If, for example, a female patient begins to exhibit an adverse reaction to the treatment, such as the growth of excess body hair, the testosterone level in the medication will be reduced to eliminate those reactions. The same holds true for men who experience breast development or other sex-related changes as a result of the medication's estrogen content. Patients who exhibit some of the typical side effects of cortisone-type drugs will have the amounts of prednisone in their medication decreased, or appropriate increases in one of the sex hormones will be made to counterbalance the negative effects of the steroids. Generally, the adverse reactions to any of the elements in the compounds disappear within a short time once the proper balance among the hormones has been attained.

In addition to the importance of balancing the anti-inflammatory hormones with the sex hormones to establish a healthy protein-rebuilding environment, Dr. Liefman explored other biochemical interactions within the body which play important healing roles in arthritis. For example, he discovered that a growth hormone produced in the pituitary gland reacts synergistically with estradiol and testosterone to stimulate bone growth. He looked at the health of the pancreas to determine whether adequate insulin was being produced to ensure the efficient breakdown of sugar within the body, because without proper sugar metabolism, the body lacks sufficient energy to build and repair bones.

HBT also incorporates principles of nutrition and stresses the importance of regular exercise. The diet recommended in HBT eliminates junk foods such as sugar and sugar products and salty and processed foods such as luncheon meats and canned goods, fried foods, and refined foods. The diet is essentially moderate in protein and emphasizes high-fiber complex carbohydrates in the form of fresh fruits and vegetables, whole grains, and legumes. Vitamin and mineral supplements are used to bolster the patient's immune system and enhance the body's natural healing abilities. For instance, vitamin D is important for strong and healthy bones because it regulates the absorption of calcium from the stomach into the bloodstream, which carries it to bone tissue. Vitamins C and A are important for the maintenance and repair of collagen, the gluelike substance that holds the tissues together and is essential for joint and muscle stability. Vitamin E and B-complex vitamins are important for bone growth. Among the minerals, adequate supply and absorption of calcium, phosphorous, and magnesium are essential for the formation of healthy bones, while zinc and selenium are important immune system nutrients.

Exercise is also an important adjunct to HBT and is recommended to restore joint and muscle mobility and function as well as muscle mass lost during periods of inactivity. However, patients generally are told not to exercise until they are free of pain, swelling, and stiffness and feel confident enough to engage in it. Walking may be the first exercise; then, as patients improve, they can be given specialized exercises for the hands, knees, fingers, shoulders, and other areas which may have been affected by arthritis.

The medical establishment has basically ignored, attacked, or criticized HBT therapy even though its basis is drugs already widely used by physicians. All Dr. Liefman did was combine certain commonly prescribed drugs to maximize the benefits and minimize the side effects of each component drug. The balanced hormonal approach to arthritis did, however, do one unorthodox thing: It challenged the rigidly held position of the medical establishment that arthritis is an incurable disease. Was it for this reason alone that, before his death in October 1973, Dr. Liefman faced considerable opposition from the American arthritis community and was actively prosecuted by the FDA?

THE PATIENTS

Here are some of the results arthritis patients have had over the years from using HBT:

MALCOLM

Malcolm had his first attack of arthritis when he was 21 years old. By the time he was 44, the pain had become constant. Deformities started to appear in the joints of his shoulders, hips, knees, upper and lower spine, and sternum. He was diagnosed with Strümpell-Marie disease (spondylitis), a form of arthritis which causes such severe deformities in the spine that the patient is literally doubled over.

Malcolm also had severe iritis, an inflammation of the eyes which is not uncommon in rheumatoid arthritis patients, and extensive retinal hemorrhages were found in both eyes. During the year before his treatment with HBT, he was taking 12 to 14 aspirin tablets daily, was receiving cortisone injections in his knee once a week, and had tried another medication which had no effect.

Malcolm began treatment with HBT in August 1962 after reading the Look magazine article in May. He experienced almost immediate relief. According to his physician, his arthritis had almost disappeared and his eyes were normal. When he was unable to get his medication in 1968, his symptoms began to return, but they subsided upon resumption of the HBT. About his treatment, Malcolm wrote years later:

"In August 1962, when I started the medication, I weighed 149 pounds and was using a cane. I could not turn my head and could do no physical work. Today I weigh 190 pounds (I am 5 feet 11 inches tall), show absolutely no sign of arthritis, and maintain an active schedule 7 days a week. I have had my blood checked three times, and each time I have been pronounced to be in top physical condition.

"I would like to add that in 1961 I was in the hospital for tests and observation. X-rays showed that my hips were so clouded with calcium that the joints could not be seen, and five vertebrae in my back were fused. I was told that in about 5 years I would be so bent, I would not be able to sit in a wheelchair. About 5 years ago, for my own information, I had a set of x-rays taken and was told that my back and hips were in better condition than the average person's."

CYNTHIA

At age 19, Cynthia began to experience the symptoms of rheumatoid arthritis. Initially the arthritis was confined to her jaw and elbows, but over a period of 2 1/2 years, while she was undergoing treatment by a traditional physician, the arthritis spread to nearly every part of her body. Five years later Cynthia was so crippled with pain and stiffness that it took her a half hour to get out of bed in the morning. The morning after she started HBT, her pain had almost disappeared except for some stiffness and soreness, which also went away during the following 3 days. About her condition and her subsequent treatment at the Arthritis Medical Center in Fort Lauderdale, which administers HBT, Cynthia said:

"I was getting worse and worse. When I first went to my doctor, I had it just in my jaw and elbows. After 2 1/2 years, I had it in just about every place except my hips and knees. I couldn't turn my head at all.

"The doctor actually told me once that he felt really bad, that he had tried everything and didn't know what else to do, and that I had better go to the crippled children's center in Palm Beach. To tell a young woman that.... I just wanted to drive off a bridge. But I thank him for saying it because if he hadn't, I don't think I ever would have tried this place. I did it in desperation."

At the time Cynthia started HBT she was taking 30 aspirin tablets a day, which were causing headaches, ringing in her ears, and ulcers. She was spending approximately $1,000 a month on painkillers alone. While Cynthia found that she bruised and bled more easily after starting HBT, she notes that she had the same symptoms while taking large doses of aspirin. However, while the aspirin and other treatments did nothing to arrest the progression of Cynthia's arthritis, a day after she started treatment with HBT, her pain virtually disappeared, and it returned only when she forgot to take her medication. At present Cynthia is pain-free and works out three times a week at a health spa. She continues on her medication, but in much smaller doses than when she started treatment with HBT.

JUNE

June suffered from severe crippling arthritis for 2 years before starting treatment with HBT. Over that 2-year period June received almost every form of traditional arthritis treatment available: gold injections, penicillamine,

Butazolidin (phenylbutazone), small doses of prednisone, and 16 aspirins daily. June says that she was spending over $100 a week for medication alone. In the meantime she kept getting worse, and when she started HBT, she says, "I was immobile in my hands and shoulders. It was at that point that I thought, What's the use of living? I couldn't even turn my head." Additionally, her liver, stomach, and kidneys were damaged by the large doses of medication. She was forced to give up her business because she was too weak and in too much pain to work. Her medical bills were ruining her financially. The second day after June received HBT, her pain disappeared. June says about her progress with HBT:

"I woke up and I could move my ankles, I could move my hands and my feet. When I stood up, the pain wasn't there. I said to [my husband], 'My God, there's been a miracle.' It got better and better, and I guess within 2 months I didn't even know I had rheumatoid arthritis. I got a bicycle, and I started dancing again and going to the beach again. It used to be if I lay on the sand, I couldn't get up again."

June continues to be pain-free, leading a normal life, and her medication has been reduced by more than half the initial amount.

DR. THERON RANDOLPH AND DR. MARSHALL MANDELL: ENVIRONMENTAL ALLERGIES

Environmental medicine, also called clinical ecology, was developed by Dr. Theron Randolph in the 1940s and 1950s when he observed early in his medical career that food allergies and sensitivities to environmental chemicals were a major contributing factor in a wide range of diseases, including arthritis. Dr. Randolph also noted that the causal relationship of allergy to disease was a very individualized phenomenon: One person could eat beef every day and never have an adverse reaction, while another person could develop a food allergy to beef even when consuming it only on rare occasions. Similarly, people with an allergy to the same product did not necessarily manifest the same symptoms. One might break out with hives, while another developed depression, and still another became arthritic. Dr. Randolph also found that seemingly innocuous chemicals found in the home, workplace, or school could in certain individuals trigger symptoms ranging from mental problems to aching joints to chronic fatigue.

The work of Dr. Randolph was applied to arthritis by Dr. Marshall Mandell, a physician from Connecticut and one of the country's leading environmental medical specialists. He has found that a considerable number of patients who come to him with arthritis or arthritislike symptoms are in fact suffering from a form of environmental allergy such as the ones outlined by Dr. Randolph. According to Dr. Mandell, "The basic process that underlies many cases of arthritis is a completely unrecognized or unsuspected allergy or allergylike sensitivity to substances that are part of daily life, including the food we eat, the liquids we drink, including the water supply, the chemicals that are deliberately or accidentally introduced into a diet, and the various forms of chemical pollutants in the indoor and outdoor air that get into our bodies." From his clinical experience, Dr. Mandell has found that more than half the patients he treats who would be confirmed arthritics by standard medical diagnostic techniques can be helped by means of simple dietary or environmental changes.

THE TREATMENT

"My approach and that of my colleagues in the field of environmental medicine and clinical ecology, supplemented by the benefits of nutritional therapy, begins by looking at the person who is predisposed to having arthritis to see if there are identifiable substances in the diet and environment which can trigger or cause the episode of illness," says Dr. Mandell. "We deal with demonstrable cause-and-effect relationships. What we do is study the patient.

"First, we take a carefully formulated history which is designed to help identify people who have problems with foods, with various chemicals, with pollutants, and perhaps with seasonal airborne substances. From this, we are able to get a fairly good idea of what we're dealing with."

Before patients are tested for food or environmental allergies, Dr. Mandell often will have them fast or go on a restricted diet for 4 days to 1 week to rid the body of any residue of substances suspected to be responsible for the symptoms.

"Next," says Dr. Mandell, "we test these people using a technique known as 'provocative testing' to determine their response to extracts prepared from all the foods in their diet. The most commonly ingested foods are often the culprits, so it shouldn't come as any surprise that wheat, corn products, milk, beef, tomatoes, and potatoes are leading offenders.

"The most common technique used for provocative testing is to place a few drops of the test substance under the tongue of the patient, where it is almost immediately absorbed. This is called 'sublingual' provocative testing. When we test in this manner, only small doses are used, so the effect is brief, but since the solution enters the bloodstream, the entire body is exposed. Symptoms can show up in the joints, muscles, brain, skin, or any other part of the body.

"If we are able to produce joint pain, stiffness or swelling, or redness within a few minutes after placing the solution under the tongue for absorption into the bloodstream, we know that we've found something that must be important, because we have flared up the patient's familiar symptoms—we have actually precipitated an attack of the patient's own illness.

"Many people will have what we call 'polysymptomatic illness,' meaning that many bodily structures, organs, or systems can be involved at the same time. The arthritic person's whole body may be sensitive, and this is why such patients may have a headache or fatigue or asthma or colitis, although they may not actually have any of the well-known allergies such as hay fever, eczema, or hives.

"We also find that many people react to chemicals. We have some people whose arthritis may be due in part or exclusively to the chlorine that is in the water supply, or perhaps to an artificial flavoring or coloring which is used very frequently, or perhaps to a preservative. We have people who have trouble because they are inhaling fumes such as tobacco smoke. We have people who in heavy traffic have trouble because the exhaust fumes will travel, along with the oxygen, through the walls of the lung into the circulation; once again, the whole body is exposed."

After Dr. Mandell determines the substances in the patient's overall environment which he suspects are responsible for arthritic symptoms, he double-checks with test meals of the specific substances.

"I confirm the results of our testing in the office with feeding tests," he says. "Three foods can be tested during the course of a day; however, for the test to be accurate, the food to be tested must be out of the person's system for at least 5 days. Sometimes we can get away with it for 4 days, but it is even better if that food has been completely omitted from the diet in all forms for 5, 6, or 7 days. We give patients a single food as the test meal; since we want to test the food all by itself, we don't put any ketchup, pepper, mustard, sauce, or anything else on the food. Instead of a usual portion, we allow patients to consume as much of the single food as they can comfortably eat as an entire meal....

"Then we observe them for at least 4 hours. If we're able to reproduce that patient's specific symptoms, if we can actually turn the symptoms on and off like a switch, we know that we have nailed it down, because we have demonstrated a cause-and-effect relationship that can't be questioned. Should food be the primary causative factor, we will design a diet that eliminates all of those foods. Then, depending on how well they follow the diet, the patients will be either well or sick."

THE PATIENTS

Dr. Mandell provides some examples of how allergic reactions can result in arthritis or arthritislike symptoms:

SARAH

Sarah was a rabbi's wife who began to have arthritis in her hands, but the flare-ups would take place only on Saturday mornings and then disappear during the course of the day. Using Saturday as a starting point, Dr. Mandell began to explore the possible sources of Sarah's "Saturday arthritis."

"Since she woke up with the arthritis in the morning," Dr. Mandell explains, "we knew it was not caused by something she was doing in the morning. So we went back 24 hours to explore Friday. What did she do on Friday? What did she eat? Drink? Breathe? What came into her system? Could it be, perhaps, the paraffin fumes from the candles on the table which were lit ceremonially every Friday night? Or could it be something they ate? Was it

caused by something she was exposed to when she went to temple on Friday night, perhaps from clothing just taken out of the dry cleaners? Or was it hair spray, perfume, cologne, or men with aftershave lotion? Was it that the temple had had the rug shampooed the day before the services or that the furniture was polished? I had no way of knowing, but I retraced all her activities, and then I tested her systematically.

"This actually turned out to be an easy one, and it was humorous, because the great 'Jewish penicillin,' chicken soup, was the thing that was undoing her. When I placed a few drops of chicken extract under her tongue, within minutes the knuckles that were affected by arthritis swelled up and became painful and red. I did this on a few occasions, and so we were able to demonstrate this. It is rare to find a patient in whom a single substance is the factor, but it does happen now and then. So here is a rabbi's wife with chicken and chicken soup arthritis—Friday night ingestion, Saturday morning appearance of arthritis."

A SURGEON

Dr. Randolph treated a surgeon who became so incapacitated by arthritis that he had to stop performing surgery and restrict his medical practice to office consultations. He had developed severe arthritis primarily in the hips, knees, shoulders, and hands and had received traditional treatment for 10 years. While he derived some relief from the treatment, he still was incapacitated. He had to walk downstairs backward, no longer had the strength or dexterity in his hands to perform surgery, and lacked the physical strength even to stand at the operating table.

The surgeon went to Chicago to see Dr. Randolph, who admitted him to the hospital and immediately put him on a pure spring water fast, free of chlorine and fluoride and without any of the contamination that affects city water supplies. Additionally, he was placed in a special room where the environment was controlled. There were no air fresheners or disinfectants and no bleaches, the floor was not waxed or polished, and the personnel were not permitted to smoke or wear perfume.

Within 5 days the surgeon was free of pain. He regained some dexterity in his hands and reported that if he was a little stronger, he felt he could return to the operating room and resume his normal work. Then he was given single-food feeding tests, and Dr. Randolph discovered that when he was tested with corn (cornmeal with some corn syrup), within a matter of hours he became miserably uncomfortable with severe pain in the shoulders and hips. He had so much pain that it felt as if he had been kicked by a mule. A few days later he was tested with chicken extract, and the effect was different. While he did not experience pain right away, the chicken affected his brain. He became so sleepy that he actually dozed off. When he awoke, he was in such severe pain that he was actually crying.

The surgeon found that as long as he avoided corn and chicken, he was virtually pain-free and could resume his regular daily life.

JANET

This example not only documents the dramatic effects which can be achieved by eliminating an offending food from an arthritic person's diet, it also shows the degree of resistance orthodox arthritis doctors have to accepting this even when it has been unequivocally demonstrated.

Back in the mid-1970s Dr. Mandell sent out a mailing to rheumatologists in the northeastern part of the country, indicating that he was studying the relationship between food allergies and arthritis and was interested in studying some of their patients free of charge. Out of 90 letters, he received six responses, of which three said yes and three said no. Through one of the doctors who agreed to send patients, Janet eventually saw Dr. Mandell. He discusses her testing and the results:

"I want to emphasize that we never tell the patient what the test material is, so we completely eliminate suggestion. When we tested her with pork, she had pain almost immediately in one finger on her right hand, and this was her arthritis joint. We caused the joint to swell up and become red and painful.

"This test was repeated three times, once a week, and after the last test I told her to stay off pork for at least a week and then have a large portion of it one morning as a feeding test. Once again the same thing happened. However, when she told her rheumatologist, the man who was willing to have her come to me, he said he didn't believe it because we didn't have any controls. This is … more than pathetic, it's almost a medical crime! Here the patient had her symptom reproduced … and the doctor says he doesn't believe what has happened to her."

The ironic thing about this skepticism on the part of the orthodox medical establishment is that many of the treatments it prescribes for arthritis have never been proved either safe or effective. Gold injections are a good example. This treatment is extremely costly, has very high toxicity, and is only rarely of benefit to arthritis sufferers. Furthermore, in cases where gold does provide some relief, rheumatologists are unable to offer a scientific explanation of how it operates within the body. Nevertheless, gold continues to be endorsed by the arthritis establishment while something as simple as eliminating a food from a patient's diet, even if that food has been demonstrated to cause the patient's symptoms, is ignored or criticized as being unscientific.

DANA ULLMAN'S HOMEOPATHY FOR ARTHRITIS AND FIBROMYALGIA Homeopathy is based on the idea that the cure for an illness is similar to its cause. As a result, treatment consists of administering small doses of a very diluted natural substance that would cause the symptoms of the condition being treated if it were taken in larger amounts.

Dana Ullman is the president of the Foundation for Homeopathic Education and Research and a board member of the National Center for Homeopathy. He is the author of several books on homeopathy, including *The Consumer's Guide to Homeopathy: The Definitive Resource for Understanding Homeopathic Medicine and Making It Work for You* and *Discovering Homeopathy: Medicine for the 21st Century*. Ullman explains the homeopathic viewpoint.

"There are estimated to be 200 types of arthritis. I'm glad that [the medical establishment has] increased that number from before. [In the past,] it's been ... about 10 or 20. From the homeopathic point of view, every person with arthritis has his or her own species of arthritis. Homeopaths see disease as a syndrome.

"Before rushing into the practical stuff, I want to comment about the research behind homeopathy, specifically in light of arthritis. The *British Journal of Clinical Pharmacology*, a major pharmacology journal, published a double-blind, placebo-controlled study on the homeopathic treatment of rheumatoid arthritis; this was way back in 1980. This study showed that 82 percent of the patients given an individualized homeopathic medicine got some degree of relief, whereas among those given a placebo, only 21 percent got that similar degree of relief."

Ullman describes some of the homeopathic approaches. "One approach is the use of single remedies to treat the acute exacerbation of the problem. Acute exacerbation of the problem means an immediate problem of a short-term nature, like a flare-up of some sort. Homeopathy and homeopathic remedies can be used to allay and relieve some of the pain and discomfort that a person is having.

"A better approach, however, is using the single remedy prescribed by a professional homeopath. This provides what we call constitutional care. It's a more highly individualized remedy, not just for the acute flare-up but for the person's overall genetic health and entire health history. For the homeopath to do this, it requires a detailed interview, lasting at least 1 to sometimes 2 hours. And sometimes a homeopath doesn't prescribe on that first interview but needs more information. This type of care is probably, in my estimation, one of the more profound ways to augment the body's own immune defense system, to not just relieve a person's condition but to really initiate a healing and curative process."

FIBROMYALGIA

To explain in specific terms how homeopathy can be effectively utilized, Ullman uses the treatment of fibromyalgia as an example:

"Fibromyalgia is also called fibrositis. For those who aren't familiar with it, it's a somewhat newly defined disease. At first, there was controversy as to whether it existed or not, but now there's basic acceptance that it is a condition. It's not officially arthritis, although it is thought to be a type of rheumatism where the person experiences pain and discomfort in the joints. They can also experience fatigue and even emotional and mental changes such as poor concentration, anxiety, and irritability. There might also be an irritable bowel, headaches, and cramps. The syndrome comes on in exacerbations. The person may be fine at one point and then all of a sudden have all these symptoms.

"A study was published in the *British Medical Journal* on fibromyalgia. The researchers admitted into the study only those patients who fit the most popular homeopathic remedy used to treat the acute stages of fibromyalgia. It's a remedy called rhus tox [*Rhus toxicodendron*], which is poison ivy, believe it or not. [With] actual poison ivy, not only [does] an overdose cause skin eruptions, but if taken internally, and I don't recommend it, at least in a crude dose, it can and will have effects upon connective tissue that make the person feel extremely stiff, recreating many of the symptoms that people experience when they have not only fibromyalgia but even many types of arthritis.

"They found that 42 percent of the people they interviewed fit this remedy. So they admitted these people into this study. In the first half of the study, half the people got a placebo and half the people got the real remedy. Then halfway through the study they switched, and the people who got the placebo now got the real remedy, and the people who began with the remedy got the placebo. The researchers found that when people began the real remedy, the homeopathic medicine, that's when relief began. And in this type of study, which is not only a double-blind placebo study—controlled and crossover is what it's called—the researcher is comparing patients with themselves. It's the most sophisticated type of research currently being done. It cannot always be done because these crossover effects, which we notice in homeopathy, are problematic since often homeopathic remedies have effects even after the person stops taking the remedy. So, when they begin taking the placebo, they're still feeling better. That sort of muddies the water. But this study did show, very clearly, that whenever people started to take rhus tox, they began experiencing relief."

SPECIFIC REMEDIES

Rhus tox is also used in many musculoskeletal problems. It is one of the leading remedies for arthritis, carpal tunnel syndrome, and lower back pain. Rhus tox is known for alleviating the type of pain syndrome in the joints that is worse on initial motion, in other words, when the person initiates movement of a particular part of the body. When the part has been moved for some time, it loosens up and doesn't hurt as much. The people who need rhus tox also tend to have an exacerbation of their symptoms from cold and wet weather.

"One of the nice things about homeopathy is that you can talk about this broad field of musculoskeletal problems. Although initially I was talking about fibromyalgia, these remedies can be used for many of these conditions. Another remedy that comes to mind is bryonia. Bryonia is an herb called wild hops. This is not the same hops that you drink in a beer. It's a different botanical substance entirely. This is for people with various types of musculoskeletal problems where any type of motion exacerbates the condition. By contrast, people who benefit from rhus tox have this rusty-gate syndrome where they feel worse only on initial motion and then loosen up and limber up. People who need bryonia, the more they move, the worse they are. Here is a really obvious difference. That's one of the unique and nice things about homeopathy. We can be quite precise in finding a remedy that fits each person because the bottom line is that we are all biologically individual. We don't have the same type of joint disease or headache or depression or fatigue. We all have our own unique constellation, our own pattern of symptoms, and homeopathy is an exclusively effective, individualized approach to using these substances from the plant, mineral, or animal kingdom to augment the body's own defenses."

Another remedy Ullman describes is honeybee venom (*Apis mellifera*). "For those of us who have ever been stung by a honeybee, or at least we know what it's like, it's a burning and stinging type of pain, somewhat sharp. If you've ever had a bee sting, you also know that if you put ice on the bee sting, it provides some relief. But if you get near heat or you apply heat to it, it worsens the pain. Likewise, people who will benefit from homeopathic doses of *Apis* will have joint pain with swelling, much like a bee might cause, because the bee not only causes that burning, stinging pain but also causes that inflammatory redness and heat. Thus, there will be swelling that will be increased by cold applications and aggravated by heat.

"One of the known parts of folklore is that beekeepers do not seem to get arthritis very often. Part of the reason for this is that they occasionally do get stung, though they don't react the way the rest of us do because they become more immune to it. Their body has developed more sophisticated histamine responses so that when there is any type of sting, the body just deals with it very rapidly and easily. And there's something about that sting that also provides protective effects. It's as if one were taking, if you will, a homeopathic medicine. You're taking something that will cause a similar syndrome to what the arthritis causes. I don't recommend bee venom therapy, usually. I don't recommend that a person with arthritis be stung multiple times by a bee. Not that I discourage it; I [just] think there are safer, easier ways, like taking homeopathic doses of bee venom."

DOSAGES AND STRENGTHS OF HOMEOPATHIC MEDICINES

Ullman feels that it is important to understand some basics about the dosages in homeopathy and the strength of homeopathic medicines. "Don't be fooled by these extremely small doses. Don't think that just because we use small doses, you need to take more frequent repetitions of the remedy. During acute exacerbations, you do need to repeat them approximately every 2 hours in intense types of syndromes and every 4 hours in less intense syndromes.

However, the idea of homeopathy is to take as few doses as possible but as much as necessary. It's a fine balance. In other words, at times you might take it more frequently, but then as pain and discomfort diminish, you reduce the frequency of taking the remedy.

"If you look in a health food store or pharmacy, it will list the name of the medicine, usually in Latin. Homeopathic manufacturers have to be really precise on the source and species of the plant, mineral, animal, or chemical that we're using. Next to the name will be a number such as 6x or 30c. Well, x refers to the number of times that particular substance has been diluted, 1 to 10. X is a Roman numeral that stands for 10. So 6x means it was diluted 1 to 10 six times. C is the Roman numeral for 100. [If it says 30c,] that means it was diluted 1 to 100 thirty times. Thus, the C potencies are a little more dilute because they're diluted 1 to 100. But both of these potencies are widely sold and widely effective, and generally we recommend that people who are not professionals in homeopathy should not use medicines higher than the thirtieth potency. The sixth potency, the twelfth, and the thirtieth are quite fine, quite effective. Although the two hundredth and the thousandth are even more effective, you have to be more knowledgeable about these remedies because the higher the potency used, the more precise the prescription must be.

"Another choice is not just the use of single remedies but various combination homeopathic remedies or formulas. These are mixtures of homeopathic medicines, usually two to eight of the most common remedies for a specific ailment, such as arthritic pain, back pain, PMS, allergies, sinusitis, and headaches. You see these in health food stores and pharmacies these days. Although these are not part of what would be called classical homeopathy and although they are not as precise as prescriptions, they are a user-friendly and quite effective means of providing help and relief to people, akin to using a single remedy for acute care.

"These formulas do not provide constitutional treatment. They do not really cure a person of their underlying problem. But they do provide wonderful relief. I do recommend that people consider using formulas when they cannot find the single remedy that they need or do not know how to find that remedy. Or they may know how to find the remedy but it is not immediately available, as is often the problem.

"There is a place for both single-remedy homeopathy, professional homeopathy, and formula homeopathy. In fact, in speaking of formula homeopathy, in terms of some injuries and trauma, I personally believe that people will experience—and I have observed this myself—even more rapid relief of an injury from using a formula of some sort. Because when you have an injury, you often need to give the person arnica [wolfsbane]. But at some other point, you need to give the person another remedy for the specific ailment. If it's a nerve injury, you give hypericum [St. John's wort]; if it's a connective tissue injury, you might give rhus tox or ruta [Ruta graveolens]. The bottom line here is that eventually anyone involved in homeopathy will need to give several remedies to the person. And I say, well, why not give several remedies together? A colleague of mine is a homeopath and a podiatrist. Every other day or so he conducts surgery on patients with various types of foot disorders, and he always gives a combination of homeopathic remedies, and he has systematically observed that people heal better from a combination rather than just a single medicine given sequentially. I do want to acknowledge that there is some controversy over these formulas, but as far as I'm concerned, the controversy should be null and void."

Betty Lee Morales's Nutritional Approach

Betty Lee Morales is a longtime advocate of a natural approach to health and disease prevention, and contributing editor of *Let's Live* magazine. She says that detoxification and rebuilding of health with an improved diet can prevent and treat arthritis.

"I work with people who are ready to do almost anything just to get a little relief," Morales says. "They don't even expect reversal, but sometimes they do experience it."

Morales uses the case of her sister to illustrate her approach. "One of my sisters was married to a professor at a leading university who was very skeptical of anything to do with diet and nutrition. When my sister developed rheumatoid arthritis, she also had five other diagnosed diseases, including high blood pressure, elevated cholesterol, and heart trouble. Her husband took her all over the world; they went everywhere looking for a magic cure. After they had spent over $40,000, she not only failed to get better, she was actually worse. They returned home and got a practical nurse to come in. She could not even wait on herself.

"Finally, when she reached the bottom of the barrel, she called me and said, 'Well, I would like to try the natural methods way to see if I can get some relief.' At that time she was on about five or six prescribed drugs and obviously had many problems from them: digestion, assimilation, constipation. I said that I would be very glad to help her. Then she said, 'I'll take these things, but I don't want my husband to know.' I said, 'Hey, back up a minute.' Although it broke my heart, I told her that I could not help her until she had suffered enough and was willing to do whatever she needed to do, especially since not all of it was going to be pleasant. I explained that she was going to have to examine her life closely and detoxify from years of faulty diet.

"Detoxification is a very important part of regaining health and maintaining it. I also told her that she could not do this on the sly without her husband knowing about it because it becomes a way of life. It begins with what you eat, the way you live, even the way you think, and you certainly cannot do it living in a house with another person and not have that person know what you are doing. 'In fact,' I said, 'he should be doing it too.' Then she got hysterical and said, 'Well, he's not open to it.' But I had to tell her that I couldn't help her by telling her to take these things, which are not drugs. The first thing you need to do is to start educating yourself. I sent her a few books, and I said, 'When you've read some of this and you are willing to say that you will really try anything, I'll give you three months. Then I will be happy to help.'"

Morales's sister reached the point where she was bedridden. She could not go to the bathroom alone, nor could she hold a glass of water or a cup of tea. "She called for me, and I went over. They live in a beautiful home and there is no problem with money, but when I outlined the things that were needed, both she and her husband said, 'Does it really cost that much?' I requested that they buy a juicer, the kind that grinds and presses, because it gives the maximum nutrition. I also wanted to bring in a practical nurse who was trained in this type of thing. I told them to think it over.

"They talked it over and decided that they would try it, so I sent over a juicer and 25 pounds of organically grown carrots. I gave instructions to the practical nurse to throw out everything in the cupboard that was opened and was refined or processed. Anything that was in cans or closed containers was to be given to Goodwill. I made it very clear that nothing was to go into that home that I didn't send in. I got rid of all the salt and sugar and all the easy-mix stuff— this was all a trauma to them because it costs money and nobody likes to throw away money. But I told her that she had to go the whole way or not at all."

Morales put her sister on a 7-day detoxification program to cleanse the small intestines and the bowel. "She had coffee enemas every day for about a week. She had nothing but the juices, potassium broth, water and herb tea—no solid food for 7 days. We broke the fast carefully. She had a massage every day, and I made sure she was taken outdoors at least once a day. I also had the nurse read different things to her every day so she would understand what her body was going through.

"Before she started the treatment, I sent her to a laboratory to have complete blood tests, and then after the cleansing, I had her do the same tests again.... Not that it was necessary in this case, but I knew that if she didn't see the results confirmed by a medical laboratory, she wouldn't believe them. Her cholesterol count was 535, which is incredibly high. Her doctor had told her that she was a walking time bomb. He was keeping her on drugs, but the cholesterol did not go down, although her liver problems increased."

Dramatic results were seen in a matter of weeks. "Three weeks later on this program—remember, this is a woman who could not get out of bed alone—she got up one day, went out to her own car, and drove down to the city to have her hair done," Morales says. "That's very typical of women and probably of men. As soon as they start to feel better, the first thing they want to do is look better. She wanted to have her hair done and get a facial and a manicure. It was a great morale booster. When her husband came home from the university, he did not know his own wife because she was up, was beginning to fix a juice cocktail, and they were so delighted that I never had more arguments or problems out of them. But she also felt so well that she decided not to wait the full 6 weeks to have the other tests done; it had only been 3 weeks. She went back to the medical lab and asked to have all the tests done over. She wanted to send her doctor a copy because she still was under the care of a medical doctor who had told her, 'These health food things won't hurt you, but they won't help you. It will only cost you some money, but you can afford it, so go ahead and do it.'

"When she had the second batch of lab tests done and sent to him, he wrote her a letter in which he said, 'If you are going to pursue these quack remedies, I can no longer be responsible for your health, and I am dismissing you as a patient.' She called me up crying and said, 'I don't even have a doctor in case I need one.' She was still laboring under the horrible fear that this doctor had laid on her by saying that she could have a stroke or heart attack at any minute.

"We continued with the program. Within a total of 3 months, she was able to go on a South Pacific cruise with her husband. Today you won't meet two people who are better advocates of the nutritional way of living. They have gone 90 to 95 percent holistic and no longer feel that they have to be under the wing of a doctor who does not recognize nutrition."

DR. LAURIE AESOPH'S SIX-STEP NUTRITIONAL APPROACH Dr. Laurie Aesoph is a naturopathic physician as well as a medical writer. She has authored more than 200 articles on topics ranging from nutrition to herbs and homeopathy, and she also is a senior editor of the *Journal of Naturopathic Medicine*.

Dr. Aesoph describes her views on the relationship between food and arthritis prevention and treatment.

RESTORATIVE FOODS

"Many, many studies tell us that what I call restorative foods, which merely are the good foods we should be eating anyway, [such as] whole grains, fruits, and vegetables, are what we need to insert in our diet. The studies show not only that good diets help out with arthritis but that specific types of food seem to have healing qualities. For example, the oils from different fish have an anti-inflammatory and pain-relieving benefit for arthritis patients. Many fruits, vegetables, and even spices double as herbs. You can use those specifically for different arthritis symptoms.

"In an article printed in *The Lancet*, a British medical journal, in 1991, researchers put their patients on a cleansing diet. But eventually what they did is switch them over to a lacto-ovo-vegetarian diet in different stages, and they had a group that was their control, their placebo, which just ate as normal. They found that even on the lacto-ovo, where people are eating vegetarian diets but also eating eggs and dairy, the benefits continued throughout that year and at the end of the year. So here's evidence where we know that diet is helping.

"Even the Arthritis Foundation is admitting this. There are enough studies that they are taking notice. They have always said that of course, if you're overweight, there is stress on the joints, so if you have something like osteoarthritis or what we call degenerative joint disease, that's going to aggravate and wear out your joints. But they are also looking at studies involving food allergies and cleansing and fish oil, and of course the purines are involved with gout. And diet has always been a large part of treating gout."

STRESSOR FOODS

Dr. Aesoph asserts that it is equally important to minimize what she calls stressor foods from the diet: "Basically, the stressor foods are what set the stage for joint degeneration and breakdown to occur. And just to give you an example of what these foods are, look at the fat category. I want to remind [people] that fats per se are not bad. In fact they're essential, and there's something called essential fatty acids that we need to have—the fish oils fit into that category. But the trans-fatty acids—hydrogenated vegetable oils, for example, and margarine—[contain] too much saturated fat. Those are the sorts of things that are stressor foods and that we should be avoiding. Alcohol doesn't do us any good, nor does caffeine. Refined carbohydrates, such as sugars, flour, white rice, the different sweeteners, the artificial sweeteners such as aspartame and saccharine, processed foods, of course, and the additives and chemicals that are added to our foods are other things that we should also be avoiding.

"When you eat stressor foods, a lot of them really deplete the different nutrients: vitamins, minerals, and all the other phytochemicals and nutrients that we're discovering are in our foods. These, of course, are essential for general body function. Now, arthritis isn't just restricted to the joints. We've discovered that there is a link between the joints and different body systems, and so the immune system is involved. Rheumatoid arthritis is actually what we call an autoimmune disease, where the immune or defense system of your body is attacking yourself. So if you don't have the vitamins and minerals, your immune system isn't going to function as well as it can. Also, with regard to the intestinal tract, it's also vital that it function properly for all sorts of different conditions. When that isn't functioning right, it will aggravate an arthritic condition. I mentioned that if you are overweight, that will stress the joints. If you tend to eat stressor-type foods, that tends to play into or add to conditions of obesity. Also, we talk about stress in our lives, and I really believe that foods that are not complete in nutrition and aren't as whole as they should be are a stress on the body. So that doesn't help your body function any better.

"Also, if you are eating a lot of cooked or processed foods, they tend to be lower in the enzymes that help us digest our foods. There have been numerous studies done where when people eat a diet that is largely composed of cooked foods, their digestive systems, the pancreas, different organs that contribute digestive enzymes to the gut, have to work a little harder, which makes it harder to digest, and then that adds to your gut being a little thicker than it should be, and then that aggravates the arthritis down the road. So, you can see that there are direct and indirect effects that these stressor foods have.

"When you use natural medicine and conventional medicine, it doesn't need to be an either-or situation. You can also use nutrition to cut back on the medication that you're using. You can think of it as a compromise and perhaps gradually get away from the drugs. Also, if you happen to be on steroids, [such as] prednisone, if you plan to cut back and use nutrition, you need to work with your doctor on that. That's something you don't want to cut out cold turkey. The nonsteroidal anti-inflammatory drugs are not as much of a problem. But when going off any prescription drug or steroids, talk to your doctor first."

THE PROGRAM

Dr. Aesoph outlines her nutritional program:

1. Cut out all the stressor foods. You want to eliminate anything that is harming your body or undermining your body's functions and really setting the stage for joint problems to develop. These foods not only weaken the joints but impinge on their ability to repair themselves as well. These are also the foods that add to excess weight, which can overburden the joints. Some of these foods are also high in purines, which tend to aggravate gout.

2. Cleanse the body with a real whole-foods diet and start to add the restorative foods. This helps repair the gastrointestinal tract, which is an imperative part of healing arthritis. At this point you should be starting to learn how to incorporate healthy eating habits and what foods to choose.

3. Test for and then begin to cut out allergy foods.

4. Rebuild damaged joints and overall health by refining your choice of restorative foods. Sea cucumber at 1,000 milligrams may help, as can manganese at 25 milligrams and the bioflavonoid complex. Glucosamine sulfate and chondroital sulfate, both at 500 milligrams, can also produce phenomenal results. Flax at 1,000 milligrams from the omega-3 fatty acid group re-establishes normal fluid and osmotic pressure, the synovial fluid in those joints. Taking an alpha lypoic acid, the best all-around intracellular antioxidant, actually fights free radical damage inside the cell. Then you have a very powerful healing mechanism to get your joints circulating nutrients and oxygen and expelling carbon dioxide and waste products as they should. There are many supplements: minerals, vitamins, and herbs. Other ones that you can add are ginger, cumin, and cayenne. Cayenne cream can be rubbed on arthritic joints because it depletes substance p, which decreases pain.

5. Decrease weight, if that's a problem, because it is a stress on the joints.

6. Eliminate any stress by learning to eat properly, such as by chewing your food properly and eating in a relaxed way.

DR. DAVID STEENBLOCK: ARTHRITIS AND ATHEROSCLEROSIS Because of the susceptibility of the joints to the accumulation of toxic material that can scratch and irritate the inner linings, leading to the pain and inflammation that characterize arthritis, an analogy has been made between arthritis and atherosclerosis (degeneration of the arteries). In both diseases corrosive substances scratch the inner linings of the body part involved, causing irritation that can lead to degeneration. These substances can come from toxic material in the bowel that gets into the bloodstream. They can also come from food. In the case of atherosclerosis, these foods include cholesterol, fats, and fried foods, which, when they get into the blood, scratch and irritate the very sensitive inner linings of the blood vessels. The same substances can also pass from the blood into the joint space and irritate the inner linings of the joints.

According to Dr. David Steenblock, this correlation between arthritis and atherosclerosis is one of the reasons why a low-fat, low-cholesterol, high-fiber diet has been useful in treating arthritis. "Many patients on this type of diet," he says, "show substantial improvement because the fiber cleanses the colon and removes many of the toxic bacterial waste products, which frees up the blood system and makes it more pure. This in turn allows the toxic materials to be eliminated from the joints, and so the joints themselves can begin to heal."

HIGH-FIBER DIET

Dr. Steenblock also explains how a diet that eliminates processed foods and focuses on the consumption of high-fiber natural grains, fruits, and vegetables works specifically in the treatment of arthritis:

"We want to eliminate white sugar and white flour products and processed foods and foods which contain food additives because these processed foods cause abnormalities in the state of health of the intestine. When you eat processed foods with little fiber, the bacterial content of the colon changes from the so-called good bacteria, which are *Lactobacillus bifidus* and *L. acidophilus*, to organisms that are anaerobic such as anerococci and streptococci and organisms that generally are not healthy and produce many toxic substances themselves. When these toxic substances are present as a result of eating a diet high in refined food and lacking fiber, these toxins pass through the bowel into the blood. Also, refined foods, because they are so easily digestible and do not require work by the intestine, cause the muscle wall of the intestine to atrophy, or become thinner. This thinness of the wall allows more toxic material to pass through the bowel into the blood. Once it is in the blood, it can pass easily into the joints and cause more problems.

"The use of the high-fiber natural diet counteracts this trend because the fiber changes the bacterial content of the colon back to normal, and this eliminates many of the toxic materials, the carcinogens, and the mutagens that are formed otherwise, which are well-documented causes not only of osteoarthritis but also of cancer of the colon and atherosclerosis. The fiber also strengthens the bowel wall, making it thicker and healthier, and this creates more of a mucosal barrier between the colon's interior and the blood. Thus the diet should be more of a natural and raw foods diet if you want to get a good result."

Dr. Steenblock does warn, however, that people who have spent an entire lifetime eating refined, fiberless foods must approach a change to a raw, high-fiber diet with caution (excess dietary fiber can, for instance, cause calcium and zinc to be washed through the system so that calcium and zinc deficiencies result) in order to give their intestinal tract time to strengthen. A good physician with a solid background in nutritional therapy should be consulted before any drastic dietary changes are made.

CHELATION THERAPY

While atherosclerosis and arthritis often exacerbate each other, treatments other than diet that are directed at one condition often are beneficial in treating the other. For example, Dr. Steenblock discusses how chelation therapy, an intravenous chemical treatment commonly used for atherosclerosis and heart disease, can also benefit arthritic patients:

"One of the problems with osteoarthritis is that the capillaries of the synovium have become rigidified, or more rigid than they should be, as a consequence of the aging process and of atherosclerosis. This limits the blood flow through these joints; therefore, the heat that is produced when the joint is put in motion cannot be taken away because the circulation is poor. As a result, pain occurs when you exercise, and conversely, when you are resting, the blood flow through that tissue is poor and toxic materials accumulate and can cause pain. Anything that increases the diameter and the blood flow through these capillaries will aid in the restoration process. This is where chelation therapy is very valuable because it actually gets into these small blood vessels and capillaries and removes the cross-linkage of the collagen and elastin. This makes these small blood vessels more pliable and elastic, gives them more diameter so that more blood can pass through them, and thus helps in the healing process."

CHONDROITIN SULFATE

Dr. Steenblock also uses chondroitin sulfate as part of his treatment. Over the past decade, chondroitin sulfate has been used in both Europe and Japan for the treatment of osteoarthritis, rheumatoid arthritis, and atherosclerosis. he explains. "Again, there is a great similarity between osteoarthritis and atherosclerosis in the sense that both result from the wear and tear caused by irritative substances in the body. We need to protect these collagen surfaces from the irritative substances that circulate in the blood and ultimately get into the joint.

"Chondroitin sulfate appears to be one of the best treatments for both arthritis and vascular disease. When you take it orally, it actually enters into the body through the intestinal tract and will selectively go to the joints and all the areas of damage in the blood vessels. It not only acts preventively but also will help reverse the diseases that are present."

Dr. Steenblock says that while chondroitin is a promising treatment, it is not a miracle cure. "The treatment is not the sort of miracle drug type of treatment where you give the person one pill and get immediate results. What we are dealing with is a natural substance, and it takes time for these natural substances to create the result we are looking for, namely, healing of the injured areas." He says that it may take from 2 to 4 months to see results.

Dr. Steenblock adds, "There is another substance, which is derived from the New Zealand green lip mussel. There are a number of trade names for it. This substance is also a mucopolysaccharide, and it is effective in treating osteoarthritis as well as rheumatoid arthritis. It is available in most health food stores.

"These mucopolysaccharides can also be used preventively to heal the small nicks and irritations that occur routinely in the blood vessels and joints. They immediately seal these little cracks and crevices so that they do not get larger. Our bodies are not really capable of doing that on their own, and we need to help them along...."

25

Osteoporosis

Osteoporosis (the word means "porous bones") is a serious problem in which the skeletal system weakens and fractures easily. It may be accompanied by pain, especially lower back pain, loss in height, and body deformity. More females than males become afflicted, with postmenopausal women being at greatest risk. Osteoporosis is attributed to the gradual loss of calcium. In women, this loss begins in the mid-30s at a rate of 1 to 2 percent a year, and can increase during menopause to a rate of 4 to 5 percent a year.

More than 10 million Americans have osteoporosis. The disease is responsible for more than 1.5 million fractures a year.

In the past, osteoporosis was thought to be an inevitable part of the aging process, particularly in women. Now most of us know that it is treatable and, more important, preventable.

Causes

According to naturopathic physician Dr. Jane Guiltinan, the most likely candidates for osteoporosis share a number of characteristics:

Northern European ethnic origin

Small frame

Family history of osteoporosis

Diet high in meat, caffeine, sugar, refined carbohydrates, and phosphates (found in sodas and processed foods)

Cigarette smoking

Alcohol use

Sedentary lifestyle

It may surprise some people to learn that dairy foods, while rich sources of calcium, can also contribute to the condition of osteoporosis. Registered nurse and acupuncturist Abigail Rist-Podrecca notes, "When I was in China, we noticed that no dairy was used. We expected to see a high incidence of osteoporosis, rickets, and other bone problems. In fact, we saw the lowest incidence. In the West, dairy is used a lot and osteoporosis is rampant. Something is not quite right here." Two main factors responsible for the Chinese not getting osteoporosis, she learned, are diet, weight-bearing exercise, and acupuncture.

Diagnosis

In the past, osteoporosis was not diagnosed until the condition was so advanced that patients began to break their bones. Today, however, bone mineral density testing is being used to detect the disease and those at risk for developing it. The National Osteoporosis Foundation recommends that every woman over the age of 65 have a bone density test. For people under 65, the test is recommended if there are risk factors for fracture, such as excessive thinness, cigarette smoking, a previous fracture in adulthood, or a family history of fractures.

Bone density testing is noninvasive and takes only a few minutes to perform. It provides a measurement known as a T-score. T-scores can indicate normal bone density, low bone density, or osteoporosis.

Conventional Approach to Treatment

For people with T-scores below specific levels, conventional treatment involves the use of prescription medications. Synthetic estrogen is the traditional drug of choice for postmenopausal osteoporosis and its prevention, but controversy surrounds its safety and effectiveness.

Naturopathic Prevention and Treatment

The first step in osteoporosis prevention is noting whether or not you are at high risk for the condition, says Dr. Jane Guiltinan. Obviously, certain risk factors cannot be changed, but many can be addressed, and will prevent the destructive effects of the disease.

Diet

A diet that is low in animal products and high in plant foods promotes bone growth and repair. Green, leafy vegetables contain vitamin K, beta carotene, vitamin C, fiber, calcium, and magnesium, which enhance the bones. Other calcium-rich foods include broccoli, milk, nuts, and seeds. Sesame seeds have high calcium content. The Chinese, who as mentioned earlier have low rates of osteoporosis, use sesame often in their foods, and cook with sesame seed oil.

Foods to avoid include sugar, caffeine, carbonated sodas, and alcohol, as these contribute to bone loss. Chicken, fish, eggs, and meat are also contraindicated. These are high in the amino acid methionine, which the body converts into homocysteine, a substance that causes both osteoporosis and atherosclerosis.

The official recommended dietary requirement for calcium for people at risk of osteoporosis is 1,000 to 1,300 milligrams per day. I recommend that women over 25 take in approximately 1,000 milligrams in supplement form and an additional 500 to1,000 milligrams from the diet. For those over 40, supplements of 1,500 to 2,000 milligrams are needed. Women on estrogen replacement therapy require between 1,200 and 1,500 milligrams.

In addition to calcium, the following nutrients are critical for keeping bones strong:

Magnesium (800–1,200 mg in citrate form)
Vitamin D (400 IU)
Vitamin C (1,000 mg)
Vitamin K (100 mcg)
Beta carotene
Selenium (75–150 mcg)
Boron (3 mg)
Manganese (5 mg)
Strontium
Folic acid (1 mg)
Silica
Copper
Zinc

A balanced vitamin/mineral supplement will provide most of these nutrients. It is best to take zinc separately, however. Otherwise, it can have an adverse effect on vitamin and mineral absorption.

Natural Hormones

Research indicates that natural progesterone from wild yams is safer and more effective than estrogen in that it builds strong bones and has no harmful side effects. Dr. Jane Guiltinan notes that "Estrogen minimizes calcium loss from bones, but progesterone can actually put calcium back into bones." Natural progesterone can be taken in pill form. It also comes in a cream form. Half a teaspoon should be rubbed into the skin over soft tissue and the spine, twice a day, for 2 weeks out of every month.

DHEA, a precursor to estrogen and testosterone, is important in the prevention of numerous chronic conditions associated with aging. As we get older, there is often a drop in DHEA. If blood levels are low, 5 milligrams a day can safely be taken as a supplement.

Herbs

Herbalist Susun Weed recommends horsetail, taken as a tea every day, to restore bone strength and density. She adds that dandelion root tincture will promote absorption of calcium. The micronutrients important for bone flexibility and strength are found in the greatest abundance in seaweeds, dandelion, and nettles, and in organic vegetables and grains.

Exercise

Dr. Howard Robins, former director of the Healing Center in New York City and coauthor of *Ultimate Training* and *How to Keep Your Feet & Legs Healthy for a Lifetime*, stresses the importance of weight-bearing aerobic and weight-lifting exercises for osteoporosis prevention.

Aerobic exercises use major muscle groups in a rhythmic, continuous manner. Weight-bearing aerobic exercises such as brisk walking, jogging, stair climbing, and dancing produce mechanical stress on the skeletal system, which drives calcium into the long bones. Non-weight-bearing aerobic exercises such as biking, rowing, and swimming are not as helpful in osteoporosis prevention, but they do promote flexibility, which is useful for people prone to arthritis.

People "need to perform aerobic exercises anywhere from three to five or six times a week," says Dr. Robins. "You need a day off every third or fourth day so that the body can heal and re-energize."

"Most women stay away from weight training because they are afraid of developing huge muscles like Arnold Schwarzenegger," says Dr. Robins. "The good news is, that won't happen. No matter how hard you train, you will never get huge muscles as a woman unless you take steroids to alter your body's metabolism."

Not only is weight training safe, it is important for preventing osteoporosis. As muscles are pulled directly against the bone, with gravity working against it, calcium is driven back into the bones. It also stimulates the manufacture of new bone. This adds up to a decrease in the effects of osteoporosis by 50 to 80 percent. People need to do weight training two to three times per week for 15 to 30 minutes. All the different muscle groups should be worked on. Twenty-four hours should lapse between sessions to rest muscles. For women, an exercise program should be started long before the onset of menopause.

A complete routine is more than aerobic and weight training exercises only. It incorporates warm-ups at the beginning and cool-downs at the end of a routine. Warm-ups are not to be confused with stretches. Rather, they are gentle exercises that produce heat by getting blood to flow into the muscles. To warm up leg muscles, for example, one could lie down on one's back and move the legs like a bicycle, or walk gently in place. Moving the arms and joints gently in all their ranges of motion will warm up the upper body. Warming up the body helps prevent injuries.

After exercise, when the body is loosest, stretching is performed. Stretches are long, continuous pulls, not bounces. Bouncing only tightens the muscles and can lead to injury. Dr. Robins's book *Ultimate Training* describes a holistic workout in detail. Aromatherapist Ann Berwick adds that essential oils enhance a warm-up and cool-down routine. "Before exercise, use warming and stimulating oils, such as black pepper, rosemary, ginger, and sage. Additionally, eucalyptus helps to deepen breathing. After exercise, you can apply a blend of lemon, rosemary, and juniper. These help to carry away waste products and to ease any stiffness."

Yoga

Yoga prevents osteoporosis by building and fortifying bone mass, keeping muscles strong and flexible, improving posture, and helping balance and coordination. Physical therapist and yoga teacher Bonnie Millen explains why this is important: "With yoga, the old adage 'Use it or lose it' applies. Building and maintaining bone mass is most important for preventing osteoporosis. Remember, bone is alive. Yoga is unique in that it incorporates weight bearing on the upper extremities. This is important because many wrist, forearm, and upper arm fractures occur when people reach forward with outstretched arms as they are falling.

"Also important is building and maintaining muscle strength and flexibility. Let's keep the muscles strong so that they can receive the stress before the fracture happens. Also if the body is strong and flexible, it can cushion falls when they occur."

What about posture? "Good posture improves overall functioning and prevents osteoporotic fractures of the spine," Millen says. "I teach yoga to a lot of older women who tell me they are afraid of getting a dowager's hump. This is where the body slouches forward and there is a hump on the back. Just take a moment to get into that posture where your chest caves in and your shoulders slump forward, with your head looking down toward the floor. Try to raise one arm up as if you wanted to touch the ceiling, and see how high the arm comes up. Now let the arm down and come into a nice seated posture, as if someone were going to take your picture. Sitting very tall, raise your arm up and see how high it goes. You can see from that little exercise that the slouched posture really decreases your range of motion. That makes it difficult to function. This is why you want to keep a good posture.

The dowager's hump can create additional problems. Millen explains, "By placing great pressure on the spinal vertebrae, the dowager's hump often leads to compression fractures of the spinal column. This is very painful, as you can well imagine, and you do not have to do anything special for it to happen. Just going up and down stairs or taking a step can cause breakage."

Yoga also helps to improve balance and coordination. "When you are balanced and coordinated, there is less chance of your falling in the first place," Millen says. "You are quicker to respond. And that can help prevent fractures."

Millen points out that there are several styles of yoga but that all systems have foundation poses that address the above needs. Here she outlines a few basic postures:

DOWNWARD-FACING DOG. This posture strengthens bone mass in the wrists and arms. In this pose, you stand and bring your hands to the floor so that the space beneath you is triangular. One part of the triangle is from your hands to your hips, and the other part is from your hips to your heels. The space on the floor between your hands and your feet is the third part. As you hold the position, you will feel that you are bearing weight on your arms.

WARRIOR POSES. These poses increase muscle strength and flexibility, as well as balance. Here you are standing with your legs 3 to 4 feet apart, depending on your height. With your legs apart, you work at the hip to turn one leg out to the side. The other leg is turned slightly inward. That really works the hip muscles, which is important in helping to prevent the all-too-common osteoporotic hip fracture. The arms are either held out to the side or up over the head, depending upon which warrior posture it is.

COBRA. This is a back-bending pose that helps posture and gives flexibility and strength to the paraspinals, the muscles of the back of the spine. To begin, lie face down on the floor. Using the back muscles, sequentially lift the head and chest away from the floor.

SIMPLE STRETCH FOR CHEST MUSCLES. This is another exercise for improving posture that is especially helpful for women who tend to slouch forward. Take a blanket and fold it to resemble a box of long-stemmed roses. Lie down on this bolster, making sure that your head and your entire spine are completely supported. Place your arms out to the side or up to form a V-shaped position with the palms facing up toward the ceiling. Just allow gravity to relax the shoulders down to the floor (Shoulders should not be on the blanket). Breathe deeply. That will expand the intercostals, the muscles between the ribs. This is important because the intercostals become constricted with slouching. That, in turn, decreases lung capacity and causes all the organs to become compressed. This is a wonderful pose where you don't have to actually do anything. You just allow gravity to work for you and your breath to move through you.

Millen says that the best time to begin yoga is before osteoporosis sets in: "The time to begin a yoga practice, or any exercise, is not when you've gotten to menopause, and all of a sudden you realize, 'Oh my gosh! I'm at risk for osteoporosis.' You need to build bone mass throughout your whole life so that you have bone stored up. It's like preparing for retirement. You build up bone mass through exercise, you eat right, you maintain a healthy lifestyle. Then, when you reach your menopausal years, you've got a good store of bone mass to help protect you."

Body Rolling

This technique, developed by Yamuna Zake, a bodyworker in New York City, uses a 6- to 10-inch ball in a series of routines designed to elongate muscles and increase blood flow in all parts of the body. As you relax your body weight onto the ball, the ball applies pressure onto bone, stimulating even bone that has begun to ossify to "wake up." "To me," says Zake, "bone is like dried fruit. Just as a raisin plumps up after you put it in water, when bone is stimulated and becomes alive it undergoes a subtle change, acquiring a supple quality.

"Studies have found that, by stimulating bone, weight-bearing exercise can prevent and possibly reverse osteoporosis. Weight bearing is nothing more than pressure exerted on bone. Body Rolling is actually a mild form of weight-bearing exercise in which the pressure is never more than the person's own body weight."

Acupuncture

As mentioned earlier in this chapter, in China, osteoporosis is the exception rather than the norm. When it is present, acupuncture is used. Acupuncturist Abigail Rist-Podrecca explains how this works: "The Chinese use an electrical stimulus along the spine. The electrical impulse actually helps the bone-stem cells, which are the reproductive cells of the bone, to reproduce, thereby strengthening the bone mass. It was very exciting to see this because we have some Western studies proving that peripheral stimulation by electricity, especially in the long bones in the leg, help this process also." She adds that women low in calcium need to take this supplement so that the body has the raw materials for making bones denser. When weight-bearing exercises are added, the benefits are remarkable.

Homeopathy

Homeopathy can be used as an adjunct to the nutritional and lifestyle factors discussed above. Among the remedies to consider are the following:

CALCAREA PHOSPHORIC. This may help where the bones are weak, soft, curved, and brittle. It can be given for a long period of time.

CORTICOID. Homeopathic corticoid is for painful posttraumatic osteoporosis, especially when it affects the hip. Consider this remedy for an elderly person who has fractured her hip because of osteoporosis.

PARATHYROID. For diffuse pain in the bones, especially the long bones. Walking is very painful. Often, there is pain in the ankles, hips, and knees.

Regarding the appropriate potencies for these substances, homeopathic physician Dr. Ken Korins says, "For acute conditions, meaning they come on suddenly, and they are very intense, use a 200c potency. That is a very dilute potency, but energetically speaking, it is very powerful. For more chronic conditions, where you will be giving the remedy for a longer period of time, you might want to start with 12c or 30c. In general, the remedies should be taken as three to four pellets placed under the tongue. Take them on an empty stomach. Wait 15 to 20 minutes before or after eating. Avoid coffee and aromatic substances, such as mints, perfumes, and camphors, which can interfere with their effectiveness. Also, it is a good idea not to touch remedies with your hands because any residues from perfumes or other substances can interfere with their energy properties."

26

Repetitive Strain Injuries

n all the hoopla that has accompanied the manifestations of the computer revolution—from the original PCs to the World Wide Web—not much attention has been paid to how the installation of computers in offices has physically affected their users. What is talked about is how jobs that were grimy, dirty, and physically grueling, like those in steel mills and automobile plants are being replaced by jobs in service industries—for the less educated, flipping burgers and for the more educated, sitting in offices at terminals processing and moving information.

Those who are infatuated with the world of computers see this exchange— back-breaking labor in the mills traded for work in sanitary, air-conditioned offices—as all to the good. However, although there are undeniably benefits to workers from this exchange, they do not necessarily fall in the area of occupational health and safety. It is undeniable that the owners and managers of plants that manufactured heavy industrial equipment were notorious for disregarding toxic chemicals and other dangers in the workplace, but it is also true that the managers of many light industries have exposed people to years of looking into computer screens and rattling out numbers on keyboards without ever taking a look at the possible health effects of this labor.

One of the better books to profile these effects on both physical and mental health is Barbara Garson's *The Electronic Sweatshop*. She moves up the job ladder, starting with data-entry clerks and moving up to Wall Street traders and Pentagon officials, in order to show how their lives are impacted negatively by working with computers. In her interviews, she hears consistently about loss of autonomy and ill health. This chapter will look at a common type of health problem experienced by people whose jobs involve a lot of time at a computer terminal: repetitive strain injuries, and particularly carpal tunnel syndrome.

The Scope of the Problem

Dr. Timothy Jameson, the author of *Repetitive Strain Injuries: Alternative Treatments and Prevention*, is a graduate of Los Angeles Chiropractic College and a certified chiropractic sports physician. He notes that many people today have repetitive strain injuries. These injuries, he points out, "can affect every structure of the body, which is what sometimes makes them so hard to treat. Most people will start off with simple muscle fatigue, such as affects people who work on computers or on assembly lines. The muscles fatigue because of the overexertion, that cumulative trauma."

To continue to put stress on already fatigued muscle will eventually lead to problems with the connective tissue, or fascia, that forms a sheath around muscle. The fascia responds to repeated stress on the muscle by becoming harder and thicker. It can start getting "sticky" and begin to bind to the muscle and other neighboring tissues. The muscles and fascia become tight and restricted. Eventually, the nervous system gets involved.

A recent study in Great Britain showed that the sensory nerves, the nerves that pick up perceptions from the hands, the skin, and so on, are affected by repetitive strain. They are damaged by cumulative trauma. Cumulative trauma can also affect the tendons that connect muscles to bones. When this happens, the tendon and the sheath that holds the tendon may become inflamed. (When this occurs in the wrist, you have carpal tunnel syndrome.) This condition may lead to problems with the bursas, sacs that protect the joints.

These problems may even involve the spine, according to Dr. Jameson. "People with this type of injury tend to have a lot of pinched nerves that lead down to the arms. The process is very complex."

Dr. Jameson adds that repetitive strain injuries can be extremely serious. "You become very limited in your ability to do any type of work, especially repetitive work. In severe cases, people cannot work at all, cannot even get dressed in the morning. They cannot do the things they normally would do."

Dietary Factors

If you are doing things that can lead to repetitive strain injury or are already suffering from this disability, there are foods you should cut from your diet. The number one items to avoid, which are major precursors of joint pain, are refined sugars, particularly high-fructose corn syrups. These increase sugar within the body, which sets off the whole process of the insulin reaction, with release of prostaglandins, which starts the inflammatory reaction.

Dr. Jameson recommends the book *Enter the Zone* by Barry Sears as a good source of information on proper nutrition. The book "goes into depth on how to prevent an inflammatory reaction. If you look through the aisles of the grocery store, you'll see that something like 50 percent of the products sold there use high-fructose corn syrup as an ingredient. The body has a lot of trouble digesting that. I know of cases where people cut it totally out of their diet, and their repetitive injury subsided within a few days."

Processed meats, such as corned beef, salami, and hot dogs, are very tough for the body to digest and can trigger an inflammatory reaction. Some of the more saturated oils, such as corn oil, palm oil, safflower oil, and butter, should also be avoided. Margarine, too, is bad. Many people think margarine is better than butter. However, margarine, because of its trans-fatty acids, is actually worse for the body than butter.

Vitamins and Minerals

Dr. Jameson recommends a number of supplements. "I would recommend vitamin C, which is very important for tissue healing, starting out with about 1 gram and going up to about 3 grams a day.

"Also very important are the B-complex vitamins. These are used for nerve regeneration and nerve healing."

Minerals are another important supplement that can help in cases of repetitive strain injuries. As Dr. Jameson puts it, "You should never underestimate the power of minerals to rejuvenate cellular tissue." He puts his patients on a complete mineral regimen, with either colloidal or chelated minerals.

"A lot of people—especially people in jobs that involve heat, a lot of sweating, in the summer—are sweating out many of the minerals in their body. So if they are doing a lot of cumulative work and sweating they are depleting their body's mineral's resources." A list of the minerals and vitamins that Dr. Jameson finds useful for preventing and treating repetitive strain injuries follows. "I usually prescribe these substances in pill form," he notes, "but you can also get all these things in food."

CALCIUM. Calcium is very important for muscle activity and for bone growth; it is also a muscle relaxant. Take about 800 milligrams a day of calcium, a little more if you are pregnant or postmenopausal.

MAGNESIUM. Magnesium is also important for muscle relaxation and for coenzymes. It is required for the functioning of about 80 percent of the enzymes in the body. Good sources of magnesium are vegetables and whole grains. Dr.

Jameson recommends starting out with about 200 to 300 milligrams of magnesium a day. He says. "That's a small amount, considering that magnesium is not well absorbed. However, I always like to start my patients out with small amounts to see how they react."

MANGANESE AND ZINC. Dr. Jameson says that zinc, in particular, is really important for enzyme function and for cellular healing. He recommends about 20 or 30 milligrams a day. Zinc is found in fish, meat, and poultry.

SELENIUM. Selenium, another valuable substance, is found in fish, wheat germ, and garlic. Take 50 to 200 micrograms a day in the pill form.

VITAMIN E. Vitamin E is a very important antioxidant; Dr. Jameson recommends 200 to 400 international units (IU) per day.

BETA CAROTENE. "Beta carotene," Dr. Jameson remarks, "is a compound found in vegetables of a yellow-orange or dark green color. Carrot juice is a great source of beta carotene. I recommend that patients drink carrot juice to get a natural, fresh form of the compound."

COENZYME Q10. Dr. Jameson says coenzyme Q10 is particularly important for patients with underlying heart disease. It's also important to maintain cellular energy, which is vital in cases of repetitive strain injuries.

PROTEOLYTIC ENZYMES. These enzymes "scavenge around the cells and rake up any cellular debris, aiding the healing process." Dr. Jameson explains.

CARTILAGE GROWTH FACTORS. Dr. Jameson adds, "There is also some good research now on the cartilage growth factors glucosamine sulfate and chondroitin sulfate. I recommend them for patients who have a great deal of joint discomfort—joint pains, irritation of the elbow, the spine, or the hands and fingers."

Herbal Remedies

Certain herbs help the body relax, which is important in overcoming some repetitive strain injuries. Although Dr. Jameson doesn't have specific dosage recommendations, he offers these ideas. "Valerian root can be used for reducing muscle spasms. It should be taken toward the end of the day, because it's a relaxant. You wouldn't want to take it throughout the day, because it might affect your ability to perform. Garlic is a natural antibiotic as well as antifungal. Some of these muscular problems can stem from an underlying fungal problem, something we also see in fibromyalgia. A third valuable herb is ginkgo biloba, which increases circulatory function and brain function and enhances memory. It helps the blood flow get down to the extremities. Cayenne has also been found to help increase circulation. And ginseng is great for stress relief."

Homeopathy

In addition to vitamins, minerals, and herbs, homeopathic remedies can be of service. Try the ones you find in health food stores that are recommended for muscle and joint injuries and for rheumatoid arthritis.

Carpal Tunnel Syndrome

Carpal tunnel syndrome, a widely recognized type of repetitive strain injury, is a common disability affecting office workers who sit at computer terminals. It is important that workers at risk for carpal tunnel syndrome not only follow the suggestions we make here but also learn to sit and type with the correct posture and to use ergonomically designed chairs and keyboards.

CAUSES The direct cause of carpal tunnel syndrome is the effect on the tendons of the lower arms of day-in, day-out use of the same muscles and nerves to perform a repetitive task. The result is numbness, tingling, and pain that worsens at night. It's a miserable disorder.

Dr. Ray Wunderlich is board certified by the American Academy of Pediatrics and the College for the Advancement of Medicine, practices preventive medicine in St. Petersburg, Florida, and is the author of many books, including *The Natural Treatment for Carpal Tunnel Syndrome*. When treating a case of carpal tunnel syndrome, he starts by looking for contributing factors. For women, he asks immediately, "Is she taking birth control pills?" The pill, in essence, "puts you in a simulated state of pregnancy, and we know that pregnancy is one of the risk factors for carpal tunnel syndrome. Birth control pills also diminish the nutrients in the body, some of the water-soluble vitamins. Moreover, many women who take them become bloated. They develop minor degrees of fluid retention." The carpal tunnel is a narrow space in the arm, which becomes too narrow if the tissues are swollen. Women who are taking birth control pills and who perform tasks likely to lead to carpal tunnel syndrome should consider some other form of birth control.

Two other contributing factors, says Dr. Wunderlich, are hormone replacement therapy (HRT) and thyroid deficiencies. With regard to HRT, Dr. Wunderlich says, "If the estrogen preparations are not in balance with the progesterones, this can cause problems."

Dr. Wunderlich finds that 75 to 80 percent of his patients have some kind of thyroid disorder. He says, "On top of the repetitive movement of their jobs, many people have thyroid disorders, which contribute to the syndrome and may be hard to diagnose. To pin this down, look for a pale, puffy person, edematous, which is to say retaining fluid. When there is swelling, especially in connective tissue and in the nine tendons that run through that carpal tunnel, that medial nerve in the tunnel is often screaming for more room."

Another background factor may be low adrenal states, which may occur for a variety of reasons. People who overwork themselves, who take caffeine and/or sugar, who have bombarded their body with these substances and are now faced with repetitive tasks and sedentary living, may wind up with low-functioning adrenals. In the workplace, they develop various allergies, sometimes combined with low blood pressure. These people often have swollen tissues, which contributes to the problem.

Then, of course, there is diabetes. Type II diabetes in particular is often accompanied by edematous conditions. This may not be readily observed, Dr. Wunderlich cautions. "It may be microedema rather than pure edema. The ankles may not be swollen, for example, or the lungs congested, but the tissues may be slightly swollen.

"When the blood sugar is too high—which is almost a definition of diabetes—osmotic pressure rises. As we know from high school, osmosis is what controls the body's fluid pressure. The fluid should be in the blood vessels and in the lymph tissues. When it's outside in the body tissues, as happens in high blood sugar states or after we eat a lot of candy or, sometimes, fruits or juices in excessive quantities, the tissue may become water-logged. This too can cause problems in that narrow carpal tunnel. The medial nerve is screaming with numbness and irritability and pain every time we move our fingers."

Food allergies are another potential contributing factor to the development of carpal tunnel syndrome—and many other disorders. The repetitive, monotonous diets that so many people consume, especially with high-protein antigens—such as milk, cheese, and sometimes eggs—often produce food allergies. And a hallmark of the allergic response is swelling. Although the swelling is on the microlevel, the little cramped carpal tunnel reacts to the swelling, causing pain.

But even if you are not allergic to what you're eating, if you're on a typical American diet, you may have problems. "The 140 pounds of sugar per person, per year, that the average American still eats is one problem," Dr. Wunderlich says. "We're not talking about a long time ago. It's still happening. And there are also the salt-laden diets, which could be improving as people are counseled by alternative nutritionists to take high-potassium foods over high-sodium foods. There are also animal foods, which are high on the inflammatory scale—they tend to accentuate the inflammatory cascade, or series of chemical reactions through which inflammation develops. Animals are on top of the food chain, and that is where all the refuse accumulates, all the toxic chemicals that get into the animals' fat. This is especially true if the animals are domesticated and not wild, which is the case with most of our animal food sources." Thus if you are not following a pristine, organic diet, which the majority of people are not, you may be contributing to the risk of carpal tunnel syndrome or worsening an already existing condition.

Finally, Dr. Wunderlich says, there are "the chemicals in the workplace. When you are sitting at your computer, you may be bombarded with pesticides they have sprayed around your place—every month they come in and do that, or every 2 weeks if they see a lot of roaches. All of this adds to the toxic load as background factors."

CONVENTIONAL TREATMENT By the time a person with carpal tunnel syndrome consults a physician, the condition is often in a quite advanced stage. According to Dr. Wunderlich, "The person often has atrophy of the muscles and irreversible or nearly irreversible nerve damage. The doctors operate, often with excellent results. So it's very appealing." However, this is a drastic therapy and will result in a life with further impaired function.

For less severe cases, conventional medicine's procedure is less felicitous. "What ordinary medicine does is give pain relievers—aspirin, Tylenol, ibuprofen, and other nonsteroidal anti-inflammatory drugs, which in the long term are all counterproductive, damaging the gastrointestinal system, producing leaky gut, as well as actually destroying cartilage. But those are the standard therapies that are offered."

ALTERNATIVE TREATMENTS Dr. Wunderlich's program is short, sweet, and sensible. "The number one approach in treating this problem," he states, "is detoxification. We do a vitamin C bowel flush. That's the first step for bowel tolerance." The vitamin C flush gets accumulated toxins out of the body. Follow this up with the second step, taking your favorite bulking agent, rice powder or psyllium, for example. "Number three," he mentions, "is to support the liver. I like artichoke and thistle compounds. Maybe 100 milligrams of thistle, three times a day, and 500 milligrams of artichoke leaves three times a day. Those are basics, plus water.

"I also use infrared heat to have people sweat, carefully monitored, of course, so there is exchange of body fluids. Also, exercise is important. I do running."

In his program, then, he emphasizes detoxification of the body, shifting to a sensible vegetarian diet, exercising, and improving stress management.

It is a question of priorities, Dr. Wunderlich concludes. "Many people have kids, two jobs, and so forth, so they think they do not have time. But you have to sort out the priorities, which we are not doing. You have to have good air and an appropriate amount of sleep. You need to avoid toxic foods. It is also important to have regular bowel movements, and you have to use your body appropriately for you, hopefully in some sweating way."

The advice that Dr. Wunderlich gives about carpal tunnel syndrome also applies to people who have any type of repetitive stress syndrome. Ultimately, we need to make our workplaces more livable. This will involve the improvement of human interaction and of the machines we surround ourselves with. If we upgraded our environments as obsessively as we upgrade our computers, we might have very few occupational disorders with which to cope.

27

Temporomandibular Joint (TMJ) Dysfunction

The temporomandibular joint (TMJ) is a hinged joint that opens and closes the jaw. There are two such joints at either side of the head. The jaw is part of a wider system, the craniosacral system, which extends from the skull to the lowest segment of the spine. Disruption at any level of the craniosacral system can result in TMJ dysfunction.

Causes

The two most common causes of TMJ problems are poor bite and stress. Poor bite may be the result of new dental work that affects tooth alignment. Sometimes braces shift the palate, which affects the jaw.

TMJ dysfunction affects larger numbers of women than men due to stresses brought on by hormonal changes. Dr. Deborah Kleinman, a chiropractor who works with TMJ patients, explains: "There are various stress factors we can talk about that are specific to women. First, we have premenstrual tension. This further weakens an already weakened system. I know women who only have a problem with their jaw 3 days before their period. As soon as their period comes, their pain goes away. This tells me that there is a weakness in the system and that hormones push the body past the point of being able to compensate for it.

Hormonal changes also occur during pregnancy. "Hormones loosen the pelvis so that the woman is more flexible during delivery. And pregnancy creates structural changes through weight gain and the loosening of ligaments. These changes can further aggravate TMJ dysfunction.

"With nursing, postural changes can play a big role. Nursing places stress on the upper back muscles, especially if the woman doesn't use the proper pillows or if she gets lazy and slumps over while feeding her baby. These upper back muscles insert into the occiput, which is part of this craniosacral system. The occiput is the bone at the bottom of the skull. Tightening or pulling on the occiput can affect the head, neck, and TMJ."

The hormonal changes that occur during menopause also play a role in TMJ dysfunction.

Symptoms

Pain can be isolated in the joint itself or it can radiate to the face, neck, ear, and shoulder. Headaches may be a part of the picture. There may be a nagging toothache, even though the tooth is healthy. A person with TMJ problems may find it difficult to open the mouth all the way. Inflammation of the muscles around the joint may cause a spasm in those muscles, locking them open. Clicking, grinding, or popping noises may accompany chewing or movement of the joint.

Craniosacral Therapy

Cranio means "skull" and *sacral* refers to the "sacrum," which consists of the lowest five vertebrae of the spine. Craniosacral therapy is founded on an understanding of the relationship between these structures and several points in between, including the TMJ. Dr. Kleinman, who uses a specific form of craniosacral therapy called the sacro-occipital technique, explains: "A chiropractor like myself who uses this technique understands that there is a balance between the nervous system and the musculoskeletal system, and a relationship between the pelvis and the sacrum and then the head and the cranium. Between both structures rests the spine, the shoulders, the neck. All of these structures react to shifts in the pelvis and the cranium. The TMJ is part of that." She adds that a stable pelvis balances the body and works in harmony with the cranium. This allows information to flow to the brain smoothly.

Dr. Kleinman says that with TMJ the first step is to have a doctor perform a series of tests to determine whether structural stresses exist, and, if so, where. Once the structural stresses are identified, treatment can begin. Dr. Kleinman explains: "We place wedges or blocks under the pelvis. The muscles will relax and contract around these levers in an unforced way, based upon what these levers tell the brain. Then we incorporate breathing techniques to assist the brain in making musculoskeletal changes. This reestablishes the proper craniosacral flow." Sometimes secondary manipulations are necessary to readjust parts of the spine that lie between the pelvis and cranium that get knotted up as a result of compensating for the pelvis and the cranium. Cranial adjustments, made specifically to the temporomandibular joint, also help to reestablish proper balance.

Other Physical Therapies

Isotonic exercise, done regularly, can help some cases of TMJ dysfunction. In addition to jaw exercise, self-treatment for TMJ problems may include jaw awareness, in which the patient tries to notice and avoid clenching and grinding the teeth, as well as biting on gum, ice, or fingernails. Eating soft foods and avoiding resting or sleeping on the stomach can also help, as can learning to rest the jaw and to adopt proper jaw posture. Other potentially helpful techniques include self-massage; relaxed rhythmic opening and closing of the jaw; alternating moist heat (15 minutes) with ice (2 to 3 minutes) to increase circulation; cool sprays and cryotherapy; bite guards; and splints. Surgery should be a last resort when dealing with TMJ problems.

Another physical therapy that can help relieve TMJ problems is Body Rolling, a technique developed by bodyworker Yamuna Zake, author of *Body Rolling: An Experiential Approach to Complete Muscle Release.* "Many of the muscles that run up the back and insert in the skull, as well as the muscles in the front of the neck, have attachments between the head and the chest. Thus the amount of tension in the muscles of the back, front, and sides of the neck can affect the level of contraction of the sutures (joints) and muscles of the cranium, and specifically the TMJ," she explains. In Body Rolling, a 6-inch-diameter ball is used to apply traction that lengthens and releases muscles. "The degree of tension in the TMJ is controlled by the tension maintained in the neck. By working the neck muscles with the ball to keep them at maximum length and minimum tension level, you can help reduce the buildup of tension in the TMJ." Zake has designed specific routines that use the ball to release the front and back of the neck, as well as an around-the-neck routine that helps break the holding pattern of tension that distorts head and neck alignment.

Nutrition

Nutritional supplements may help in treating TMJ problems. Some of the most useful are listed here.

CALCIUM AND MAGNESIUM. These minerals are essential for proper muscular function and have a sedative effect.

B-COMPLEX VITAMINS. Take 100 milligrams of B-complex vitamins three times a day. B-complex vitamins are essential for combatting stress.

PANTOTHENIC ACID. The appropriate amount of pantothenic acid to take is 100 milligrams, twice daily. B-complex vitamins, like pantothenic acid, are for combatting stress.

COENZYME Q10. Coenzyme Q10 is another stress fighter.

OTHER SUPPLEMENTS. L-tyrosine and vitamins B_6 and C will improve sleep quality and alleviate anxiety and depression. It is also important to take a multivitamin and mineral complex.

PART FIVE

Foot and Leg Care

The film *Raise the Red Lantern* concerns the problems of a bride who marries into a polygamous household in early 20th century China. Although it is basically a tragic story of rivalry between the husband's four wives, it does have a few lighter moments. The newest wife, played by Gong Li, learns that whichever wife the husband temporarily favors receives more gratifications than the others, such as better food, more attention from servants, and so on. This includes, as one of the most prized features, the right to a foot massage. Of course, the reprehensible ancient Chinese practice of foot binding probably accounts for some of the respect given to foot massage. However, Western audiences see nothing but humor in the sensuous pleasure Li obtains from the massage, not recognizing, as this section will show, the value of massage, which should be part of the regimen of anyone who wants to have and maintain healthy feet and legs.

Massage is just one way to have healthy feet and legs. It is also necessary to choose good shoes, exercise properly, and have the right attitude toward your extremities. After discussing the components of keeping your feet and legs in good health, this section will look at some of the typical injuries and disease conditions that attack our lower extremities—and suggest remedies. We also include a special focus on sports injuries.

28

Healthy Feet and Legs For a Lifetime

In the modern world, our feet are at a disadvantage. Long ago we used our feet, along with our hands, to swing from trees. Our toenails were helpful for maintaining a strong grip on the bark of trees. When our feet weren't taking us through the treetops, they were taking us along the ground—with our hands doing the other half of the work. Through many generations our feet gradually adapted to carrying our weight alone and walking miles across soft, grassy earth.

Even now, our feet have not fully adapted to bearing our entire body weight, and they are far from adapted to walking on hard surfaces like concrete. They are still evolving, growing longer and wider, in response to the hard surfaces we pound them on. The bigger the area of the foot, the more the weight of our bodies and the pressure of the concrete is dispersed, and the less trauma to the foot. This evolutionary change is happening rapidly: Each new generation has feet larger than those of their parents. You can even see the change reflected in the sample shoe sizes displayed in stores. Where the ladies' sample size used to be a 5 or 6, it is now more likely to be a 7 or even an 8.

Get Familiar With Your Feet

If you were shown pictures of 10 pairs of feet, including your own, could you pick yours out? Many people couldn't. If you want to pamper your feet, you first have to recognize their features and be aware of the changes they go through at different periods of life. Let's start with the foot's "normal" shape. (Don't worry about normality too much, though. Nature offers wide variations and what my be "abnormal" for some is perfectly normal for others.)

Take a look at the line of your foot. Does your foot appear to be twisted, or is it straight? If you trace your foot on paper, you may find it easier to see. Look at your toes. The first should be nearly straight, the second through fifth curving slightly. The shape of the normal foot is smooth, with no lumps or bumps. Is your heel well-rounded and smooth without bumps? Are your arch and instep high or low? If you notice your arch is dropping, then you know something is changing, and you should have it checked. If you have smooth heels now but later see a bump on one of them, you know something unusual is happening. This is significant: If you know what the normal shape of your foot is now, then you'll be alert to any changes that are taking place.

Does your skin look and feel normal? Is it soft, supple, and evenly colored? Skin color should be uniform, with no red marks. What is the texture of the skin? Do you normally have hair on your toes or not? A minute detail like a disappearance of hair from your toes can alert you to a circulation problem.

Now with a full-length mirror, watch yourself walk. What is your normal posture? Is your head erect and your shoulders straight? If your head and shoulders are slumped too far forward or held back too rigidly, the rest of your body will be thrown out of line. Your chest should be slightly out, stomach slightly in. Look at the upper body as a unit. It should be held squarely over the pelvis, which should be in line with your legs. Do you throw your hips or your upper body forward when you walk? Too much of a forward thrust can create an imbalance, which can cause back, hip, knee, ankle, or foot problems.

Look at your feet as you walk. Each foot should strike the ground on the heel, just slightly to the heel's outside, then twist slightly in. At that point, the foot should start to twist up again until "toe-off" occurs. This may sound complicated, but if you walk slowly and mindfully for a minute, you can determine your normal pattern.

You can heighten your awareness even further by observing what is normal for other people in walking. If you think you have posture problems, it would be worthwhile to consult a professional to help you diagnose, correct and control any difficulties. Professional treatment can help you return to or maintain your normal gait, which can prevent foot and leg problems further down the line.

Feet From Infancy to Old Age

As we age, what is normal for our feet and where difficulties are likely to occur will change. So, along with knowing what is normal now, it's important to know how our feet are going to change as they move through time.

INFANTS The rotated-out positioning of a baby's legs stems from the thighbone's outward rotation. The rest of the leg and foot structure follows suit. Babies' feet are supposed to point outward. Dr. Howard Robins, my consultant for this chapter, often sees worried parents who say, "My baby's feet are twisted out. How will he walk?" Out-toeing should correct itself naturally, normally disappearing by the time the child is 2. But in-toeing, pigeon-toedness, is not normal and will not correct itself.

In-toeing is easy to spot in adults: Feet point toward each other as the person walks. It's harder to check for in-toeing in a baby who is not yet walking. If you notice your baby's feet turn in rather than out, ask your pediatrician to take a look. The younger the child is when you spot such a problem, the easier it will be to correct.

What about the baby's hips? An easy way to check for normal hip placement is to turn the baby over on his or her stomach, face down, and look at the creases behind the thighs. Do they line up evenly from side to side or are they out of line with one another? If they seem significantly off, the pediatrician should be consulted. Also check the "anchor sign." This is the double curve running from the crack down the baby's buttocks and through the two highest creases on the top of the thighs. It should be well formed with the line straight down the middle and evenly curved on each side. As in the case of in-toeing, any hip dislocation should be treated immediately.

If you know how the skin on your baby's feet and legs normally looks and feels, then discoloration, inelasticity, or dryness will alert you to the need for care. At any sign of inelasticity or dryness, give your baby a foot massage with oil. If the condition hasn't cleared up after a couple of days, consult your doctor.

Besides knowing what is normal for your infant's feet, you also have to respect their feet by using good hygiene. Proper footwear is necessary for good hygiene. Since babies don't walk, shoes are not needed. In fact, chances are that if your baby develops a toenail problem, it's because he or she has been wearing the wrong kind of footwear. If you want to keep your child's feet warm, use booties or socks.

Proper foot hygiene includes washing and massaging baby's feet, as well as clipping toenails. No soaps should be used on baby's feet and legs unless they are dirty. Otherwise, only warm water on a daily basis is necessary, since your baby is hardly likely to get dirty enough to need a soap bath, which dries the skin. In the bath, make sure to clean between the toes as well as washing the baby's feet. When you dry, gently pat over the whole foot rather than rubbing vigorously.

Babies love massage and their feet and legs can benefit from it. After drying the baby's feet and legs, gently rub in a little sunflower, safflower, or soy oil, using the same technique you would use on your own body. (Later, we will describe adult massage.) Massaging is especially useful for dark skinned babies whose skins tend to be drier than those with lighter skins.

TODDLERS Once your baby starts to walk, the outside edge of the child's foot should be almost straight. If you notice it turning in, have his or her feet checked.

A simple exercise can complement a physician's treatment toward correcting this condition. Sit in front of your child while the child is lying on his or her back. Grasping the baby's heel in one hand, place your thumb and index finger on each side of the foot along the borders of the sole, so the toes lie between these fingers. Very gently place pressure on the outer side of the foot to straighten it. Hold the stretch for 15 to 20 seconds. Doing this exercise five or six times in a row, twice a day, can help move the bone structure back into the proper position, avoiding later problems.

The out-toed effect should have disappeared by the time the child has begun to walk. If out-toeing persists after age 2, bring it to the notice of your doctor.

As your child begins to walk, you may notice he or she has flat feet. This should not cause worry since your child's foot structure will be developing over the years and that includes developing the arch that is right for the child's weight and body type.

You also might worry if it seems your toddler is not toddling as early as the children of other parents are. Your child will walk, when, and not until, the musculature in his or her feet and legs is ready to do the job. There is certainly no rush, and trying to make your baby walk before his or her time is foolish. Nationally, the average age for the first step is16 months. However, to see a child beginning to walk at 20 or even 24 months is not unusual.

As far as selecting the child's shoes, remember the "rule of half thumb." There should be at least a half thumbnail's length—an eighth to a quarter of an inch—from the end of the child's longest toe to the end of the shoe. Toddler's shoes should be flexible so they respond to the movements of the foot. The shoe should actually bend with the ball of the foot, so he or she can "toe-off" properly. As for socks, cotton is best because it allows the toddler's feet to breathe and is less likely to irritate the skin than a synthetic.

Shoes and socks are important to wear. Even in the house, the child should wear socks or slippers. Even a tiny hair can penetrate a child's delicate skin, causing pain, redness and infection.

OLDER CHILDREN You might notice that your child seems either knock-kneed (with legs too close together) or its opposite, bow-legged. Both conditions can occur within "normal" development but if either condition seems to hamper your child's movement, then see your doctor.

Keep an eye on the skin of your child's feet and legs. If it becomes dry, give an oil or skin cream massage for a night or two after bathing. By now the toes should be lying straight, and there should not be any new twists or bends. The arch should be fully developed.

Going barefoot results in one of the biggest foot problems for children: picking up foreign bodies that penetrate the skin. Because an older child tends to be very active, a running shoe is highly recommended. However, if your child is involved in many different sports, you would be wise to purchase basketball or baseball shoes, since running shoes are made for unidirectional activity, and they may trip up a child who is making quick turns and darting off in all directions. In any case, most children this age have little use for a leather-soled dress shoe. They need the adequate support, easy movement, and protection found in a lightweight canvas or nylon shoe.

ADULTS AND THE ELDERLY We will consider adult foot care in the sections immediately following. If you are over 60, observation and maintenance are more important than ever. At this stage any change in your feet or legs can point to a larger problem. For instance, swelling in the feet can indicate general edema. Since your feet are at the far end of the circulatory system, they can give you signals as to what is happening in your system as no other organ can.

Good hygiene is central. Daily bathing is not imperative, particularly since you may be susceptible to dry skin. Because of the dryness, moisturizing should be stepped up to twice a day, morning and evening, with the same oils we recommended for infants. You might want to massage your feet twice a day when you moisturize because it stimulates circulation. Later we describe the 10-Minute Morning Massage, which is applicable here.

Before and After Your Exercise

Along with eating sensibly, getting proper rest, and having a positive outlook on life, exercising is essential to living in optimal health. Although we cover exercise in other parts of this book, in this chapter our focus will be on the proper care of the feet in situations ranging from formal exercise programs and sports to plain old fun on the beach. We will also outline a walking program.

Later in this chapter we will talk about sports injuries, but at this juncture let us look at preventive measures. In playing sports and in training, it is important to be in touch with your body. Your body is always giving you feedback. Any lack of awareness of this feedback can leave you prone to injury.

Proper warm-up and stretching before beginning any type of workout is crucial for preventing injuries to the legs and feet. The best way to warm up the leg muscles is with the Robins Six-Step Exercise.

WARMING UP: THE ROBINS SIX-STEP EXERCISE Lie down on the ground with your legs straight in front of you. This exercise is to be done with a slow, rhythmic, continuous movement. Counting with a beat will give you the proper rhythm for the exercise. It is to be repeated five or six times in a row on each leg. Do not alternate legs but do one at a time.

STEP ONE: Slowly bring your heel toward you.

STEP TWO: Bring your knee to your chest, without using your hands.

STEP THREE: Straighten your leg up in the air so the knee is straight (even if this means lowering the leg slightly).

STEP FOUR: Lower the straight leg about halfway to the ground.

STEP FIVE: Slowly let your heel come down to the ground.

STEP SIX: Straighten your leg out again on the ground. This exercise will get the heart rate up slowly and gradually increase circulation to the muscles.

REAR LEG STRETCHES To prevent rear leg muscle injuries, use two gentle stretches. First, while you're lying on the ground on your back, taking one leg at a time, bring a knee under your leg and help pull your leg and knee into your chest. Never put your hands in front of the knee as the hands may slide up and cause the kneecap to jam into the thigh. When you pull the knee to your chest, it should be a long, slow pull, never letting it bounce outward. After 20 seconds, allow the leg to go straight out again. Then repeat the exercise. Do this three to five times per leg. This stretches the hamstring and gluteal muscles of your upper leg.

The second exercise is for the calf muscles. This is done by sitting up and a grabbing a towel or belt and slinging it around the bottom of your foot. Grab one end of the belt with each hand. Sit with your back and head straight and your arms straight in front of you. Do not let the arms bend at the elbow joints. Lean backward and allow your body weight to pull your foot toward you. Next, let go of the towel with one hand and your foot should flop forward to where the other foot is resting since you aren't using muscle power to pull the foot. Do this exercise three to five times per leg.

WINDING DOWN After completing your workout, there are two valuable active stretches you can do to help wind down. For both, face the wall, standing as close as you can get, with feet and legs a shoulder-width apart and palms placed flat on the wall at face level. Take a step back, keeping both feet pointed perpendicular to the wall. In the first of the two stretches that use this stance, the rear leg is kept straight. As you stretch, try to keep your rear leg, knee, hip, and shoulder all in a straight line and do not allow your heel to come off the ground. Lean toward the wall and support yourself with your entire arm and forearm. Hold the position for 20 seconds. You should feel the stretch from behind the knee all the way down to the heel. After the allotted time, push out from the wall to relax.

In the second wall stretch, allow the rear leg to bend slightly forward at the knee. This will work another portion of the rear leg muscles. You will feel this stretch more in the belly of the calf muscles and behind the heel bone. This should be done three to five times per leg, not alternating but taking one leg at a time.

To stretch the upper rear leg muscles, the hamstrings, place your foot on a stool, chair, or table. Straighten your leg, then pull your foot forcefully toward your body, and hold it that way. Keep your back straight and arms straight out in front of you. Let your fingertips lift as you lean forward gently. By lifting your fingers and arms up as you lean, you will find that your back stays straight so it is unstressed. Pulling your foot toward you has created a strong stretch on the rear leg muscles.

The iliotibial band of muscles extends from the hip to the thigh. To stretch these muscles, stand with shoulder against a wall, then step away from the wall with both feet. Gently let your hip lean in toward the wall. This causes your body to move in the shape of the letter C, gently stretching the iliotibial band muscles. Do this stretch three to five times.

It is not necessary to do this stretch often unless you have problems with these muscles.

Remember, overstretching can also lead to injury. A stretch should be slow and continuous, lasting from 10 to 30 seconds. A stretch that is too long or overextends the muscle or that involves choppy, bumpy motion can lead to injury.

Walking As Exercise: The Elements of a Good Walking Program

Only recently has walking been recognized as an excellent exercise for everyone. What we want to spend a few minutes talking about is not the walking to the store each of us does every day, but a walking exercise program. To condition our hearts and circulation, tone up our muscles, and generally keep our body systems functioning at optimum capacity, walking has to be undertaken systematically and conscientiously. It must be done daily. If you're elderly or out of shape, however, you might start by walking for 3 or 4 days in a row, then taking a day off to let your body rest.

As with any other route you take in exercising, embark on walking in a gradual, controlled way. You'll need to build up the length of time you walk, from perhaps 10 minutes a day at the beginning to perhaps 30 minutes to an hour when you're in shape.

A big help when you start out is to keep a notebook of your physical signs. As with other aerobic exercise, progress is to be measured by pulse rate. First you'll have to establish what your optimum heart rate for exercise should be. Subtract your age from the number 220. Multiply the result by 60 to 75 percent, which gives you the range of heartbeat you should be able to reach as the goal of your walking program. Then take your pulse rate when you are sitting down. The best place to take your pulse is at your wrist or temple. If you take the pulse at your wrist, use the lesser fingertips to feel the pulse, not your thumb since it has an artery whose pulse can interfere with your reading. The fingertips are placed on either side of the two grooves found on the underside of the wrist near the outer edges. You may take your pulse for a minute or for as little as 10 seconds, multiplying by six to obtain the beats per minute. Record your pulse rate in your notebook.

As you walk, stop every 5 or 10 minutes to take down your pulse rate. This will give you an idea of the effect the exercise is having on your heartbeat and circulation, and how close you are getting to your target pulse rate. When you get home, record in your notebook the highest pulse rate reached during exercise.

It is important not only to increase the length of your daily walk systematically, but also to increase the pace of your walk. With increased exercise, your heart rate will tend to decrease. Therefore, to reach your desired goal, you must exert yourself to increase the challenge to your heart and circulation. If you are elderly or disabled, you may be unable to do this. In that case, compensate by increasing the length of time you walk. The longer and faster you walk, the more conditioning you get.

Build up slowly in terms of time and pace to a peak program. If you're using time as your guide, add about 10 percent more to the time you walk every 2 weeks. For instance, if you start by walking 20 minutes a day, after 2 weeks, add 2 minutes more. If distance is your guide, increase by the same 10 percent each 2 weeks. This allows safe stress buildup in the bones and muscles and lets the heart adapt to the stress that's being placed on it.

GETTING READY Wear a comfortable shoe that fits so as to cushion and protect your foot. A running shoe is ideal since it is made for the same unidirectional motion as walking. What you don't wear is as important as what you do. Don't carry anything—not even a purse. Any weight at all can throw your posture off. Wear clothing that allows heat buildup to dissipate quickly. Cotton undergarments are good because they allow the moisture on your body to evaporate.

Running shirts and jogging pants are good to walk in as long as they are constructed from materials that will absorb and dissipate perspiration. In the winter your outer clothing should be made of wool, which breathes while keeping you warm, while the clothing next to your skin should be cotton or polypropylene. Also wear something to keep your face warm as well as gloves and mittens.

It's best to walk on a somewhat empty stomach. Try not to eat for 2 or 3 hours before walking, just so your body won't be burdened by trying to digest and walk at the same time. However, you should be completely hydrated. Drink 8 to 10 ounces of water every hour before you go. This measure ensures your body won't overheat as fast while you're walking.

A warm-up is essential. Start by relaxing your mind and body. Try to let any tension and stress go. This paves the way for loosening your muscles. Once you've relaxed, stretch for 5 or 10 minutes, utilizing some of the stretches we outlined earlier. After the stretches, loosen up. Move all your joints, from the neck down. After shaking your body, spend a minute on each foot, massaging it, kneading it, flexing all the joints by hand. This prepares the feet for a good walk.

Plan your route before you leave. Decide where you are going to be walking, what terrain you will be traveling over. Try to avoid areas of rough terrain.

WALKING STYLE The first thing to be aware of when walking is your posture. Your body should be erect, with head up, shoulders back, chest out, stomach in. Avoid being slumped, stoop-shouldered or hunchbacked. Don't look straight down at the ground.

Walk with a regular cadence. Walking at a slower rate to begin helps you warm up your body. After 5 or 10 minutes of walking slowly, you can work up gradually to the actual speed you want to maintain. There's no need to take big, long steps, which can actually throw off your balance. Instead, to increase your heart rate, increase the cadence, that is, the number of steps you take in a given interval.

At the beginning of your walk, as you are building up to your optimum pace, you will have lots of energy. However, if you get winded or tired, you should slow down. Easing off helps build up your wind, restoring your tissues by getting more fresh blood into them to wash away waste products and increase the energy flow. When you feel stronger, you can go back to a quicker cadence. At that point, you will be able to maintain your faster speed for a longer period of time. Again, remember to make a record of your walk in your notebook so you can see the progress you are making.

As you walk, a natural swing of the arms from front to back is important. Not too tight, not too loose is the rule. For example, never hold your hand in a tight fist, but don't let it fall totally slack at your side either. Just hold your fingers lightly together, with the thumb resting on top of the index finger. If your arms are swinging this way, your shoulders will be relaxed as well.

As far as the lower half of your body goes, you should be swinging your legs from the hips forward, allowing the heel to strike the ground before the ball of the foot, slightly on the outside. If you find yourself bouncing up and down and walking on your toes, your rear leg muscles probably need to stretch. It will be better, though, to do that after you walk rather than before or during the exercise.

The way you breathe is as important as the way you walk. Abdominal breathing is best. Breathe through your nose and let the breath go out through your mouth. Take long, deep breaths that fill up the upper and lower portions of your lungs. This type of breathing naturally forces your stomach to expand when you inhale. Breathing this way gets the most oxygen possible into your system quickly, increasing your strength and stamina during the walk.

If you start to get winded and need to breathe faster, do so. If you get too winded, stop and take a few deep, cleansing breaths to reoxygenate your tissues. Then continue your walk.

If you develop cramps in your legs, stop, massage the muscle and let the cramp dissipate. Then continue. If you feel the cramp starting again, stop again. Cramps may be caused by waste products building up in your tissues when not enough blood and oxygen are getting to them. By massaging the ailing tissue, you break up some of the spasm in the muscle tissue and increase circulation. This helps wash away the waste products, re-energizing the tissue.

AFTER THE WALK After your daily walk, you'll want to stretch both rear and front leg muscles. For the rear muscles, you can use the stretches described earlier. The muscles in the front are important since they may actually be weakened by walking. You can do this by sitting on a countertop or firm tabletop. Slowly extend your foot until the leg is perfectly straight. You should be in an L shape with your back straight. Hold that for 10 seconds and let your leg come back to a bent knee position. Repeat this from 10 to 20 times for each leg.

After your walk, rehydrate your body by drinking plenty of fluids. You may want to eat a light meal after your pulse rate is normal.

THE BENEFITS OF WALKING By walking in this way, consciously and with discipline, not only are you benefiting the entire muscular system, you are burning excess fat and reducing overall body weight while gaining balance, stamina, strength, and endurance. Moreover, you'll be improving your ability to relax emotionally. The extra oxygen coursing through your brain raises the levels of serotonin and endorphin, morphinelike but natural substances that allow a state of relaxation to occur.

This is a program well suited to dieters. Recent studies have determined that if you are exercising at 70 or 75 percent of your maximum heart rate (as indicated according to the calculation described earlier), you are taking in enough oxygen to burn fat rapidly. Your body will turn to the fat for fuel to supply the energy needed for your walk, using it for about 70 percent of that supply. If you are walking above 75 percent of your top heart rate, your body will turn to the glycogen (starch) stored in the muscles and tissues and burn that as well. So if you want to lose weight, shoot for getting your heart rate into the 70 to 75 percent range.

Footwear Basics

Whether you are embarking on a walking program, participating in sports, or just trekking to the subway on the way to work, you need to have the right shoes. In this section, we will look at what criteria to use in buying shoes, which shoes are the best for different sports, and which are a must to avoid. In general, what we have to look at in every shoe is fit, material, and style.

IF THE SHOE FITS... First remember the "rule of thumb." For infants, a half thumb was sufficient, but for adults there should be a thumbnail's length between the end of your longest toes and the end of the shoe. This ensures adequate toe room. Your foot slides forward from an eighth to a quarter of an inch each time you take a step, so the rule of thumb is important. You don't want to jam those toes with every step.

Next, the width. The foot width is usually measured across the ball of the foot. If you want to tell whether a shoe you are trying on is the proper width, first, stand up. Take your thumb and roll it across the leather on the top, across the ball from one side to the other. You should be able to see the leather wave, almost as if you could pinch it between your thumb and forefinger. That's adequate width. If your big or little toe joints press out on the shoe when you're standing up, it's too tight.

Next check the width at the heel. Good shoes are wider up front and narrower in the heel. The top of the shoe shouldn't rub against toes that are higher than others. If the shoe rubs, you're inviting corns. Also be sure that if the shoe is leather, the leather is soft enough to flex and bend with your foot.

MATERIALS AND CONSTRUCTION For the upper part of the shoe, the best material is leather, which will let your foot breathe, allowing perspiration to escape and letting the shoe dry overnight. As far as insole and inner materials go, the more natural, the better. Synthetic materials cause your feet to heat up, leading to a buildup of sweat that can cause problems for your feet as well as accelerate the breakdown of your shoes.

While leather soles were once considered ideal, with the hard surfaces we are forced to walk on today, thick rubber soles or ones made of a synthetic material are best. They save wear and tear on your feet in a way that leather simply can't.

The back part of the upper shoe, which surrounds the heel and comes along the side of the foot about midway forward, is called the "counter." The counter is usually made of a rigid material, often some form of plastic. For dress shoes as well as regular walking shoes look for a firm counter because your feet need that support.

Heels should never be totally flat. A heel height of approximately 1 inch, with a slight wedge construction, gives the average person the best prevention against leg, foot, and lower-back problems. Whether the heel is rubber or leather does not make much difference. A rubber heel has the slight advantage of absorbing more stress when the heel strikes the ground.

STYLE CONSIDERATIONS For dresswear, it is best to choose slip-on shoes. For walking around, however, you will do better with strap and lace shoes, which don't allow the foot to move around in the shoe quite so much. If you walk a lot on the job, you'd be better off in an oxford than in a slip-on.

If you want the ideal shoe for everyday life, for walking and standing still, choose a running shoe. This applies to everyone, whether or not they run.

Running shoes are more shock-absorbing than the average leather shoe or any other kind of sports shoe. They are built with a wedge. The wide-flared heel gives good ankle and knee stability by preventing the foot from moving around inside the shoe. Running shoes not only shock-absorb the forefoot but the heel-strike as well, reducing the amount of pressure that will go through to the foot and leg.

SHOES TO AVOID

HIGH HEELS: These can wreak havoc on your feet by shortening the calf muscles, hamstrings, and buttocks, which will often lead to lower-back, knee, and ankle trouble. If you have to wear them, do proper stretching exercises after you wear them to compensate for the stress on those muscles.

BOOTS: Boots are not made for walking on concrete. They are suited for farmers or wranglers who spend their time on soft earth. They do not hold the foot securely. The movement they allow can lead to instability. If you wear them for dress, choose a pair with a little less than the thumbnail you would allow plain shoes. Too much room will allow too much slippage and the possibility of blisters. On the other hand, don't give yourself too little room or you will end up with corns on your toes.

SANDALS: Wear them on the beach not on the block. The same goes for moccasins and deck shoes. In the city, with their thin soles, they just transmit huge amounts of stress and force into your feet that can end up really hurting them.

RUBBER THONGS: Unlike sandals, my recommendation for these is that they shouldn't even be worn at the beach. The synthetics in them can cause skin irritation when they react with the perspiration on your feet. At the beach, they may catch in the sand and you end up with a twisted ankle. The thongs between your toes can cause blisters.

Special Considerations for Sport Shoes

Three factors determine what shoes are right for your sport: the motion it requires of your feet; the surface you will be playing on; and the shape, flexibility, and other idiosyncrasies of your feet and legs. Finding the right shoes after having pondered these three factors is largely a matter of trial and error.

The point of this section is not to recommend particular shoes, which change season by season as manufacturers incorporate improvement and a new understanding of what works best for individual sports. The best source of this type of concrete consumer rating is probably the magazines devoted to particular sports. They usually review new shoe models. Another potential reservoir for information is the salespeople in the stores that cater to customers who practice the sport in which you are involved.

RUNNING, JOGGING, AND WALKING A running shoe is suited to the few sports, such as running, jogging, and walking, in which an athlete sets out in one direction—forward. Where most other sports require players to move in all directions, the runner always goes straight ahead. The runner's shoe must be one that keeps the foot and leg facing forward, so the runner doesn't twist the knee or ankle and has a cushioned landing. This is taken care of in running shoes by a flared heel. The heel helps control your rear foot and knee as they leave the ground, keeping the leg's unidirectional movement stable.

At the same time, the width of the heel absorbs the impact of your foot against the ground. This is crucial since with each step you take your heel may have to endure three to four times the force of your body's weight as it hits. Running shoes have a special shock-absorbing wedge, called a midsole, between the rubber bottoms and the upper of the shoe. You can see the sides of this midsole when you look at a good running shoe. It's usually a lighter colored wedge of material that gives the bottom added thickness. Some of these midsoles are firm, others emphasize compressibility. In general, if you have fairly rigid feet with high arches, you need maximum flexibility together with high compressibility and shock absorption. If your feet are softer you can tolerate a more rigid shoe, since your feet already are designed to absorb some shock.

If you are using the highly compressible, impact-absorbing midsoled shoes, there is one thing to be aware of. These shoes lose their compression ability rather quickly, which may be gone before the sole shows any real signs of wear. If you have high arched feet that demand this type of shoe, you'll have to buy running shoes more frequently than your less arched competitors. To be specific, if you are a serious runner, covering 10 to 20 miles a day, your shoes will lose their compressibility after 6 weeks. You may hate to toss what look like still new shoes, but giving your feet the protection of zippy new sneakers as soon as the old ones lose their bounce is your best insurance you have to keep your feet and legs healthy.

Running shoes shouldn't cost an arm and a leg, but don't buy the cheapest available either. Usually, within the $40 to $60 range you can get a decent pair. Another tip: Don't try to buy your running shoes in a regular shoe store. Go to a good running-wear store that specializes in footgear and equipment, and carries a wide variety of shoes up to the top of the line. That way you can try on the best and compare them. Most of these stores will let you walk around for a decent period in the shoes you think you like best. Gary Murke, winner of the first New York Marathon, and now owner of Super Runner's Shop in Manhattan, even lets customers jog up and down on the sidewalk in front of his store to see how the shoes feel. He knows how frustrating it is to buy shoes without knowing whether you will feel good running in them.

As far as fit goes, remember the points already made in this section about the rule of thumb and checking width. Note also, that you shouldn't be trapped into thinking that you wear a certain size and that's it. In a running shoe, you may need a half to a size and a half larger than your street shoes.

For very wide feet, try shoes from New Balance of Boston, Van's of California, and Saucony of Massachusetts. If your feet are narrow, see if you can find shoes made by Brook's, New Balance, or Van's.

RACQUET SPORTS For racquetball, tennis, squash, paddleball, and other racquet sports, another factor comes into play in selecting your shoes. Because you need to be able to twist and turn when necessary, you should avoid the flared heel of the running shoe, as it will trip you up when you try to move to the side. You want simple shoes that conform to the shape of your foot and are adequate for the terrain on which you will play.

For tennis, especially when you are playing on a concrete court, an impact-absorbing, a padded sole wouldn't hurt. As opposed to running, where most of the weight falls on the heels, in racquet sports you have to be on your toes, literally, since it's the ball of your foot and toes that take most of the floor shock. Unfortunately, most tennis and racquetball shoes sold today are not as good for the feet as they should be. The soles are thin and the shoes offer little in the way of compressibility. However, a few manufacturers are starting to adopt a wedge construction that incorporates a layer of impact-absorbing material. If you play often, it would be worth your while to shop around until you found these shock-absorbing shoes.

As in running, if you have very wide or very narrow feet, you may have trouble finding shoes you can wear. However, New Balance has brought out wide widths for racquet sport shoes and, hopefully, other companies will follow this lead.

OTHER SPORTS Traditional basketball sneakers, which many players still prefer, lace all the way up the ankle. Researchers have found the canvas "high-top" ankle section is actually too flimsy to give the support most players need. For most people involved in this sport, we recommend a regular, low-cut sneaker. You can buy sneakers that are specially designed for basketball but, in truth, any sneaker designed for multidirectional movement will do the job.

For baseball, too, normal sneakers will do. Some players feel, because baseball is played outdoors, they play best with a rubber spike, which can dig into the earth, giving them added traction. If you want to wear spikes, that's fine, but try to avoid shoes with long, thick spikes or metal-tipped cleats to reduce the chances of hurting another player.

Some people swear by the special cycling shoes that are now manufactured. They say these shoes are superior because they fit well into the toeclips (which are on the pedals to keep your feet from slipping off) and they transfer force more readily to the pedals. In my opinion, unless you're a serious competitor, just about any flat-bottomed shoe will do, such as tennis or racquetball sneakers. You can even wear running shoes, since the flared heel is of no disadvantage to a cyclist who uses no sideways motion. It is worth remembering that in running the main force falls on the heel, whereas in cycling force falls on the forefoot, so a shoe with added forefront shock-absorbing qualities would be preferable.

The metal cleats of golf shoes don't carry the same risks as those worn on baseball shoes since you don't slide into other players on the putting green. The only risk these cleats pose the wearer is that the player may get caught in a pot-hole walking between shots. The cleats on golf shoes are not for efficient walking but so that the golfer has traction and stability when swinging the club.

As an alternative to golf shoes, you can wear almost any athletic shoe, though you should avoid running footwear, which would limit rotary movement of the feet and ankles.

Socks for Sports

It may sound silly, but the socks you're wearing can make all the difference between enjoying yourself and playing your best, and being uncomfortable, cranky, and off your game. In sports and exercise, even little things count and that means you should pay attention to things that seem insignificant, like socks.

The primary purpose of socks is to keep your feet comfortable and as dry as possible. Socks that are too tight bind your feet. Socks that are too large bunch up, causing blisters and skin irritations.

The best socks for most sports are made of cotton or cotton/Orlon. These materials are good because they act like the wick of a candle (hence the attribute of these socks called "wicking"), which draws perspiration up and away from your feet, leaving them relatively dry and sweet-smelling while you work up a sweat. Synthetics, especially nylon, do the opposite. They insulate your feet, leaving them sticky, sweaty, hot, and, most likely, smelly. Smelly feet are not just to be avoided because they bother your locker room partners. Smelly feet are a sure sign that large numbers of microorganisms are breeding on the surfaces and in the warm, moist crevices of your skin. The best preventative is not to wear synthetic socks, though a thin band of nylon elastic to hold up the socks is acceptable.

In winter, for sports such as ice skating, skiing, and hockey, you will want the warmth of wool, but you also need something with the ability of cotton to wick away perspiration. So wear two pairs of socks: a thin undersock of cotton and a warm outer sock of wool.

Year-round, the best color for socks is white. Colored socks contain synthetic dyes. If your sweat mixes with and dissolves the dye from your socks, you may not only find your skin is tinged with the color of the socks, but that it itches and smarts because your skin has reacted adversely to the dye.

Change your socks at least once a day. If you perspire a lot, change whenever your socks get wet. Whatever you do, never wear a pair of socks twice in a row without having washed them. Fungus and bacteria grow at an alarming rate in sweaty socks.

Foot Massage

We have already talked about the high value Mainland Chinese place on foot massage. Massage can be used to treat injuries as well as to reduce the tension that causes back pain, muscular tenderness and tightness, headaches, swelling in the legs and feet, and weakening of the immune system. Regular massage from one to three times a week can help prevent and safely treat these problems, as well as reduce the strains of athletic performance.

To understand how massage is beneficial we must think about what happens when our muscles or tendons are injured or overtightened. First, the muscle and tendon fibers contract. They become brittle and inelastic, and hence easy to tear. This tightness causes electrochemical changes in the salts found within and outside each muscle-tendon cell. As a result, fluid gathers around the cells, and trapped protein molecules cluster and grind together. A swelling forms around the cells made up of lymph and protein molecules. The return flow of lymph throughout the lymphatic circulatory system is blocked. This disruption puts pressure on the nerve endings, causing pain in the muscle.

Massage reverses this process. It breaks up the clusters of protein cells that block the flow of lymph fluids. Electrochemical balance is restored. Finally, the muscle-tendon fibers relax. When these fibers are relaxed, energy is consumed and utilized more effectively. High blood pressure caused by constriction of arteries from tight muscles is often reduced. The circulation to injured cells returns to normal, bringing in nutrients and removing toxins and waste products. As muscles relax, tension and anxiety are reduced.

There are some basic principles and techniques that will help you get the most out of massage. Following are two massage routines. The first, designed to take from 6 to 10 minutes, is easy to do by yourself. It is an ideal wake-up tonic for your feet and legs in the morning or to soothe them after a long day. The second, more in-depth massage will take between 30 minutes and an hour. It is best administered by a friend and is meant for maximal therapeutic benefit.

THE 10-MINUTE MORNING MASSAGE The best preparation for any foot massage is relaxation. Take a nice hot bath to relax your muscles or, if you don't have time for that, just lie down on the floor, close your eyes, and "let yourself go" by taking long, slow, deep breaths for 3 to 5 minutes. Open your eyes slowly. Now that you are relaxed, you can start the massage. It helps to have an oil like sunflower, safflower, or soy oil—which moisturizes the skin at the same time—on hand.

If you are fortunate enough to have someone massage your foot and leg, the best position is to be lying on your back. If you must do it yourself, sit up with your back supported against a wall or firm chair. This will prevent back strain. Start at the toes and work your way back to the heel and then up the leg. First, manipulate all of the joints in your toes. Flex them one at a time in each of the toes—the metatarsal joints, the bunion joints, and the ones further back. Then flex the ankle joint by rotating your foot in a circle to loosen the whole area up.

The best way to rotate your foot is to cross your legs, hold the leg of the crossed one just above the anklebones, and relax the foot completely. The point here is not to use the muscles of your foot to rotate it—that wouldn't be very relaxing—but to use your hands and let your foot just flop. Just take the front portion of your foot and slowly turn the whole thing in small, slow circles. Go first in one direction, then in the other. Alternate directions for at least a minute. This loosens up and lubricates your ankle joint with synovial fluid, a clear liquid manufactured in your joints to lubricate the cartilage. Synovial fluid also softens your ligaments—those panels of tissue that make your joints stable—and keeps them pliable. So, getting the fluid into the joints on a regular basis is a good way to prevent sprains. As we age, the natural production of synovial fluid lessens, making it especially important to lubricate the joints.

After you've rotated each foot for a minute, gently massage the musculature of each foot, top and bottom. You can use your fingertips to knead the feet with varying pressure. Move them in circles. Use the heels of your hands, or your whole hand, to gently squeeze and knead the muscles. Don't be afraid to use pressure, unless you are very sensitive. Massage should start with the toes and work all the way up the leg to the thigh. To do it properly, spend at least 3 to 5 minutes on each leg. That may seem like a long time, but it's really not very much time for preventing injury to your feet and legs by keeping them pliable.

IN-DEPTH FOOT AND LEG MASSAGE A complete massage of the legs and feet will take between 15 and 30 minutes per side. Put aside the time. Why rush such a pleasant experience? Missing any section of tissue or point of energy blockage may minimize the positive effects of the effort. Always be in touch with your body's sensations, and communicate them to the person massaging. This will allow the person to concentrate on areas and points that need it most.

A quiet room with dim lighting will be most relaxing. A noisy, bright room will tend to work against the stress-reducing benefits of the massage. The room temperature should be warm enough to prevent a chill. While scented massage oils are generally available, cold-pressed safflower or sunflower oil is less costly and will usually work as well. You may add your own fragrance if you wish.

Massage is best performed in five simple stages. In each stage, begin with the tip of the toes and work up. This will encourage proper lymph circulation and energy flow. Never start with the legs and work toward the toes, as this can block flow.

STAGE ONE breaks up swelling in the muscles and tendons and encourages fluids to flow out of the muscle fibers and into the lymph channels. This is accomplished by short, fast, light stroking of the fibers toward the heart. When muscle fibers are sore or tender, this stroke may hurt slightly. After only 20 or 30 seconds, however, the discomfort will probably diminish. Much of the pain is caused by trapped fluid between muscle cells. This stroke should be repeated for up to 1 minute along the whole length of the muscle. Begin at the bottom of the foot and work back toward the heel. Next go to the top of the foot and work from the toes to the ankles. Continue this process from the ankles to the knee both in front and in back of the lower leg. Next work from the knee to the hip. This process directs the flow of the extra lymph fluid toward the major collection area in the groin. If a particular areas hurts more to the touch spend more time on it, but always be very gentle.

STAGE TWO uses very firm, long, slow strokes. As in Stage One, begin at the toes and stroke first toward the ankle, both on the top and bottom of the feet. Next stroke from the ankle to the knee, and finally from the knee to the hip. Use the palm of your hand and the area between your thumb and index finger. It is very important to add more and more pressure with each stroke to help force out the extra fluid from the muscle fibers. If a particular area is very painful, go back to Stage One for that area before continuing. At this stage lotions or creams will allow the hand to slide easily over the skin. If no lubricant is used, the skin may begin to feel tender and irritated. The smooth sliding action is important to help relax the muscle fibers, and can help reduce anxiety and general tension. This stage may take from 5 to 15 minutes per leg to complete.

STAGE THREE requires slow, careful pressure applied to each point on the foot and leg, beginning at the toes and again working toward the hip. You may use your thumbs, fingertips, or both. Press down gently and feel for a firm, small lump of tissue (often the size of a pea) under the skin, deep in the muscle or tendon, as well as around it. The pressure should be straight down. These points follow the patterns of acupuncture points called meridians. Not all the places along these lines will be painful. If there is no pain or discomfort, move to the next place on the skin. As you come closer to active points, discomfort will mount, often changing to pain when you are over an active point. It is important to breathe deeply. Shallow breathing blocks lymph flow, while deep breaths pump fluids up to the center of the chest as well as reduce the pain the acupressure may cause.

Press for 10 to 30 seconds over each very painful point. Press for only 1 or 2 seconds over nonpainful points. Press each painful point three times, trying to go deeper each time. Picture each painful, firm spot as a balloon that you are trying to pop. When the point is broken, it will no longer feel firm, though it may still feel painful to the touch. People are often surprised to feel these points as they had no idea that they were there.

Charts are not necessary. Discomfort and pain will lead you to the correct places as a Geiger counter leads to radioactive material. The vast majority of points will be found on the bottom of the feet, including in the toes, as well as on the calf and rear thigh. Few exist on the top of the foot and the front of the leg, so don't waste too much time there.

STAGE FOUR is performed by rubbing transversely—across the muscles or tendon fibers—with very fast, short strokes. Increase the pressure gradually. This stroke can help break up adhesions, a form of internal scar tissue on an injured or overused muscle or tendon. Breaking up adhesions returns normal elasticity and a normal range of motion to the muscle or tendon. Spend more time over the most painful areas or points, using your fingertips as well as the palm of your hand. The time it takes to complete this stage varies depending on individual need. Begin with the toes and work your way up to the hip.

The amount of time spent massaging your feet and legs is determined by several factors. If your muscles are tight, injured, or lack adequate blood circulation for any reason, more time should be devoted to massage. How much time will be determined by such factors as who is massaging you, how much free time you have available, the cost if done professionally (the charge is usually by the hour), and the patience, perseverance, and fatigue of the massager. A maximal therapeutic effect is probably obtained somewhere between 15 and 30 minutes per foot and leg, or 30 to 60 minutes total.

STAGE FIVE repeats Stage One, completing the circle of massage therapy.

29

Common Foot and Leg Problems

In the previous chapter, we outlined the way to maintain your feet and legs in the best possible health. Preventing problems by being aware of your extremities, eating right, exercising, purchasing the right footgear, getting enough rest, utilizing massage, and living with as little stress as possible will keep you as fit as possible.

Nonetheless, even the healthiest individual can sustain and injury or illness. This chapter will look at some of the common problems that occur in the foot and leg area, beginning with those that affect everyone and then moving to sports injuries particularly.

Dry Skin

Dry skin on the feet is very common, especially among elderly people who often have poor circulation. If your circulation is bad, that means there is a reduction in fat secretion by the feet's sweat glands, which in turn leaves the skin dry. The decrease in blood flow to the feet also leads to dryness.

Dark-skinned people tend to have drier skin than light-skinned people do. If you have dark skin, avoid using any soap on your feet at all. If you must use soap, make it one of the super-fatted ones—soaps with added oils that are low in alkalis. Among soaps of this type are ones made by Dove, Neutrogena, and Alpha Keri. It's still best, though, to use warm water without soap.

If dry skin is a problem, take the time after your bath to give your feet an oil rub, using soy, sunflower, or safflower oil. Let your skin have a minute or two to absorb the oil while you rub. Then wipe off the excess. If your skin is really dry, try Herbal Salve One (described at the end of this chapter), two or three times a day. At the same time, make a point of avoiding irritating chemicals.

Besides the dry skin oil treatments, try increasing the circulation of your feet by undertaking a cardiovascular exercise program such as the walking routine described in the previous chapter. Vitamins, especially A, D, C, E, and chelated zinc, are helpful in controlling any skin inflammation or problem such as dry skin.

Blisters

Anybody who has ever taken a long hike in the wrong shoes knows all about blisters. When the skin gets irritated, it gets inflamed. To soothe the inflamed area, a natural healing fluid, lymph, flows into the tissues. The fluid puts pressure on the nerves, which can be painful. The best treatment for blisters is prevention. With good hygiene, proper exercise, and appropriate footgear, blisters will never develop.

If you already have a blister, use the following procedure. First gently wash the area with soap and water. Next, wipe it liberally with rubbing alcohol. Clean an ordinary needle by allowing it to soak in alcohol for at least 15 minutes. When the skin and blisters are prepared, remove the needle from the alcohol and use it to create an opening near an edge of the blister. Allow the fluid to drain by gently pressing the blister with a gauze pad. Apply Herbal Salve One over the entire blister and cover it with a sterile gauze pad. Never rub the salve into the blister. If the blister refills, repeat the process.

Calluses and Corns

A callus is a thickening of the skin on the bottom of the foot, usually in a pressure area like the heel or the ball. It is never "normal" and should not be ignored. If you have a normal foot structure, the fat pad that is under your foot should prevent callus formation by acting as an impact absorber. But if the bone structure of your foot is moved out of position, more pressure is placed on dropped metatarsal heads, causing calluses to form across the balls of your feet. (The metatarsals are five long bones that run on the top of the foot to the toes and correspond to the bones on the back of the hands.) If your heel strikes the ground at an improper angle or if you are heavy, calluses can also form.

Calluses are easy to treat by taking a warm-to-hot foot bath every night. Don't use soap, which dries the skin. When you're finished, use pumice stone or an emery board to gently scrape the skin smoother. Then rub oil into the skin until you can see it is absorbed. You might also invest in impact-absorbing insoles to reduce pressure. If these methods don't work, consult your doctor.

Corn is such an innocent name for those hard, round yellow lumps that sometimes grow on people's feet. Corns, which may form either on the tops of your toes, at the tips of your toes, on the sides of your feet, or even inside a callus, are a symptom of intermittent rubbing. They might be caused by extra extensions of bone—calcium deposits—pressing on your skin from the inside of your shoe or from the ground pressing on your skin from the outside. They can even be traced to a bed sheet tucked too tightly. Indeed, patients in nursing homes often develop corns and calluses from this pressure. The delicate skin on your feet can't take too much pressure and so it thickens, growing a protective lump at the point of pressure.

If the corn grows too large, and the source of the pressure has not been relieved, it becomes part of the problem your body was attempting to solve in the first place. The simplest treatment for corns is to reduce the pressure from the outside. You can do this by wrapping lambs wool around high-pressure areas or by using shock-absorbing insoles. You can also work on your corns by pumicing them down after a long bath. But steer clear of over-the-counter corn removers, which have the same danger of burning your healthy skin as do wart removers. You may need a doctor's advice if the corns are persistent.

Skin Infections and Inflammations

FUNGAL INFECTIONS Athlete's foot, the most common fungal infection of the foot, develops as a result of excessive perspiration and the ensuing sensitivity to a fungus that is actually always present on the skin. That should lay to rest the idea that you pick up athlete's foot from the floor of the shower or locker room, left there by other infected individuals. The fungus is already on your feet, it just suddenly gets out of control.

The most common place for fungal infections is between the toes. Along the bottoms of the feet and the soles are other typical locations.

These infections can be chronic, subacute, or acute. The chronic infection looks like dry skin. The skin may peel and itch. In a subacute infection, there may be a breakout of little water blisters. In the more acute infection, there are also breaks in the skin that can become secondarily infected by bacteria. An infection this acute is usually extremely itchy.

While fungal infections are not contagious, they can spread on your own foot until the entire sole is covered.

For an acute infection, the best treatment is to wrap the foot lightly in a gauze bandage, elevate the foot and leg, and use a wet-dressing treatment with Herbal Solution One (explained at the end of the chapter). Pour the solution onto the gauze and let it dry completely. Then wet it again. This treatment should dry out the inflammation. Follow this procedure for 24 to 48 hours. If the acute stage has not subsided by then, consult a professional.

If you have a subacute infection, you do not need the evaporative dressings. Instead you should use Herbal Salve One (also explained at the end of the chapter) three or four times a day. Rub a small amount in until it disappears, wiping away any excess. If there are fissures in your skin, protect them by wrapping them lightly in a cotton gauze bandage. Keep your feet as cool and dry as possible during the treatment. The subacute stage should be resolved in 3 to 5 days.

The chronic infection is the hardest to treat. Most people don't recognize dry skin as a fungal infection at all. To heal a chronic infection, use the salve three or four times a day. If the condition has not cleared up in 6 to 8 weeks, you will need to talk to a physician.

While you are treating your infection, it might be helpful to apply powder to the skin on your feet. However, do not apply powder to the insides of your shoes, because the perspiration from your feet will cause it to cake and become a new medium for fungus to grow.

You can use vitamins and minerals to help with the healing. A good program for that includes vitamins C, E, A, and D, and chelated zinc. If you've ever had a fungal infection, taking vitamins and minerals daily is a good preventative measure.

Nails, too, are part of the skin and can suffer a fungus reaction, which causes them to blacken or thicken. There is no lotion, salve, or other outside chemicals to treat this condition. One treatment that will help is vitamin therapy. Vitamin E taken orally and applied topically to the skin around the nails can improve the quality of your nails. Never apply the vitamins directly to nails themselves. Put it lightly around the nail on the skin and wipe off any excess. The only nonsurgical way to get rid of fungus nails is through a drug, griseofulvin, prescribed by a doctor.

WARTS It is quite common to get warts on the bottoms of your feet. A wart is a virus that gets inoculated into your system through a break in your skin. This is a problem you can pick up in the locker room.

Once this tricky virus is inside, it secretes an enzyme that prevents your immunological system from detecting it. Therefore no antibodies are produced as a defense. The body calls up a second line of defense, surrounding the virus with skin cells to prevent it from spreading.

The majority of warts disappear after about 2 years. It is not exactly understood why, but its seems that the body eventually works out what is going on and develops an antibody or other means to eliminate the wart. But if a wart has existed for at least 2 years, then it should be treated with other means, particularly if it is causing discomfort.

In trying to eradicate a wart, it is important not to overuse over-the-counter remedies. Most contain acid to dissolve the wart, but this can dissolve the skin in the area as well. Professionals use these acids in a different way. They put on a little to cause a skin irritation that will awaken antibodies that will rush to the area and eventually kill the wart.An innovation in recent professional treatment is the surgical laser. This method is often very effective, but does have drawbacks. There is no guarantee that the wart will not return.

CONTACT DERMATITIS Contact dermatitis is another skin condition that can affect the feet. It can be caused by something as simple as a chemical in your socks. Your skin reacts to the irritation, becoming red and inflamed. Little blisters may form or the skin may crack. This problem can occur on any part of your foot.

Your first task is to find out why it is happening, that is, what is irritating your foot. Wash your socks with warm water only, using no soaps or detergents, since these contain alkalis that can irritate your skin. White cotton socks should be worn to eliminate the risk of being bothered by the chemicals in colored socks and synthetics. Change your socks regularly. If your shoes may be causing a problem, change them. Even the most natural leather has been treated with tanning agents that can irritate. The glue that holds the leather together may also be giving you problems. Orthopedic shoe stores carry hypoallergenic shoes, made without the chemicals known to irritate the feet. These may represent the answer.

While you are trying to track down the cause of your difficulty, you can start working on eliminating the problem you already have. Elevate the foot and leg, wrap the foot in gauze, and start applying the evaporating wet dressing, using Herbal Solution One. After 24 to 48 hours of this treatment, the condition should have subsided to a subacute stage. If that's happened, discontinue the wet dressings and switch to the herbal salve, applying it three or four times at day. If the foot is itching, rub the area with an ice cube for several minutes.

IMPETIGO Impetigo is one of the only truly contagious foot conditions. It is usually found in children and starts with a crack in the skin, which leads to a bacterial infection, usually around or between the toes. In the acute stage, it must be treated by a doctor.

In the milder stages, you can approach impetigo with the following methods. Dress the foot lightly in gauze and use Herbal Solution One to draw out the infection and inflammation. The child should be kept off his or her feet as much as possible with the leg elevated. If the condition has not improved after a day or two, go to the doctor.

Other Skin Problems

Psoriasis is a skin condition that commonly affects the feet and lower legs. It is not a disease but a condition—the body's way of ridding itself of negative energy such as tension resulting from problems at home or at work.

The symptoms of psoriasis are patches of reddened, irritated skin, with white scales. If you scratch one of these patches, it will bleed. The best treatment is Herbal Salve One four times a day, particularly if your case is mild to moderate. For a severe case, where there is a lot of thickening on the soles of the feet, it's necessary to rub the salve into the feet at night, covering them with a plastic bag to help hold the salve's moisture in all night. While you're using the salve treatment, it's a good idea to cushion the tissue on the bottoms of your feet by wearing shock-absorbing insoles in your shoes or even flexible protective athletic shoes. Another good idea is to wear cotton socks, so as not to be bothered by the irritants found in synthetic materials.

The best ultimate treatment for psoriasis is to recognize you are taking your problems out on yourself, so you should try to relax. Change your attitude toward your problems, and loosen up.

MORTON'S NEUROMA This is a particular type of tumor. Pressure on the ball of the foot can sometimes result in pinching of the nerves that run between the metatarsal bones. The pressure that results in inflammation of the nerves will first create burning or tingling sensations in the ball of the foot, running up to the toes. If this condition is allowed to continue untreated for months, the fat around the nerves can congeal into a benign tumor, which is called Morton's neuroma. This neuroma is best treated by not allowing the pressure to create it in the first place. It can be relieved with massage and comfortable shoes. Once it has developed, however, it can only be treated by a doctor.

INGROWN TOENAILS Ingrown toenails are another common problem, especially among teenagers and young adults. If you let an ingrown toenail go without treatment, by the time you finally see a professional the treatment may be extremely uncomfortable because the nerves are particularly sensitive here. If treatment is sought early, surgery on the nail will be less painful. So it is important to seek professional care as soon as you realize you have an ingrown nail. Surgical lasers offer an effective means of removing ingrown nails and permanently preventing their recurrence.

INSECT BITES Insect bites can be especially irritating to the feet. Treat them as soon as possible by rubbing the area with ice, which will prevent the release of histamines that cause swelling and itching. Rubbing the area for several minutes also prevents the toxins that were injected by the bite from spreading because it slows down circulation. Repeat the ice treatment every 10 or 15 minutes. You need to seek a doctor's aid only if the bite might be from an insect that transmits disease. If it's a typical bite, ice followed by an evaporating wet dressing such as Herbal Solution One will draw out the inflammation, and that is all that is necessary.

Circulatory Complications

Circulation is the ground of everything we have talked about so far. It feeds your bones, your muscles, every cell in your body with blood. If there isn't enough blood, your tissues will not get sufficient oxygen and nutrients to keep them healthy.

Regular aerobic exercise can prevent arterial and venous disease from getting a "foothold" in your system. Because muscular contractions assist both arteries and veins in keeping a regular blood flow, you build up the health of the conduits by using your muscles. If you don't exercise, you are contributing to the breakdown of circulation. With age, the circulation to the feet and legs becomes less efficient; therefore, the older you get, the more important it is to do some kind of exercise to aid this circulation.

Exercise is also important if you spend a lot of time sitting down. Sitting for long periods can cause a vasospasm, closing off blood vessels and diminishing the circulation. Getting up and walking around the room for 30 seconds every 15 to 20 minutes will help break up vasospasm and restart normal circulation.

The way you eat is also important. If your diet is heavy in fats and cholesterol, you are inviting fatty deposits to develop in the arteries. If you smoke you are also inviting problems. Nicotine is a vasoconstrictor. It causes the nerves to make the blood vessels contract, which stops the flow of blood in some areas.

Let's look now at some specific problems of circulation that can affect the feet and legs.

ARTERIOSCLEROSIS The arteries, which bring blood from the heart to the extremities and the rest of the body, have an elastic quality. If that elasticity is not being maintained because the artery is not getting enough oxygen or nutrients, the artery deteriorates, inviting calcium deposits. This results in hardening of the arteries, or arteriosclerosis obliterans, which keeps the artery from expanding enough to allow a sufficient flow of blood down to the feet and legs. The result of this can be pain in the legs and feet, loss of mineral content from the bones, muscle spasms, and muscle cramps.

The seriousness of arteriosclerosis in the legs and feet can be assessed by seeing how many blocks you can walk before the charley horses begin. These cramps are clinically called claudication pains.

If you suffer from this symptom, you know the only way to stop the pain is to stop walking. A rest allows your heart to pump enough blood into your feet and legs to wash away the waste products that have been clogging up the muscle and causing it to contract. Massage can help too. However, one of the only ways to overcome this problem is exercise. Exercise sends large amounts of blood into the feet and legs, forcing the arteries to open and close widely, forcing them to become more elastic.

Changing your diet can also help. If you have been heavy on the cholesterol, eating a lot of meat and dairy, fatty deposits in your arteries may be one cause of the problem. Taking at least 1,200 international units (IU) of lecithin daily is one of the best ways to control fatty deposits nutritionally, along with cutting down on the fat in your meals.

PERIPHERAL DIABETIC NEUROPATHY The arteries take the blood from the heart while the veins bring it back to the heart for another go-round. In between are the smaller capillaries, which ferry the oxygen and nutrients down into the individual cells and take the waste products out, eventually leading back into the veins.

When there is poor circulation through the capillaries to the nerves in the feet and hands, it can result in peripheral diabetic neuropathy (PDN). PDN is related to diabetes, which can bring on the condition faster than it would for a nondiabetic. (See chapter 44 for a full discussion of diabetes.) One of the results of diabetes, which stems from the inability of the pancreas to produce insulin, is that there are high levels of sugar in the blood. A high level of sugar contributes to the damage of the nerves that results in PDN.

Peripheral diabetic neuropathy is often first detected by symptoms in the foot. There will be excessive sweating as well as sensations of burning, pins and needles, tingling, itching, and numbness. In the most severe cases, the skin may break down into abscesses and ulcers underneath the foot.

Keeping your blood sugar down to normal levels will minimize peripheral neuropathy and regular exercise will maintain adequate vascular circulation throughout the body. This should be aerobic exercise, which uses major muscle groups in a rhythmic and continuous way.

THROMBOANGITIS OBLITERANS Another circulatory problem that affects the feet and legs is thromboangitis obliterans (TAO). It is restricted to people who smoke tobacco. The nicotine in tobacco causes the nerves that control the blood vessels to misfire, shutting them down at the wrong time. Since nicotine affects individuals differently, this condition may be minor for some people but cause drastic changes such as gangrene in others. The obvious solution is to stop smoking.

RAYNAUD'S PHENOMENON Another condition where the sufferer's nerves are misfiring and wrongfully contracting the blood vessels is called Raynaud's phenomenon. It largely affects women and anyone who is easily stressed and deeply emotional. It results in a lack of circulation in the feet and hands. People who are extremely sensitive to the cold are also affected by it.

This phenomenon is even more difficult to treat than some other circulatory problems because it is partly caused by psychological susceptibility and so calls for counseling to teach the sufferer how to control his or her energy by handling problems more constructively.

If you have Raynaud's, be sure to wear proper shoes and socks in the winter to keep warm and even dress warmly in the summer. You can also approach the problem nutritionally. Take vitamin E in doses of 800 international units (IU) three times a day, a half hour before you eat. Vitamin E counteracts Raynaud's phenomenon by dilating the blood vessels, which gets more blood to flow to your feet and legs. Niacin can help in the same way. Vitamin C will work to strengthen arterial walls, while lecithin helps cleanse the fatty buildups on the walls.

FROSTBITE Frostbite shuts down the capillaries. The capillaries are small and those in the toes are the smallest in the whole body. When the foot is very cold, it reacts by cutting off these tiny blood vessels to conserve heat. If the vessels are closed long enough, frostbite results.

Warning signs of frostbite are a painful burning sensation followed by numbness. You may notice not only that the skin on your feet and ankles is cold, but it may be mottled purple and white as well.

The first step when you've seen these warning signs is to rewarm your feet, slowly and gently, in lukewarm water of between 90 and 100 degrees. Circulation will return slowly. In a half hour, the feet will be warm enough for you to assess the damage. If little damage has been done, applications of vitamins A, D, and E (in ointment form) would be helpful. The skin should be protected with a layer of cotton or lambs wool and kept warm. If there's more extensive damage, indicated by injured skin that turns black and continued pain after rewarming, do not try to treat yourself but go to the hospital for immediate attention.

If you know you have a problem with becoming cold, try to protect yourself before you go out. Protect the skin with vitamin A and D ointment or some Vaseline in a thin, even layer all over your foot. Wear cotton undersocks and wool oversocks. An insulating insole can keep the cold from reaching your foot from the ground.

Keep moving when you are outdoors. The more you move, the more the blood circulates. It's when you stop moving that you are at risk.

VARICOSE VEINS Varicose veins, a common condition that usually affects the lower extremities, is the result of damaged valves in the veins. Normally, these tiny valves ensure that the blood flowing through the veins will fully return to the heart. But when these valves are injured, and do not open and close properly, some of the blood runs backward in the veins, pools, and finally engorges the vessels. Varicose veins are large, contorted, unsightly, and sometimes even painful.

Three mechanisms help return blood to the heart, says Dr. Leon Chaitow, a naturopath, osteopath, and acupuncturist from England, writing in an article on the HealthWorld Online website (www.healthy.net): the action of muscles through which veins run, the pulsation of arteries that run alongside veins, and the movement of the diaphragm during breathing. Thus, he says, poor breathing function and lack of exercise, as well as various mechanical stresses, such as those resulting from occupations that require long periods of standing, will make venous return less efficient. Other factors that can increase the chance of developing varicose veins are inadequate fiber, vitamins C and E, and bioflavonoids in the diet; increased pressure in the pelvis, as from chronic constipation.

Another cause of varicose veins, says Dr. Chaitow, is thrombophlebitis, a condition in which the veins are obstructed due to clot formation or an aggregation of platelets and fibrin, which restricts blood blow, causing inflammation and damage to the veins.

Herbalist David L. Hoffman lists several other reasons why the walls of the veins receive inadequate support, resulting in varicose veins: obesity, genetic predisposition, advancing age, tight clothing, and pregnancy.

There are ways to help relieve varicose veins, mainly by doing what you can to keep your blood flow up, in spite of the fact that the veins are not doing their job properly. Exercise on a daily basis is one of the keys to helping this condition. By helping the blood flow, you are counteracting some of the problems due to the damaged valves. Another way to ease the problem is to sit with your feet and legs elevated, waist-level or higher, whenever you possibly can. By doing that, gravity can help the blood move back to your heart.

You can also wear support stockings. Many types are available but we recommend you buy them at a pharmacy or surgical supply store, where the items will be better quality. If you have a severe problem with varicose veins, you might look into custom-made surgical support stockings. In this country, two companies, Jobst and Sigvaris, make them. If you can't afford support stockings, sometime an Ace bandage will give you the support you need. Wrap a 3- or 4-inch bandage around the leg where the varicosity is a problem. This may require wrapping your legs from the toes to the groin if the problem is severe.

Certain foods and supplements may strengthen the integrity of the vein wall. These include dark-skinned fruits and berries, such as blueberries, cherries, and purple grapes. Vitamin C with bioflavonoids, especially quercetin or bilberry, improves elasticity, so that blood can return more effectively to the heart.

Dr. Chaitow also recommends vitamin E, in a daily dose of 500 to 800 international units (IU), which is thought to help develop other channels of circulation, thus relieving the pressure in the veins. Vitamin E can also be applied directly to leg ulcers. Selenium, which works together with vitamin E, should also be taken daily in a dose of 50 micrograms. Essential fatty acids in the form of 500 milligrams of evening primrose oil and four to six capsules of EPA (eicosapentaenoic acid) a day will help decrease the likelihood of inflammation and lower the viscosity of the blood. Finally, he says, it is essential to consume enough fiber to keep the bowels functioning well so that no straining occurs.

Astringent herbs, such as horse chestnut, witch hazel, gotu kola, and butcher's broom, are good to take, although the first two should not be used when pregnant or lactating. Naturopathic physicians often recommend 1,000 milligrams of butcher's broom, two to three times daily, for pregnant women in their third trimester who are troubled by varicose veins or hemorrhoids.

Another factor to consider is dietary support for the liver. This is because a congested liver backs up venous circulation and places additional pressure on the veins, which can then damage valves. Foods such as beets and artichokes and herbs such as milk thistle and dandelion can improve liver circulation. At the same time, it is important to refrain from substances known to cause liver damage, such as drugs, alcohol, and other harsh chemicals.

David Hoffman offers the following lotion, which can be used as necessary to relieve irritation:

8 parts distilled witch hazel
1 part horse chestnut tincture
1 part comfrey tincture
Rose water, if desired

PHLEBITIS Phlebitis is a common adjunct to varicose veins. When the blood doesn't flow up properly because of varicosities, it starts to clot. If blood starts to clot in varicose veins, phlebitis, or inflammation of the veins, results. The overall condition is very dangerous because the clot may loosen and flow to the heart, causing a heart attack, or to the brain, where it will cause a stroke.

The phlebitic area is easy to discern because it is hotter than any other part of the body. A warm compress might prove useful. Just take a kitchen towel, soak it in warm water, wring it out, and place it on top of your elevated leg for 5 to 10 minutes. This will help dry out some of the inflammation in the veins, skin, and tissue, yet it is not hot enough to induce the clot to dislodge.

Another symptom indicating phlebitis is pain in the affected area. The skin in the troubled area becomes dry, itchy, and brittle. It may even crack and peel. Any superficial break in the skin over a varicose area in the leg must be treated promptly to avoid an ulcer. Apply Herbal Salve One to the spot three or four times a day, then cover it with sterile gauze.

Although the outer manifestations of the condition are not that bad, phlebitis requires great care. Total bed rest in which you stay in bed for 2 weeks is the best treatment. You shouldn't even get up to go to the restroom as any movement may dislodge the clot.

Sports Injuries

For athletes in any sport, the feet and legs are particularly vulnerable to injury. Here are some tips about foot and leg injuries that are common to athletes, arranged by affected area.

TOENAIL INJURIES Toenail injuries are common in athletes who wear poorly fitting footgear. If your shoes are too tight, when you run, jump, slide, dance, skid, or skate, your toenails will jam against the end of the shoe, resulting in bleeding under the nail. When the blood dries, you have a black nail. If this happens often enough or seriously enough, your toenail will fall off.

However, if you have the right shoes and you're still plagued by black toenails, your problem may be fungus related. A fungus toenail can look a lot like one injured by being stubbed. If fungus is your problem, refer to our earlier discussion of Fungal Infections.

TOE JOINT INJURIES Toe joint injuries plague athletes of every sort. These joints are very easy to jam. All you have to do is jump onto a toe that happens to be bent under your feet. If the pressure is sudden enough, you will feel a sharp stabbing pain and hear a snapping sound.Probably you've torn a tendon or ligament. Even if the tissue is only partially torn, it can take 6 weeks or longer to heal. With this kind of injury, you must stop playing immediately, get off your foot, and elevate it. Apply an icepack to keep the swelling down. Do this on and off for 24 hours. Then start moving the toes to prevent adhesions or scar tissue from forming.

When you're ready to get back to your sport, tape the injured toe with half-inch tape. Don't tape it too tightly or circulation will be impeded. Just wrap it gently so there is some compression. If it's necessary to tape a neighboring toe, do that as well. The point of taping your toe is not only to strengthen it, but to provide a built-in alarm. If your toe starts to swell again, you can feel it and will know to get off your feet before you are injured again.

But how can you tell if that snap was not a tendon or ligament pulling but an actual bone breaking? A broken bone doesn't just swell, it also turns black and blue. Look for black and blue marks even further up the foot than where the suspected broken toe is. When the bone breaks, so do a lot of blood vessels. If you think a bone is broken, go to a doctor.

METATARSAL JOINT INJURIES The metatarsal joints of the foot are like the knuckles of the hand. Because they are joints, they also have tendons and ligaments that will tear under stress as well as bones that will break.

You'll know the metatarsal joints are injured if you have sharp, stabbing pain and, perhaps, a cracking snap, and swelling. If you've broken a bone, it will likely be evident from the black and blue marks. Treatment, too, is similar to that given a toe. Use elevation, ice, and an Ace bandage or compression dressing.

Injury to the joint under the big toe is popularly know as "judo joint," since aficionados of this sport often suffer from it. Basketweave strapping of the toe can help here as a way to prevent swelling, aid the healing process, and allow for a certain amount of joint movement even though the area is taped.

A stress fracture, a complete or partial breaking of the bone, can also appear at these joints. This one is different from the type of fracture caused by sudden, intense force. You can recognize this injury by the fact that you feel intense pain from the joints when you are working out, but it disappears if you stop the exercise. This fracture will heal by itself if you decrease your workout to about half your normal time and intensity. If this doesn't work, then take a 2-week break, and restart your exercising gradually.

A march fracture, so called because it frequently afflicted soldiers in World War I who marched too long, affects athletes who work out too heavily at the beginning of the season on bones that have been relatively idle. Your foot will hurt and the pain is continuous, not decreasing when you stop your workout. For this you will have to see a doctor who will set the bone and tell you to rest up a couple of months before you return to play.

ARCH INJURIES There are two common types of arch injury. The first is a simple strain. This usually occurs in people with sharply arching feet. Flat-footed people are immune to it. They may suffer from the second problem, plantar-fasciitis, or inflammation of the sheet of fibrous muscle tissue that runs underneath the foot.

Both conditions call for the same treatment: extra arch support. Athletes should tape the ailing foot. Shoe inserts are not enough. Taping the foot for extra support is a temporary but useful way of relieving the pain.

Use either flexible cloth adhesive tape or elastic adhesive tape, 1 1/2 to 2 inches wide, cut into 8 to 10 inch strips. Then reinforce the arch as follows. Place one edge of the tape about 1 1/2 inches up on the top of the outside of the foot just in front of the outside ankle bone. Pass the tape under the foot, pulling gently on the tape as you lay it against the skin. The tape should gently lift the arch of the foot up to prevent it from flattening. The tape should end up on top of the inner side of the foot, just before the tendon that goes to the big toes. Never cover this tendon, as it will stop it from moving and could result in tendinitis. Overlap the first strip of tape with another approximately 1/2 inch and continue with additional strips of tape until the entire bottom of the foot in the arch area is covered with overlapped tape. It is important to protect the skin from the negative effects of prolonged taping by using a special solution sold in surgical supply stores.

HEEL INJURIES The heels are vulnerable to stress fractures when they are overused. The symptoms are the same as with metatarsal fractures: pain that increases when you exercise, decreases when you stop. Treatment is also the same. Give your heels a rest by reducing or stopping the exercise temporarily.

Heelspur syndrome, another common problem, is characterized by fluctuating pain. You feel it when you start to play, but then it goes away only to flare up a few minutes later. This condition, if untreated, will only get worse. The periods of relief will get shorter while those of pain extend.

Heelspur syndrome is caused by a bone spur, a mass of bone and calcium deposits actually growing on the heelbone and protruding from the heel. The pain comes from the irritating rub of this extra bone on the tissues surrounding it. If an athlete has all the symptoms of heelspur but an x-ray can't find a trace of it, then this may be a case of acute plantarfasciitis, described earlier.

In either case, your best bet is to take pressure off the heel so that the spur will not continue to grow or the muscle will heal itself. To get rid of the pressure, get some sort of padding for your shoe, either a professional orthotic device or even a simple horseshoe-shaped foam rubber pad cut to the shape of the heel.

Another simple and useful tactic to use against the pain is to stretch out your calf muscles. Sometimes your rear leg muscles tighten and contract in reaction to the spur, because they're trying to lift the heel off the ground faster than normal in reaction to the pain. If you stretch those muscles, you can break the spasm and reduce the pain in your heel.

ANKLE INJURIES Almost everyone seems to sprain ankles, the most vulnerable of joints. You're especially prone to such sprains if you turn your feet slightly inward as you take a step. You can determine if you do this by taking a look at one of your old pairs of shoes. If the insides of the heels are more worn down than the outsides, you're "pronating." When this happens, the ligaments on the outside of the ankle tend to shorten. At the same time, those on the inside are stretched to the limit. Under this situation, it only takes a little extra pressure for the ligaments to rip.

The easiest way to prevent these sprains is to stretch as part of your warm-up. Sitting down, cross one ankle over the other knee. Using the hand on the same side of your body as the ankle that's crossed, grasp your ankle just above the ankle bone and hold it steady. Then let your foot relax completely. With the other hand, slowly rotate the foot in circles, first in one direction, then in the other for at least 30 seconds each. Now gently twist the entire foot inward at the ankle. This stretches the outside ligaments. Hold it in that position for 10 or 15 seconds, then relax. Now twist the foot out for 10 to 15 seconds. Now treat your other ankle to the same stretch.

If you're prone to ankle sprains, another good preventive measure is to wear an ankle brace. A simple elastic band will give your weak ankle an extra margin of support.However, what if, after taking all these precautions, you still get a sprain? First elevate the foot. Then wrap the ankle in an Ace bandage and apply ice. Do this for 1 or 2 days. Then begin to gently move the ankle again, while keeping up the ice applications to keep the swelling down. This way your joint will retain its normal range of motion with minimization of scars and adhesion.

ACHILLES TENDINITIS The Achilles tendon, a ropelike tendon behind the lower half of the lower leg, is formed by the two tendons that emerge from the two large muscles of the calf. It extends down the leg, inserting into the heelbone behind the ankle. It may become inflamed and can tear at any number of attachment points. Both of these conditions are known as tendinitis.

To relieve this condition, put a heel lift in your shoe on the side that was injured. Try a quarter inch of felt or other shock-absorbing material. If you are careful, the tendon should be healed in about 6 weeks.

If this condition recurs, use the old-shoe test we discussed in the section on sprained ankles to see if you turn your ankle inward as you walk. This can complicate or even cause tendinitis. An orthotic device can help you keep your ankles from turning it. Also keep stretching your calf muscles daily.

LOWER LEG INJURIES Like the metatarsals, the lower leg bones are subject to stress fractures. Commonly this will occur in the upper or lower portions of the bones. The symptoms of the fractures are increased pain during exercise with a diminishment of that pain when you rest. Rest, ice, and elevation are suggested. Also reduce or lay off exercising for a while as the area heals. A full orthotic, made of thermoplastic, can be useful. This controls the foot from heel-strike to toe-off, allowing only normal ranges of motion, rather than the excessive ranges of motion that helped cause the fracture.

Lay people use the term "shinsplints" for any pain in the front of the lower leg. Actually this term covers a number of possible problems including "anterior compartment shinsplints," inflammation of the muscles and tendons; and "posterior compartment shinsplints," caused by the muscles pulling away from the bone. In either case, a bone scan will be needed to properly diagnose the condition.

If you suspect this condition, either in the front or rear position, use rest, elevation, and ice packs for a few days. Then do plenty of stretching and exercise for the rear leg muscles, which are partly to blame in almost every case. Before getting back into working out, check with a foot specialist to see whether you have a foot imbalance that could be corrected. Return to exercising slowly and carefully.

How to Prepare and Use Herbal Remedies

Following are the instructions for preparing and using the herbal remedies mentioned in this section. They are only some of the tools you can use to keep your legs and feet healthy and vigorous in a natural way.

HERBAL SALVE ONE

1 qt. cold-pressed safflower, sunflower, or canola oil1/2 oz. comfrey leaves1/2 oz. goldenseal root1/2 oz. peppermint leavesVitamin E (d-alpha tocopherol)

capsulesVitamin A (B-carotene) capsulesVitamin D capsules from a vegetable sourceMason jar of the type used for preservesCheeseclothMix the oil, comfrey leaves, goldenseal root, and peppermint leaves in a large pot. An electric pot is best. Heat the mixture at a very low temperature. You must be able to test the oil by placing your finger in it without burning yourself. The oil should only be warm, never hot (at about 150 degrees Fahrenheit). Start the process early in the morning as you must allow the mixture to cook for 12 to 24 hours. The purpose of this procedure is to leach out the natural herbal-healing elements without destroying them with excessive heat. Cold-pressed oil is best because it contains vitamins, such as vitamin E, and minerals, which help in healing and can be destroyed by extraction processes that use high heat. After the oil has been cooked, strain it through clean, fresh cheesecloth, which you may want to boil first to kill bacteria. Strain it twice to remove impurities that could become abrasive to inflamed or damaged skin. Add to this the contents of the vitamin capsules.

It is wise to add at least 25,000 to 50,000 IU of each vitamin. You can pop open the capsules using a round toothpick. Mix the vitamins in well with the oil. Note that the oil will probably have taken on a green color from the herbs during the cooking process.

If the salve is kept refrigerated in the mason jar, it will last up to 6 months. The vitamin E in the oil and from the capsules will help act as a natural preservative. It is a good idea to buy a small ointment jar from the pharmacy or health food store, which can hold half an ounce or one ounce of salve. Thus, a small amount can be kept at room temperature for daily use and the rest refrigerated to maintain its potency.

This salve must be used three times a day. Gently rub in a small amount. Wipe away any excess salve that doesn't absorb into the skin. Discontinue use if any skin irritation develops. This antifungal, antibacterial salve is ideal for fungus infections, cuts, scratches, bee stings, and so on. Never use it on deep wounds or cuts nor around the eyes.

HERBAL SOLUTION ONE

1 qt. boiled water1/4 oz. comfrey leaves1/4 oz. goldenseal root1/4 oz. peppermint leaves1 qt. Mason jarCheesecloth Make a tea by adding the ingredients to the boiling water. Allow the mixture to stand, covered, for 30 minutes. Carefully strain the mixture with the cheesecloth, twice to remove all the leaves. Allow the solution to cool to room temperature. Never use it boiling hot. The solution may be kept in a closed jar for 48 hours before being discarded. The amount of ingredients may be reduced proportionally.

Wrap the area to be treated with sterile gauze or bandages. Pour just enough of the solution onto the gauze to thoroughly saturate it. Allow the gauze to completely air dry. Repeat the process as often as necessary.

The solution is antifungal, antibacterial, and mildly astringent. Used as described above, it brings infection in the skin to a head, reduces itching and inflammation, and dries up oozing skin caused by abrasions, fungal infections, and so on. Be warned, however: Never soak your feet in a basin of the solution, and discontinue use if skin irritation occurs.

PART SIX

Heart, Blood, and Circulation

W.B. Yeats' poem, "The Circus Animals' Desertion," concludes, "I must lie down where all the ladders start / In the foul rag-and-bone shop of the heart." His metaphor is meant to suggest a mature person's heart that has been lacerated by romantic and political betrayals. However, given the lifestyles of many Americans who fill the arteries around the heart with plaque and debris, we might take the poem literally. With heart disease being the number one killer, we are certainly driven to ask if there is any way to clean up our foul hearts.

A sufficient supply of blood and oxygen is critical to the body. In the case of heart attacks and angina, blood flow is severely reduced through atherosclerotic and occluded arteries leading to the heart. Strokes, which can cause severe brain damage, may be brought on by the inability of the oxygenated blood supply to pass freely through the arteries leading to the brain.

Peripheral diseases—those affecting less vital parts of the body farther away from the heart and brain—are caused by the same mechanics. Poor blood flow through the legs can cause intermittent claudication. Patients with this problem are frequently unable to walk more than a few feet before stopping because of the pain.

Arteriosclerosis provides a sad but clear example of how cardiovascular disease is closely interwoven into the fabric of lifestyle and diet. It is estimated that by age 3 practically all American children have arteries that are lined with fatty deposits—the initial stage of arteriosclerosis. As this condition becomes advanced in the adult years, it can lead to associated degeneration. This may take the form of atherosclerosis and arterial occlusion, angina and heart attacks, peripheral disease of the legs, and strokes.

A less severe and more generalized indication of insufficient blood flow through the circulatory system is lethargy. This is fatigue that may be created by various degrees of oxygen reduction in the bloodstream. When fat-laden blood cells cannot pass through many of the tiny capillaries in remote parts of the body, the body is deprived of a portion of its required oxygen supply and feels tired and sluggish. Even a single meal of greasy meat and heavy dairy products may make the body respond with this tired, drained feeling. After one has rested sufficiently and the fat starts getting digested through the system, the blood begins to thin out and flow better. When more acceptable oxygen levels are restored, a person's energy level rises. Eating this way habitually, though, may result in a constant feeling of sluggishness—a condition of chronic fatigue.

We are now gaining a greater understanding that these conditions are not irrevocable. A Harvard study released in 2000, which analyzed data from more than 86,000 women over 14 years, found that those who followed all of the now-standard health recommendations—from eating properly to exercising—reduced their chances of heart attacks, congestive heart failure, and stroke by 82 percent. It's becoming more and more apparent that changing diet, reducing stress, stopping smoking, getting exercise, and using natural therapies can reverse heart and circulatory problems and put you back on the road to good health.

30

Heart Disease

In nearly every year for which we have records, heart disease has been the number one cause of death in the United States. Every 33 seconds an American dies of heart disease. In 1999, an estimated 1.1 million Americans had a new or recurrent coronary attack.

Causes and Types of Heart Problems

"Overall, there are 247 risk factors that can damage the heart," states Dr. David Steenblock, a complementary physician from California. "A risk factor is anything that injures the inner lining of the blood vessels that supply the heart with oxygen and nutrition. Any agent that injures this inner lining, such as tobacco, air pollution, food additives, high blood pressure, and gasoline fumes, can initiate atherosclerosis, the so-called hardening of the arteries. Then the accumulation of such things as cholesterol, calcium, scar tissue, and fat causes atherosclerotic lesions, which gradually go on to occlude, or block, the arteries to the brain and the heart. When the arteries to the brain [the carotid arteries] are blocked you have a stroke, and when the arteries to the heart [the coronary arteries] are blocked, you have a heart attack."

High blood pressure (hypertension) which affects some 50 million Americans, increases the risk of heart attack and stroke. Dr. Michael Janson, president of the American Preventive Medical Association and author of *The Vitamin Revolution in Health Care* says, "High blood pressure can be the result of dietary habits; lack of exercise; high stress; being overweight; having too much caffeine, sugar, alcohol, or, in particular, salt in the diet. In the past few years, some reports have said that salt does not make much of a difference for most people. The fact is, that's not true. Even a slight elevation in blood pressure is enough to increase the risk of heart disease."

Among the more recently identified potential risk factors for heart disease are high levels of the amino acid homocysteine, high fibrinogen (a blood-clotting protein), and certain viral and bacterial infections. An elevation in the level of C-reactive protein, a substance in the blood that indicates the presence of inflammation, is also thought to be involved.

Dr. Janson describes other common heart ailments, some of which are precipitated by atherosclerosis.

In angina pectoris, he explains, "clogged arteries leave the heart muscle with inadequate oxygen. As everyone knows, muscles hurt when exercised beyond their oxygen capacity. When not enough blood flows from the coronary arteries to the heart muscle, people experience pain in the chest. Sometimes they feel pain in the jaw, the shoulder, or even the wrist. Often they do not realize that this is referred pain coming from the heart itself."

Congestive heart failure is another common heart problem. "Hardening of the coronary arteries can lead to a number of other problems," Dr. Janson explains. "When heart muscle tissue functions inefficiently, more blood comes in than is pumped out. In other words, with each beat the amount of blood being returned to the heart is more than the heart muscle can handle. Fluid backs up, and other tissues, such as the lungs and legs, can get congested. Congestive heart failure leads to shortness of breath, water in the lungs, and swelling of the ankles."

Symptoms

Heart disease is a gradual process that takes years to develop into a serious condition. At first there are no warning signs. If the coronary arteries become severely blocked, a person may experience shortness of breath or chest pressure and pain (angina pectoris) that is relieved by rest. Other signs of an impending heart attack may include lightheadedness, sweating, nausea, and pain spreading to the shoulders, neck, or arms. Unfortunately, many people are unaware of or overlook these signs: 50 percent of all people who have heart attacks wait 2 hours or longer before seeking treatment, and many die before reaching the hospital.

Diagnosis is an important first step. Before any one begins a cardiovascular health program, a doctor should take the following factors into account: family history, blood pressure, cholesterol level, weight, and stress electrocardiogram (ECG) tests. After assessment of the person's risk factors, the program can begin.

Conventional Treatment

Conventional treatment of heart disease often involves the use of medication to address symptoms such as high blood pressure and high cholesterol. Every year, about 1 million Americans undergo surgery such as coronary bypass and angioplasty (in which a balloon catheter is used to open clogged arteries) to restore their hearts.

Dr. Janson believes the general public is being misled into believing that medications for high blood pressure are safe and always necessary: "We all hear advertisements on the radio telling us to stay on these medications for life. They say that no symptoms tell you whether or not your blood pressure is high. Therefore, if you are taking medication for high blood pressure, you must stay on your medication and never, ever stop. That so-called public service announcement is really a sales pitch from the drug companies that make the medications. We know that these medications actually cause more heart disease and that they create side effects in addition to the high blood pressure."

Dr. David Steenblock warns, however, that patients who depend on medication to control high blood pressure should not self-discontinue: "Many people have this idea that since the doctor is not getting at the cause of their high blood pressure, it is somewhat illogical for them to take their blood pressure medicine. True, doctors often do not have the answer. Still, if you fail to take your medicine and your blood pressure gets out of control, you can develop heart disease and go on to have a stroke."

The Complementary Approach

The solution here is to work with a complementary medical physician until your heart health is restored. In some cases, medication may be needed long term, even for a lifetime, but no one can fail to benefit from improving lifestyle and diet. The following sections can serve as guidelines.

Diet

We all know that "eating right" can reduce the risk of heart disease. Just what does this mean?

REDUCING FATS The power of a vegetarian diet in a cardiovascular health program was recognized in a now-famous study by Dr. Dean Ornish. The Ornish study placed heart patients on a protocol of healthy vegetarian foods, daily aerobic exercise, and relaxation. At the end of a year, a significant number of patients showed improvement in their heart condition, and in some the disease was even reversed.

Dr. Paul Cutler, a complementary physician from Niagara Falls, New York, says, "Medicine in general owes Ornish a great deal of gratitude. He showed that a drastic reduction of fats was most important. I believe that the total dietary fats should be well below the typical average of 40 percent. Modern nutritionists are saying 30 percent. I try to get fat content down to 10 percent of the total calories. I see improvement in angina just by reducing the fats to that degree."

There is not much controversy about what is wrong with the standard American diet with its high amounts of animal proteins, saturated animal fats, dairy products, deep-fried foods, and refined carbohydrates. The average American diet consists of 43 percent fats and 14 percent proteins and the rest is mainly carbohydrates. The average daily intake of cholesterol is 450 to 500 milligrams. But there is controversy over the proper foods for those with heart disease. There are over 60,000 dietitians in the United States, and they have been a primary source of information on what a sick person should eat. After all, physicians graduate from medical school with only an hour or two of learning about nutrition. However, even though dietitians are well-trained, there is a split in the field. Only a very small percentage of dietitians believe the standard American diet plays a large role in causing the diseases we are beset with, including heart disease.

The American Heart Association recommends that we cut fat intake to 30 percent, with only 10 percent of this in the form of saturated fats (fats found particularly in land animals, palm and coconut oils, and hydrogenated vegetable oils). We have been told that margarine, made from "polyunsaturated fats," is good for the heart and will lower cholesterol. That is simply not true; margarine is loaded with the fatty acids that contribute to heart disease. Instead of margarine, use olive oil, canola oil, or flaxseed, almond, safflower, sunflower, or soy oil. Of these, olive oil would be at the top of my list. But don't have margarine.

No more than 10 percent of the oils you eat should be polyunsaturated fats, such as those found in some vegetable oils, including corn and cottonseed oils. According to the American Heart Association, we should get the rest from monounsaturated fats such as olive oil and take in less than 300 milligrams of cholesterol each day.

While the dangers of saturated fats to heart health are well known, Dr. Ray Peat, a distinguished scientific researcher in Eugene, Oregon, says unsaturated fats can be just as damaging: "Many people have been soaking their bodies in unsaturated vegetable oil diets for years. As a result, every time they get hungry or face stress, their blood sugar falls, their adrenaline rises, and these unsaturated fats are drawn out of storage. Once released, they immediately start poisoning the lining of the blood vessels and all the cellular energy-producing systems. In 1960, this effect was demonstrated by a group in England which saw that adrenaline, either natural or synthetic, caused damage to the circulatory system. It turns out that this occurs after unsaturated fats become mobilized. They hit the lining of the blood vessels, where they cause lipid peroxidative damage."

Dr. Janson adds that people should avoid foods such as sugar, salt, white flour, white rice, and particularly any shortening or hydrogenated vegetable oils found in products like margarine and vegetable shortening: "Whenever you see vegetable shortening, hydrogenated vegetable oil, or partially hydrogenated vegetable oil on a label, avoid that product. These are not foods. In fact, I consider margarine an industrial waste product that is fashioned to resemble food."

HEART HEALTHY FOODS Dr. Janson continues, "The diet should be high in complex carbohydrates, including whole grains, beans, vegetables, and fruits. Remember, flavonoids, which are plant pigments, are present in fruits and vegetables and in some beans and grains. These are very protective, and most of them are not available as supplements.

"I think the diet should be largely vegetarian, although a number of studies show that fish also reduces levels of heart disease and cancer. Fish may or may not be the reason for this. It may be that eating more fish means eating less chicken and meat. Cutting those foods out of the diet helps cut down on heart disease."

Broccoli and other vegetables are the first foods to turn to. We eat broccoli and all kinds of produce, seeds, legumes, and grains to get our beta carotenes and maybe vitamin C, but they also contain important phytochemicals. These phytochemicals include beta carotene, alpha carotene, ascorbic acid, ash, boron, caffeic acid, calcium, chlorophyll, chromium, citric acid, copper, glycine, iron, linoleic acid, lysine, magnesium, niacin, oleic acid, phosphorus, potassium, riboflavin, selenium, thiamin, tryptophan, and zinc, among others. These chemicals have all kinds of healing properties. Chlorophyll, for instance, helps purify the blood and acts as a detoxifier.

You can lower your blood pressure by eating vegetables such as garlic, broccoli, and asparagus. You should have at least five servings of vegetables and three of fruits each day, raw, steamed, or juiced. Once you start, you will notice a world of difference in your overall vitality. Other valuable heart foods are rice and beans, which are complete proteins rich in fiber and B-complex vitamins.

Many people grow up with the pernicious myth that if it is not an animal protein, it is not a complete protein and so is not really nutritious. I did studies at the Institute of Applied Biology that proved conclusively that beans, legumes, and all grains contain complete proteins just like animal proteins, without the saturated fats. They are not high in calories and are rich in vitamins, minerals, and essential oils.

Nuts, despite their high fat content, are being found to have some important benefits as well. Not only do they provide protein, they also contain nutrients that can protect against heart disease, high blood pressure, and stroke. The protein in peanuts, hazelnuts, and walnuts, for example, is a good source of arginine. This amino acid is noted for its ability to produce nitric oxide, which helps blood vessels to widen and may stop or even reverse plaque buildup. These nuts also contain folate, which has been found to lower blood levels of homocysteine. High levels of homocysteine are associated with increased blockage in the arteries.

A recent Harvard study of 86,000 nurses found that those who ate more than 5 ounces of nuts a week were 35 percent less likely to develop heart disease than those who rarely ate nuts. Other studies have reported similar findings.

Exercise

"Aerobic exercise and an improved diet should go hand in hand," notes Dr. Paul Cutler. "Aerobics help the good cholesterol go up significantly, which in turn helps remove cholesterol from arterial walls after the cells are through with it so it is less likely to form plaque." Exercising aerobically means getting the heart rate up three or four times a week. A doctor can help determine how much exercise is needed.

Dr. Michael Janson adds that people should stretch before and after an aerobic workout: "The stretching has another benefit in that it relaxes the body and keeps people limber and more flexible. That makes it easier to continue an aerobic exercise program."

Exercise is, however, not a panacea. Some people mistakenly assume that cholesterol can be burned off by exercise and activity and that as a result, people who engage in athletics and body building can eat more meat and eggs without suffering ill effects. There is no scientific basis for this notion. To the contrary, studies have shown that good conditioning and muscle tone do not necessarily put a person in good cardiovascular condition.

Dr. Julian Whitaker refers to "studies done on marathon runners in South Africa in which five of them died of heart attacks. These were conditioned long-distance runners. They all had cholesterol levels of 270, 290, etc. They were very fit but not very well."

Supplements

Supplements provide wonderful support for the heart and sometimes help eliminate or reduce dosages of medication. Antioxidants help protect the heart from free radical damage, also known as oxidation. Antioxidant nutrients include vitamin E and vitamin C (see below), beta carotene, and selenium. Free radicals damage the tissues lining the arteries, which leads to atherosclerosis and plaque deposits. Antioxidants, particularly vitamin C, can prevent this from happening by protecting the lining of the arteries. The following are nutrients you should know about. In addition, two other beneficial supplements are chondroitin sulfate A and evening primrose oil (1,500 mg/day).

L-ARGININE. L-arginine is an amino acid that has been receiving well-deserved attention in the medical literature for its ability to produce nitric oxide. Nitric oxide benefits the arterial walls in several ways. It helps the smooth muscles in the arterial walls relax, promoting an antianginal, antihypertensive, and antistress effect. Additionally, research shows that l-arginine reduces the activation of platelets, the small bodies that can initiate arterial spasm and plaque development. Other studies show that l-arginine slows plaque development and even reverses small amounts of plaque buildup. "I've seen it work," says Dr. Cutler. "Taking 2 to 3 grams of l-arginine per day has quite a marked antianginal effect. L-arginine now is a must in my protocol for nutrients. Usually I start with about 1,000 milligrams per day, and raise the levels if that amount isn't helping."

L-CARNITINE. The heart muscle needs to burn fat for energy, and l-carnitine allows this to happen. Dr. Janson explains, "l-carnitine gets fat into the little engines inside the cells called mitochondria. These little mitochondrial engines are where fat is burned for energy. Your heart muscle needs to burn fat for energy, and the only way it can get the fat into that little engine is with the amino acid l-carnitine. At the same time, that inner mitochondrial membrane requires another nutrient to burn the fat: coenzyme Q10." Dr. Janson recommends that people take 500 milligrams l-carnitine two to three times a day. You should take l-carnitine along with vitamin E, because they work together synergistically.

CHROMIUM PICOLINATE. Chromium picolinate has been shown to be beneficial both for the heart and for blood sugar levels.

COENZYME Q10. Coenzyme Q10 is a nutrient that should be taken by anyone who has heart problems or who wants to avoid getting them. Along with l-carnitine, it helps prevent angina and protects the heart muscle by letting it burn fat for energy more easily. It also improves heart health by reducing blood pressure and arrhythmias. As an antioxidant, it prevents the damage to blood vessels that leads to hardening of the arteries. Therapeutic levels are between 50 and 150 milligrams for mild heart disease. More severe heart disease may respond to 200 milligrams.

LECITHIN. Lecithin is made from soy. Not only does it keep the arteries strong and healthy, but it helps emulsify fats, helps the brain, and is good for memory.

MAGNESIUM. Magnesium increases blood flow by allowing muscles in the arterial wall to relax. Usually 500 to 1,000 milligrams are needed.

MAXEPA. MaxEPA, a combination of EPA (eicosapentaenoic acid) and DHA (docosohexaenoic acid), also known as fish oil, is part of the omega-3 and omega-6 fatty acids found in salmon, sardines, and mackerel. Since many people do not eat these fish, they should be getting these fatty acids in fish oil. The recommended daily dose is 500 to 1,000 milligrams. Clinical and epidemiological experience as well as scientific studies have found that people who eat a lot of fish have less heart disease than people who do not.

NIACIN (VITAMIN B3). A 15-year study on the effects of niacin published by the American Heart Association in the mid-1980s connected the use of niacin to a significant reduction in heart attacks and death from heart disease. Long-term niacin use has also been associated with decreased rates of cancer. Niacin should be taken under medical supervision, since it can affect liver function.

TAURINE. Taurine, an amino acid, is another important antioxidant that helps prevent atherosclerosis. Additionally, it can avert heart failure by improving the strength of the heart's contraction. That increases the outflow of blood from the heart and reduces congestive heart failure. Generally, 500 milligrams are taken twice a day.

THYROID SUPPLEMENTS. Thyroid supplementation may normalize high cholesterol, according to Dr. Ray Peat: "high cholesterol indicates a thyroid hormone deficiency. A clear demonstration of this was seen in the 1930s in patients whose thyroid glands were surgically removed. After the operation, cholesterol levels became abnormally high, but they returned to normal with thyroid supplementation." He adds that thyroid extract is linked to fewer heart attacks: "one of the foremost American researchers in the field, Broda Barnes, wrote *Solved: The Riddle of Heart Attacks* after finding that patients in one group had far fewer heart attacks than did patients in another group. All the low-heart-attack group did differently was take thyroid when they needed it."

VITAMIN B1 AND OTHER B VITAMINS. Vitamin B_1 (thiamine) is the most important B vitamin for the heart: 25 to 50 milligrams daily are recommended. Dr. Janson adds, "other B vitamins, such as folic acid and B_{12}, can help lower blood levels of homocysteine, a risk factor for heart disease."

VITAMIN C. If there is one vitamin everyone needs to take every day, it is vitamin C. If you have a cold or flu, you may require 50,000 milligrams for quick recovery; for heart disease, you may require substantially more. Get over that old-fashioned idea that all you need is one glass of orange juice to get the necessary vitamin C. Now we have thousands of studies of the valuable properties of vitamin C, which can help with everything from cancer to heart disease and diabetes. I would take 500 to 1,000 milligrams, five times a day. Vitamin C washes out of the system, so you need to take it throughout the day. Two well-known specialists in coronary heart disease recommend that their patients take vitamin C before going to bed at night because they find it helps prevent heart attacks during sleep and in the morning, which is when the majority of heart attacks occur.

VITAMIN E. Vitamin E has several functions. Aside from being a protective antioxidant, it reduces the stickiness of the platelets, little blood fragments that initiate blood clots. This effect is helped by the addition of essential fatty acids and garlic to the diet. Minimizing free radical damage and keeping platelets from clogging the arteries give arteries a chance to heal and recover. There is more room for oxygen to flow through the arteries to reach tissues. It is estimated that between 400 and 800 international units (IU) are useful in preventing stroke. You may go higher, up to 1,200 or 1,600 units, unless other medical conditions preclude a higher level. I believe we would cut the incidence of stroke by 20 percent, saving 50,000 to 100,000 people a year, just by having everyone take this little, inexpensive supplement.

Herbs

In addition to the herbs listed below, consider taking barberry, black cohosh, and butcher's broom.

BUGLEWEED. Bugleweed is a remedy for heart palpitations and elevated blood pressure. It may also alleviate anxiety, since elevated blood pressure is frequently associated with a rapid pulse rate, anxiety, and agitation.

CAYENNE. Capsaicin, the active ingredient in cayenne, helps the heart in many ways. It stimulates circulatory function, lowers cholesterol, reduces blood pressure, and lessens the chance of heart attacks and strokes. By decreasing blood levels of fibrin, it also reduces the risk of forming blood clots that cause heart attacks and strokes.

GARLIC. Among its many benefits, garlic helps lower blood pressure and decrease cholesterol. When combined with vitamin E, it lessens the frequency of blood clots in arterial walls, which in turn helps prevent heart attacks and strokes. The recommended amount is 500 milligrams or more of deodorized garlic taken twice a day.

GINKGO BILOBA. Ginkgo biloba helps improve small blood vessel circulation.

HAWTHORN BERRY. Hawthorn is an overall heart tonic that works against arrhythmia (irregular heartbeat), angina, high blood pressure, and hardening of the arteries. It aids circulation and ameliorates valvular insufficiency and an irregular pulse. Hawthorn berry can also correct acid conditions of the blood. It can safely be taken every day.

MISTLETOE. Mistletoe is a cardiac tonic that stimulates circulation. Fifteen drops of tincture taken three times a day or three cups of tea daily can help lower blood pressure and alleviate heart strain. Mistletoe should not be overused, nor should the berries be eaten.

MOTHERWORT. Motherwort helps stabilize the electrical rhythm of the heart. The amount taken should be monitored by a doctor.

WILD YAM. Wild yam stimulates production of DHEA. Low levels of this hormone have been related to higher incidences of heart disease.

Chinese Herbal Therapy

Letha Hadady, one of the leading herbalists in the United States, says most Americans do not go to the doctor when they are a little sick; they wait until they are really suffering. They may have chest pains or difficulty breathing, but they generally don't go to the doctor nor, of course, to the herbalist. They say, "I'm tired; I'm under stress," and ignore it. That is a problematic approach because some of the underlying problems of heart disease are the ones they are complaining of: fatigue, stress, and poor digestion. Poor digestion and fatigue lead to cholesterol buildup, which leads to pain and heart congestion. People try to breathe more deeply and reduce stress when they experience these early symptoms, but that does not help. But changing your diet, taking herbs and foods that reduce cholesterol, will definitely help.

Hadady's clients often have conditions that they believe are unrelated to heart disease; but her special training as an herbalist enables her to see a connection to the heart. Mind, body, and spirit are interconnected, and the heart is affected by all of these things. Depression, for example, is related to a weak heart. Insomnia, poor concentration and palpitations are all signs that poor circulation could be affecting the heart.

Many Western doctors will say that herbs have not been tested. But when you go to a public library or consult an on-line medical search and reference service such as Medline, which is available free to any interested person, you find 3,500 studies on Chinese herbs alone. The majority of the research is done in Asia.

Quite a number of these remedies are available in health food stores, by mail order, or in your local Chinatown. The ingredients are always in English or Latin on the back.

Hadady points out that one of the major underlying problems associated with heart disease is fatigue. Chinese doctors link the heart's health to the strength of the adrenal glands—not an obvious connection. Hadady states, "If I had a patient complaining of fatigue and being overweight, I would suspect heart problems—if not then, somewhere down the line, so I would work on the adrenals. To strengthen the adrenals, you can get the herbal preparation from Chinatown called Goldenbook. It adds to immune energy and will help with kidney and heart problems. We strengthen what is weak so the heart will not falter."

Hadady explains that clove is a strong stimulant. A pinch in the late after-noon will act like coffee. Coffee is a major problem because it increases painful, sluggish circulation in the gastrointestinal tract that affects the whole circula-tion, meaning that the heart will not run smoothly. A pinch of clove will replace coffee better than anything else can.

Siberian ginseng, a blend of various ginsengs, is beneficial. The ginsengs are adaptogens; that is, they help us maintain energy as well as aid us in living under a high level of stress. They support the nervous system. Raw Tienchi gin-seng, one that Americans are less familiar with, comes in powdered form. A half teaspoon in cool water, taken every day, will reduce cholesterol and pain around the heart.

One Chinese remedy that is especially valuable in relation to heart pain and blood vessel congestion is *dan shen wan*, which combines salvia and camphor. The camphor dilates the blood vessels while the salvia increases the heart's action. Another valuable remedy is *guan xin su he wan*, which contains frankin-cense. Both frankincense and myrrh improve circulation. Frankincense increas-es blood flow around the heart. You can take it once a day to prevent heart attack. It can be chewed and swallowed. Hadady recommends it even if you have no heart symptoms. It has healthy ingredients such as liquid amber and sandalwood, which keeps the esophagus and chest cool.

Yans shen jia jiao wan is a combination of ginseng and other herbs that free the circulation of the blood in the brain. This is not just for victims of heart attack but also for those with stroke and hemiplegia (paralysis of one side of the body). People with high cholesterol and those at high risk of heart trouble can take one dose a day as a preventive measure.

Baoxin wan is a remedy for heart attacks. If you feel faint and experience pain and weakness, you sniff it like a smelling salt. If the pain is great and you feel the onset of an attack, take it orally. It includes ginseng and liquid amber. It treats the congestion of the blood vessels around the heart and opens up the blood vessels.

Some of the underlying problems leading to a heart attack, such as excess weight and cholesterol, are well countered by herbal remedies. One preparation whose name is self-explanatory is Keep Fit, Reduce Fat. The ingredients are ginseng, hawthorn, and other herbs that are good for the heart. Hawthorn, a slightly bitter, slightly sour berry, works as a digestive. You can take a capsule of Keep Fit after meals. Cholesterol is reduced, and the muscle of the heart is made stronger.

Evening primrose oil is another useful herb for reducing cholesterol. Chinatown is an excellent place to purchase this remedy since the prices are apt to be considerably lower than those for comparable items in health food stores.

Another popular remedy in Asia is green tea, which has been reported in the popular press as being very good for reducing cholesterol. "This is a good alternative to other caffeine teas," Hadady notes, "because the caffeine in it is very low. It gives the satisfaction of a bitter tea while reducing cholesterol."

Bojemni slimming tea protects the heart. It includes hawthorn. *Xiao yao wan*, a digestive remedy that boosts circulation and combats depression, contains ginger, mint, and other herbs; it eases the flow of bile, eases the digestive process, and reduces chest congestion.

Digestive Harmony is an American-made product that contains Chinese herbs, one of many such products that are now on the market and sold door to door or through mail order. "This is part of a trend now," Hadady explains, "a very important trend in herbalism, of using Asian herbs manufactured with American standards. Digestive Harmony can be ordered from Oakland, California. It will ease the underlying troubles related to heart disease.

"Remember that depression is in part a heart problem," Hadady goes on. "The heart is not just a digestive center, but is related to our emotions. Depression is rightly associated with heart disease since it affects the heartbeat. When we are not happy and our emotions are not smooth, we feel it in the heart.

"Some remedies that combat depression come to us from China. Coschisandra strengthens the energy level and keeps us from losing the energy we have. It is good for both the adrenals and the heart. It fights against poor memory, poor concentration and depression. Also try *anshen bu nao pien*, available in all the Chinatowns in the United States. It is for depression, blood deficiencies and heart-related problems such as panic and anxiety.

"Also useful is *mao dong qing*, which is the Chinese name for holly, and it comes in capsule form. It is for chest pain and prevention of heart trouble. You can take several of these capsules each day as a preventive. If you already have heart problems, it reduces cholesterol, congestion, and pains.

"In general," Hadady concludes, "Chinese remedies for the heart also treat not just pain, but also emotional problems: sadness, anxieties, and other mental suffering."

Chelation Therapy

Chelation therapy, which is being administered to hundreds of thousands of heart disease patients, is proving quite successful and is considerably safer and substantially less expensive than bypass surgery. It is not new, having been in use for over 40 years.

Chelation involves the infusion into the bloodstream of the amino acid EDTA. The EDTA bonds with toxic metals and calcium and carries them out of the bloodstream through the kidneys, slowing or reversing some plaque formation in the arteries and thus retarding the degenerative process. EDTA enhances blood flow, permitting more essential oxygen and nutrients to circulate and be absorbed by the body. As chelation therapy is more commonly used, chelation specialists feel that it will become the most important heart disease therapy offered in the future.

As Dr. Steenblock describes it, "EDTA binds with calcium that has deposited in artery walls and is excreted from the body through the kidneys. In addition, it breaks down scar tissue and allows the arteries to become softer. In other words, it takes the hard out of hardening of the arteries."

When deciding whether or not to administer chelation therapy, Dr. Cutler tests patients for heavy metal buildup. "I look for elevated iron and copper levels in the blood. I also measure something called the serum ferritin, which reflects artery tissue levels of iron. If I start chelation, as the iron levels come down in the blood, there are also clinical improvements in angina and exercise tests. And there are angiogram and treadmill test improvements as well.

"If I do not find any abnormality in these metals, I do what is called a challenge, which means I give one chelation treatment, collect urine for 24 hours afterward, and observe the metals that come out. Based on these results, I make the decision as to whether I want to chelate the person."

Dr. Steenblock, who has administered chelation therapy for more than 20 years, uses the treatment more extensively. He explains why it is so valuable for most individuals: "In their 40s most people develop some degree of atherosclerosis due to cholesterol, scar tissue, fat, and calcium, which accumulate in the artery walls.

"You have to try to prevent all these risk factors by keeping your diet low in fat and cholesterol and by exercising, thinking properly, avoiding chemicals, and taking antioxidants to protect the inner lining of the blood vessels. In addition, you can break down scar tissue and remove calcium with chelation.

"Studies show that if you start chelating in your 40s, you can actually reverse all the atherosclerosis as soon as it starts to develop. If you have done things that have not been perfect in your life—you haven't eaten right, you have been under too much stress, you have smoked—by the time you are 40, you will have some degree of atherosclerosis. Chelation can reverse this process and keep those arteries more pristine.

"By the time you are 60, the amount of calcium that has been deposited in your arteries is 10 times what you had in your arteries at 10 years of age. Al Fleckenstein, a leading cardiovascular drug researcher, says in one of his books that the amount of calcium present in the walls of the arteries is the single most important risk factor in the development of atherosclerosis. In other words, as calcium accumulates in the arterial walls, it promotes the development of atherosclerosis; atherosclerosis develops because you are gradually accumulating this calcium. If you can remove the calcium somewhere between the ages of 40 and 60, you can change that ratio, reverse the whole process, and put off the development of atherosclerosis for a number of years. That's for prevention.

"Of course, if you have outright disease, you can be helped as well. I have been doing chelation since 1977, so I have treated thousands of patients, and most do not come for prevention. They come for treatment of disease. They come in with angina or claudication [lameness due to leg pain]. With chelation, most of the time these symptoms disappear. If they do not, it is usually because the person has advanced disease and needs more than the standard 30 treatments. When people who are 75 or 80 years old come in with advanced disease, I tell them that they need to start out with 30 treatments—that's one treatment twice or three times a week. They wait a month or two, and then come back and do another 30. This process continues until we clean out these arteries because it takes time to reverse all of the terribly occluded blocked arteries that develop over many, many years of bad living."

See chapter 32 for more on chelation therapy.

Stress Management

Virtually all the authorities agree that if you want to get a handle on heart disease, you have to deal with stress. Stress or distress is a major problem for the American psyche.

For a long while we have known that stress is a contributor to heart disease, but only recently have we begun to understand the physiological basis of the connection.

Richard Friedman, Ph.D., of Harvard Medical School, remarks that when we are confronted with stressful situations, most of us try to oversolve the problem. We constantly try to fit square pegs into round holes, and when we find that is not going to work, we turn inward, brood, and look for ways to dissipate stress, frequently by acting inappropriately, such as overeating, drinking, or taking inappropriate drugs or medications. This contributes to the disease process.

Dr. Friedman says there is a link between stress and cardiovascular disease. When we are stressed by a fear of physical or psychological danger, the body exhibits a fight-or-flight response as it prepares to deal with an enemy. Very recent research indicates that the body readies itself not to bleed if it is cut or injured, which makes a lot of sense from a biological and evolutionary perspective. However, if the threats are psychological and you have a bad diet, you may be going through stressful incidents 20 or 30 times a day, triggering the fight-or-flight response. Each time this happens, the body prepares not to bleed by making the blood platelets stickier. This internal clotting takes place every time you get angry, whether on a supermarket line or in a traffic jam. Over time this continual clotting can contribute to plaque buildup in the arteries.

Stress also contributes to heart disease by increasing free radical damage to tissues and increasing spasms in the arterial walls.

When you are exposed to a biochemical or psychological stress, a host of changes take place in addition to platelet stickiness. The body's ability to fight off viral and bacterial infection is lessened by the weaknesses induced by stress. Stress compromises the immune system's ability to fight off opportunistic diseases.

There is some good news, though, about our ability to fight off the debilitating conditions that lead to a heart attack. Dr. Friedman notes that just as continued stress leads to a weakening of the system, there is an opposite effect, one that has been labeled by his colleague at Harvard Dr. Herbert Benson as the "relaxation response." Eliciting this calming response on a daily basis makes it less likely that you will have high blood pressure or arteriosclerotic plaque buildup or a heart attack down the road.

The relaxation response should be combined with other behavior modifications to create a healthier response to stress, and all these techniques should be combined with the best medical care. That is the way to optimize your health.

Dr. Friedman tells us how the relaxation response is induced: Use whatever strategy you have available to let go of any muscle tension you may be experiencing. Make sure your muscles are loose and your jaw lets go. After you feel a bit more comfortable, focus your attention on your breathing. If you find yourself having any distracting thoughts, do not let them bother you or take you away from the process. As soon as you have a distracting thought, simply say to yourself, "Oh well," and return to a concentration on your breathing and to a thought or image that allows you to stay calm, peaceful, and relaxed. Become aware of the cool air coming in your nostrils and the warm air going out. Keep this up till you are deeply relaxed.

Other ways to overcome stress are exercise, deep breathing, visualization, *tai chi*, yoga, meditation, *qi gong*, mantras, massage, Reiki, biofeedback, and aromatherapy. An essential oil blend of *ylang ylang*, lavender or peppermint, and marjoram added to oil and applied during massage helps calm the system and may even lower blood pressure.

Treatment of Helicobacter Pylori

Dr. Paul Cutler says that recent research links the *Helicobacter pylori* bacterium to high incidences of heart attacks and strokes. "*Helicobacter pylori* causes ulcers and chronic gastritis. Most practitioners are well aware of the higher incidence of stomach complaints in patients with heart disease. Apparently, this little bacterium, which comes from contaminated foods, burrows its way into the stomach wall. In its attempt to fight off the body's defenses, it produces toxins that initiate plaque development and thickening of the blood. This points to a strong correlation between stomach ulcer disease and coronary artery disease."

Fortunately, this problem is simple to cure, says Dr. Cutler: "You can use one particular type of honey that is high in hydrogen peroxide or cider vinegar, bismuth, and extracts from licorice. Or you can take a 1-week course of three antibiotics to kill this bacteria, probably 97 percent of the time. It is very gratifying as a physician to see not only stomach symptoms but angina improve, sometimes dramatically, with the treatment of this common bacterial parasite."

Homeopathy

Dr. Ken Korins explains how his specialty, homeopathy, seems to get results with heart disease: "Homeopathy works by giving very small doses that are extremely individualized to the person's symptoms and physical state. These doses work by means of a type of vibration or energy that stimulates the body much as acupuncture does."

Many traditional practitioners dismiss homeopathy. These physicians say this therapy has never been proved by randomized, double-blind studies in the way more scientific procedures have been. Dr. Korins argues that is absolutely incorrect. He tells us that a 1991 *British Medical Journal* article by Kleijnen reviewed 107 clinical studies of homeopathy. About 80 percent of them found that homeopathy had positive effects. Many of these were extremely rigorous studies. A double-blind study in the *Journal of Pediatrics*, for example, showed extraordinary results from homeopathy.

What kinds of heart problems improve with homeopathy? Hypertension is one. Homeopathy can also help people recovering from congestive heart failure, cerebrovascular accidents, arteriosclerotic heart disease, and a wide range of other conditions.

In classical homeopathy, the specialist selects a single remedy. Korins elaborates: "We don't rely on a lot of tests and the high technology that goes with them. We prefer to look at what symptoms a person has and how they present themselves. For example, if a person is having angina, tightness, a squeezing sensation, a remedy such as songea or cactus, which is extremely effective in treating angina, is called for. Sometimes there is a congestion in the head, a hot feeling when the blood pressure goes up. The prescription there might be gloline.

Qi (Chi) Manipulation

An Asian treatment that has some success with heart patients is the manipulation of *qi (chi)* energy. This term refers to all the nonliquid, biological energy that circulates through the body. Dr. Jeie Atacama uses *qi* to accomplish healing. He estimates that in 20 years of practice he has helped between 3,000 and 5,000 people. Rebalancing *qi* energy can help greatly with heart disease by rebuilding the body's health and restoring its self-healing powers.

This practice works exactly like acupuncture. It does not use needles, but it shares with acupuncture a focus on the meridians of the body. In a technique he learned from his father, Dr. Atacama uses his fingers directly on the patient's skin. U points are found on either side near the base of the spine. One point is connected to the large intestine, which is part of the body system particularly in touch with the *qi* energy. The treatment session should be done three times a week for as many weeks as are called for by the condition. If the problem is cramps in the leg due to poor circulation, 10 sessions will get rid of the problem.

Healing practices such as *tai chi* and *qi gong* depend on channeling internal *qi* energies to rebalance the body.

Psychological, Social, and Spiritual Factors

Most healing programs focus on physical modalities. We look at diet, exercise, supplements, and substances to avoid, but people are beginning to understand that more subtle factors have a powerful influence as well. Dr. Ron Scolastico, a spiritual counselor and author of *Healing the Heart, Healing the Body*, believes that the process of remaining healthy involves four important elements: "The first element is our physical life, which most people know a great deal about. The second element looks at our mental life. It is becoming clearer and clearer that our thoughts promote or hinder health and in some cases actually cause disease. The third element addresses our emotional lives. Feelings, particularly love, have a profound effect. The fourth element addresses spiritual factors. I believe those energies come from the soul, which is an incredible source of power, love, and wisdom inside each of us."

Dr. Scolastico says we must draw on each of these factors as needed. Sometimes we must take physical steps such as seeing a doctor and taking medications or herbs, but sometimes that is not enough. "For example, one of my clients developed congestive heart failure after a painful divorce, along with pericarditis, which is an inflammation of the membrane surrounding the heart. She failed to respond to medical treatment, and her condition began to worsen. As I worked with her, she realized that she had lost touch with her soul. The divorce had wreaked such havoc in her emotional life that she could no longer feel love.

"Every day for 6 months she took an hour to connect with her soul. By doing this, she was able to regain a feeling of deep love for her body and herself. Today she is symptom-free and believes that without inner work she might be dead. So, many times, we need not only physical treatment but mental, emotional, or spiritual work to augment that process."

To promote health at every level, Dr. Scolastico advises the following:

➤Connect with your spiritual nature. Religious or not, we need to accept the existence of some benevolent, healing force larger than our personality and physical being. Once we realize we are never alone or abandoned, amazing changes can happen.

➤Be mindful of your thoughts. We all have negative thoughts, but this alone does not cause illness. Swallowing them and engaging them does. We must learn to release negative ideas. This work takes time, and we should not be hard on ourselves when our thoughts are less than perfect.

➤Follow the physical principles of health. Living in a healthy way includes eating the right foods, exercising, and getting enough rest, play, and social activity. Giving to others has a beneficial impact on health.

➤Create love in your life every day. This is perhaps the most important principle of all. Research shows that love affects every aspect of our beings, including the physical. When we feel love, all body systems work better. The endocrine system produces beneficial hormones. Muscles relax, so that the flow of oxygen to the cells increases. Immune system function is enhanced. When we are filled with self-love, our health is strongest and our lives improve all around. Recent studies show that teaching self-esteem improves academic performance and promotes emotional stability and greater health.

"A powerful way to enhance self-love," advises Dr. Scolastico, "is to notice when you are creating negative thoughts and feelings about yourself. Then consciously create an experience of love for yourself right at that moment, using the power of the word to augment the process. You can say, 'I just noticed I'm creating these negative thoughts and feelings about myself. I now choose to use my imagination, my creativity, and my will to create an inner experience of love for myself right now, in this minute.'"

Another way to build love into our lives is to set aside time each day for building loving energy. Dr. Scolastico says, "For at least 5 minutes, use your mind, open your heart, and create love in your feelings. You can do that by imagining a person you love. Let your feelings for that person fill you as you bring that loved one fully into your thoughts and feelings. Let the corners of your mouth lift up in a smile. Just let your heart swell with love. You won't need a scientific test to prove the benefits."

Equal in importance to self-love is the love we share with others. Connecting with family, friends, and community gives us a sense of belonging that is invaluable to our well-being. Recently, a link between social bonds and heart health was reported in *Natural Health*. The magazine summarized 30 years of research on the town of Rosetto, Pennsylvania, and concluded that the most important risk factor for heart disease is a lack of community and intimate relationships. In this town, people lived in three-generation households with grandparents, parents, and children. There was a lot of interaction among families and much participation in community organizations. The incidence of heart disease was virtually nil even though residents ate high-fat diets and did not go out of their way to exercise. In fact, there was less coronary heart disease in Rosetto than in any other population in the United States.

Herbal Pharmacy

Plants containing phytochemicals with antihypertensive properties, in order of potency, include the following:

Viola tricolor hortensis (pansy)
Sophora japonica (Japanese pagoda tree), bud/flower
Oenothera biennis (evening primrose)
Lactuca sativa (lettuce)
Cichorium endivia (endive)
Vigna mungo (blackgram)
Chenopodium album (lamb's-quarters)
Raphanus sativus (radish)
Portulaca oleracea (purslane)
Brassica pekinensis (Chinese cabbage)
Avena sativa (oats)
Amaranthus sp. (pigweed)
Chrysanthemum coronarium (garland chrysanthemum)
Anethum graveolens (dill)
Taraxacum officinale (dandelion)
Spinacia oleracea (spinach)
Cucumis sativus (cucumber)
Brassica chinensis (Chinese cabbage)
Allium cepa (onion)

Plants containing phytochemicals with antiarteriosclerotic properties, in order of potency, include the following:

Cucumis melo (cantaloupe), cotyledon
Juglans regia (English walnut)
Persea americana (avocado)
Cucumis sativus (cucumber)
Carthamus tinctorius (safflower)
Prunus armeniaca (apricot)
Papaver bracteatum (great scarlet poppy)
Helianthus annuus (sunflower)
Juglans cinerea (butternut)
Lagenaria siceraria (calabash gourd)
Bertholletia excelsa (Brazil nut)
Papaver somniferum (opium poppy)
Sesamum indicum (sesame)
Pinus edulis (pinyon pine)

Cannabis sativa (marijuana)
Cucumis melo (cantaloupe), seed
Cucurbita foetidissima (buffalo gourd)
Nigella sativa (black cumin)
Oenothera biennis (evening primrose)
Pinus gerardiana (chilgoza pine)

Plants containing phytochemicals with antiarrhythmic properties, in order of potency, include the following:

Lactuca sativa (lettuce)
Portulaca oleracea (purslane)
Coptis chinensis (Chinese goldthread)
Cichorium endivia (endive)
Avena sativa (oats)
Vigna mungo (black gram)
Raphanus sativus (radish)
Chenopodium album (lamb's-quarters)
Brassica pekinensis (Chinese cabbage)
Anethum graveolens (dill)
Amaranthus sp. (pigweed)
Spinacia oleracea (spinach)
Cucumis sativus (cucumber)
Coptis japonica (huang lia)
Chrysanthemum coronarium (garland chrysanthemum)
Taraxacum officinale (dandelion)
Phaseolus vulgaris (black bean)
Strophathus gratus (quabain)
Brassica chinensis (Chinese cabbage)

Plants containing phytochemicals with antianginal properties, in order of potency, include the following:

Catharanthus lanceus (lanceleaf periwinkle)
Carya glabra (pignut hickory)
Carya ovata (shagbark hickory)
Chondrus crispus (Irish moss)
Portulaca oleracea (purslane)
Phaseolus vulgaris (black bean)
Papaver somniferum (opium poppy)
Avena sativa (oats)
Vigna unguiculata (cowpea)
Spinacia oleracea (spinach)

Tephrosia purpurea (purple tephrosia)
Ammi visnaga (visnaga)
Trichosanthus anguina (snakegourd)
Glycyrrhiza glabra (licorice)
Prunus serotina (black cherry)
Nyssa sylvatica (black gum)
Juniperus virginiana (red cedar)
Rhizophora mangle (red mangrove)
Symphoricarpos orbiculatus (buckbush)

Plants containing phytochemicals with anti-ischemic properties, in order of potency, include the following:

Portulaca oleracea (purslane)
Ipomoea aquatica (swamp cabbage)
Panicum maximum (guinea grass)
Viola tricolor hortensis (pansy)
Moringa oleifera (ben nut)
Asparagus officinalis (asparagus)
Elaeagnus angustifolia (Russian olive)
Frangula alnus (buckthorn)
Ipomoea batatas (sweet potato leaf)
Bertholletia excelsa (Brazil nut)
Ribes uva-crispa (gooseberry)
Linum usitatissimum (flax)
Fagopyrum esculentum (buckwheat)
Ipomoea batatas (sweet potato root)
Capsicum annuum (bell pepper)
Capsicum frutescens (cayenne)
Pisum sativum (pea)
Lens culinaris (lentil)

Plant containing anti-infarctal phytochemicals include *Jateorhiza palmata* (calumba), root.

Full Alternative Therapy Programs

DEAN ORNISH'S PROGRAM FOR REVERSING HEART DISEASE The Ornish Program has four main components:
    1. Moderate, supervised exercise.
    2. Stress management, involving stretching exercises, some yoga poses, and the teaching of relaxation and meditation techniques.

3. Low-fat, vegetarian diet with no animal products and no added fats.

4. Group support sessions where patients meet to learn more about their problems and act to express themselves.

The main focus of the program is to modify risk factors known to increase the dangers of coronary disease. It is not that different from a general medical program. The goals are to reduce weight, lower cholesterol and blood pressure, control diabetes, stop smoking, and control stress.

In a 1989 study reported in the British medical journal *Lancet*, two groups of heart patients were followed. One group adhered to the Ornish guidelines, and the other took the regular medical treatment for coronary disease. One year after starting the Ornish program, there was a reversal (improvement) of the coronary artery disorder as measured by an angiogram. In a follow-up study of the same group 5 years into the program, a PET (positron emission tomography) scan (then a state-of-the-art procedure) demonstrated that there was still a significant improvement in blood flow to the heart. This follow-up study was published in September 1995 in the *Journal of the American Medical Association* (JAMA).

"One thing we emphasize to patients who enter this program," registered nurse Deborah Matra says, "is that they need to regard what is required as a prescription from their doctor. They need to stick with the diet and exercise, do the stress management routine daily, stay with it as they would honor a doctor's prescription."

THE HEALING CENTER: INTRAVENOUS VITAMIN AND OZONE THERAPY The Healing Center in New York City takes a holistic approach to healing. They use state-of-the-art techniques—vitamin C drips, dietary counseling, acupuncture, massage therapies, chelation, and body therapy—and they have had magnificent results.

One patient, John, talks about his experience: "I'd say that I'm 95 percent responsible for my ill condition, out of sheer laziness and neglect. I weigh about 600 pounds, and I realize I am apt to get various diseases because of my weight. I have already suffered some: high blood pressure, fatigue, severe viral and bacterial problems, and edema of the right leg that causes cramps. I have trouble flexing the joints."

In the African-American community to which John belongs, there is, unfortunately, a high incidence of death from coronary heart disease and far too many cases of high blood pressure. John notes that much of his disease arose from faulty lifestyle habits: growing up eating too much fat and a lot of meat and drinking alcoholic beverages, all of which undermine health.

Dr. Howard Robins described his work when he was at the Healing Center. "We try," he said, "to let the body heal itself from all its injuries and weaknesses. We do not focus on one illness, but on the body as a whole. This is how holistic medicine was originally formulated.

"We have a medical doctor who assumes charge of the patient's medical condition, a homeopathic practitioner; a nutritionist who does extensive nutritional counseling with each patient on vitamins, herbs, and minerals; an acupuncturist who also prescribes Chinese herbal remedies to strengthen a weak organ system; and a dentist who removes mercury amalgam fillings, which cause fatigue and weaken the immune system. We also have a chiropractor who rebalances the back structure to create better innervations so the nervous system won't misfire and damage the organ system. Since all the body's systems are interconnected, we need to put everything back in order."

Dr. Robins's particular specialty was intravenous vitamin C and ozone therapy. He explained that in vitamin C therapy a person is built up very rapidly to large doses, to the 100,000-milligram range and eventually to the 200,000-milligram range. High levels of vitamin C cleanse the artery walls of calcified fatty plaques. EDTA is added in the drip, which melts the calcium bonds to the walls so the plaque is freed and the EDTA and vitamin C can wash it out of the body. Then the solution cleanses and heals the scars left by the low-density lipoproteins, healing the walls so that plaque will no longer adhere to them.

In ozone therapy—called major autohemotherapy—about 300 cubic centimeters (cc) of blood is drawn and an oxygen-ozone combination is mixed into it. The blood is then infused right back in, which takes about 30 minutes. The ozone helps oxidize fatty plaques, in a sense liquefying them and removing them from the walls, while making the red blood cells more flexible so that they can slip through the clogged arteries. This last measure is very important in preventing the need for bypass surgery and getting rid of angina pain.

Dr. Robins traced ozone therapy back to World War I. It was found that men who had been burned by mustard gas, injured, or shot and were kept in the back of the hospital tent, where the electric generators for the field lights were, were getting well. Eventually, doctors realized that the cause of the improvement was the ozone gas created by leakage from the generators. That began the work on ozone as a means to heal and prevent the amputation of limbs that had developed gangrene. "We've seen some miraculous results of ozone therapy at the Healing Center, for it's one thing that really does work."

DR. JULIAN WHITAKER'S NUTRITION AND EDUCATION PROGRAM Dr. Julian Whitaker was on the medical staff at the Pritikin Center. Nathan Pritikin helped millions of people by prescribing a diet that eliminates refined carbohydrates and animal fats and putting patients on a strict but moderate exercise regimen. In 1979, Dr. Whitaker went on to found the Whitaker Wellness Center in Newport Beach, California. He has expanded the Pritikin program, adding special vitamin supplements and eliminating most, if not all, animal protein from the prescribed diet.

Dr. Whitaker runs an intensive 5-day nutritional and educational clinic designed to teach people dietary and exercise guidelines that can help them prevent or overcome heart disease. Many patients attend the clinic as an alternative to major surgical procedures and/or drug therapy. They are frequently able to avoid these invasive and toxic treatments; more important, in the long run they establish or regain a healthful lifestyle and vitality that they had assumed was beyond their grasp.

Dr. Whitaker's treatment is as much a matter of education as of actual therapeutic intervention. Patients learn what they can do about their conditions so that the responsibility becomes theirs. Once patients understand how nutrition, vitamin supplementation, and exercise can help stop and even reverse most heart conditions and cardiovascular diseases, they must be resolute in applying this knowledge to their own lifestyles. They make these changes a routine part of each day.

"Heart disease," Dr. Whitaker states, "is not really as much a disease of the heart as it is a disease of the artery." The arteries carry blood to the heart at a uniform rate of flow, and if that flow is interfered with—speeded up or slowed down—the heart must adjust its activity to compensate for the change. If the arteries become clogged, the blood supply to the heart may be insufficient to the point where "the heart muscle begins to die in sections. These are what we call heart attacks, when a section of the heart muscle does not receive enough oxygen and simply dies."

It is important to understand that the heart itself usually remains healthy until the arteries are damaged. If the arteries become too rigid or are obstructed by clots and occlusions, they are not able to get the blood supply to and from the heart at a steady, healthy rate. "Heart disease" patients must be taught first and foremost how to repair and maintain the cardiovascular system in general rather than the heart specifically.

THE PROGRAM

Dr. Whitaker considers the three major risk factors to be elevated cholesterol levels, elevated blood pressure, and cigarette smoking. Other high-risk factors he looks for are obesity, diabetes, and lack of exercise. These are important but "are not as strong or as predictive as the other three."

Once patients understand the basic causes of their problems, the Newport Beach Program is geared to teach them how to deal constructively with the situation. Naturally, patients who smoke must give up the habit. Then they learn how to structure a diet that will attack the root causes of the disease as well as the symptoms. While surgical and drug remedies may relieve symptoms temporarily, they do not deal directly with the underlying causes of disease and rarely effect an actual cure or reversal of the dysfunction. Dealing effectively with the actual disorders leads ultimately to the disappearance of symptoms. This can be very exciting if you are one of the millions of people who have long suffered from cardiovascular problems that traditional physicians consider insurmountable without radical and invasive intervention.

ELIMINATING ANIMAL PROTEINS

Early on, Dr. Whitaker's patients are taught about reducing fats in their diets. Dairy products and processed meat are the chief culprits here. Eggs especially should be avoided by those with heart and cardiovascular diseases. Just like meat, eggs are directly related to elevated cholesterol levels, leading to damage and corrosion of the epithelial tissue lining the arterial walls.

People who continue to consume meats, cheeses, eggs, and other animal proteins, says Dr. Whitaker, cannot seriously reduce their overall body fat. Strangely enough, even animal products such as yogurt that may have no fat or cholesterol trigger an internal reaction that treats them as if they did simply because they are animal products.

Dr. Whitaker estimates that by getting away from animal proteins, "you shift from 49 percent fat down to around 15 percent fat, and you shift your carbohydrates from 40 percent up to maybe 65 to 75 percent. This will dramatically lower blood cholesterol if the shift is made accurately. The drop in the cholesterol level should be anywhere between 15 and 30 percent. It will also aid in weight loss, triglyceride control, and blood pressure control."

One can effectively reduce the intake of animal proteins by adding more carbohydrates to the diet. Dr. Whitaker explains that with animal proteins, which have only two sources of calories—fats and proteins—it is still necessary to add carbohydrates for a balanced diet. However, carbohydrates contain all three caloric sources—fats, proteins, and carbohydrates—and therefore can replace animal proteins. Instead of bacon and eggs, you might have a whole-grain cereal or bread with fruit. Pasta and rice and bean dishes such as bean tacos and burritos along with vegetables and a high-fiber salad with plenty of calcium-rich dark greens constitute a fine substitute for the standard meat and potatoes. There's nothing wrong with potatoes in and of themselves, but by the time they are smothered with butter, sour cream, and ketchup, they become fatty and high in cholesterol.

By turning away from meat and dairy products while increasing the proportion of fruits, vegetables, legumes, grains, breads, cereals, and pastas, heart disease patients replace high-fat, high-cholesterol foods with high-fiber, powerhouse-type foods. This switch lowers the patient's blood cholesterol levels, while the additional fiber will help clean out whatever fat and cholesterol are already clogging the system. Even foods containing significant amounts of fat, such as nuts and oils, can be used in moderation.

Olive oil, a monosaturated fat, "seems to be less deleterious to the system," Dr. Whitaker states, "than some of the polyunsaturated fats, such as corn oil and sunflower oil, which are common in our food processing. Greeks and Italians, who eat substantial amounts of olive oil, have been found to be in better health than, for example, Israelis, who eat a substantial amount of corn oil and sunflower oil."

In the case of nuts, some are better to consume than others. Walnuts, for example, have substantial amounts of omega-3 fatty acids, which are very beneficial for cardiovascular health. Peanuts, however, may contribute to sluggish blood flow related to serum cholesterol levels.

Besides the quality of the fats heart patients consume, it is crucial for them to reduce the overall quantity of fats. Dr. Whitaker insists that "you need to reduce the fat intake by about 50 percent of what the American population is eating now to be at what I consider to be the upper limit of fat intake."

One reason why many people do not change their lifestyles sufficiently to establish good health is that they are encouraged by their doctors to maintain the average range of white blood cells, cholesterol, and triglycerides. Dr. Whitaker believes that his patients deserve better than this. He tries to get them to establish healthy, not just average, levels of these heart disease culprits. They do this through exercise and socializing, proper vitamin and mineral regimens, and the reduction of animal fats in the diet, replacing them with complex carbohydrates.

INCREASING COMPLEX CARBOHYDRATES

Carbohydrates are preferred to fats because they do not have the high cholesterol levels that fats have and do not deposit sludge in the arteries, interfere with normal blood flow, or damage the inner arterial walls. Carbohydrates are high in fiber, vitamins, and minerals, all of which promote overall cardiovascular health. They also do not convert into fat very readily, although many people believe, partly because of misinformation from the scientific community, that carbohydrates are fattening.

Dr. Whitaker explains: "It is very difficult for carbohydrates to actually put fat weight into your system; some studies have shown that carbohydrates are not converted into fat nearly as rapidly or as efficiently as many scientists used to think. The conversion of carbohydrates into fat takes more energy than is actually present in the carbohydrate molecule trying to be converted, so the body just doesn't do it. The primary thing that really deposits fat into fat is fat itself. Often, when people add carbohydrates to their diet, they add them to an already increased fat diet. Generally, when I put people on an increased carbohydrate diet, they will almost always lose weight, and they will call begging me to give them something to stop the weight loss if they are truly following a 70 to 75 percent carbohydrate diet. Believe it or not, the high-carbohydrate diet we use causes a weight loss that creates a problem."

It should be made clear that Dr. Whitaker does not recommend an increased intake of all carbohydrates. A lot of carbohydrates, particularly simple and processed carbohydrates, are nothing but junk food. Processing breaks down their fibrous cellular structures and robs them of much or most of their vitamin and mineral content. Cakes, jams, sugared fruit juices, baked goods, highly processed breads, and bleached flours and flour products are examples. Often the only thing left in these foods is sugar. The carbohydrates espoused in

Dr. Whitaker's program are unprocessed, unrefined, and wholesome complex carbohydrates such as whole grains and fresh fruits.

VITAMIN AND MINERAL SUPPLEMENTS

Vitamin and mineral supplementation is another significant part of Dr. Whitaker's program. Vitamins A, B$_6$, C, and E are especially important, along with the minerals selenium, calcium, magnesium, and chromium.

Between 25 and 50 milligrams of vitamin B$_6$ may be used. Some B vitamins, such as niacin, are used in large doses much as a drug is used. "If there is an elevated cholesterol and triglyceride level which doesn't respond adequately to our diet," Dr. Whitaker explains, "we will use niacin at a rate of 500 to 700 milligrams per meal." This is strictly a therapeutic dose and should be used only in conjunction with a physician's prescribed treatment.

Vitamin C is of particular significance in maintaining the sound structure of arterial walls since it promotes strong, healthy connective tissues. "In my opinion," Dr. Whitaker says, "early on the most important vitamin, if there is a single one, would be vitamin C."

It is especially important that the patient's blood remains thin and free-flowing, and this is where vitamin E plays a role in Dr. Whitaker's treatment. Vitamin E is an anticoagulant that keeps blood platelets from clumping together so that they can pass easily through narrow openings and small capillaries. It is also an antioxidant, protecting the arterial cells from damage from free radicals.

Dr. Whitaker also uses MaxEPA, a blood thinner and anticoagulant that acts somewhat like vitamin E. MaxEPA, he says, "is beneficial to a patient who has an elevated level of triglycerides plus elevated cholesterol. We use large doses of it at that stage. We will use large amounts per meal to drop the triglyceride and cholesterol level." He goes on to note that MaxEPA is ineffective in lowering cholesterol levels when very low levels of triglycerides are present. Dr. Whitaker warns that MaxEPA alone is not a "panacea for lowering the cholesterol," as some sponsors have made it out to be, but is very effective when integrated with an overall treatment program.

Mineral supplementation is equally important. Magnesium has been found to be deficient among heart patients, up to 50 percent lower than in noncardiac patients studied recently at the University of California. To restore the mineral to acceptable levels, Dr. Whitaker uses injectable magnesium for angina patients. Diuretics, which are commonly prescribed to lower blood pressure in patients with cardiovascular disorders, deplete magnesium as well as potassium. While most physicians are careful to replace the potassium lost during diuretic treatment, few replace the magnesium. This can cause further complications, especially since the loss of magnesium affects serum calcium levels. This is part of the reason Dr. Whitaker believes that "diuretics, and the way they are currently used, are making a lot of people worse instead of better."

WHY CONVENTIONAL THERAPIES DO NOT SUCCEED

Dr. Whitaker believes that technology has been confused with science. Just because it is possible to do a coronary bypass or angioplasty does not necessarily mean that it always makes sense to undertake it. Bypass surgery involves severing the artery before the blockage and rerouting the blood flow through an unblocked blood vessel taken from the leg. "It has been conclusively demonstrated," he states, "that bypass surgery fails to reduce mortality rates for 75 percent of heart patients who undergo the procedure." While failing to cure many heart disease victims, such surgery frequently puts the patient at needless risk, with 0.3 to 6.6 percent of such patients dying after the surgery. Still, Americans spend between $2 billion and $3 billion a year on coronary bypasses.

Similarly, catheterization has an insufficient scientific basis in Dr. Whitaker's opinion, yet thousands of catheterizations are done almost routinely. Catheterizations are used to detect arterial blockages and open them up, often in conjunction with a balloon angioplasty or a bypass. Angioplasty, a procedure in which a catheter is snaked through the arteries to open up blockages, has been hailed as a great technological feat. However, it has a death rate of 3.5 percent and a conversion to bypass rate of 15 percent, and the whole procedure must be repeated in more than one in three cases because it does not work the first time.

An obvious problem with this routine approach to dealing with heart disease is that the catheterization itself—sticking a catheter inside the heart—can cause harm. To perform this exploration without good reason is dangerous, yet it is commonly done to patients who do not have life-threatening conditions and frequently don't even suffer from chest pain.

Moreover, the results of catheterization are not dependable. Dr. Whitaker explains: "Studies were done comparing the blockages found in patients who had been recently catheterized and had died from some other cause, and they did an autopsy within 30 days of the catheterization. When they looked at the arteries at the autopsy and looked at the angiogram picture and the way it was read, they found very little correlation. Even more alarming is the fact that different doctors viewing the same catheterization had different opinions concerning the exact location of the blockage. Studies at the University of Iowa showed that blood flow measurements taken during surgery were quite different from what had been indicated by the angiogram."

DR. JOHN MCDOUGALL'S DIETARY PROGRAM According to Dr. John McDougall, traditional therapies may be introduced in crisis situations, but the body benefits most from the restoration of normal biochemical balance. The standard American diet, he feels, has lost its ability to maintain that balance. A natural diet, free of animal protein and consisting of small amounts of food eaten many times a day, can help restore it. His vegetarian diet helps not only people with heart disease but those who suffer from cancer, arthritis, and obesity.

Dr. McDougall, author of *The McDougall Program: Twelve Days to Dynamic Health*, believes that the American public needs to be informed about the best diet available, not just a moderate or prudent one as recommended by the American Heart Association. Since nutrition has been given so little attention in medical school curricula, few doctors know how to prescribe diets appropriate for specific conditions. They tell their patients to cut down a little on fat, add a bit of fiber, and so forth, but patients with heart disease have their lives on the line and need much more informed direction.

BACKGROUND

Dr. McDougall began taking dietary histories of his patients to see if he could get some clues to helping patients who were not being healed by the traditional treatments. He took dietary histories of every one of his patients for 3 years and was amazed by what he found.

Practicing in rural Hawaii, he had a unique opportunity to study an isolated group of sugarcane plantation workers through several generations. The first, older generation was made up of Japanese, Chinese, and Filipinos who had come to Hawaii in their teens or early childhood. Their children, grandchildren, and great-grandchildren were natives of Hawaii and had a very different background in terms of lifestyle and diet.

The members of the older generation possessed far superior health to that of the second, third, and fourth generations despite all having been in the same location and the same industry for years. The members of the first generation were trim and hardy, still vital and vigorous even in old age. The younger generations, by contrast, were commonly obese or at least overweight, plagued with diseases that Dr. McDougall had been taught were primarily genetic: diabetes, colon cancer, heart disease, and high blood pressure.

Clearly, genetics was not the issue here. The only variable Dr. McDougall could establish was dietary history. The members of the older generation were primarily vegetarians, consuming very few high-fat, high-cholesterol animal products such as eggs, cheese, and milk and instead eating mostly rice and vegetables. The younger generations, raised in Hawaii instead of Asia, had become accustomed to the American diet of animal products and meats, highly refined and processed foods rather than whole foods, and sugar- and salt-laden snacks. Dr. McDougall came to realize that diet is a far greater factor in the incidence of degenerative disease than he and others in his field had been led to believe.

He also noted that, in a broader perspective, throughout history it has always been those in the upper, rich, privileged classes who have been plagued by the degenerative diseases. The royalty of past centuries were the people who had the means to enjoy rich diets replete with fats, including dairy and meat products. The feast was a routine part of their privileged life, and gluttonous eating was a major source of socialization and entertainment. The poor peasants who tilled the earth from sunup to sunset could afford to eat only what they themselves grew—grains, vegetables and potatoes—a simple diet high in starch, complex carbohydrates, and fiber. This "poor man's diet" was largely responsible for the fact that the peasantry rarely suffered the degenerative diseases so common among the elite: heart disease, diabetes, gout, and the like. The diet rich in saturated fats, cholesterol, and salt might have been fit for a king, but it certainly did not keep the king fit.

Dr. McDougall pondered the fact that for hundreds and even thousands of years the general populace had not depended on high-protein foods such as meat and dairy products for their daily nutritional needs. In New Guinea and South America whole civilizations revolved around sweet potatoes; the Indians of North America were hunters for whom meat was only an occasional treat, the main diet being primarily corn-based. For Asians, to this day, rice has been central. Europeans originally ate high concentrations of grains, breads, and, later, potatoes. Africans consumed mostly grains and beans. In Mexico and Central America, rice, corn, and beans provided the main sustenance. In the Middle East, wheat, sesame seeds, and chickpeas have been the traditional mainstays of the diet. Even today in many of these parts of the world meat is consumed infrequently.

THE PROGRAM

Dr. McDougall says that practically everyone who participates in his 12-day live-in program is able to get off drugs and experience drastically reduced cholesterol, triglyceride, and blood sugar levels by the end of the 12 days. This is not a quick cure, however. The disorders plaguing these patients may have been arrested, but true reversal and restoration of coronary and arterial health take months to accomplish. The special diet used in the program is not a temporary one but must be continued for as long as the patient wishes to avoid re-establishing heart disease and vascular dysfunction. In other words, the new eating habits are not really a diet but, along with a structured and progressive exercise program, constitute a whole new lifestyle.

DIETARY CHANGES. In the McDougall program, people with heart disease are taught how to let go of their high-fat diets and how to choose and prepare high-quality complex carbohydrate meals that are high in starch and fiber. At breakfast, coffee, ham and eggs, and white buttered toast with sugar jam might be replaced by oatmeal with strawberries. A whole-grain bread without the fat-laden butter, maybe topped with a real fruit jam instead of sugary jam or jelly, might be paired with herbal tea or a hot beverage derived from grains rather than coffee beans.

Patients are taught to distinguish simple from complex carbohydrates. The simple sugars may be called glucose, fructose, maltose, or lactose: they are found in honey, corn syrup, milk, molasses, maple syrup, and fruit juices. They provide the body with quick-burning fuel which does little to sustain energy levels evenly or over an extended period of time. In a processed state, they do not even retain their fiber and nutrient values and become little more than highly concentrated sugars full of calories with little nutritional value. These types of carbohydrates should be avoided, but not as much as the fats and animal products.

Complex carbohydrates, in contrast, provide a very slow burning fuel that is stored in the muscles and provides a steady energy supply throughout the day. Potatoes, rice, and vegetables such as peas, corn, and asparagus contain ideal forms of carbohydrates.

Dr. McDougall offers a variety of suggestions regarding starch-based meal planning, preparation, and variation using a carbohydrate-centered diet: "The foods we suggest are corn, pasta, rice, most vegetables, grains, and all fiber-rich foods. For breakfast, you can have oatmeal or other hot whole-cereal meals, grains, waffles, and pancakes. For lunch, you can have all kinds of soups, such as lentil soup, bean soup, tomato soup, onion soup, or pea soup, as long as you make the soup yourself. Main entrees for dinner can be spaghetti with marinara sauce, curry vegetable stew, brown rice casseroles, baked potatoes, bean burritos without lard or oil, Indian curry dishes, and all kinds of Chinese and Japanese dishes. You can have all these foods as long as they are not processed in any way and are made fresh.

REDUCING HIGH BLOOD PRESSURE. Besides the symptoms of their diseases, many people suffer greatly from the medications they take to treat those diseases. Dr. McDougall relates, "We take people who come in on medications for high blood pressure, and they just want to get off those medications because the side effects are so horrendous. They may even be on 10, 12, or 15 medications. It's rare that we can't get them off."

Here is an example of such a patient: "I had an accountant come into my office and state that he was on 20 drugs and wanted off them. Actually, he was on 12 high-blood-pressure pills, one diabetes pill, and several heart pills. After 4 days on a healthy diet consisting of no salt, low-fat, and no cholesterol, he was off all his medication; his blood sugar, which was 235, fell to 168; and his blood pressure, which started at 190/110, became 150/70."

Dr. McDougall says that conventional medicine treats high blood pressure "by lowering it, which makes as much sense as giving aspirin to someone with an infected toe. We've lowered the fever but have not cured the infection. When there is a sign that the blood vessel system is diseased, we use blood pressure pills to eliminate the sign, but the disease stays. What we should do is deal with the cause. So far only a half dozen people in our program have not been able to eliminate blood pressure medications. Over the last 10 years, I have treated over 7,000 people.

"Let me tell you about a minister at the church I've gone to for several years. This young man, who is only 32 years old, had blood pressure problems for 10 years and had been taking blood pressure pills for 2 years before I saw him. He was recently married and was having problems with sexual function. He was being treated by a doctor who gave him the standard line: 'You're on pills for high blood pressure; we don't know what causes the problem, and you'll be on them for the rest of your life with no chance of getting off them.' He finally decided to see me, and when he asked what could be done for him, I told him to stop taking the blood pressure pills and told him how to do this (he was taking the kind that can't be stopped immediately). He changed his diet. This was over a year ago, and his blood pressure went down from the high level of 160/95 to 110/70 in 2 to 3 weeks. He lost 30 extra pounds he'd been carrying around since his teenage years, and he's absolutely drug-free and feels wonderful. He still sees the doctor who told him he'd never get off blood pressure pills and gloats a bit as the doctor takes his blood pressure and finds it perfectly normal. The doctor's response to all of this is, 'It was a coincidence.'"

Dr. McDougall says that this sort of "coincidence" occurs in more than 90 percent of cases where patients have changed their diet dramatically.

DR. ERIC BRAVERMAN'S APPROACH TO HYPERTENSION Dr. Eric Braverman has published more than 60 papers in peer-reviewed journals and is the author of numerous books, including *Hypertension and Nutrition: The Amazing Way to Reverse Heart Disease Naturally*. Like Dr. McDougall, Dr. Braverman believes that a general wellness program that combines a proper diet, supplementation, and exercise is the best way to treat hypertension. The diet he recommends combines these elements with a special nutrient formula designed to lower high blood pressure and then help maintain good cardiovascular health.

Dr. Braverman believes that the primary cause of hypertension and heart disease is the accumulation of heavy metals such as lead, aluminum, and cadmium that produce arterial hardening as people age. With that hardening comes an increase in blood pressure because an aging body is no longer as flexible as it once was. This problem is compounded by the loss of estrogen, progesterone, testosterone and DHEA, depending on a person's sex, and the loss of growth hormone. According to Dr. Braverman, the danger of hypertension and heart disease begins at a blood pressure level that exceeds 120/80, and in some cases, the risk level may be 110/70.

Not surprisingly, the first step in Dr. Braverman's approach to treating high blood pressure is a diet that adds potassium and restricts sodium and cholesterol intake. Regarding the ongoing debate about the cholesterol content of eggs, Dr. Braverman asserts that high cholesterol usually has more to do with the other elements in the average person's diet than with eggs being the central culprit. As he puts it, "The average person is still eating white flour, junk food, and garbage essentially. So cholesterol intake will throw off cholesterol levels. But as a rule you're making 90 percent or more of the cholesterol in your body, and it's triggered by the diet. So, if you're eating a Null diet or a Braverman style diet, then the eggs are going to be a good food for you as long as you're not allergic."

NUTRIENT FORMULA Dr. Braverman also advocates the following nutrient formula to lower hypertension: 200 milligrams of garlic, 200 milligrams of taurine, 50 milligrams of magnesium, 10 milligrams of potassium, 20 micrograms of selenium, 4 micrograms of zinc, 20 micrograms of chromium, 50 micrograms of niacinimide, 50 milligrams of vitamin C, 50 micrograms of molybdenum, 50 milligrams of vitamin B_6, and 1,000 units of beta carotene. "Then," he says, "you just multiply that from about 5 to 10 to get a balance of those. Those are what I call the poor hypertensive nutrients.

"We've worked hard on a supplement called the heart or hypertensive supplement. On the basis of the research I did, we put all these nutrients in one pill, so you could lower your blood pressure naturally with one vitamin that you could take a lot of. However, one doesn't have to do that. There are many ways to take these supplements, but it's clear now that supplementation is one aspect of lowering your blood pressure."

OTHER PARTS OF THE PROGRAM

Despite the fact that supplementation is a useful tool in lowering high blood pressure, Dr. Braverman stresses, "The defeat of high blood pressure is a transformation of being and lifestyle." A person who exercises, keeps his or her weight down, generally maintains a low-fat, low-salt diet, and gets useful supplementation preferably through diet, but alternatively in pill form, will be better off for it in the fight against heart disease."

Other possible ways that Dr. Braverman suggests to lower hypertension include the use of borage and fish oil; relaxation; meditation; an electrical stimulator that has been FDA-approved for anxiety; melatonin; and last but not least the revolutionary role that retreats to healing centers and wellness programs can play in people's lives when they are trying to precipitate a long-term lifestyle change.

Dr. Braverman explains: "Many, many individuals can go to health retreats, go on juice fasts, go on new dietary regimes, start cleansing techniques, and exercise, and they reverse their blood pressure, their weight, their blood sugar. Even I continue to underestimate the revolutionary nature of the wellness movement which says to the drug company and the drug managed care hospital network, no."

Choosing a Therapy

Five years ago, I suggested to a leading cardiologist that the use of vitamin E, stress management, exercise, dietary changes, power walking, and proper supplementation would make a vast difference in the prevention and treatment of heart disease. He looked at me and responded, "No way. It's not scientific. It won't work." Today *JAMA*, *New England Journal of Medicine*, *Medical Tribune*, *Lancet*, and many other major medical journals recommend the same treatments that doctor disparaged 5 years ago. Thanks to the pioneering work of Dr. Dean Ornish and others, the concept of alternative treatment is less controversial and people are now willing to accept these treatments if they seem to offer the best possibility of health. Hopefully, in the future we will not have to reject any form of treatment, but accept the best features from each as they lead to better health.

Having reviewed the material in this chapter, you should know enough about the available alternatives to radical surgery and drug treatment to decide whether you prefer to seek traditional, alternative or complementary care for cardiovascular distress. Whatever sort of care you seek, you should monitor the progress you are or are not making to determine whether it may be feasible to abandon one course and embark on another.

31

Stroke

Strokes are the third leading cause of death in the United States. Every 60 seconds, someone dies of a stroke. Strokes are also the leading cause of adult disability.

There are two different types of strokes: hemorrhagic stroke, which is a rupture in a blood vessel, and ischemic stroke, which is caused by a blockage in the blood vessels. The result of both types of strokes is a lack of blood flow to the brain and consequently insufficient oxygen for brain function.

Symptoms

Symptoms of stroke include dizziness, blurred vision and loss of sensation, slurred speech, loss of bladder control, and partial loss of hearing. A person should seek medical help immediately if he or she experiences one or more of these symptoms. Often a stroke will be accompanied by paralysis of an arm or leg on one side of the body. Strokes can cause swelling of the brain, stupor, and coma.

Enzyme Therapy

Dr. Anthony Cichoke is a leading medical researcher in the field of enzyme therapy. Dr. Cichoke has taught at the University of Minnesota and the University of Rochester Medical School and is the author of hundreds of articles and seven books, including *The Complete Book of Enzyme Therapy*.

Dr. Chichoke uses enzyme therapy to boost the immune system and detoxify the body. "Enzymes are catalysts," he explains. "Anything that is alive has to have enzymatic activity—whether it is in the grass outside or whether it is in your body. Enzymes are critical for every cell of our body. Nothing can go on in the body without enzymatic activity. Without enzymes there would be no breathing, no digestion, no growth, no blood coagulation, no reproduction. "Enzymes, he says, fight strokes by acting "as sort of a 'Roto Rooter' that helps break up cholesterol and toxins in your body.

"Strokes can be treated systemically with enzymes. They are used as digestive aids; they improve the absorption of other nutrients, herbs, health foods, whatever, Enzymes aid absorption and metabolism at the cellular level."

Dr. Cichoke has his patients take enzyme supplements orally between meals. He recommends enzymes such as bromelain, papain, trypsin, chymotrypsin, pancreatin, and microbial proteases, all of which have primarily proteolytic enzyme activity. Dr. Cichoke describes how enzyme supplements pass through the gut into the small intestine, where they are absorbed into the circulatory system. "These are all enzymes that work in the bloodstream and the various organs as well as at the cellular level of the body."

Enzymes aid in detoxification at the cellular level in various organs and in the bloodstream and digestive tract. He explains why it is important to have a well-ordered circulatory system: "The blood must get to the cells in order to bring nutrients to the body, and blood needs to help take the waste products away from the cells. Further, enzymes help break up the cholesterol and fibrin in the blood vessels." Dr. Cichoke pictures a blood vessel as a stream or river, with little curves and eddies. These curves fill up with fibrin and cholesterol, which clog blood vessels so the blood and oxygen can't get through.

"Proteolytic enzymes help to break up the fibrin and cholesterol and allow the body to eliminate these waste products. Enzymes also improve circulation. They help keep the bloodstream normalized." He explains that it is important to have a balance between blood coagulation and blood thinning. "Enzymes help to keep this critical equilibrium in order."

Enzymes also help break up free radicals. "As part of the aging process, and also as a result of stress and illness and injuries, the cells of our body tend to oxidize—they rust. Think of the body's tissue as if it was like a lovely leather jacket. When you first buy that leather jacket it's soft and pliable. But then, as it gets older the leather oxidizes and it becomes cracked and hard. As we go through life, our body tends to oxidize. When you take antioxidant enzymes, such as superoxide dismutase, catalase, glutathione, and peroxidase, they fight free radical formation and work as antioxidants."

Enzymes can also dissolve large blood clots, which can cause strokes. Dr. Cichoke says that enzymes are currently being used both in and out of hospitals to break up blood clots and also to break up fibrin formations. "In hospitals, some enzymes used for this purpose are brinase, which comes from Aspergillus oryzae, streptokinase, which is of bacterial origin, and urokinase or prourokinase, which is actually from human urine."

Dr. Cichoke tells a story about a stroke patient in Portland, Oregon, who was treated with these enzymes. "They had given up on him. But as a last-ditch effort, 9 hours after the stroke, they began to give him urokinase. Not only did he regain consciousness, he also regained the ability to move his arms and his legs. After 6 weeks of rehabilitation therapy he went home."

Dr. Cichoke cites an article in *The New York Times* science section of February 9, 1999, which stated, "Enzymes offer hope for reducing devastation from strokes." Currently, Dr. Cichoke notes, the Cleveland Clinic in Cleveland, Ohio, is using prourokinase to fight strokes. He stresses the importance of proteolytic enzymes as well as antioxidant enzymes. "I suggest taking 200 micrograms of antioxidant enzymes three times a day between meals and 8 to 10 tablets of combination enzymes three times a day, also between meals. If you take bromelain, take four to six tablets of approximately 230 to 250 milligrams every day.

"I know this can be fairly expensive," he goes on, "but how much does health mean to you? In 1960 medical services were 5 percent of our gross national product; by 1990 this figure was over 12 percent. We eat too much fat and too many refined carbohydrates, we smoke too much, we get virtually no exercise, and we overeat. For this reason, exercising, having a positive mental attitude, and eating fresh fruits are all very important. And enzyme supplementation is critical."

32

Chelation Therapy

For the past 40 years, one of the most promising and exciting healing therapies has been ignored and attacked by the medical establishment. This treatment, called chelation therapy, could be saving hundreds of thousands of lives a year and improving the quality of life for millions more by treating heart disease, stroke, diabetes, peripheral vascular disease, memory loss, and damage due to smoking, drinking, and environmental toxic exposure to heavy metals.

Hundreds of thousands of people have undergone the therapy, more than 400 doctors now use it, and more than 4,000 scientific articles have been written on various aspects of the process. Chelation is safe and effective when properly administered, and yet it has been kept from an objective review until now because it threatens the economic stability of the multibillion dollar cardiovascular and coronary bypass industry, which profits from the very illnesses that chelation treats.

An example of the difficulties involved in completing clinical studies on chelation took place some 15 years ago. During the mid-1980s, the Food and Drug Administration (FDA) approved two careful clinical studies on chelation to be conducted at the Walter Reed Hospital and Letterman Army Hospital, with the results to be published upon their completion. The studies were halted in 1991 during the Gulf War; following the war, however, the studies were never resumed due to lapses in funding. Other physicians and medical organizations attempting to acquire both approval and sufficient financing for clinical studies on chelation today have run into similar roadblocks.

Mainstream doctors, for the most part, still ignore the possibilities of chelation treatments despite its good track record with patients. There are no better experts on the therapy's safety and effectiveness than the pioneering doctors who administer it and the patients who receive it. This chapter tells the story of such doctors, and of their patients, all of whom have well-documented records to prove the extent of their improvement from chelation therapy.

What Is Chelation Therapy?

Chelation therapy is a safe, easily administered alternative to drugs and surgery in the treatment of heart disease and other illnesses. The term is derived from the Greek root "chele" meaning claw, and refers to a molecule that is able to grab onto, deactivate, and remove a mineral from the body. The process involves the infusion into the bloodstream of the amino acid EDTA, which moves through the blood vessels and removes excesses of iron, copper, and various other metals that are implicated in the formation of plaque. As the plaque is reduced, and through a variety of other biochemical mechanisms, blood flow all over the body improves.

Dr. Michael B. Schachter of Suffern, New York, former president of the American College of Advancement in Medicine (ACAM), explains how chelation works: "We know that EDTA removes metals and that it is not metabolized in the body at all. It just comes in, grabs a mineral, and goes out through the urine. In so doing, it brings about a number of profound reactions in the body that result in the therapeutic effects. For example, as people age and as disease occurs, we get an accumulation of calcium in and around the cells of the soft tissues, and the EDTA helps to remove this excess calcium from the wrong places. In other words, we like calcium in our bones but we don't like it in our arteries and our joints, and EDTA helps to get rid of that. It also helps stop excessive free-radical formation, which results in destruction of cell membranes and serves as a common pathway for diseases such as multiple sclerosis, arthritis, cancer, arteriosclerosis, and so on. So, EDTA does a number of very remarkable things in the body."

The History of Chelation

Chelating agents were first used by the German textile industry in 1935 to remove calcium from hard water, which was staining and ruining fabric. After considerable research, a synthetic amino acid known as ethylene diamine tetraacetic acid (or EDTA) was found to be excellent for that purpose. So chelation's first use was a commercial one.

Soon afterward it was discovered that chelation therapy could promote healing by removing heavy metals from the body. During World War II, when an antidote for poison gas was being sought, it was found that chelating agents could be helpful by chelating arsenic, an essential component of some poison gases. One chelating agent that was particularly helpful was BAL or British antilewisite. After the war, chelation therapy was used in the treatment of radiation poisoning, for heavy metals like strontium and uranium. Later it was found that EDTA could effectively and quickly help in cases of lead poisoning.

At the same time, an unexpected benefit of chelation was discovered. In the early 1950s, Dr. Norman Clarke, Sr. reasoned that since EDTA binds to calcium, it might benefit patients with coronary atherosclerosis. He began to explore this phenomenon, and it soon became apparent that his original hypothesis was correct. Dr. Clarke published a number of studies showing that patients with various forms of cardiovascular disease improved. In Dr. Clarke's landmark article published in the *American Journal of Cardiology* in August 1960, he stated the following:

"For several years we have been administering intravenously to patients with advanced occlusive vascular disease 3 to 5 grams of EDTA. An accumulative experience with several hundred patients has demonstrated that overall relief has been superior to that obtained with other methods. In occlusive vascular disease of the brain there has been uniform relief of vertigo and the signs of senility, even when advanced, have been significantly relieved. In summary, the treatment of atherosclerotic vascular complications with the chelating agent EDTA is supported by a large volume of information."

A CONTROVERSIAL TREATMENT Unfortunately, Dr. Clarke's research and future chelation work were dealt a heavy blow shortly after his article appeared. The treatment was attacked by nearly all components of the medical industrial complex: physicians, professional organizations and journals, government regulatory boards, and insurance companies. In 1969, Abbott Laboratories' patent on EDTA ran out and the company decided not to invest in further research. At the present time, the Food and Drug Administration (FDA) has not approved chelation therapy for use in treating cardiovascular and degenerative conditions. However, once a drug is approved for one purpose by the FDA, physicians are permitted to use it for other indications provided that there is some medical justification for the unapproved use. EDTA has been approved for use in lead and heavy metal toxicity, and so is able to be used for other ailments.

Opponents of the procedure say that chelation therapy is dangerous. In fact, there is no evidence to support this claim. When you compare the risks from surgery to the possibility of having adverse effects from chelation, it almost boggles the mind as to why doctors are constantly pushing these surgical modalities before trying something like chelation. Studies published in the *Journal of the American Medical Association* (JAMA) and elsewhere have shown that most patients getting bypass surgery should not have received it. Yet the numbers continue to increase: from 1979 to 1996, the number of bypass procedures in the U.S. soared some 425 percent.

Dr. John Sessions, who has given the treatment to thousands of patients over a period of nearly 15 years remarks that no one has ever been harmed by the treatment when given in the proper way by a physician trained in its administration. "I have seen some of the most astounding and gratifying results. Specifically, my father had about 10 treatments and was then able to get rid of his walker and walking cane. In 30 treatments he went back into his business, raising cattle and farming, and bought new equipment."

Dr. Sessions believes that some of the controversy also dates back to early research done in the field when chelation was given to people without nutritional supplementation. Since chelation therapy removes many important nutritive minerals from the body, some of these early patients became deficient in zinc and other minerals during the course of treatment.

Another concern that some physicians have about chelation is how it affects the kidneys. In fact, published articles substantiate the fact that chelation actually improves deficient kidney function when administered properly. Dr. Sessions confirms this in his experience with dialysis patients in whom at first "the kidneys were functioning at 5 percent" and after treatments, "they were able to cut down on their dialysis to one and two times a week. In addition, their lifestyle improved to where they could go back to exercising and having a more acceptable lifestyle."

How Chelation Helps the Heart

Chelation therapy helps the heart in a number of ways. First, it cleanses the body of toxic material and moves the calcium out so that normal contractions can resume. Dr. Murray Susser of Santa Monica, California, says that according to the work of Hans Selye calcium goes to the site of an injury and acts like an internal scab. When you heal the calcium goes away, but if you keep on injuring yourself, like smokers do with cigarette smoke every day, it builds up and arteriosclerosis forms around it. EDTA can go in and take out that calcium, and when accompanied by a change in lifestyle it can reverse some of the effects of continued injury.

Another way chelation can help the heart is through the injection of magnesium along with the EDTA. More magnesium helps the coronary arteries to relax and open up so that a greater amount of blood can flow through them.

In the long term, EDTA also acts as a calcium binder. As serum calcium decreases, the body responds by secreting parathyroid hormone, which helps mobilize calcium from abnormal soft tissue sites and move it into bones where it is needed. In this way, chelation can be an indirect treatment for osteoporosis.

In addition, by acting as a calcium channel blocker, EDTA may cause the blood pressure to go down. High blood pressure medications may become unnecessary over time.

Dr. Kirk Morgan, director of the Morgan Medical Clinic in Louisville, Kentucky, has been using chelation on heart patients with hardening of the arteries since 1982 with 90 percent or better improvement. His article, "Myocardial Ischemia Treated with Nutrients in Intravenous EDTA Chelation:

Report of Two Patients" documented the results of two patients with exercise induced angina pectoris. After the administration of less than 40 treatments, electrocardiographic heart tracings (EKGs) were taken. They showed abnormalities to become normal on repeat stress testing 15 months after beginning the treatment. Both patients demonstrated total resolution of symptoms and renal function did not deteriorate in either subject. The article concludes, "Though only two such cases are described, there is increasing evidence that chelation using EDTA is a relatively inexpensive, effective, safe, and even preferential, but often neglected technique for medical management of cardiovascular and related diseases."

Most other studies in this area show equally dramatic results. Dr. Albert Scarchilli was involved in a study of 19,187 retrospective cases of patients with peripheral vascular disease. It was revealed by thermoscan that 87.5 percent of all patients who received chelation therapy showed significant improvement.

Dr. Michael Janson, author of *The Vitamin Revolution in Health Care*, has used nutrition and dietary supplements in his practice for the past 20 years. He says that pain from angina pectoris is relieved in 90 percent of the heart patients who receive chelation therapy. He gives an account of one patient's condition before and after treatment:

"Before treatment, this man could not walk from his golf cart to the tee to do his golfing and he told his buddies he was not going to be with them next year. He noticed some friends of his getting better and went to their doctor. He said, "Doc, I don't know what you are doing for these people but I have got to have some of it." After chelation, he is free from angina. He is golfing a full golf course and walking the course now instead of taking the cart."

The number of infusions necessary to correct a cardiovascular problem varies. According to some physicians, circulatory problems due to blockages in small arteries show more rapid improvement than blockages in larger arteries. Therefore, it is not uncommon to see someone with significant blockages of the larger arteries to require 50 to 100 infusions before really getting better. A rough rule to apply is that the further from the heart the blockage is, the slower the response rate will be. In other words, coronaries respond the earliest, carotids second, and arteries in the legs third.

Removal of Toxic Heavy Metals

Heavy metal toxicity is a growing problem. Heavy metals can get into our food if the food is grown near a polluted area. They can be found in our drinking water, and in the air we breathe. Dr. Murray Susser sums up the situation: "The average civilized human being now has a body burden of lead which is 1,000 times greater than people had 500 years ago. We are all, to some extent, lead poisoned, some much worse than others."

As mentioned, chelation therapy is approved for the removal of these heavy metals. However, mainstream medicine would like not to see it used except when levels in the body are very high. Many alternative practitioners believe that toxic substances like lead are dangerous, have no biological function, and do not belong in the body no matter what the level. Unfortunately, heavy metals do not show their tremendous burden to the body until a great deal of harm has already been done. Only when damage is in its acute phase will symptoms like headaches and dizziness appear. When chelation therapy is used it usually lowers the level of toxic metals in the body significantly after only 5 to 10 treatments. In one man's experience:

"I went to Dr. Yurkovsky with many complaints. I had some days where my thinking was foggy and I felt like a car with a clogged fuel filter. It was as if my brain wasn't getting enough oxygen or enough blood. And I kept losing weight.

"Dr. Savely Yurkovsky discussed the weight loss as a possible malabsorption and as a possible result of heavy metal toxicity, maybe from mercury which was suppressing pancreatic function. He asked me about my amalgam fillings and when I told him that I had a lot of them, he suggested I take them out.

"I had a chelation test where you get one treatment followed by a 24-hour urine test for heavy metals, and I was found to be high in cadmium, mercury, and lead. Then we started a program of chelation, and after 25 treatments all the metals were down within what is called a reference range. In addition, I had my amalgam fillings out. As a result I have started to gain weight and I feel much better.

"It was a good experience all around and I am continuing with the treatments even though I am below what is considered a dangerous level because my doctor has encouraged me to get all the metals out."

Other Conditions Treated with Chelation

Dr. Serafina Corsello, a chelation practitioner, notes that unlike coronary bypass operations, which work only on the heart, chelation therapy can benefit the entire circulatory system: "You often have atherosclerotic plaque of the little vessels of the kidneys even before the heart is affected and this weakens the body's cleansing process. By regulating the amount of EDTA accordingly and adding vitamin C to repair the tissues, the little vessels of the kidneys will get cleaned out. Then we can increase the amount of EDTA, and ultimately clean the whole vascular system, the heart, kidneys, liver, pancreas, and brain."

Chelation is especially helpful to people with diabetes since diabetes generally involves the arteries. The blood sugar simply happens to be an indicator of how rapidly the disease is progressing. Chelation will open up insulin receptors and can decrease the body's need for extra insulin.

Chelation also improves circulation to the brain. It can prevent the onset of a stroke or aid in alleviating the effects of one.

Tens of thousands of people have been successfully treated with chelation for intermittent claudication, a type of peripheral vascular disease involving poor circulation in the legs that produces pain in the calf muscles upon walking. Dr. Michael Janson reports his experience with peripheral vascular disease: "We have seen dramatic results with people who have vascular disease to the legs where they had sores from diabetes or other causes. Some of them had ulcers that had not healed for up to a year. But these ulcers healed during chelation therapy."

Chelation therapy has also been used in people with Alzheimer's disease, migraine headaches, scleroderma, gangrene, macular degeneration, hypertension, arthritis, impotence, kidney calcification, high cholesterol, and multiple sclerosis. Dr. Edward McDonagh's Kansas City, Missouri, clinic even had success with people who had been poisoned by Agent Orange in Vietnam.

Chelation as a Preventive Therapy

Chelation may help prevent disease simply by removing the toxic substances that interfere with our natural physiological processes. According to Dr. Martin Dayton: "I have been doing chelation therapy for approximately 10 years now, and I have found that people who go in for treatments fare better years later. I think the reason why is that it removes toxic material and therefore helps the body repair itself and function better."

Dr. McDonagh has noted a decreased incidence of cancer in his patients who received chelation therapy: "We have treated approximately 20,000 patients and of those cases we should have seen thousands of cases of cancer develop by this time according to the national statistics. However, we have not seen them. We have probably seen three, four, or five cases total in the [nearly 30] years that I have been doing chelation therapy. I think it boils down to the fact that once you stimulate the immune system back to a normal position, the body can heal itself. The body has tremendous powers of rehabilitation even with advanced cases where people were told their conditions were hopeless."

According to Dr. Trowbridge of Humble, Texas, chelation helps correct the problem at the cellular level: "Calcium builds up around the little energy batteries, called mitochondria, within every cell of our body. What happens is a little change here and a little change there add up to an injury pattern. The work of Peng in 1976 showed that if you take a heart that is injured and you flush it with EDTA, calcium will get out of those energy batteries and they will work better so that your heart is stronger. This is molecular medicine, which will actually change the way people get old and die."

Many chelation practitioners utilize this treatment on themselves. For example, Dr. Corsello, who has been using chelation therapy in her practice for 10 years, says she uses it on herself to prevent the formation of atherosclerotic plaque. "Chelating physicians do practice what they preach, so I utilize this on myself preventatively. My patients see me going around with the bag and pole, and when they wonder where I get all my energy and stamina in spite of the multiple things that we have to do, the answer is in chelation therapy."

Effectiveness of Chelation Therapy

After chelation therapy most people are given functional tests to see how much their arteries have reopened. One of Dr. Sessions' patients had an arteriogram after bypass surgery that showed that he was still occluded in all the arteries. After chelation therapy he was able to pass a treadmill test with flying colors, which means he was getting enough circulation back to the heart muscle to carry on the strenuous activity.

Other patients elect to go back for an arteriogram to see if all the plaque is gone, with differing responses. Some will develop marked collateral circulation around the blockage, which gets the needed blood supply to the heart or other area even though the entire blockage has not disappeared. This is because chelation therapy does not always work like a Roto-Rooter treatment. What it is doing, however, is helping the body to re-establish the proper amount of blood flow to any given area of the body.

Ultrasonography, thermography (the measurement of temperature on the surface of the skin), MRI angiography, and echocardiography are among the other methods that can be used to determine the effectiveness of chelation.

Nutritional Supplementation Following Chelation

Chelation therapy will not be effective if the patient will does not make other positive lifestyle changes. It is important to remember that no one modality is so good that it can function as a cure-all in overcoming a toxic burden. Diet and nutritional supplements can help to correct deficiencies and keep the body as healthy as possible, Exercise and stress management also are necessary.

Dr. Kirk Morgan advises his patients with adequate kidney function to drink a lot of good quality water. He also suggests a diet high in fiber and the avoidance of animal fats."I simply tell [my patients] to think of cereal for breakfast, vegetables for lunch, and beans and lentils at supper," he says. "I ask them to keep the fat down in the diet similar to what Pritikin has said and I ask them not to skip meals, particularly the overweight patients. In addition I suggest exercising. I try to teach them to count grams of fiber and grams of fat, so that they will get some idea of how much fiber and how much fat their various choices have."

In Dr. John Sessions' practice all patients are given an organic multivitamin that is well absorbed and well tolerated. Then a hair analysis is done, and a history and physical findings are taken into account. In this way patients can be treated on an individual basis. Some patients need more zinc, others more selenium. Dr. Sessions also uses fish oil supplements for improving circulation, and antioxidants to reduce free-radical activity.

In the view of Dr. Michael Janson, recent research has revealed that supplementation is essential to anyone undergoing chelation therapy. In his opinion, "Chelation is not the only answer to vascular disease. It's just an important addition to the other therapies that I think are important."

Dr. Janson goes on to emphasize, "We have to recognize that when we pull out metals from the body, we also pull out nutritional elements that are very important for health, like zinc and manganese. So an important part of the approved protocol for chelation is to give certain dietary supplements along with the intravenous treatments, not at the same time, not in the IV, but as a separate oral treatment where people take these supplements to improve and enhance the effectiveness of chelation."

Dr. Janson, who has himself been a recipient of more than 65 chelation treatments, recommends that the following supplements be taken in conjunction with chelation therapy: zinc, vitamin B_6 or pyridoxine (if there isn't enough vitamin B_6, repeated chelation treatment can cause a skin rash), and manganese. Dr. Janson also recommends at least 4,000 milligrams a day of vitamin C; 800 to 1,200 units a day of vitamin E, 100 to 250 milligrams a day of coenzyme Q10, and 1,000 milligrams twice a day of taurine.

According to Dr. Janson, the B vitamins have been shown to lower the level of a substance in the bloodstream called homocysteine. High levels of homocysteine have been associated with increased blockage in the arteries. The B vitamins that are important for dealing with this problem include B_6 or pyridoxine, folic acid, and B_{12}.

Checks and Balances: Making Sure Chelation is Properly Employed

Many doctors as well as a lot of clinics are administering chelation therapy. Unfortunately, some of these individuals have no background in cardiology and are not board-certified in this area. The American Board of Chelation Therapy is one organization that certifies physicians who have attended the training in chelation therapy offered by the American College for Advancement in Medicine (ACAM).

According to Dr. Martin Dayton, chelation is a serious treatment that is not to be used by someone who has not been properly trained. Chelation should always be employed in conjunction with kidney analyses, calcium magnesium studies, a mineral balance analysis, and a general physical examination. Administration of the technique by someone who is not board-certified and does not have proper training in chelation therapy is highly irresponsible. Dr. Dayton states, "It's alarming what's going on. We have doctors that are setting up chelation clinics similar to fast food restaurants.

He continues, "It is very important to know that chelation is simply a tool that should be used in a larger scheme of things, a larger health strategy, to balance the person, to get rid of the toxic material that prevents normal function and repair, to add those things that are necessary, so we can obtain optimal health."

Patient Stories

I was going through a period in life where a lot of my friends, who are in the over 50 age group, were experiencing heart attacks, angina, and associated symptoms. That prompted me to think about my own condition, so as a precautionary move I took a thallium stress test. To my surprise, they found a blocked major coronary artery. The hospital recommended at that time that I do an angioplasty. First they do a catheterization angioplasty and they open up the artery. I felt that was an invasive procedure. I discussed this with Dr. Corsello, who suggested I try chelation for a year or so. She said I could always have the angioplasty done later because it was not yet at a serious stage and I was in good condition from running. I agreed. In fact, I had wanted to take chelation therapy for another reason: as a dentist I had been exposed to a lot of heavy metals over the years.

I went through a year's chelation therapy. During that year I had a tremendous increase in my energy level. I had younger looking skin, and I felt younger, and everybody said I looked great. A year later I went back for another thallium stress test and to the doctor's surprise the blockage was no longer there. I have had two successive thallium stress tests since then with the same results. I have maintained a schedule of having chelation therapy once or twice a month since that time and my heavy metal level has decreased almost 80 percent. I feel great.

Some of my patients have used chelation and the results are equally positive. It alleviates tiredness and it restores the immune system. I have even seen people suffering from Lyme disease have equally good results. Other people who were intoxicated with heavy metals have all had very favorable experiences. We had one person with Epstein-Barr who was walking around with a cane for years because nobody was able to ascertain what he had or give him a definitive treatment. He calls me up every month to thank me.—Dr. Bush

I had a blockage in the bend of my leg. My leg circulation was so bad that I could hardly walk. After running an arteriogram on me the doctor said I should take an aspirin a day. Then I went to Dr. Sessions and I have had no trouble since. I have had 95 chelation sessions and I can walk now. My legs don't hurt me like they did and I can do almost anything I want to. I believe that Dr. Sessions' chelation therapy kept me from having my leg amputated. Also, I was right on the verge of a stroke when I went to him and he straightened that out. I am over 81 years old.—Claude

33

Anemia

Anemia is a health condition characterized by red blood cells deficient in hemoglobin, the iron-containing portion of the blood. Hemoglobin enables the blood to transport oxygen from the lungs and circulate it throughout the body and to carry away carbon dioxide. The listlessness, pallor, and shortness of breath in an anemic patient reflect a lack of oxygen and buildup of carbon dioxide in the tissues.

Causes

Dr. Dahlia Abraham, a complementary physician from New York City, describes three major classifications of anemia, each of which is associated with a specific cause:

EXCESSIVE BLOOD LOSS. This can result from conditions such as hemorrhoids and a slowly bleeding peptic ulcer, or in association with menstruation.

EXCESSIVE RED BLOOD CELL DESTRUCTION. Dr. Abraham explains, "Normally, old and abnormal red blood cells are removed from the circulation. If the rate of destruction exceeds that of manufacture of new cells, anemia can result. A number of factors can cause excessive red blood cell destruction, such as defective hemoglobin synthesis, injury, and trauma within the arteries."

NUTRITIONAL DEFICIENCIES OF IRON, VITAMIN B12, AND FOLIC ACID. This is the most common type of anemia, with iron deficiency the most frequent.

Dr. Abraham further explains, "People require extra iron during growth spurts in infancy and adolescence. Pregnancy and lactation are other times when women need iron supplementation. During the childbearing years, many women experience anemia caused by an iron deficiency."

Do supplements help? "Supplementation may not solve the problem because many people have difficulty absorbing iron," Dr. Abraham says. "They lack enough hydrochloric acid, the stomach acid that helps the body assimilate iron. This is common among the elderly, who generally produce less hydrochloric acid." Chronic diarrhea also may cause of decreased iron absorption.

A defect is absorption is the most common cause of a vitamin B_{12} deficiency. Dr. Abraham remarks, "Vitamin B_{12} must be liberated from food by hydrochloric acid and bound to a substance called intrinsic factor, which is also secreted in the stomach. For B_{12} to be absorbed, then, an individual must secrete enough hydrochloric acid and enough intrinsic factor." For this type of anemia supplements of vitamin B_{12}, hydrochloric acid, and intrinsic factor may help.

A deficiency in folic acid may also cause anemia. Alcoholics and pregnant women are particularly at risk. "Folic acid is vital for cell production in the growing fetus and prevents birth defects, such as neural tube imperfections," Dr. Abraham says. "This is why prenatal vitamins must contain this nutrient. In addition, a number of pharmaceutical drugs, such as anticancer drugs and oral contraceptives, can drain the body of folic acid."

Dr. Pat Gorman, an acupuncturist and educator in New York City, explains anemia and other blood disorders in women from an Asian perspective: "In women, blood has an actual cycle that rises and falls every month. There is a building phase that occurs for about a week after the menstrual period. Then there is a peak phase where the blood reaches its richest moment; that's the moment you ovulate. This is followed by a storage phase. (If you are pregnant, the blood is stored.) A week before the period, you go through a cleansing phase where your organs release toxins into the blood. That's the week before your period, when you can go through a PMS hell if the toxins are not being properly released. Next is the purging of the actual period."

Using this philosophy as her framework, Dr. Gorman holds that women become anemic when they are out of touch with their monthly cycles. In a fast-paced society, one of the major reasons for this condition is that women do not rest at the appropriate times: "Women work all the time. They show no vulnerability and just keep on going no matter what. There is no respect for the actual rhythm of the cycle. I believe that we need to bring back the menstrual hut. When you are bleeding, you need to stop working for a day or two. I know I am saying things that sound impossible, but if you have anemia—and 60 to 70 percent of the women I see do—you need to face the fact and work with it."

She adds that another major reason women become anemic is that they approach pregnancy incorrectly: "There is a law called the one-month, one-year law. After a pregnancy is terminated, whether by abortion, miscarriage, or birth, one month of absolute rest is needed. Women say, 'That's not possible. I just gave birth, but I have other children. I have to take care of things.' The Chinese say this is a straight road to a severe anemic problem.

"The one-year aspect is the avoidance of pregnancy for at least another year. Women who try to conceive and who then miscarry often frantically begin again. They need to build up the blood for an entire year's cycle before trying to conceive again. It is very difficult for me to help anxious patients relax and understand that this is the way to overcome anemia and to have a really healthy baby."

Additionally, Dr. Gorman warns that birth control pills are unhealthy because they disturb the integrity of the blood's cycle. They trick the body into believing that it is continuously pregnant by locking blood into its storage phase. By eliminating the cycle of building, peaking, storing, cleansing, and purging, oral contraceptives create many problems.

Symptoms

The general symptoms of anemia are weakness and a tendency to tire easily. When there is a vitamin B_{12} deficiency, the symptoms may also include paleness; shortness of breath; a sore, red, swollen tongue; diarrhea; heart palpitations; and nervous disturbances.

Diagnosis

According to Dr. Abraham, the treatment of anemia is dependent on proper clinical evaluation by a physician. Too often, physicians assume that anemia is caused by an iron deficiency, but this is just one possible reason. "It is absolutely imperative that a comprehensive laboratory analysis of the blood be performed. Do not be satisfied when your physician offers a simple diagnosis of anemia," she warns. "Insist that your doctor investigate the underlying causes."

While Dr. Gorman agrees that clinical studies help confirm the diagnosis, she adds that Asian physicians are trained to detect anemia and other blood disorders through observation: "In Chinese medicine, you examine the body. Look at your tongue. Is it pale? Look at your lips. Are they pale? See if the mucous membranes under the eyes are pale. These signs indicate whether you are anemic."

Dietary Remedies

Green, leafy vegetables are high in iron and folic acid. It is best to purchase organic vegetables, since pesticides interfere with absorption. Eating vegetables raw or lightly cooked preserves their folic acid content. Soy or shoyu sauce, miso, and tempeh are rich sources of vitamin B_{12}.

Proteins should be eaten every day, preferably vegetarian proteins such as those from grains and legumes such as rice and beans or oatmeal with soy milk. When animal protein is eaten, it should be from fish. Caffeine and alcohol are detrimental to healthy blood and should be eliminated.

Supplements

According to Dr. Abraham, iron, vitamin B_{12}, and folic acid should be prescribed as needed. Additionally, hydrochloric acid and intrinsic factor are often required to aid the absorption of these nutrients.

Naturopath Dr. Tori Hudson, in a column in *Prevention* magazine, advises that iron citrate and iron aspartate are forms of iron supplementation that are less likely to cause constipation. She suggests taking 1,000 to 3,000 milligrams of vitamin C with the iron to enhance absorption.

Herbs

Dr. Janet Zand, a naturopathic physician, acupuncturist, and doctor of Oriental medicine in Los Angeles, in an article posted on the HealthWorld Online website (www.healthy.net), suggests an herbal program that anemic women can use to build the blood. It is meant to accompany iron and iron-synergistic nutrient supplementation as directed by a health care practitioner. Dr. Zand bases her herbal regimes for women on the shifting hormonal balance over the 4 weeks of the menstrual cycle.

During all 4 weeks of the cycle, red raspberry leaf and *dong quai* are used to build blood and balance hormones. These herbs can be taken as a tea, tincture, capsule, or tablet three times a day. Then, during the specified weeks, one also takes the herbs specified below:

FIRST WEEK. Take yellow dock leaf (*Rumex crispus*) and chlorophyll as a tea or tincture three times a day.

SECOND WEEK. Take American ginseng (*Panax quinquefolius* root), a blood builder, as a tea or tincture three times a day.

THIRD WEEK. Take nettle (*Urtica dioica* leaf) and chlorophyll as a tea or tincture three times a day.

FOURTH WEEK. Take alfalfa (*Medicago sativa* leaf), with chlorophyll as a tea or tincture three times a day.

Ayurveda

According to Swami Sada Shiva Tirtha, founder of the Ayurveda Holistic Center in Bayville, New York, in an article on the center's website (ayurvedahc.com), practitioners of Ayurvedic medicine consider anemia an imbalance of the blood that can have a number of causes. Too many sour, salty, or hot foods; drinking alcohol; poor nutrition; injury; excessive menstruation or bleeding; liver disorders; pregnancy; excessive sexual activity; and fevers are all factors that can cause a disorder in the kidneys, blood, and *ojas* (life force) and lead to anemia.

Swami Sada Shiva recommends certain foods that help build blood. These foods include organic milk, pomegranate or black grape juice, boiled black sesame seeds, molasses, and Sucanat (whole cane sugar). Otherwise, people should follow the diet that is appropriate for their body type, according to Ayurvedic guidelines. Ayurveda uses meat as a medication only when anemia is extremely severe.

Women should use blood-building herbs after the menstrual period. To properly assimilate iron supplements, take them with ginger or cinnamon. You can take two or three teaspoonfuls of *chyavan prash* twice daily with warm milk as well as turmeric and ghee.

Aloe vera gel and triphala are very gentle laxatives that regulate the bowels and thus can help remove excess bile from the liver, a common reason for thinning of the blood. Other Ayurvedic herbs used to treat anemia are saffron, *shatavari, manjishtha,* and *punarnava.*

Patient Story

I was born in Nicaragua, and I used to be a very healthy person. But in June 1993 I went to the emergency room. My hemoglobin was down to 2.8; the normal count for a woman is between 12 and 14. There I was with aplastic anemia, meaning that my bone marrow was not making any blood cells: no red cells, no white cells, no platelets. I almost had no blood.

The doctor said that my sickness was idiopathic, meaning that they didn't know what caused it. They said that one possible cause was the use of an antibiotic. But the only time I had ever taken one was 15 years earlier. Another possible cause was exposure to chemicals or pesticides. A lot of towns in Nicaragua are surrounded by cotton plantations where cotton growers use a lot of pesticides to spray their crops.

In July 1993 I was referred to a bone marrow transplant unit and was put on a medication, a kind of chemotherapy. After 1 month of treatment, the medication failed to work. Then the doctors wanted to do a bone marrow transplant. I have seven siblings, and so I had donors, and one of them was a perfect match. But I had reservations. A bone marrow transplant is very costly. Also, you get bone marrow that is working, but because of the chemotherapy or radiation, your liver, kidneys, pancreas, and so forth, pay a terrible toll.

Before my sickness I was following a macrobiotic diet. I was starting to use Oriental and alternative medicine, and I knew about the power of the body to heal itself. I decided to stay on my macrobiotic diet and was able to more or less clean myself of the chemotherapy. During this time I did not even get a cold. I didn't sneeze through all my sickness.

I was clean, but my blood counts were still very low. I needed a transfusion every 10 days. The transfusions were very helpful, and I was grateful to be able to get them. But through transfusions I was also receiving a lot of genetic and other information completely foreign to my body. I could not control what the person who donated that blood was eating. So I was trying to clean my body of toxins, and I decided to look for help.

I went to a naturopath who helped me a lot. Then I read an article on Ayurveda. It said that Ayurveda is very specific, even with the use of grains and vegetables. There are grains and vegetables that are not appropriate for your body type. In early February 1994 I went to an Ayurvedic doctor. He gave me a very gentle treatment consisting of diet, aromatherapy, massage, and meditation. After 3 weeks of following that treatment, my blood count went up for the first time.

I keep up with this treatment still. My last checkup at the hospital showed normal white cells. Red cells were a little bit low. They were 3.83, and the normal count is 4. But they are increasing day by day. My energy level is excellent. I went back to work 3 months ago and am now leading a completely normal life. I am very grateful to Ayurveda.—Yolanda

PART SEVEN

Allergy, Asthma, and Environmental Illness

Technological advances in our society have been accompanied by unprecedented challenges to our bodies and our health, and have caused an overload on our immune systems that can produce a condition called environmental illness. In the1970s and 1980s environmental medicine specialists—allergists who view a person's whole environment as having the potential to create an immune system response—realized that allergies contribute to illnesses and diseases that traditionally had been left out of discussions of allergic responses. Migraine headaches, depression, and arthritis are just a few of the conditions that were found to be allergy-related. While clinical data have supported this work, many traditional allergists and immunologists believe that there is insufficient theoretical explanation of these phenomena to accept them as scientifically valid.

Dr. Stephen M. Silverman of Port Washington, New York, says that thousands of substances in our food, water, and surroundings are responsible for environmental illness: "The first thing you must realize is that what you eat can have a tremendous effect on your immune system.... Along with what you eat, you must consider what you drink. Most people are being exposed to tap water, whether directly from the sink or outside when they buy a cup of coffee or tea. Probably one of the highest exposures to carcinogens comes from this source.

"Among the other factors that can set you up for illness are the things you put on your body. I am talking about cosmetics, moisturizers, and hair sprays. We know through medical applications of the nicotine and estrogen patches that what you put on your skin will be absorbed into the bloodstream. If you were to take a look at the ingredients in your cosmetics, hair sprays, and underarm deodorants, you would see that they are loaded with chemicals. You have to realize that when you use these chemicals every day, they eventually get into the bloodstream. When you think about it, is it possible that these chemicals have no effect on your immune system? It's almost impossible.

"In addition, there are environmental factors. One of the most important rooms to be safe in is the bedroom. If you happen to have a carpet that is outgassing, by which I mean releasing chemicals at a very low level, and some of those chemicals are suspected carcinogens, despite how well you may be eating, you are going to get sick from that carpet. When we sleep at night, we are supposed to detoxify. Your body attempts to purify itself at night of any additives or toxins in foods that you may have eaten. If you have a toxic bedroom where the carpet, the paint on the wall, or a mattress loaded with formaldehyde is releasing gas, and if you're reacting to these chemicals, then 8 hours a night, instead of restoring your immune system, you may be causing it severe damage."

According to environmental medicine specialist Dr. Marshall Mandell, "There is absolutely no question that environmental factors play a major role in many diseases; where they do not actually start the disease, they can complicate it. Anything that makes your illness worse is important for you to know about."

Conventional physicians and traditional allergists simply recognize only a very limited range of symptoms. If their patients aren't sneezing or itching, they will not recognize the possibility that an allergy may be present. But logically, once a doctor recognizes that minute flecks of animal dander or pollen in the air can produce marked symptoms, is it so difficult to see that chemical toxins in meat or milk or air pollution, among a host of other possible causes, might also have an adverse effect? Simply put, the human race has evolved over millions of years and has adapted to most of the conditions on this planet. But many of the pollutants and toxins we are dealing with have arisen over the last 30 to 50 years. Our bodies just haven't had time to evolve in response to these changes in our environment. Unless we act sensibly by at least recognizing this discrepancy, we may cause great damage to ourselves and our environment.

34

Environmental Illness

Environmental illness was first recognized three decades ago, but mainstream medicine still generally disregards this syndrome. When patients come in with the symptoms of sensitivity to a toxic environment, doctors often do not know the correct protocol. Standardized blood tests appear normal, leading doctors to assume that no problem exists.

Another problem is that most doctors today are not trained to work with a disease that affects the whole body. Heather Millar, author of *The Toxic Labyrinth* and former sufferer of environmental illness, notes, "In the medical community we have created a world of specialists. Physicians are now neurologists, cardiologists, rheumatologists, and so on. We have gotten away from the old-fashioned approach. We no longer have general practitioners. Before, you would go to a doctor's office and tell him your history from start to finish. He would look at you as a whole individual, checking the psychological as well as the physical aspect of the body. Only then would he make an assessment.

"Now technology has compartmentalized the body. The neurologist looks only at the symptoms of numbness, tingling, and headaches. The rheumatologist looks only at arthritis, joint pain, and aches. The infectious disease doctor looks only for infection. What happened to me was, I would go in and give a detailed history of what was happening. The doctor, according to his specialty, would look only at one specific area. He or she did not want to hear about the other symptoms I had.

"What we are failing to realize with all this supertechnology in medicine is that the body works in harmony. You do not have one body system that works separately from something else. They all work together. So if you are having symptoms in one system, you are probably having symptoms elsewhere."

Diagnosis

In her book, Heather Millar has a checklist to help people determine whether they may be suffering from environmental illness. These are some questions she asks people to consider:

> *Do I have a toxic lifestyle?*
> *Does my environment contain chemicals that could be making me sick?*
> *Do I feel ill at work?*
> *Do I feel ill at home?*
> *Do I live in a new home?*
> *Have I recently painted or installed a new carpet?*
> *How much plastic do I have in the home?*
> *Does my neighborhood contain chemicals that could be making me sick?*

"Discovering the cause of the problem is a detective process," Millar says. "It involves taking a close look at your home, workplace, and neighborhood.

"Start with your home. You may ask, 'Why didn't we have these problems before? We always painted our house and put new carpet in.' What I'd like to suggest is that technology has changed a lot of chemicals and manufacturing processes. Since the 1980s we have added more synthetics and are now seeing their effects. A lot of these products emit gas. The newness smell is a gas that is coming off. Basically, it's a chemical soup that is very hazardous to our health. Also, since we live in energy-efficient buildings, we do not have the ventilation needed to lessen the concentration or these gases.

"Plastics present further problems. They have a lot of these estrogen-mimicking properties. Softer plastics have more toxicity. We used to live with metal, wood, and glass. These are far safer alternatives. When replacing plastic with wood, consider the type of finish on it. Does it smell?

"Then look at the workplace. Ask yourself, what are you doing as an occupation? Are you working with chemicals on an ongoing basis? Or are you working in an energy-efficient office building that was recently renovated? Is it currently being renovated? Does it have no open windows? Do other people in the office frequently get colds and flu or feel unwell?

"Finally, examine your neighborhood. Where do you live? Do you have chemical manufacturing in your backyard? Is there some kind of toxic incinerator nearby? What is in your water supply? What kinds of pesticide regulations does your neighborhood have?

"You may react differently to toxins in your environment than your coworkers do. For example, in my workplace, which was extremely toxic, my symptoms were mainly neurological. Other colleagues were diagnosed with chronic fatigue. Still others experienced asthma or fibromyalgia, which is an aching of the muscles. We react differently depending on our genetic predispositions."

Fortunately, there are physicians who do recognize the illness, and there are tests available to pinpoint the condition. Occupational health doctors and environmental physicians prescribe tests that look at solvent levels in the blood. They look at pesticide levels in the blood and check mineral levels, which are usually low in people who suffer from chemical exposures.

Four Clues to Proper Treatment

Dr. Michael Schachter, a clinical ecologist, or environmental medicine specialist, identifies four contributing factors which he considers key in his examination and in determining a course of therapy: the quality of nutrition generally and the identification of any nutritional deficiencies, infections, psychological stresses, and toxicity. According to Dr. Schachter, the course of therapy should be determined by the condition of the patient in regard to these four criteria.

Dr. Schachter is also concerned with improving the oxygenation and energy utilization of the body at the cellular level. Anything we can do to improve that process is going to strengthen the immune system and thereby help reduce a person's tendency toward sensitivity and reactions. Thus, Dr. Schachter encourages the use of oxidant therapies, but only up to a point, since oxygen in too great quantities can have a damaging effect. The key here, as in virtually every area of health, is balance.

The first and foremost oxidant therapy must be aerobic exercise. Keeping in mind that oxygen is the main nutrient of the body, it is easy to understand that as we improve oxygenation, we improve the body's ability to detoxify and enhance the immune system. Beyond exercise, a number of new nutrients are available to enhance oxygenation, such as germanium and ubiquinone, as well as a variety of traditional oxygenation techniques.

Vitamins and minerals are another key component in Dr. Schachter's approach. He sees vitamin A as a major protective factor that guards against both chemical sensitivities and infections. Thus, cod liver oil, which parents once gave automatically to children, is indeed an excellent preventive medicine with its high concentrations of vitamins A and D. In treating children with recurrent ear infections, Dr. Schachter has found that by simply enhancing their diet, removing most of the sugar and refined foods, and adding a spoonful of cod liver oil, the ear infections can be controlled and prevented in many cases. Other useful vitamins include vitamin C, vitamin B_{12}, and vitamin E, which is an antioxidant. Selenium and beta carotene are also important antioxidants. Vitamin B_{12} can help counteract the adverse effects in the body of pesticides in the environment. Moreover, while conventional physicians may test for vitamin B_{12} levels in the bloodstream, normal levels may be present in the blood while there are deficiencies at the cellular level.

According to Dr. Schachter, infections are a key factor in going from troubled to good health. Frequently, infections will yield to nontoxic treatments.

Take *Candida*, for example. Patients who have repeatedly used antibiotics, include a lot of refined carbohydrates in their diet, and may have been exposed to steroids or birth control pills tend to develop a chronic overgrowth of *Candida*, a yeastlike, funguslike organism which we all have in our bodies. In certain cases the infection will give off toxins which may impair the immune system and produce a variety of symptoms. Some of these symptoms will be the result of food and chemical sensitivities that have been aggravated by the infection.

Dr. Schachter has found that starting the patient on a special diet that excludes refined carbohydrates, especially sugars and alcohol, and includes various nutrients, especially certain fatty acids that inhibit *Candida* growth, will go a long way toward controlling the infection in many cases. He also notes that garlic has strong anticandidal properties.

Chronic viral syndromes are another key problem. A previously healthy individual suddenly gets a flu and instead of recovering completely experiences frequent fatigue, exhaustion, swollen glands, sore throat, night sweats, anxiety, and loss of appetite. However, conventional testing shows nothing definite. More sophisticated testing may show exposure to various viruses, but the main problem here may be that the person's immune system just isn't responding as it should. Dr. Schachter has obtained excellent results in patients with this profile by using nutrients to bolster the immune system. Intravenous vitamin C may be used, along with germanium and a variety of other vitamins and minerals given orally. In cases of herpes virus, for example, he may use high doses of the amino acid lysine, which has antiviral effects for the herpes virus and certain other viruses. For short treatment periods, he may administer as much as 10 to 15 grams of lysine per day.

Psychological stress is another key factor, according to Dr. Schachter. Environmental medicine specialists, he warns, must be careful that in emphasizing the importance of the physical environment they do not underestimate the importance of psychological factors in determining the strength of an individual's immune system.

As for toxicity, Dr. Schachter feels that hydrocarbons and other chemicals are already playing a major role by damaging our immune systems, as are heavy metals. He sees chelation therapy as a valid treatment to detoxify our systems of the effects of heavy metals. Chelation therapy has also shown impressive results in patients with cardiovascular disease.

Detoxifying the Body

Without detoxifying the system, all other steps to repair the body will be to no avail.

Dr. Zane Gard, an expert in toxicology, explains some methods of detoxification that have had impressive results in the reversal of environmental illness:

"Heat stress detoxification includes wood saunas, hot sand packing, steam baths, and sweat lodges. The history of these approaches goes back several thousand years. Careful supervision is required. Heat stress detoxification can be effective but requires knowledge of toxins and their potential effects on the body. If it is not administered properly, there can be a lot of complications, and the patient can actually end up worse.

"The biotoxic reduction program was designed with the toxic-chemical-syndrome patient in mind. It is a comprehensive, medically managed program that addresses toxicology, psychology, neurology, pathology, and immunology. The program must be followed 7 days a week, 3 to hours a day, for a minimum of 2 weeks. It would be nice to have off on Saturday and Sunday, but patients actually regress 1 or 2 days every time they take a day off during the first 2 weeks. So it has to be every day during that initial period.

"The program consists of increasing niacin, aerobic exercise, sauna therapy, and other therapies as necessary. With those who have neurological damage, other therapies will be needed, including a therapy that stimulates the myelin sheaths of the nerves to regenerate. As a result, many peripheral neuropathies completely reverse. In over 80 peripheral neuropathies, including multiple sclerosis (MS), we have only two patients who did not fully recover.

"In a study of patients in our program, the average blood toxin levels after 21 days of therapy are as follows: toluene drops from 19.3 to an average of 0.34, ethyl benzine drops from 14.7 to 0.1, xylene drops from 72.9 to 0.94, 1:1-trichloroethylene goes from 7.7 to 0.92, and DDE goes from 5.7 to 1.8. We know that DDT, which is the parent compound of DDE, will be 97 percent removed within 4 months. You continue to detoxify for a good 4 months."

Detoxifying the Environment

It is no longer enough to watch what we eat or the medicines we take; environmental toxins have become an unavoidable reality, especially for those living in densely populated urban areas. The very air that we breathe on the streets or in our homes and offices can attack our health; noise pollution and artificial lighting add to the physical and mental stress of urban life.

The myth is that you should look for the big toxin. But it's the chronic, day-in, day-out exposure to small toxins that are really the concern. It may take decades—none of these environmental toxins, even asbestos, will knock you out right away—but you may pay for your lack of awareness with lung cancer, leukemia, arthritis, or heart disease down the line. Perhaps worst are the subtle symptoms of fatigue, anxiety, and minor nagging physical problems that many of us come to accept as a normal part of life.

Elimination of the unseen substances that attack your system stealthily, over time, is half of achieving good health. If you never use any supplementary vitamin, mineral, or herb but simply eliminate those factors that depreciate your health, you should be able to live to 100 years of age in a healthy way. One group of people, nearly 70,000 in number, in the north of Pakistan at the base of the Himalayas, often live well past 90 or even 100, putting in full days of work daily until they die. It may not be possible for all of us to live in the pure atmosphere of the Himalayas—not to mention emulating the diet, activities, and social structure of these people—but we can alter our environment realistically and functionally. A good place to start is where we live.

Dr. Alfred Zann, a fellow of the American College of Allergists and the American College of Physicians, has written a book, *Why Your House May Endanger Your Health*, which explores the relationship between our homes and our well-being more thoroughly than we can here; much of the following discussion is indebted to information he shared on my radio show as well as to Dr. Richard Podell.

The Sick Building Syndrome

The "sick house" is a relatively new development. Materials and methods used to construct houses have changed considerably since World War II; an extreme example is the energy-efficient office buildings built during the energy crisis of the 1970s, about which we'll have more to say later in this chapter. But not only are houses built with more emphasis on energy efficiency—which means heavy insulation and minimum ventilation to the outside—the construction materials themselves, as well as the furnishings—carpeting, fabrics, furniture—are new, often more convenient, cheaper, lighter synthetic compounds unheard of in prewar houses. The particleboard that is so useful in modern house and furniture construction exacts a price for this convenience; it is a silent time bomb, giving off invisible, odorless—but no less dangerous—vapors years after it is installed.

Formaldehyde is a major culprit in the modern house or office building. Particleboard, new synthetic carpets, insulation, many interior paints, and even permanent-press fabrics can give off formaldehyde. It is invisible and odorless except in high concentrations, but even quite low chronic levels can cause symptoms ranging from burning eyes and headaches to asthma and depression. New houses may be built largely of materials that vaporize formaldehyde for years; the worst culprits are mobile homes, which also are often poorly ventilated.

Another important factor in a house's potential toxicity is its source of heat. Combustion-heating appliances using natural gas, oil, coal, kerosene, or wood can all create afterburn byproducts even if you can't see or smell them. Good ventilation can help but makes it harder to keep a house warm. Electrical heat, though expensive, is the safest source.

What can be done about a toxic house? Some changes can be made in the furnishings, floor coverings, and ventilation and heating systems, but often much of the problem lies in structural components which would be expensive and difficult, if not impossible, to alter. Building your own house or having it built with attention to all the materials used is one solution if you can afford it or have the time and skill. If you are looking for a place to live, consider an older home. Prewar houses were often constructed of bricks, plaster, and hardwood, not the chemically treated plywood, composite board, and other synthetic materials used almost universally now. If synthetic materials were used in an older house, they will have had years to emit their toxins. Often a house built before the energy crisis will allow more air circulation. Ceilings are often higher, allowing fumes to rise away from the inhabitants.

There may be disadvantages in an old house, however; molds and mildews may have accumulated over the years. Old carpet is a fertile ground for mold as well as accumulated dust, animal hair, and whatever toxins have been tracked in or sprayed over the years, but it can often be pulled up to reveal a hardwood floor. Outdated heating systems can usually be replaced without too much trouble.

If moving or rebuilding your house is not an option, you can still do a lot to detoxify your home. We'll identify the weak spots room by room.

THE GARAGE An attached garage is like a toxic waste dump stuck to the side of your house. Many garages have heating and cooling systems that lead directly into the house; anything that can be absorbed through any crack or ventilation system will end up in the house. What's in the garage? The car, of course, and gasoline. Gasoline vaporizes. The afterburn fumes caused by inefficient burning of gasoline are mostly carbon dioxide, which has no odor and is invisible. Breathing these fumes results in headache, dizziness, and mood swings. (Think of people stuck in traffic jams, breathing the afterburn of all the cars around them for hours at a time.) When you park a hot car in the garage and close the door behind it, the hot oil in the engine is volatile and gets into the air. Park the car outside and wait for it to cool off before you bring it into the garage.

Other things you may keep in the garage—paint thinners and removers and turpentine—also vaporize easily and stay in the air for months at a time. If you smell a rag that was used for paint thinner 3 months ago, you will see that it is still giving off these fumes. Try to minimize the number of these substances in your garage. If you must keep them, use a small shed or garbage can outside the garage to store them. And the garage should be ventilated out, not into the house, with a suction fan. There should be no ducts from the garage into the house.

Your garage is probably where you keep chemicals you use on your lawn and garden: pesticides, fungicides, or herbicides, for instance. In the first place, do you really need them? Look at it this way. If it's going to kill an insect, a plant, or a mouse, it's a toxin and it can affect you, your pets, and your children. If you spray a weed killer on your lawn and then walk around on the lawn, you will repeatedly be bringing it inside on your feet. It doesn't just go away. Think of all the things you bring in on your feet and think, for instance, of your kids playing on the carpet, perhaps putting things into their mouths that have been on it.

Taken individually, none of these things is going to kill you, but be aware that everything you spray outside is likely to be in the air you breathe or will make its way back into your house and settle there. There's no real need to run this risk: We can use diatomaceous earth and natural biological controls or just weed without spraying.

THE BASEMENT A typical basement in a private home is often damp. People like their lawns unencumbered by debris that might wash down from the gutters of the roof through the downspout, and so the downspout is kept close to the house. Thus the water runs off the roof, down the downspout, and into the ground directly by the foundation of the house. You might just as well run this water directly into the basement, since its walls are rarely waterproof. A little dampness in the basement is enough to support a healthy growth of mold, which can then permeate the house. A forced-air system of ventilation, which has ducts running to the basement, will create a vacuumlike effect that will suck particles of mold into the system, to be dispersed around the house.

Many people react to mold whether it is eaten or inhaled, a point that is obvious to anyone who begins to sneeze as soon as she or he walks into a damp basement. More insidiously, though, mold that is inhaled even in small quantities cross-reacts with mold that is ingested in food. This effect, known as concomitancy, means that a small quantity of inhaled mold that in itself would hardly cause a noticeable reaction will enhance sensitivity to foods that contain mold.

Any food made by fermentation can induce this reaction. Wine and vinegar are fermented fruit juice, cheese is fermented milk, yeast in bread ferments, and even mushrooms are in the mold family. Thus, it is easy to ingest mold three times a day, exacerbating our inability to tolerate the mold which has circulated upward from a damp basement. Obvious symptoms are sneezing and watering eyes, but allergic symptoms can also be systemic, making them harder to pin down to a specific source. Fatigue, headaches, depression, and even arthritis can have a basis in chronic allergic irritation.

In addition to water coming into the basement from the downspout, groundwater can roll down a hill toward the house, which then serves as a dam. You can raise the earth around the house to divert its flow away from the house. If a high water table is the problem, a sump pump is needed. Thoroseal, a dense cementlike material, can be applied to the outside block foundation as caulking to keep water out.

If the basement is still damp, a dehumidifier can help, but these work well only above a temperature of 50 to 60 degrees Fahrenheit. Chemicals such as baking soda are only temporary measures. The best way to remove the mold is to scrub the area with sulfur water. The basement can be hosed down and the water removed with an industrial vacuum.

THE KITCHEN What's the most dangerous toxin in most kitchens? Gas. You should always have a vent in the kitchen; it has been shown that cerebral allergies are often directly attributable to the gas burnoff of pilot lights on stoves, which leak constantly. If you often have headaches and suspect that they are more common when you're spending time in the kitchen, try disconnecting your stove when you're not using it. If this makes a difference, you should consider replacing the gas stove with an electric one. Not only gas ovens are a health risk, though. Microwave ovens can leak; a defective microwave creates a very unhealthy environment within about 8 feet around it.

The freon in the condenser of the refrigerator is a highly volatile, dangerous chemical. It is a very good idea to replace refrigerators that are more than 10 years old.

The refrigerator contributes to another seldom considered form of pollution found especially in the kitchen: noise pollution. You should be able to tolerate background noise of about 30 to 35 decibels. Noise higher than 50 decibels becomes uncomfortable. Above 80 decibels, you become substantially irritated, and noise above 100 may cause ear damage or central nervous system overstimulation. The compressor in most refrigerators is up to 60 decibels. You don't appreciate this until you turn on a refrigerator when everything else is totally quiet. But think of a kitchen with a television or a radio on, things cooking, telephone conversations—you can't even hear the refrigerator, and the noise level may be up around 100 decibels. The kitchen is one of the most stressful places because of this level of background noise. Even if you are unable to replace appliances such as refrigerators and air conditioners with less noisy ones, you can cut down on the number of noisemakers you are using at the same time.

Street noise can be irritating in any room. Noise-buffering double-fold drapes can keep noise down as well as insulate.

Mold and mildew are common invisible toxins in a kitchen. When was the last time you changed the water tray in your refrigerator? Under the condenser coil is a tray to collect water, but it can also collect all kinds of mold. Mold spores are in the air all the time, and you're inhaling them. If you're sensitive and your immune system is low, you'll feel it: Your eyes will get puffy, your nose will clog, and your throat will get sore. Keeping this area clean and dry could make a big difference.

Look under your kitchen sink; you'll be amazed at the range of toxic chemicals you keep there, so close to your food. Cleansers, for instance, especially ammonia-based products, often vaporize easily. Ammonia is very toxic and will stay in your blood for hours after you've smelled it. When you wax the kitchen floor, the floor wax will evaporate and you will breathe it in. Try to install floors that will not need waxing, but if you don't want to tear up your current floors, you might want to settle for a matte finish rather than a high sheen if you have to constantly apply volatile chemicals to get that sheen. As with the weed killers and insecticides in your garage, there are alternatives to chemical cleaners in the kitchen. Apple cider vinegar and hydrogen peroxide mixed half and half in cold water do the same job as ammonia. This preparation will clean windows and glassware perfectly, too.

Roach sprays are very stable. They can last for months and vaporize constantly. A dog or cat licking the floor can pick them up directly. A safer alternative is to use boric acid. You can mix it with sugar as a bait, but be sure pets and children can't reach it; line all the counters and fittings underneath with a strip of this no thicker than a pencil. This mixture is not volatile and is safe as long as it's put only in inaccessible places. Diatomaceous earth is safe and works well too. Or use the roach motels that use resin instead of poisons.

Aluminum-based cookware in which the aluminum can come into contact with food should not be used. Aluminum has been implicated in Alzheimer's disease. It is a heavy metal that lodges in the blood, brain tissue, and central nervous system, where it can cause motor problems. Aluminum foil is all right to store cooked food but should not be used in cooking, where it can oxidize in microscopic amounts. You can't see this, but it can get into your food and your body. Teflon and all other nonstick coatings should also be avoided. They easily scratch or flake off with age, getting into food as well as exposing it to the often inferior metal underneath.

Water from the kitchen tap may contain over a thousand chemicals, including those which the government puts in, such as fluoride; traces of herbicides and pesticides that have leached down into the water supply from fields; and traces of metal, rust, and molds from the inside of your pipes. Most water filtration systems can remove only a portion of these; the finer particles, including toxic chemicals such as pesticides, come through. If you live in a polluted area and your water supply is from underground streams, buy bottled water. I would buy plain distilled water. You get minerals from food; you don't need them from water. Since 72 to 74 percent of our bodies consists of water, we should be sure it is the purest water possible.

THE BATHROOM One of the most common causes of allergy is what we put on our bodies: soaps, deodorants, and cosmetics. We use these things day in and day out, rarely thinking about their effect on us. For example, women who wear lipstick every day and lick their lips are absorbing chemicals never meant to be eaten. Perfumes vaporize and get breathed in. Read the ingredients of your antiperspirant; most likely it contains an aluminum-based compound that can be absorbed through the skin and carries the risks of aluminum outlined above. You can minimize these sources of toxins by using natural soaps and shampoos made out of vegetable ingredients, a nonfluoride toothpaste such as Dr. Bronner's or Tom's, and mouthwash you can make yourself with a little ascorbic acid in water. (See chapter 68 for a full discussion of holistic dentistry).

It's important to air out the bathroom after a shower or bath and let it dry out. A window fan to evacuate the moist air is a good idea. Bathrooms are too often closed up most of the time and can be like little chambers that trap the perfume, deodorant, and cleaning fluid fumes in a small space. Odor disguisers such as pine- or lemon-scented aerosol sprays are worse than useless; the odor is a molecule floating around in the air that can be removed only by letting the air escape. Products that claim to take away odors only cover them up with a chemical that probably smells worse and is certainly worse for you.

The "disinfectant" cleaners so popular for bathroom tiles and tubs are virtually useless. To disinfect something, you have to boil it for 20 minutes, but within 1 minute it will be covered with germs again. Those germs are not going to kill anyone despite the fear tactics used to market these cleaners. Their heavy aromatic odors are often more of a problem than the germs; pine, for example, is a resinous material that is quite troublesome to allergic or sensitive people.

Never store medications in the medicine chest; it's hot and humid in the bathroom, and this can cause them to go bad. Store medicine and vitamins in the refrigerator.

As in the kitchen, look around the bathroom and think about potential toxins: cleaners for the tiles and sink, toilet fresheners, and so on. Do you need all those things? Can you substitute natural, nontoxic products?

THE BEDROOM We spend a third of our lives in the bedroom; if you live 72 years, that means 24 years in bed. An ecologically ideal, safe place to spend all this time should be as free of dust as possible. Many bedrooms have wall-to-wall carpeting, which is an ecological disaster. Carpeting is toxic in several ways. Whereas new synthetic-fiber carpeting contains chemicals, such as formaldehyde, which will vaporize for a year or more, old carpets collect dirt, yeast, fungus, and mold. Dust mites live in rugs. Through an electron microscope these mites look like tiny dinosaurs; their diet is chiefly composed of the shed human skin cells which are another large component of dust. House dust mites can be wafted into the air by currents and breathed into the lungs. People who are allergic to them react as they do to cat or dog dander. Like dander, they can get into your eyes and make them red and puffy.

Think about ripping up your old carpet and putting in nice hardwood floors. They're easy to maintain and nontoxic. The Japanese have never had polyvinyl fluoride or no-wax floors; they use natural resins on wood, and some of these floors are 500 years old. If you feel you must have carpets, buy wool or natural fiber rugs with natural dyes. Stay away from synthetic carpets. And learn to vacuum efficiently. Most people just zip the vacuum over the carpet; by the time the dust has had a chance to get up through the nap into the air, the vacuum has moved on and has only raised the dust. You've actually increased the pollution in the air. Run the vacuum very slowly over the carpet, giving the dust you raise time to get into the vacuum.

You may be sleeping on foam-filled synthetic pillows and using synthetic-fiber pillowcases and sheets. Replace them with down-filled pillows and comforters and pure cotton sheets. Be aware of what you're putting in your sheets when you wash them; bleaches and fabric softeners are potential irritants. Many manufacturers of bedding use chemicals to which many people are allergic to fireproof the material. The way to test for this is to sleep on bedding that is not treated to be fireproof and see if your symptoms disappear. Again, if you feel better when you are sleeping away from your house on vacation, it should alert you to the fact that something in the bedroom is causing trouble.

Sleeping on clean sheets that are changed frequently reduces possible reactions to dust and dust mites. When you wash bedding, it's best to avoid perfumed detergents, antistatics, and softeners and look for biodegradable brands. Bleach should be oxygen bleach, not chlorine, which leaves an irritating residue. Miracle White, made by Beatrice Food Company, works well. If you suspect that a pillowcase, for example, is bothering you, wash it with a simple unscented detergent, rinse it three or four times, and try it again to see if the problem goes away.

Even your closets can affect your health. Mothballs emit a dangerous gas. Try a mixture of rosemary, mint, thyme, ginseng, and cloves that has the additional advantage of smelling good.

AIR QUALITY If you ever see the sun slant into a room at a certain angle, you know how much dust and smoke are in what you thought was clear air. It's there all the time. An air purifier with a negative ionizer is the best way to eliminate airborne toxins: spores, dust, cigarette smoke, hydrocarbons and pollutants from the street, cat hairs, and positive ions. The ionizer bombards the room with negative ions that attach themselves to the positive ions of pollutants, which then drop to the ground and can be filtered out by the filtration system.

Humidifiers are fine for improving air quality as long as you use distilled water in them. Otherwise mineral deposits from the water will end up all over your carpet, floor, and furniture.

PLANTS One efficient and natural air-quality *improver* is living greenery in your house. The more plants in your environment, the better. A large number and variety of houseplants will increase the oxygen level in the air. Green, nonflowering varieties are best, since they will not give off pollen. Plants are also a great natural air pollution filtration system. They help maintain humidity levels and a proper electricity balance in the air. They also create a living energy field that we can share and be invigorated and calmed by.

LIGHT Your visual environment is more important than you might realize. If you feel tired, ill, or depressed inside in the winter, especially if you live at a high latitude where the days are very short, and if you spend most of your day indoors, you may be suffering from seasonal affective disorder. In this condition the hypothalamus of the brain is deprived of full-spectrum natural sunlight—most artificial lights use only a part of the spectrum. The best solution is to allow plenty of natural light into your house; use double-glazing rather than small windows or heavy drapes if insulation is a concern. Try to spend time outdoors or arrange your activities so that you're near a window.

If getting more daylight is beyond your control—the days are short, your house is dark, and you must stay indoors—the situation can be improved with full-spectrum light bulbs. Full-spectrum incandescent lighting works on a completely different principle from that of fluorescent lighting (discussed in the section on the workplace below) and is more natural for the eyes. These bulbs are available in health stores in all sizes; using them in your office as well as in your home can make a big difference in your energy level and mental state.

HEAT In cold areas we shut down for the winter, closing and sealing the windows to avoid ventilation from the outside. These practices contribute to the toxic state of the air inside.

Oil heaters often burn inefficiently and release unburned oil fumes into the house. An afterburn catalyst that is available on the market now can recycle these fumes, creating a clean air burn. Electric stoves are not a problem. Gas or oil space heaters are one of the worst offenders. Dry radiated heat can dry up your nose and skin. Wood-burning stoves may seem rustic and natural but can be one of the worst sources of indoor pollution.

In forced-air combustion heating systems that use gas or oil, a little pinhole not infrequently develops between the heat exchanger, which is next to the combustion chamber, and the air going past it to be heated. As the air that you're going to breathe goes around that heated chamber, it sucks in the partially combusted gases. You may not even perceive this in the air, because it's at a very low level, but over a 6-month period this air can produce severe illness. Therefore, you must have your forced-air system checked out electronically for these pinholes every year. The smell test is not satisfactory. If you don't do this, you're at risk.

THE WORKPLACE The energy crisis of the 1970s led to a generation of very well insulated but poorly ventilated office buildings. People who work in these buildings often complain of fatigue, nasal congestion, dizziness, and a host of other mysterious symptoms, yet there has been clear-cut documentation of toxic levels of pollutants in very few cases. The levels of toxins in these buildings are rarely high enough to provoke official alarm, but they are high enough to cause fatigue and illness through long-term, chronic exposure. Even low levels of organic chemicals, pesticides, formaldehyde, carpet cleaners, and tobacco smoke can affect those exposed to them for a long enough period.

The individual pollutants can be located and reduced, but the single most important factor is ventilation. Monday is the worst day for headaches and stress, at least partly because the ventilation systems have often been shut down over the weekend; you're breathing old, stale air. The ducts of your office air venting system probably haven't been cleaned in years. Dust and molds have built up inside them and are coming out into the air you breathe when the system is restarted. Ask the maintenance people to clean them; if they won't, get a heavy-duty charcoal filter and put it in the vent with a thick white insulation pad over it. These filters can be bought inexpensively at any hardware store. In 1 week the insulation pad will be covered with black particles large enough to see.

If it's noisy where you work, wear earplugs. You can also make your desk more pleasant with a small portable ionizer. The ionizer can actually fit in your pocket and is also useful in airplanes or on the dashboard of your car.

The fluorescent lighting often used in offices flashes on and off rapidly and constantly, placing great stress on your central nervous system. Although you are not consciously aware of this very rapid flickering, your eye and nervous system are overstimulated by it; 2 or 3 hours of work under fluorescent light can have the effect of three or four cups of coffee. At a certain level of overstimulation the central nervous system will shut down, and you will find yourself deeply fatigued. Replace the fluorescent lighting at your desk with a lamp that uses incandescent bulbs and use the natural full-spectrum lightbulbs described earlier. It's best to have an office with a window or skylight for true natural lighting; if you don't have one and can't arrange it, it's especially important to have natural—and sufficiently bright—lighting.

Stay away from the photocopier at the office as much as possible; it uses volatile chemicals. Don't leave typewriter ink or correction ribbons lying around open; put them in a sealed plastic bag when they are not in use. An exhaust fan on the ceiling will help draw away vaporizing fluids.

Patient Story

I started becoming ill a year before I realized what was happening. At first I just thought I was tired. I was having trouble getting out of bed. I was dragging myself to work. I would come home feeling exhausted. Sometimes I had asthmalike symptoms and couldn't quite catch my breath. I wondered why this started all of a sudden when I was 30 years old, because my understanding was that most people develop asthma as children. I attributed these symptoms to working and living a fast-paced lifestyle, and I ignored them. One day my wrist started to ache for no apparent reason, which made me wonder if I was getting arthritis. But I ignored that as well and thought it would go away. I had these warning signs for a year before collapsing at work in September 1993.

I had woken up feeling as if I had the flu but thought I was well enough to go to work. I had gone shopping with my mom that morning and had had difficulty walking up stairs. When I arrived at work, I realized that I was feeling quite unwell and that I would be able to work only part of my nursing shift. At the end of the first hour, I needed to go home because I was too ill to walk down the corridor and deliver medications to my patients. It was then that I returned to the nursing station and collapsed. I could hear, but I couldn't move. I felt as if I were paralyzed. I couldn't communicate with the other nurses who came to attend to me.

They took me to the emergency room, but I started to feel better and went home. I decided that I had the flu and that I would be better in 3 days.

Three days of flu evolved into a year and a half. During this time, I experienced many difficulties. The problem with environmental illness or chemical sensitivity is that you have a wide array of symptoms that come and go. You don't really know where to start and what connections to make. These are some of the symptoms I experienced.

Flu symptoms plagued me every day and became worse with time. As time passed, I was having more difficulty getting out of bed and walking around the house. I was extremely tired. No matter how much I slept, I just could not seem to get enough sleep. Even small tasks that shouldn't take much energy overwhelmed me. Cooking a meal was too much to even think about.

I also started having disturbed sleep. Despite my fatigue, I would wake up between 2:00 and 4:00 each night with numb hands. Sometimes I would have an incredible thirst. And sometimes I would wake up shaking as if I had a very high fever.

At one point I lost sight in my right eye. This happened for a short time but was extremely frightening nonetheless. All of a sudden, the vision in my right eye became completely silver, as if I were trying to look through a piece of tinfoil.

I had headaches with stabbing pains in my temples and a burning sensation in the back of my neck that made it difficult to turn my head. If you try to drive a car or move to do something, you realize how important it is to have range of motion in your neck.

The next month, I started to experience food allergies. It started with a few things. First I wasn't tolerating wheat very well and stopped eating it. Then I noticed that I did not feel well after drinking coffee and milk, so I eliminated them also. As the months progressed, I was unable to tolerate more and more foods. By January, I was virtually down to two foods: lamb and yams. By February, I lost my tolerance for everything. I was caught in a vicious cycle. I knew I needed to get nutrition in order to turn my health around, but eating these foods would make me even sicker.

As I became increasingly ill, my sense of smell became more and more acute. All of a sudden perfumes were a problem. I absolutely hated going to the department store and passing the perfume counter. I couldn't stand the smell of car exhaust either. I even avoided the hardware store because of the strong smell in there. Going to public places became difficult, as many people wear scented products such as clothes washed in scented laundry detergents, perfumes, and aftershaves. I would walk into a room, and if someone had perfume on, I would suddenly feel like I had the worst flu. My shoulders and muscles would start to ache. I would feel short of breath. I would get a headache.

A heightened sense of smell is part of the illness. People who are not affected need to understand what is happening when individuals with environmental illness ask, "Please do not wear that fragrance because it makes me feel sick."

I also started to have ringing in my ears. That would come and go, so I never could associate it with any particular event. Sometimes it would affect one ear, sometimes both. It was bothersome trying to have a conversation with somebody and trying to hear that person over the ringing in my ears.

Additionally, I felt dizzy. I had days when it was even difficult for me to stand up and navigate my way to the bathroom. Several times I fell over.

One of the most disturbing symptoms that I had was difficulty concentrating. I could no longer read something from start to finish. It would take me three to four tries to read material I should have comprehended in the first reading.

I also noticed that I was forgetful. Previously I had had an exceptional memory. All of a sudden I noticed that I couldn't remember things that were extremely important. At age 30 I was wondering if I was getting the beginning stages of Alzheimer's disease, the loss of memory was so apparent. Some days my memory was better than others, and some days my ability to concentrate was better than others.

Then there were the panic attacks. My heart would race while I was driving my car on the interstate. I did not understand why I felt better on residential streets. Later, I realized that I had difficulty on the interstate because the exhaust was so much more prevalent there. Every time I was exposed to exhaust, my heart raced; I felt anxious and had difficulty concentrating.

I also felt extremely anxious in shopping malls. I have since learned that there are extremely high levels of chemicals in shopping malls, such as formaldehyde, emitted by new building materials. These synthetics are highly toxic. What I couldn't understand was why I felt anxious at some times and not others. The reason was that some shopping malls are less toxic than others, and some stores, because of the types of merchandise they carry, are also better than others.

The day I collapsed at work was the last day I worked as a nurse. I kept assuming that within a month I would feel better and go back to my job. One month rolled into two, two months into three, and three months into a year and a half.

Being a nurse, I felt that I would receive the support I needed. After all, I was a medical person myself. What I experienced instead was how a patient feels when he or she is told that nothing is wrong. I had always been on the other side of things. I found this new perspective extremely alarming.

The medical community has become technologically based. Everything relies on a diagnostic test. I would go in, and they would run a gamut of tests. As with most people with environmental illness, the standard tests would come back negative. The doctors would then tell me that there was nothing wrong. This was disturbing because I was extremely ill. I was so sick that I could hardly get up off the couch. Nor could I make myself a meal. Going to the bathroom was an effort. How, on a diagnostic test, could I look perfectly normal?

When the doctors could not diagnose me, they said that I was suffering from stress. But this was not the case. Before I got sick, my life was wonderful. I had one of the least pressured jobs I had ever had, and I was enjoying what I was doing. At the end of a contract I would go on vacation to Europe for a month. I was about to get married. My life couldn't have been better.

Stress is becoming the catchall diagnosis in the medical community. We must ask why so many people in our society are being told that they have stress, panic disorder, anxiety, and depression. That category is growing larger and larger. People have to ask, Why is this happening in our society? Is something chemical bringing this on? Do we need to make changes in the environment?

If you are feeling some symptoms of toxicity, it is time to take action now. Don't wait until you end up, as I did, in a wheelchair, bedridden, and completely intolerant to food.—Heather Millar

35

Food Allergies

I t is a classic case of over-reaction. Your body incorrectly senses that the food that has just been eaten is a foreign substance to be repelled. Cells begin to exhibit diseaselike symptoms as they react and over-react to the food.

Allergists conservatively estimate that up to 15 percent of the population suffers from a minimum of one allergy, frequently one that is serious enough to warrant medical attention.

Symptoms can range from a mild tension headache or irritability to criminal actions and full-blown psychotic behavior. Most common are fatigue, headache, insomnia, rapid mood swings, confusion, depression, anxiety, hyperactivity, heart palpitations, muscle aches and joint pains, bed wetting, rhinitis (nasal inflammation), urticaria (hives), shortness of breath, diarrhea, and constipation. Reactions can be immediate following exposure to the allergen or delayed for many hours after contact.

Allergic symptoms are so diverse that the reactions can occur in virtually any organ of the body. Reactions in the brain or central nervous system may lead to behavioral changes and to paranoia or depression. A response in the gastrointestinal tract may translate into bloating, diarrhea, or constipation. Different food combinations can cause multiple reactions in the same person. If a person has an allergy to wheat that manifests itself in the brain, while their gastrointestinal tract is sensitive to milk, they may experience both fatigue and irritable bowel syndrome from a breakfast of whole-wheat toast and milk.

All forms of a potentially offensive food can cause an allergic reaction, not just the whole form. Corn sugars and syrup, including dextrose and glucose, for example, will cause symptoms in many corn-sensitive patients. In many instances, researchers find, corn sugars will cause a more immediate reaction than will corn starch or corn as a vegetable.

Environmental medicine experts, also known as clinical ecologists, say that one reason people are developing sensitivities to certain foods is their widespread occurrence in our diets in both the natural and processed forms. Just because you only rarely treat yourself to corn on the cob, for example, doesn't mean you're not eating corn every day. On a typical day you might eat corn flakes, a corn muffin, and processed food products containing both corn starch and corn syrup. Also, many of the daily vitamin C supplements are derived from corn.

Types of Food Allergies

The foods we eat most frequently are also the most common causes of allergies. These include milk, wheat, corn, eggs, beef, citrus fruits, potatoes, tomatoes, and coffee. Food allergies can fall into several categories:

FIXED FOOD ALLERGY: Each time you consume a specific food, you react. For example, whenever you eat beef, a reaction occurs.

CYCLIC FOOD ALLERGY: This is the most prevalent type of allergy. It occurs when you've had an abundance of a particular food. If exposure to the food can be reduced to no more than once every 4 days, little or no reaction occurs. The food, in other words, can be infrequently tolerated in small amounts. So, in a cyclic allergy, a person can remain symptom-free as long as he or she eats the offending food infrequently.

Of course, other factors can influence the degree of this sensitivity. Infection, emotional stress, fatigue, and overeating can increase susceptibility. The condition of the food (raw or cooked, fresh or packaged) may also be an important factor. Pollution, the presence of other environmental allergens, or marked environmental temperature change can also help trigger or subdue a reaction. A food eaten by itself may be tolerated. But if it is combined with other foods at the same meal, an allergic response may develop. The length and severity of the symptoms will depend in part on how long the allergens remain in your body after ingestion.

ADDICTIVE ALLERGIC REACTION: Here the person craves the foods to which he or she is allergic. In essence, the person becomes addicted to the foods. When made to go without the food, depression and other withdrawal-like effects may appear. Moreover, eating the food may momentarily alleviate the symptoms, only to aggravate them later. Over time, the symptoms of the addictive allergy may grow increasingly complex.

This type of allergy often remains hidden or masked—even to the individual who is suffering from the problem. Because of its insidious nature, the person never suspects that the foods that seem to alleviate the symptoms might contain substances to which he or she is allergic.

But allergies do not always fit neatly into one of the three categories. A fixed allergy in infancy can develop into an addictive allergic reaction later in life. Milk is a good example of such a food. When first introduced to a baby, it may cause an acute reaction in the form of hives or spitting up. However, if the parents don't recognize this as an allergic reaction and continue to keep milk in the diet, the symptoms may take on a more generalized and less obvious form.

What is first experienced by the body as an acute reaction will—in the body's attempt to adapt by assimilating the new foreign substance—lead to more chronic symptoms such as arthritis, fatigue, depression, or headaches. For example, if you drink milk or eat milk products every day, symptoms of allergic reactions may blur with your natural personality traits and may become an accepted, even unnoticed part of your everyday life.

Eventually, you may develop a chronic condition, like arthritis, migraines, or depression. Your daily dose of milk would never be suspect at this stage. Your body has upped its tolerance levels in trying to adapt. At the same time, milk's harmful effects have been subtly registered. You keep on with a daily dose of milk, your own substance for abuse, to keep withdrawal symptoms at bay. Acute reactions are gone—except when the milk is withdrawn completely. Chronic reactions have replaced them.

Hidden or masked food allergies, no different from allergies generally, tend to be to the very foods we eat most frequently. In the United States, dairy products, including milk and eggs, are high on the list. Corn, wheat, and potatoes are also common allergens, as is beef. Yeast, which occurs in many foods, is often a cause. Finally, many people have a hidden allergy to coffee.

Why Food Allergies Occur

IMPAIRED DIGESTION Most food allergies can be traced to an impaired digestive system. Proper digestion requires that the body secretes sufficient hydrochloric acid and pancreatic enzymes into the stomach to process foods. These substances break down large protein molecules into small molecules so they can be absorbed and utilized. When too few digestive juices or enzymes are secreted, the large protein molecules go directly into the bloodstream. The immune system reacts to these large molecules as if they were foreign invaders—the allergic response.

ENVIRONMENTAL AND EMOTIONAL STRESSES In addition, other stresses can affect a person's "allergic threshold." These include environmental stresses such as air, water, and food pollution; inhalants such as perfume, aerosol hair spray, or room freshener; and emotional stress. The less healthful the physical and mental environment, the less likely are our chances for achieving and maintaining a state of well-being.

Environmental pollution poses a particular problem. Over the past two centuries the barrage of chemicals introduced into our environment has disrupted the balance of our ecosystem. Residues of many toxic chemicals such as pesticides, herbicides, and insecticides are ingested into our bodies along with food additives and preservatives that are added during commercial food processing.

In many cases, the contamination of food is an irreversible result. Foods such as oranges, sweet potatoes, and butter can be dyed. Other processed and packaged goods like Jello, ice cream, sherbet, cookies, candy, and soda can contain large amounts of food additives.

Most of our commercially raised meats and poultry are riddled with residues of antibiotics, tranquilizers, and hormones. It is even common practice to dip certain fish in an antibiotic solution to retard their spoilage. A person allergic to these antibiotics and drugs may be unknowingly ingesting them continuously, provoking either long-term or short-term reactions or illnesses, the source of which might remain unidentified. It is estimated that more than 10 percent of all Americans are sensitive to food additives. But remember, even when a person eats only organically grown foods, they may still be food allergic.

In most cases, the more severe a person's food sensitivity becomes, the more numerous the allergens that induce it. One clinical study reported that the average person suffering from hay fever was allergic to five foods as well. A total picture of a person's allergen exposure, environment, habits, and history are vital for effective treatment.

The end result of repeated or prolonged sensitization of the body by recurrent allergic reactions is termed "breakdown"—the point at which diseaselike symptoms appear. They may be erroneously diagnosed as the onset of an illness. But the biochemical breakdown, although it manifests itself suddenly, was actually initiated years before by prolonged exposure to allergens.

GENETIC MAKEUP You can inherit allergic sensitivities. If both parents suffer from allergies, their children have at least a 75 percent chance of inheriting a predisposition to this hypersensitivity. When one parent is allergic, the chances of an inherited allergy remain as high as 50 percent. The child does not have to inherit the same allergic response. What is inherited is a genetic makeup that is more likely to have allergic reactions in general. For example, the mother may have chronic indigestion while the child's allergy manifests itself as acne. A mother may be sensitive to corn while her child is sensitive to yeast. Infants can develop allergies to the same foods as their mothers while still in the womb, through the placenta, or through breast milk after birth.

The Mechanisms of Food Allergy

Conventional allergists believe that the mechanism of food allergy is triggered by direct contact of the food antigens—the substances the body produces to fight the "foreign food invader"—with immune system antibodies in the gastrointestinal tract. The usually swift reaction that results is called an immune system-mediated response. This is the only kind of allergic reaction that conventional allergists recognize.

But there is a second mechanism recognized by clinical ecologists, through the absorption of the allergen from the gastrointestinal tract into the bloodstream. Circulating in the blood, allergens can react with elements other than antibodies. The resulting reaction can occur in the blood, in the nervous system, or the musculoskeletal system. Sometimes referred to as a sensitivity or intolerance, to distinguish it from a classic allergic reaction, this second mechanism can be extremely complex. However, tests to uncover these more subtle intolerances are available.

Hypersensitivity to foods can come at any time of life and continue to any age, although the onset occurs most commonly in infancy and early childhood. This is largely because the gastrointestinal systems of the very young are less efficient than in the adult. One researcher refers to the progression of allergies from childhood to adulthood as the "allergic march." Symptoms can move from one organ system to another. A child may suffer from asthma as a result of drinking milk. During teen years the allergy may take the form of pimples. Unfortunately, many people erroneously believe that they have outgrown their allergy because they no longer suffer from the original symptom. They don't consider that their current problems may have the same underlying cause. Their allergic symptoms may continue to vary throughout their lives because of an underlying imbalance that remains constant. Hyperactivity as a child may be the result of ingested food additives. In later years, these same ingredients may cause migraines and fatigue.

The Link Between Food Allergies and Chronic Disease

If food and chemical sensitivities were routinely considered in each case of chronic disease, there would be a tremendous increase in well-being in this country.

An overly analytical medical system insists instead on classifying patients into narrowly defined disease states. Environmental aspects, including a patient's diet, are considered to be nonmedical. The person's whole experience—including diet, environment, lifestyle, emotional life, and work life—may also be considered to be outside the physician's domain, although few physicians would deny that the cause of almost any patient's illness will involve one or more of these factors to some degree.

FOOD ALLERGIES AND MENTAL HEALTH It may be that up to 70 percent of symptoms diagnosed as psychosomatic are probably due to some undiagnosed reaction to foods, chemicals, or inhalants. Different allergic reactions occur. There are localized physical effects like gastrointestinal disorders, eczema, asthma, and rhinitis (nasal inflammation). There are acute systemic effects like fatigue, migraine headaches, neuralgia (nerve pain), muscle aches, joint pains, and other generalized symptoms. And there are acute mental effects such as depression, rapid mood swings, hallucinations, delusions, and other behavioral abnormalities. It has been estimated that over 90 percent of schizophrenics have food and chemical intolerances.

Researchers now believe that food allergies may directly affect the body's nervous system by causing a noninflammatory swelling of the brain, which can trigger aggression. Despite studies at various correctional centers showing clearly the connection between diet and behavior, little is being done to change the dietary standards of correctional facilities throughout the nation. Routine screening programs for food allergies and nutritional deficiencies in chronic offenders do not exist.

While many other factors—not food alone—mitigate criminal, antisocial behavior, or mental illness, a case can be made for testing for and evaluating food sensitivities in any overall treatment, prevention, or rehabilitation program.

FOOD ALLERGIES AND MIGRAINE HEADACHES Migraines are an example of a condition in which recognition and elimination of food allergens can make a tremendous difference. The trick is to recognize the possibilities.Right now, about 25 million people who consult their physicians each year complain about bad headaches. Although there are various types of headaches, about 50 percent of these people suffer from migraines. While conventional medicine has very little to offer the migraine sufferer, clinical ecologists see migraine as a disorder frequently resulting from food allergies. The nontraditional medicine offered by the clinical ecologist may offer a unique opportunity to relieve the suffering.

Headaches due to food or chemical sensitivities often can be treated simply by eliminating the allergy, once it has been identified, with an elimination or rotation diet. Yet, as a rule, food sensitivities are not investigated in the diagnosis and treatment of headaches.While the pain may sometimes appear immediately after eating a particular food, it may also be delayed until hours afterward. For this reason it is not unusual for a person to fail to identify the correlation between what they're eating and the onset of their headache. A food may even seem to relieve migraine symptoms temporarily—a classic example of an addictive allergic reaction.

Of course, allergic headaches typically occur as the result of combinations of factors, rather than from food allergies alone. Emotional stress, for example, may play a large role in triggering an episode. Thus, even when a food allergy is at cause, the specific food source may not produce the same symptoms on every occasion, depending on the array of associated circumstantial factors. In some individuals stress may be compounded when the allergic reaction triggers further emotional symptoms. A vicious cycle is created. Sudden changes in temperature or light may also affect one's susceptibility, as well as the presence of any other health problems.

Environmental medicine specialists have found that some of the foods that occur most frequently in the typical American diet are also the foods most commonly implicated in food allergy-related headaches. The list includes wheat, eggs, milk, chocolate, corn, pork, cinnamon, legumes (beans, peas, peanuts, and soybeans), and fish. Moreover, individuals with food allergies should avoid or limit their intake of fermented products like red wine, champagne, and aged cheese because of the presence in these foods of a substance called tyramine. Tyramine has been associated with migraine occurrence in some cases.

Too often, conventional medical practitioners tend not to look toward nutritional solutions in cases involving allergies, including allergy-related migraines. In part, this is because the medical training they have received does not extend deeply into nutrition. And yet, a preponderance of evidence continues to point to the importance of nutritional solutions for an increasingly wide range of health problems. (For more information on migraines, see chapter 46).

FOOD ALLERGIES AND FATIGUE Probably no allergic disorder is more puzzling and pervasive than "tension fatigue syndrome." Indeed, for many of us, varying daily levels of tension and fatigue are the norm; tranquillity and energy, the rare exceptions. To compensate, we choose artificial solutions for moderating energy, from the first caffeinated gulps of coffee in the morning to the quick sugar, caffeine, or drug fix during the day, and the alcoholic "equalizer" in the evening. The result is that energy levels are either depressed or falsely elevated most of the time. In many cases, these quick pick-me-ups are responses to allergic disorders with their roots in food and nutrition.

Next to headaches, tension fatigue syndrome is the most common manifestation of cerebral and nervous system allergy. Yet, too often, this far reaching malady is not even recognized by physicians or allergists. Its symptoms are usually assigned a psychiatric origin and treated with drug therapy or some other conventional modality when, in fact, a simple elimination and rotation diet is the best medicine.

There are several reasons for this all too common oversight. First, there are similarities between tension fatigue syndrome and psychiatric disorders. And second, there is the failure of standard scratch tests to identify many food and chemical reactions. The scratch tests simply have not been shown to be effective in the diagnosis of food and chemical sensitivities. And yet they continue to be used by allergists.

Of course, tension, extreme nervousness, irritability, depression, and emotional instability may be symptoms of psychological disorders in some cases. But too often this is the only possibility that is considered. The allergy may be due to any number of foods, and it is only through careful testing that a definitive diagnosis can be made. In all cases where such symptoms appear, food allergies should be ruled out first—before further traditional medical sleuthing occurs. This can save a lot of trouble and mistaken diagnoses.

SYMPTOMS

The symptoms experienced in tension fatigue syndrome can include fatigue, weakness, lack of energy and ambition, drowsiness, mental sluggishness, inability to concentrate, bodily aches, poor memory, irritability, fever, chills and night sweats, nightmares, restlessness, insomnia, and emotional instability. Mental depression is another common symptom, ranging from mild to severe episodes of despondency and melancholia. Generalized muscle aches and pains, especially in the back of the neck or in the back and thigh muscles may also be present, as well as edema (fluid retention), particularly around the eye, and tachycardia (rapid heart beat). Gastrointestinal symptoms often associated with this syndrome are bloating, abdominal cramps or pain, constipation, diarrhea, and a coated tongue. Chills and perspiration are also frequently experienced in association with fatigue during food testing of symptomatic patients.

The disorder can begin at any age. It can last from several months to several decades. In some adults the extreme fatigue, bodily aches, depression, and mental aberrations that come from this continuing allergic state can be so severe that they interfere with work and domestic life.

As headaches or gastrointestinal upsets caused by allergy increase in frequency, the fatigue is more likely to remain even between episodes. Fatigue soon becomes the allergic individual's major complaint. The allergic origin of the fatigue and weakness commonly remains a mystery.

It's not unusual for allergic individuals to sleep up to 15 or more hours for several successive nights to try to overcome their fatigue. Unfortunately, in most cases, these efforts prove futile. The fatigue experienced in allergic fatigue is quite different from the fatigue that naturally follows physical exertion. It cannot be relieved by normal or even excessive amounts of rest. It can be relieved only by eliminating its cause—the allergen.

DIFFERENTIAL DIAGNOSIS

Before the diagnosis of allergic fatigue can be defined, a complete medical workup should be done to exclude both organic and functional origins. This should include a comprehensive case history, complete physical examination, and diagnostic laboratory blood testing. Other causes for nervous fatigue include chronic infections and metabolic disorders, including diabetes, hypoglycemia, hypothyroidism, neurological disorders, heart disease, anemia, malignancy, and various nutrient deficiencies. Even if another disease is found, allergic fatigue may still be a causal factor. In some cases, fatigue is caused both by an allergic reaction and an underlying chronic disease state.

FOOD ALLERGIES AND OBESITY Many obese men and women believe that they are overweight due to heredity, because they have a thyroid or metabolic problem, or because they simply eat too much. They may blame their lack of self-control or become convinced that they have psychological problems. Some experts believe that roughly two out of three obese individuals suffer from some form of allergy.

Of course, allergy may be only one of several factors affecting an obese person's weight. The presence of a thyroid condition or psychological problems can cause or aggravate a weight problem. Obesity is also related to many diseases including high blood pressure, heart disease, kidney problems, and diabetes. For obese individuals with allergies, the problems of each condition may adversely affect the other. Typically, someone who is obese will have allergic responses more often than a person who is not obese does. The extra weight is a burden on the immune system, and the weaker the immune system, the greater the effects of allergies. People who are obese also may have difficulty breathing.

We store chemicals in the body in fat. Very often, allergies are triggered by a response to chemicals stored in this way. Because the obese person may naturally hold more chemicals in the body, he or she may tend to experience more frequent allergic responses. This also may explain why he or she feels worse, or has strong food cravings, at the beginning of a diet. Chemicals are stored in fat, and as the fat is burned, a large quantity of chemicals is passed into the bloodstream, often causing such cravings.

The mechanism by which an allergy can trigger obesity may be that of the hidden addictive allergy, whereby a person is addicted to the very foods to which he or she is allergic. Often, these are high calorie foods, such as chocolate, cheese, or sugar. So, the person may gain weight because he or she eats these high calorie foods too frequently.Hunger itself can be an allergic response, and compulsive eating and intense cravings for particular foods may also result from hidden allergies. In some cases, compulsive eating of the food one is allergic to may really be an attempt to stave off withdrawal-like symptoms induced by going without the food for too long. Such withdrawal symptoms might include headaches, drowsiness, irritability, or depression.

Allergies can cause weight problems if they interfere with the body's natural ability to regulate itself. As noted by Dr. Arthur Kaslow, physician and author, both humans and animals naturally attempt to maintain their bodies in a state of biochemical equilibrium known as homeostasis. Unless there is a flaw in their regulatory system, human beings will maintain their proper weight by eating the amounts and types of foods their bodies need to function properly. When the body needs food, it will send out a hunger signal. When it needs water, it sends out a thirst signal. If this mechanism breaks down, an individual may feel hungry when he or she does not really need food. It is possible that allergies can temporarily impair the cells responsible for sending out these signals.

FOOD ALLERGIES AND ARTHRITIS

Some clinical ecologists estimate that 80 to 90 percent of all cases of arthritis are either allergy induced or are allergylike reactions to some food the patient has eaten. The arthritis may also be related to an environmental factor to which the patient is sensitive, such as gas inhaled from constant proximity to a gas stove. Examining arthritics for both food and environmental allergies may help reduce current symptoms, prevent recurrences of symptoms, and minimize the damage that eventually results from joint inflammations.

Dr. Marshall Mandell has successfully treated hundreds of arthritis patients by putting them on a 5-day distilled water fast and then allowing their usual foods, one at a time, back into their diet. If a food causes the arthritis symptoms, the symptoms will return when it is reintroduced into the diet and should be permanently eliminated. (For more information on arthritis, see chapter 24.)

Testing for Food Allergies

In some cases, a comprehensive medical history will provide significant clues about a person's allergic profile. A trained clinical ecologist may find the needed information from such a medical history alone.

The skin test performed by the traditional allergist has minimal use in identifying food allergies. In some cases, however, it may be helpful. A similar test takes another approach, putting extracts of food mixed with glycerin under the tongue, instead of into the skin by injection. A technique called applied kinesiology is based on the principle that there is a reflex response between a suspected allergen and the patient's body, in the patient's muscles. In this test, a doctor offers food to the patient and then measures or evaluates the energy or muscle function after the food is ingested. Here many foods can be tested in each session. However, the results may not be highly accurate depending on the nature and experience of both the person administering the test and the person being tested.

Newer tests are being developed. Some, like the cytotoxic test, mix blood samples with food extracts and measure how many white blood cells burst. In allergy smears, samples of different body fluids or secretions are evaluated in the laboratory to look for a specific type of white blood cell. The various immune system cells may also be evaluated. In the Arest program, radioactive atoms are used to determine how antibodies respond to particular antigens.

There are also less technical tests, some of which can even be done at home. A fasting test, which should be done under medical supervision, begins by cleansing the system. Symptoms may subside, remain unchanged, or, if the allergy is an addiction of some sort, worsen by the second or third day of the fast. Then foods are reintroduced one at a time to check for symptoms.

Another test that can be performed at home is the Coca Pulse test. First find your normal pulse range, by taking it every 2 hours. Then take it again at specific, regular intervals after eating the suspected allergen. If your pulse rises more than 10 points, the food eaten last becomes suspect. The pulse is rising as a reaction to increased adrenaline in your system. The adrenaline may be released in reaction to an allergy.

Another home test involves keeping a food diary, and recording everything you eat for a week. Record symptoms and when they occur as well. After the week, look for a relationship between symptoms and food eaten.

Elimination testing is yet another approach. Eliminate the suspected allergen until symptoms clear up over a 12-day period. Reintroduce the food on an empty stomach. Usually, if symptoms are to develop, they will do so within an hour of testing. A variation on that is the elimination of all common allergens—wheat, corn, dairy foods, citrus fruits, food colorings, sugar—and foods you may crave, over the course of a week. Then reintroduce the foods, one per day. If symptoms develop, the food may be an allergen. Don't eat it for 5 more days and then reintroduce it to double-check the result.

A final home test—perhaps among the most effective and sensible of all tests—also doubles as a treatment for food allergies. It is called the rotary diversified diet. Plan a diet in which you eat no individual food more often than once every 4 days. After 5 days, start a food and symptom diary. After reviewing correlations that may crop up through your record keeping, eat any suspected food the next time it comes up in the 4-day rotation alone as one full meal. Note symptoms. Eliminate foods that stimulate adverse symptoms from your diet—permanently. The theory here is that food sensitivities become even more pronounced when a food is eliminated and then reintroduced into the diet. With this diet, your symptoms—and with them the responsible food—are clearly highlighted. This approach is also useful as a maintenance diet, enabling people who are prone to food allergies to prevent the emergence of new allergies, since they never eat any food too frequently. And even then, if a new food allergy does develop, it is spotted and quickly eliminated.

Treating Food Allergies the Natural Way

ELIMINATION AND ROTATION DIETS Elimination and rotation diets as described above can be used to treat food allergies.

NEUTRALIZING DOSE THERAPY Neutralizing dose therapy is a treatment method that is especially useful in cases of multiple food allergies, and when avoidance of chemicals and medicinal inhalants is difficult, as during the pollen season. A neutralizing dose is determined for each allergen, and when it is injected or administered under the tongue, this dilution can bring about relief from the allergic symptoms.

These treatments are administered in a series during which the dose of the allergen is progressively increased, causing a desensitization to this substance. (They work on the same theory as allergy shots or vaccines. The only differences are in the dilution of the substance and the wide variety of the substances that can be tested in this way.) Eventually, the person can tolerate contact or ingestion of the allergen with only a mild reaction or no reaction at all.

With the neutralizing dose treatment, the allergist is first determining the amount of a particular allergen that causes an allergic reaction. The physician can work with many substances that the traditional allergist would be unable to treat, including foods, chemicals, perfumes, and cigarette smoke. The neutralizing dose approach seems to be effective in 8 out of 10 patients.

Like the traditional allergy shot, the neutralizing dose can be administered by injection. However, it can also be given as drops under the tongue. Instead of taking approximately 6 months to find the optimal dose, the physician can usually determine the correct dosage in one or two sessions using this technique. Another advantage of the neutralizing dose is that the patient can be given the drops to take at home. It not only works as a preventive measure, but also can block a reaction that has already started.

BOOSTING THE IMMUNE RESPONSE Strengthening the immune system should improve resistance to current allergies and reduce susceptibility to new ones. There are several ways in which the immune system may be strengthened. Making sure you are getting sufficient amounts of rest is essential, as is regular exercise. Keeping stress levels to a minimum will also help. You must also be receiving the right nutrients in the right amounts.

Many nutrients have been found to enhance the effectiveness of the immune system. These include vitamin C, beta carotene, vitamin E, selenium, and glutathione. These are all antioxidants, which help to eliminate free radicals from the body.

Garlic has been found to be an immune stimulant, having both antifungal and antibacterial qualities. Garlic is most effective when eaten raw. It may be added to food or taken as a supplement in tablet or capsule form.

The essential fatty acids are also important to a proper immune response. Many researchers recognize the importance of omega-3 fatty acids, which are found in such oils as linseed and walnut, and in many fatty fishes, like salmon.

It has been noted that 200 to 500 milligrams of pantothenic acid plus 50 milligrams of B complex vitamins can be useful in people with allergies. Vitamin C, in addition to its antioxidant properties, also has an antihistamine effect, which may benefit those with allergies by reducing the swelling of tissue and cell membranes. One study found that people with asthma who took 1,000 milligrams of vitamin C daily had 25 percent fewer asthmatic attacks than those receiving a placebo. Another study found that asthmatic children benefited from magnesium supplementation.

STRESS MANAGEMENT A number of techniques are available to recondition the body to learn a new, more healthful way to respond to and deal with stress, including that associated with food allergies. These include progressive relaxation, biofeedback, self-hypnosis, visualizations, meditation, yoga, and tai chi. Stress management techniques can improve the digestion of allergy sufferers.

36

Asthma

Approximately 17 million Americans have asthma, including nearly 5 million children under the age of 18. The prevalence of asthma has increased 75 percent since 1980. Direct health care costs for asthma in the United States total more than $9.8 billion every year.

To what can we attribute this growing problem? Dr. Kenneth Bock, a family practitioner who has two holistic health centers in New York and is the author of *Natural Relief for Your Child's Asthma*, shares the thoughts of many when he explains:

"I think it is really because of the increasingly toxic environment in which we live. It is due to the pollution, both indoor and outdoor, the types of foods we are eating, which are nutrient empty and calorie dense, and also the stresses. I think [even] our kids are subject to our fast paced lives."

What is Asthma?

Asthma is a chronic inflammatory disorder of the airways. It interferes with normal breathing by narrowing the passages both within and leading to the lungs. The airways become narrowed as a result of spasm or contraction of muscles that wrap around them, inflammation of the airways' lining, and/or overproduction of mucus.

Asthma episodes can be triggered by a number of factors. Many people develop symptoms after exposure to allergens such as dust mites, mold, and animal dander. Asthma is frequently associated with hay fever. An infection of the nose and throat can spur an attack, as can a sudden change in the weather. For some people, asthma is triggered by aerobic activities such as jogging or cross-country skiing. During these activities, air is breathed in through the mouth. This air is colder and drier when it reaches the lungs than air that is inhaled through the nose.

Asthma can range from mild and intermittent to severe and persistent. Its severity can change over time. Many children with asthma will "grow out of it" as their bodies develop and mature.

Diagnosis

Among the most common symptoms of asthma are coughing, wheezing, shortness of breath or rapid breathing, and chest tightness. A diagnosis of asthma is generally based on a thorough medical history and physical examination. Listening to the lungs with a stethoscope can reveal characteristic sounds. A spirometer may be used to assess the condition of the airway passages by measuring the amount and speed of air that is breathed out. X-rays also may be indicated to rule out other causes for symptoms.

Conventional Treatment

Conventional doctors manage asthma by attempting to identify and eliminate exposure to the substances that may trigger the attack. If a specific allergen has been found, allergy shots may be administered. A variety of medications are used to prevent and control the symptoms of asthma. Long-term control medications include inhaled corticosteroids such as beclomethasone (Beclovent, Vanceril) and fluticasone (Flovent), cromolyn sodium (Intal) and nedocromil (Tilade), long-acting beta agonists such as albuterol, and theophylline. The quick relief medications include epinephrine and inhaled beta agonists. Children too young to use an inhaler receive their treatments in mist form though a nebulizer. Oral steroid therapy is often needed to reduce the airway inflammation associated with more severe attacks. Many of these medications are associated with side effects, but they are necessary and effective nonetheless.

In this chapter, we discuss some therapies that can be used as adjuncts to traditional medical treatment. Remember: Asthma is a potentially life-threatening condition that must be managed professionally by a physician. Always follow the doctor's orders for using asthma medications. You can supplement your program with some of our suggestions.

Nutritional Therapies

Good nutrition is an important key to controlling asthma. Yochebed Batimedt, a holistic nurse and author of *Golden Wings: A Holistic Approach to Managing Asthma*, explains.

"What we need to be doing is eliminating all junk food and eating as much organic raw vegetables, fruits, and whole grains as possible. We need to be drinking fresh fruit and vegetable juices. We need to avoid foods that contain additives and food dyes.

"Water is extremely important in preventing as well as managing asthma attacks," she says. "Water helps to eliminate and loosen mucus and it helps to cleanse the system." Batimedt also says that adding raw onions to salads and a pinch of cayenne to foods can help eliminate mucus.

What about supplements? Dr. Kenneth Bock recommends quercitin, an anti-inflammatory type of flavonoid. Quercitin usually comes in capsules of 300 milligrams. The adult dosage can be anywhere from 900 milligrams to 1,800 or 2,400 milligrams. If used in children the dosage must be adjusted. Dr. Bock also recommends use of grape seed extract in doses of 150 to 300 milligrams per day, and ginkgo biloba, 120 to 240 milligrams per day.

"Another good antioxidant herb, again when you talk about inflammatory conditions you need to have high doses of antioxidants on board, can be green tea extract in a dose of 100, 150 or 300 milligrams per day," Dr. Bock says. "Certainly, if you are going to use decaffeinated green tea extract you would like to make sure that it is also organic."

Dr. Bock has seen good results with licorice root extract in doses of 500 milligrams two to three times a day. This is not recommended for people with high blood pressure. He also recommends echinacea, 350 milligrams three to four times a day. Astragalus is another important herb, taken in doses 500 milligrams three times a day.

Relaxation and Stress Management

The rapid, heavy breathing associated with crying, laughing, shouting, or feeling anxious can trigger an asthma episode in some people. Among the relaxation techniques that may help are the quieting response and deep breathing, both of which emphasize breathing from the diaphragm. Put your hand on your abdomen as you breathe. You'll know you're breathing right if your abdomen— not your chest or shoulders—moves in and out.

For the quieting response, inhale deeply through your nose and hold your breath for 5 seconds. As you slowly exhale, think about relaxing your muscles. Repeat this two or three times. For the deep breathing technique, gently blow out all the air you can. Then count to 8 slowly while breathing in through your nose. Hold your breath for 8 seconds. Slowly breathe out through your mouth, again to the count of 8. For the next few minutes, resume slow, rhythmic breathing. These techniques may be used before, during, and after an asthma attack in conjunction with appropriate medical treatment.

Environmental Control

Eating right, maintaining a healthy lifestyle, and reducing stress is the first line of defense for most adverse medical conditions, and asthma is no exception. Maintaining a clean, unpolluted, dust-free environment is equally important.

Exposure to tobacco smoke must be avoided. Studies have shown that children who live with smokers are at greater risk of developing asthma than other children are. Melody Milam Potter, Ph.D., and Erin E. Milam, co-authors of *Healthy Baby/Toxic World: Practical Ways to Protect Your Baby During Pregnancy and Infancy*, offer a number of other suggestions for indoor environmental control, including:

➤Clean with a high-efficiency vacuum cleaner.

➤Use electrostatic air filters, charcoal filters, or HEPA filters in your heating and air conditioning systems, and clean the ducts regularly.

➤Stretch cheesecloth over the inside of air vents and change the fabric every few weeks.

➤Eliminate carpeting in favor of wood floors or other surfaces that can be easily cleaned. Even the new environmentally safer carpets will collect dust mite excrement, molds, animal dander, and other allergens and asthma triggers.

➤Install an air purifier in the bedroom and a dehumidifier in the basement and other areas that stay damp

➤Use 100 percent cotton fabric bed coverings washed in baking soda or vinegar.

➤Avoid the use of scented or chemical products.

➤If possible, choose electric rather than gas heat.

➤Clean moldy areas with baking soda solution, vinegar, Australian tea tree oil products, or citrus extract products.

➤Use plants to clean the indoor air, provided that the person with asthma doesn't react to them.

Homeopathy

Dr. Richard Cantrell says that the following homeopathic remedies may help during an asthma attack. He recommends giving doses of a remedy every hour for up to three doses, and every 2 hours after that. If there is no improvement after the third dose, move on to another remedy. Consult with your doctor before starting any alternative therapy, and always be watchful for signs of an impending emergency such as severe shortness of breath and sore throat.

SPONGIA. Recommended for dry wheezing with labored, noisy breathing. The wheezing tends increase when lying down or moving about, and subside after consuming warm food or drinks and leaning the head back.

ARSENICUM. Recommended for the person who is "fearful, restless and weak." He may be wheezing and coughing with symptoms of a cold or hay fever. He has chills and may be thirsty.

LOBELIA. Recommended for the person with a dry asthma attack, chest tightening and shortness of breath. Symptoms may be most severe in the middle of the day. Cold air makes the wheezing worse. Walking rapidly may help alleviate breathing problems.

SAMBUCUS. Can be used in children, especially those with late-night exacerbations of symptoms.

PULSATILLA. Recommended for the person with a "mild and tearful disposition" who "feels worse in warm rooms, but has little thirst." The person coughs to eliminate mucus buildup in the chest. Symptoms are worse at night, and after consuming fatty or rich foods.

CHAMOMILLA. Recommended for the person who is angry and irritable after an emotional crisis. These symptoms are relieved by cold air.

37

Allergies in Children

When people think of childhood allergies, they often think of hay fever, asthma, eczema, and hives. But there are many other areas of the body that can be affected by allergies. As Dr. Doris Rapp, a pediatric allergist and specialist in environmental medicine, informs us, "Allergies can cause headaches or stomachaches; they can affect the bladder, causing your child to wet the bed or to have to run to get to the toilet in time. Allergies can cause leg aches, muscle aches, joint aches, sleep problems, behavior problems, and learning problems. Some children will become tense, nervous, and irritable. Others will become withdrawn and unreachable, hiding in corners and pulling away when you go to touch them. Still others will become very hyperactive and aggressive.

"Most allergists—including myself for my first 18 years in practice—would not recognize this host of physical and emotional symptoms as having been caused by allergies. But I now recognize that dust, molds, pollens, foods, and chemicals can affect almost any area of the body and can cause all of the problems mentioned above in some individuals.

"Now it would be going too far to suspect that every time a child has a headache it is an allergic reaction, or that every time an adult has a bellyache it is due to food sensitivity. But currently, with conventional medical practitioners, this diagnosis is never even considered and is therefore missed too many times. People will have headaches for years and never once consider whether there might some underlying reason for the headache.

"Environmental medicine wants patients to start to take more control of their health. We want you to pay attention to how you feel. If you don't feel well, or you suddenly can't think correctly; if you're confused, or unusually irritable, or emotionally volatile; if you cry or become upset or angry for no reason; you have to start to ask, 'Why am I having this reaction now? What did I eat, touch, or smell?' Our whole society is geared to go to the medicine cabinet for a painkiller or an antihistamine when we should be geared to get a pencil and paper to record what could be causing this problem at this time.

"After we have educated the parents, they often come in to see us knowing exactly what is causing their child's problems. They can tell if it's something inside or outside the house, if it's a food or a chemical. They can pinpoint the cause."

The Role of the Immune System

A primary contributor to allergies in children as well as adults is a poorly functioning immune system. "If the immune system is inadequate," Dr. Rapp says, "we can develop allergies and environmental illness. One way to strengthen the immune system so that your child is less prone to environmental illness or allergy is by using various nutrients. A helpful resource is the book, *Super Immunity in Kids*, which says, basically: If you take the correct nutrients in the correct amounts, you can strengthen the immune system so that you are less apt to become ill from natural things such as pollen, dust, and mold exposures. You will also be less apt to become ill from exposure to infections." Throughout this book you'll find information on how healthy eating and lifestyle can boost the immune system so that the body is able to handle assaults from the outside. You'll find specific information for children in chapter 65.

Environmental Allergies

Dr. Rapp offers many tips for helping parents to determine whether a child's behavior is related to allergies or environmental factors. "Think back," she says. "Does your child say, 'When I go to school in the morning I feel great!'? Or does the child say, 'I feel great when I leave the house and by the time I get to school I don't feel right'? Or does he say, 'I feel nervous'? Or tired, or irritable, or, 'I have a headache'? If that happens, you have to think, it might be the fumes on the school bus, or what he ate for breakfast, or what he uses to brush his teeth, or the soap that he uses. You've got to think of everything that he came in contact with before he got on the bus, and then what happened when he was on the bus.

"Now, children who are sensitive to things in the school will frequently notice that their headache starts within an hour. And the headaches frequently become more intense during the day. By Friday afternoon, the headache will be much worse than it was on Monday morning or on Sunday night. At first the headaches may disappear 1 to 4 hours after your child leaves school, but later on, if there are too many exposures during the week, you may notice that they don't get better at night and that it might take the whole weekend for the headache to go away."

It's also a good idea to pay attention to your child's sense of smell. "Another clue that certain exposures are making your child feel worse is when your child can smell everything before anybody else," Dr. Rapp explains. "She smells natural gas, or smells that perfume across the room, or she can smell food cooking before anybody else. She can smell disinfectants. If these odors bother your child and she can perceive them faster than anybody else, it means that she is probably becoming sensitized to the abundance of chemicals that we have now managed to put in our food, air, water, clothing, homes, schools, and workplaces."

Your child's academic performance may yield clues about a possible allergy to something in school. "The child may get an A one day, and an F the next day in the same subject," Dr. Rapp says. "It isn't that your child lost brain cells within 24 hours, but it does indicate to me that you should investigate that school to try to find out what could be causing the problem. Is the school dusty or moldy? Are the ventilation ducts open and clean? Was the basement of the school ever flooded? Does it smell worse on damp days?

A big problem in schools is poor ventilation, especially in the winter. Many systems are old and functioning improperly. The windows don't always open. Dust, molds, and chemicals can accumulate at very high levels. More children and teachers seem to be adversely affected when they go to school.

Dr. Rapp adds, "There is nothing worse in present-day schools than some of the synthetic carpets. They are made of chemicals that cause problems. In addition, they use adhesives that are full of other chemicals that cause even more problems."

TESTING FOR ENVIRONMENTAL ALLERGIES Traditional allergy testing is conducted in a few different ways. In the scratch or puncture test, an allergen is scratched across or lightly pricked into the skin. The skin will show evidence of allergic reaction by producing a small, raised area. In the intradermal test, an allergen is injected under the skin. This test may be needed if the scratch test results are not conclusive. A blood test is another option.

"If you suspect that your child may have been exposed to neurotoxic substances—those that actually damage the nervous system—ask your doctor to send you to specialists who can tell you whether the nerve conduction time in your child's body is normal or not," Dr. Rapp continues. "They can do a variety of blood tests to find out if the chemicals that are in the carpets and the adhesives are in the blood."

"The doctor may even make an allergy extract of the air in a room that smells of chemicals. Sometimes we can actually reproduce a headache, a stomachache, or problems thinking. The doctor makes the allergy extract the same way one would bubble air through a fish tank: using a pump to bubble the room air through a salt solution in a tiny test tube. The air bubbles for about 8 hours and at the end of this period a solution remains that contains some of the chemicals that were in the air. Then an allergy extract is prepared from this solution which can be injected in the skin, or placed under the tongue. If it causes numbness in the arms, tingling in the fingers, a headache, stomachache, problems with remembering, or a change in activity or behavior within 10 minutes, we have probably collected the problem chemical from the air within the solution.

TREATMENT AND ENVIRONMENTAL CONTROL Dr. Rapp explains how an environmental medicine specialist might proceed to treat a child. "The doctor can make dilutions of the chemical solution [found to be causing symptoms] and probably eliminate those same symptoms…. In other words, if the child develops a headache in a certain room, you can put a drop of the air allergy extract under the tongue and provoke the headache in 3 to 8 minutes. Then you can give the child a 5-fold weaker dilution of that same solution and often you can eliminate or neutralize the headache in less than 10 minutes."

As with adults, the first step in managing environmental allergies is avoiding exposure to a suspected allergen or irritant. Some recommendations for what you can do at home can be found in chapter 34. What if you suspect or determine that your child is being affected by an exposure at school? "One of the things that you can insist on is that school officials check the ventilation system," Dr. Rapp says. "There are fast and easy ways to measure the amount of carbon dioxide in a classroom, which can tell you whether the ventilation is good or not. Relatively simple tests can also be done to measure for certain chemicals, such as chlorine and formaldehyde. Sometimes, because of poor cleaning of the ventilation systems in schools, the problem is dust and molds, not chemicals. Other times, they put chemicals in the ductwork while cleaning, which really causes trouble because the chemicals then circulate throughout the school, causing illness. Sometimes the intake for the ventilation system is too close to the area where all the school buses line up. The bus drivers let the engines idle for long periods, resulting in all the gasoline fumes and hydrocarbons entering the ductwork intake and circulating throughout the school."

Food Allergies

Medical literature is filled with case studies in which children experience irritability, hyperactivity, insomnia, lack of concentration, poor memory, fatigue, and lethargy. After isolating and omitting all of the allergens from their diets, these sensitive children often improve. Not only do their physical symptoms clear up, but their behavioral imbalances do as well.

Among children, the most common sources of food allergies include chocolate, milk, wheat, eggs, and pork, Dr. Rapp says. "Ideally," she adds, "your child should eat only organically grown food because it is less contaminated with pesticides, food coloring, and other chemical additives that may be causing adverse reactions. However, in some places, it remains difficult—and expensive—to buy foods uncontaminated by chemicals."

The methods used to test for and treat food allergies in adults can be applied to children as well (see chapter 35). Dr. Rapp offers some additional suggestions. "Ask your children to write down or tell you their five favorite foods and beverages. The five foods and beverages that they write are probably the foods that are most likely to cause them difficulty.... If they wrote down bread, cake, cookies, pasta, and macaroni, chances are the problem is wheat. If they wrote down ice cream, yogurt, milk, cheese, and pizza, they are probably sensitive to dairy products."

Dr. Rapp also suggests asking your children to talk about how they feel, write their names, and draw pictures before and then after eating a meal." Using a peak flow meter or other device, check their breathing patterns both before and after eating. Pulse rate can be monitored as well. "If the pulse is 80 and suddenly after eating it is 120, a food has set off a silent alarm in the child's body, which has caused her pulse to increase," Dr. Rapp says. "So check the writing, the drawing, the pulse rate, the breathing, and how your child feels and looks before a meal and then a half hour or so later. If any of these variables indicates a change for the worse after a meal, one of the foods your child ate may be the cause of the problem.

As in adults, food allergies in children can be treated by an elimination or rotation diet, neutralizing dose therapy, reducing stress, and strengthening the immune system (see chapter 35).

Patient Stories

As Alison's mother, I can honestly say that Alison was born crying. She cried for the first 2 years of her life. I took her to a clinic at the time and found out she was allergic to corn, wheat, and bananas, which caused her to cry every day, all day long. I took her off those foods, and she became a normal, happy 2 year old. She did well for quite a while until she got a problem with a vitamin deficiency, which caused her to be uncontrollable. I couldn't do anything with her. If I wanted her to get dressed she would scream, rant, and rave. It would take me 3 hours just to get her dressed.

After reading an article on vitamins, I put her on vitamin supplements. That's when we realized that she hadn't smiled in 6 months. Then she was fine again, until 2 years ago, when she started to scream at me all the time, day in and day out, no matter what I wanted her to do, over absolutely nothing. She would scream at me that her shoes were wrong, her hair was wrong. It would take me all day long just to get her into the shower. At this point she was 10 years old. She should have been bathing on her own. I would go pick her up at school and when she was 70 feet away from me, she would scream,

'Mom, you are early!' And she would go on and on about why I was early. The next day she'd look at me and she'd scream, 'Mom, you are late!' And she would scream the whole way home, until she went up to her room and I would go off somewhere else to get away from her....

Dr. Buttram diagnosed my daughter as having food allergies to corn, potatoes, chicken, egg yolks, rice, and chocolate. They put her on these sublingual drops and now I have my normal, happy daughter back again. It was a dramatic change. She had become extremely difficult to live with.... Some days were worse than other. Now I know that on the days she had a combination of foods or a lot of the foods she was allergic to that she was at her worst. The way that I figured out it was food again was because every once in awhile we would have a great day or two and every once in awhile her diet just happened to not include these things. Then she would be fine. But the next day she'd be right back again with the behavior—totally out of control for long periods of time.

When my mother found out about Alison's behavior, she told me that I myself had been an absolutely horrendous child. Now that Alison had been diagnosed, she understood that I had had food allergies too. Now I understand that children's behavior problems are not always due to what the parent is doing with the child, as far as discipline is concerned. I've had a lot of children; I've been a foster parent for years. When Alison first started this behavior I tried everything in the book and nothing worked. And the thing that told me that something was controlling her, instead of her doing this, was the fact that we would have good days. And it didn't matter what we were doing on a bad day. If I would sit and play with her all day long, and it was a bad day, we would have a bad day. And discipline meant absolutely nothing, because something was controlling Alison. It was a chemical imbalance in her brain that was controlling her because she had absolutely no control over what she did. It was like the food was controlling her. I related it to the behavior of a manic-depressive or a paranoid schizophrenic who has no control over what they are doing....

I feel bad that Alison was so miserable for so long. There are so many kids out there that are this miserable. There are kids in learning disability classes and the parents just don't look any further than their nose. Some parents do make an effort and take their kids to standard allergists who test them, but those doctors may not be able to locate the problem. A friend of mine took her child to a regular allergist who tested him for all the standard things and said he was fine. But he never tested him for half the things to which Alison is allergic and the doctor never questioned the mother about the child's diet.
—Alison's mother

A patient I saw last week has three sons who came home smelling of mop oil, which is used to clean the school. The mother said that the children's clothes smelled so badly that she had to use very hot water to eliminate the smell. One of the boys developed a headache and a burning sensation in his throat. So I asked her to bring some of the mop oil and I just put it underneath his nose and let him take one whiff of the odor. Within seconds, he was complaining of a headache around his forehead on both sides of his temples and he said it was throbbing and that his throat was burning. I gave him oxygen for about 10 minutes and the headache, throbbing, and burning in his throat gradually subsided. We videotaped this reaction.

There was another child who had trouble only on the two afternoons a week when he went to school. He would be weak and tired, hardly able to stand; he couldn't hold a pencil, clung to his mother, but only on those 2 days. I sent the mother to the school and asked her to try to figure out what's different in the schoolroom that might be causing your son problems. It turned out that they used a very common disinfectant aerosol in the room, six times a day on the tabletops, to reduce infections. Then they used the same solution on the cot that he napped on. All she had to do was ask the school to stop using that disinfectant and install an air purifier, and the child improved remarkably.—Dr. Doris Rapp

PART EIGHT

Cancer Prevention and Treatment

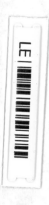

38

Cancer Overview

In today's society, cancer is epidemic and the single most important medical issue—an issue inseparable from politics and economics. Billions of dollars and an entire industry in which hundreds of thousands of people work full time are involved. The National Institutes of Health estimated that in 2000 alone, the total annual cost for cancer was $107 billion. The "war on cancer" has led to the formation of an enormous army consisting of the American Cancer Society (ACS), National Cancer Institute, and other major cancer research centers throughout the United States.

Each year, just before the ACS's annual fund-raising drive, we are bombarded with news stories of an imminent breakthrough that could change the lives of millions of sufferers. Months after the collection pots have been passed, there is still no breakthrough and the human toll in suffering continues. According to the ACS, nearly 5 million Americans have lost their lives to cancer since 1990. In 2000, more than 1.2 million new cases were diagnosed. While we are told that improvement in the treatment of various cancers is just around the corner, and while there have been gains in treating a few forms of the disease, overall we are losing the war.

Part of the reason lies in the strategy of the people who are leading the fight. Their view of the disease is determinedly myopic. To them, cancer is a localized disease represented by the tumor. By excising, poisoning, or irradiating the tumor, the traditional oncologist attempts to kill it in order to save the patient. The allocation of research funds depends on who controls this battle.

This is not to suggest that established cancer researchers are not interested in finding a cure for cancer. They are dedicated and sincere but many are equally eager, I believe, to have their cancer cure be the one that is ultimately accepted. And every company is pushing for its drugs to be the ones of choice.

The mainstream cancer community is only now beginning to recognize that a person's attitudes, beliefs, and especially diet can affect the outcome or causation of cancer. Only recently has it acknowledged that environment can be a determining factor and that cancer represents a breakdown in the body's overall immune system. Just a few years ago, for example, the Office of Complementary and Alternative Medicine (OCAM) at the National Institutes of Health established 10 research centers to evaluate alternative therapies, including one at the University of Texas that focuses solely on alternative and complementary treatments for cancer. But many traditional physicians are still reluctant to acknowledge that treatment that consists solely of removing the tumor with surgery or killing the cells in the tumor with radiation or chemotherapy may end up doing more harm than good.

Cancer Today

Cancer. A dreaded diagnosis. Especially in the past cancer meant certain death, pain, and disfigurement. People were ashamed to have the diagnosis. Evita Peron, the famous wife of Juan Peron of Argentina, died of uterine cancer in the 1950s without ever being told that she had it. This was even after surgery to try to stop the cancer. Her husband did not want her to know what she had. Yet nowadays, things have changed. Mayor Rudy Guiliani of New York City holds press conferences to discuss his diagnosis of prostate cancer and to talk about its impact on his political career. The world has come a long way since the days of Evita Peron. But cancer is still the second most common cause of death in the United States. These deaths are mostly among the middle-aged and elderly but children and younger adults are also struck down.

There is some good news. The rates of cancer death overall have been declining over the past decades. About half of all cancer patients now survive at least 5 years after treatment. People who remain cancer-free during that time have a good chance of remaining permanently free of the disease. Death rates are down because of better interventions that can now be curative. And people are taking better care of themselves, screening themselves so that cancers are diagnosed at earlier stages when they are more curable.

Unfortunately, the bad news far outweighs the good. The diagnosis of the most common cancer in men, prostate cancer, and in women, breast cancer, has increased. Whether this is because of better diagnostic techniques is unknown. Brain tumors, esophageal cancer, non-Hodgkin's lymphoma, and melanoma are dramatically increasing. Changes in the environment can certainly account for much of this.

In terms of treatment, the picture is not much brighter. The cures can be horrible. The powerful drugs can make you very, very sick. Surgery is still disfiguring. Pain is still part of the picture. Many times the cure is worse than the disease. And, after all this time with millions and millions of dollars spent on cancer research, the cure for cancer is no closer.

What is Cancer?

Cancer is a group of diseases in which abnormal cells multiply and spread. The cells no longer follow the rules for the usual orderly progression of growth and become renegades. Cancer can attack any part of the body and may spread to other parts. The sites most often affected are the skin, the digestive organs, the lungs, the prostate gland, and the female breasts.

Before exploring what happens in cancer, let's look at the life cycle of a healthy cell. A healthy cell starts out as immature and then goes through routine changes to mature. As a mature cell it performs whatever job in the body it is supposed to do and then it gets old and dies. Along the way, the active mature cell needs maintenance. There are genes in the cell that do the job of repairing mistakes and keeping the cell in running order.

So what is the outlaw cell, the cancer? Cancer occurs when the cell doesn't mature, doesn't repair its mistakes, or doesn't die. There are two types of cancer: those that form tumors and those that don't. When these outlaw cancer cells are regular building-block cells, like cells in the breast, lung, prostate, or skin, tumors occur. These cancers show up as abnormal masses or tumors because the cells are replicating out of control, heaping up into big masses, and killing the normal cells around them.

Cancers can also be in non building-block cells. This type of cancer doesn't produce a tumor and occurs in the cells of the blood. The blood cells go out of control, resulting in cancers like leukemia and lymphomas. These blood cells remain immature. They proliferate, and push out and kill the regular healthy mature blood cells. They show up in the bone marrow or clog up the lymph nodes or the spleen.

Then there is a really tricky part of cancer, and the part that can lead to death, which is when the aberrant cells migrate. They metastasize and invade other parts of the body, setting up shop in parts of the body distant from their original site. For instance, prostate cancer likes to invade the bones and brain. Breast cancer cells like the bones and the liver. The cancer cells develop the ability to spread by making special enzymes that cut through cell walls and travel through the blood.

What makes the cell go haywire? That is a very interesting question that no one can answer for sure. What can we do to prevent cancer? What can we do to fight cancer once the cells have gone out of control? There is a lot to say in response to these questions.

First off, there are poisonous elements from the environment that cause the cell to become cancerous, things like asbestos and cigarettes. But it also turns out that some people are more inclined to get cancer than others are. Genetic predisposition and environmental assaults appear to provide the powerful one-two punch.

Early Warning Signs

Among the early warning signs of cancer are a change in bowel or bladder habits; unusual bleeding or discharge; a thickening or lump in the breast, testicles or elsewhere; an obvious change in a wart or mole; a persistent cough or hoarseness of the voice; a sore throat that does not go away; and difficulty swallowing or indigestion.

Conventional Treatment

In conventional medicine, the usual treatment for cancer is surgery to remove the tumor, radiation to blast away tumors, and/or administration of powerful drugs that find and kill the cancer cells. Unfortunately, these treatments are very difficult to endure and don't always work. Surgery leads to disfigurement. Radiation leads to fibrosis (scarring). Chemotherapy essentially poisons the body in order to kill the tumor. It is toxic because it introduces a poison into the body, and it is invasive because the poison aggressively invades the cells and tissues of the body. The problem is that the poison is indiscriminate. It kills not only cancerous cells but healthy ones as well. In fact, its invasion of the body is systemic (total), not local, and therefore seriously damages the immune system. Chemotherapy drugs are very toxic to healthy cells and can make you feel really sick—your hair falls out, you can't eat, you're weak, and deeply fatigued.

Alternative Approaches

Another approach is the try to get the body itself to fight the cancer. Remember that a normal cell has its own maintenance team that repairs damage. If that part of the cell can be bolstered and reactivated, it can do its job of overcoming the tumor-forming oncogenes, reactivating the cell's tumor suppressor genes, and subduing the cancer's growth. Whenever this has occurred, the cancer goes into remission and disappears.

Taking care of yourself and living a healthy lifestyle is the best way to start. Of course, no tobacco. The number one cancer that kills is lung cancer. Of course, use sunscreen. Of course, women should perform breast self exams. Once you're middle-aged, have your colon and prostate checked out. Of course, eat a healthy diet as we have emphasized throughout this book.

Diet and Nutrition

Diet and nutritional factors are among the most important contributors to cancer development. Cancer has been linked to diets that are high in fats, animal and even certain types of vegetable proteins, and processed foods. Pesticides and some types of food additives also can cause cancer. Not only are diet and nutrition causative factors, they are also preventive ones.

Gar Hildebrand, president of the Gerson Research Organization, recommends a diet that detoxifies and stimulates cells back to health. "Doctors have long been aware that most cancer patients have an aversion to meat. They'll smell it and gag; that's a self-defense mechanism. It's absolutely essential for these people to stop taking in heavy proteins—animal proteins and sometimes even heavy vegetable proteins like legumes—for a while, just to clear up. The tumor is converting that stuff into caustic chemicals, related to the ammonia we use in our laundry machines. It's those chemicals that create damage systemwide.

"We can also detoxify the body by supplying oodles of plant chemicals, called phytochemicals. These foods can be eaten cooked or raw, and should include vegetables of all sorts, fruits, and a few whole grains. Fruit and vegetable juices are especially important. You have to flood the system with nutritious fluids such as carrot and green leaf juices. Apple juice should always be added because apples contain a material that is very good for cellular energy. If you put those juiced phytochemicals into the body every hour, these cancer patients will have their cellular enzyme systems speeded up so that the individual cells can spit up toxins."

Among the foods that are especially important in fighting and preventing cancer are alkaline foods, cruciferous vegetables, garlic, fiber, omega-3 fatty acids, chloryphyll-rich green foods, soy products, juices, green tea, mushrooms, and seaweed. Other nutrients that have been found to be helpful, often in supplement form, include:

vitamin A
vitamin B$_6$
vitamin C
vitamin E
folic acid
beta carotene
selenium
calcium
magnesium
zinc
chromium

phytochemicals
enzymes

A number of herbs have anticancer properties, including turmeric, red clover, echinacea, and ginseng.

Mind-Body Connection

Exploration of the effects of outlooks and emotions on health and disease processes has opened up an exciting area of science known as psychoneuroimmunology. Researchers have discovered that the mind, nervous system, and immune system interact with one another at the cellular level. When we feel joy, we enhance our healing mechanisms. Conversely, when we feel fear or hopelessness, we generate disease.

Dr. Carl Simonton, medical director of the Simonton Cancer Center in California and coauthor of *Getting Well Again* and *The Healing Journey*, is one of the early pioneers in this field. In the late 1960s, as a radiation oncologist, he noticed that emotional factors and patient attitudes influenced the course of treatment. His research led him to an extensive body of literature, where he learned that the three biggest mental influences on cancer are a tendency to respond to stressful situations with hopelessness, the bottling up of emotions, and a perceived lack of closeness to one's parents. This understanding prompted Dr. Simonton to look at the influence of counseling on the course of treatment. He discovered that survival times doubled, quality of life improved, and there was a better quality of death as a result of counseling efforts.

Dr. Simonton firmly believes that emotions drive healing systems and that the imagination and standard counseling can be used to increase a patient's will to live: "The emphasis of our approach is to focus on what is right with the individual. We ask, What are the person's goals and aspirations? What are the person's main sources of inspiration and creativity? What is the person's sense of purpose and destiny? As people become clearer and more connected to these concepts, they rediscover a strong desire to live. That in turn enhances their inherent healing mechanisms.

"As we explore these areas, we begin to address those things that interfere with achieving these very important aims. One primary culprit is unhealthy beliefs."

Dr. Simonton emphasizes that there is a relationship between all types of cancer and rigid thinking: "Here we tend to be controlled by beliefs about how we should be or have to be. That allows very little room for the expression of the spirit. Becoming aware of the direction in which our life force wants to go is essential for renewing vitality and healing power. It becomes important to listen to the voice within and to develop ways of enhancing that. This takes practice."

Dr. Simonton says that the way we use the imagination can mean the difference between success and failure in treatment: "In our imagination, we must think about the things we do for ourselves that are helpful. There are three areas that we need to look at: our beliefs about treatment, our beliefs about the body's ability to heal itself, and our beliefs about the disease itself. When a person is first diagnosed with cancer, if she shares the common cultural perspective, she believes that cancer is strong, that the body is weak, and that treatment is harsh. In keeping with these beliefs, a person is going to experience much in the way of undesirable side effects and less benefit. As we look at those beliefs, we find that they are not at all compatible with reality; cancer is a weak disease composed of weak cells. It is important to remind ourselves that our bodies have always been able to recognize and destroy cancer cells since before we were born. Shifting those images helps healing occur."

Combination Approaches

More patients would triumph over cancers if a combination of approaches were employed. Gar Hildebrand emphasizes the importance of utilizing any and every cancer protocol that works: "We believe that it's time we stopped living in an either/or world where orthodoxy is over on one side and the marginalized alternative professions are in the trenches and foxholes, and nobody talks. We believe it's time to get the doors and windows of communication open so that we can find the context for each of these treatments and the way they fit together. Our own experience reveals that using the nutritional approach takes a toxic load off the immune system and speeds up intracellular enzymes so that they can repel toxins and pull them from the blood rapidly. Calorie and protein restrictions and a diet high in nutrients can lead to the sensitization of a tumor. Years of experience show that diet therapy alone can produce monthly fevers, and tumors may or may not regress through those fevers. But if you stimulate the immune system when those fevers are hitting, you have a much greater chance of tumor reduction. That's why we suggest the marriage of these disciplines and the respectful recognition of the role of every aspect of anticancer medicine that's ever been developed."

In the chapters that follow, you will learn more about the role of diet in causing and preventing cancer. In addition, you will see that keeping your immune system healthy is essential, as is allowing your body to detoxify and destroy any cancer cells that start up. Some people require a rebalancing of the body's biochemical functioning, and there are nontoxic, natural substances such as antineoplastons that may help in this regard. Other alternative therapies focus on metabolic processes and take a whole-body approach to cancer by combining a number of therapies in the hope of revitalizing the entire system.

The chapters in this section provide practical information on selected alternative and complementary therapy programs, as well as a look at the critical scientific discoveries that led to their formation. There are many other alternatives not discussed here that have also shown good results. Some of these therapies are discussed elsewhere in this book, in the chapters on specific types of cancer.

The following discussion is intended for informational purposes only. If you have cancer, or suspect you have it, you must consult a medical professional to discuss your options. It is important to talk to your doctor about any therapy method you are considering or already using.

39

Cancer Therapy:
Boosting the Immune System

A weak or malfunctioning immune system is believed by many to be a primary cause of cancer. Likewise, a strong, healthy immune system plays a major
role in cancer prevention and treatment. In this chapter we detail the discoveries and programs developed by two distinguished practitioners who
focused their attention on immune-enhancement: the late Dr. Virginia
Livingston and the late Dr. Lawrence Burton.

Dr. Virginia Livingston's Therapy: Diet, Vaccine and Antibiotics

The lump in Dr. Owen Wheeler's neck was not large, but it was a lot more than
a swollen gland. Closer examination confirmed the physician's worst fears. He
had a cancer of the lymph glands that had wrapped itself around the major
arteries nearby. An attempt at surgery would be the equivalent of slitting the
doctor's throat.

As a physician, Dr. Wheeler had seen a great deal of cancer in books, in laboratories, and in his own and other doctors' patients. Now he had to choose a
treatment for himself. For him, since surgery was out, it had to be either radiation or chemotherapy. Radiation, the doctor soon discovered, would be almost
as damaging as surgery to the major blood vessels near his cancer. However, he
did not feel ready to subject himself to chemotherapy. Just a few years previously

he had watched his father die of the same type of cancer, suffering horribly from the side effects of the drugs used to combat the disease.

Like many other physicians, Dr. Wheeler refused chemotherapy when his own health was involved and began looking into alternative therapies. Ultimately, he decided to go to Dr. Virginia Livingston's clinic in San Diego, California, which featured an innovative treatment based on an unorthodox theory of the nature and cause of cancer, a theory with far-reaching implications for public health. At this clinic, Dr. Wheeler's cancerous tumor gradually disappeared.

Dr. Wheeler did not make the decision to go to San Diego lightly. He knew his life was at stake, but he also knew he was not going to undergo a Johnny-come-lately treatment of uncertain background and unpredictable outcome. He knew that Virginia Livingston was a remarkable physician whose interest in and work on cancer went back two generations.

THE DISCOVERY One of only four women to graduate from New York University–Bellevue Medical College in 1936, Virginia Livingston was one of the first women residents appointed to a New York City hospital. Her interests then were tuberculosis and leprosy. Her path to cancer research began indirectly in 1947, when she was asked for a second opinion on a case diagnosed as Raynaud's phenomenon, a circulatory condition that causes ulcerations on different parts of the body. While many of the patient's symptoms resembled those of leprosy, Dr. Livingston thought a more likely diagnosis was scleroderma, a skin disease characterized by hard, knotty patches, which can be fatal if it spreads to the internal organs.

Curious about the apparent similarity of scleroderma to leprosy, Dr. Livingston tested some smears with a special dye designed to detect the presence of tuberculosis and leprosy microbes. The tests were positive, suggesting that these scleroderma microbes were closely related to the tuberculosis and leprosy bacteria.

Dr. Livingston went on to test these organisms on chickens and guinea pigs. To her amazement, almost all the chickens died while the guinea pigs developed hardened patches of skin, some of which looked cancerous. Since cancer in guinea pigs is nearly unheard of, these results raised unsettling questions: Could this microbe from a human being cause disease in chickens and guinea pigs? Could this same microbe transmit disease from animals to humans? Was cancer perhaps infectious? Was it caused by bacteria?

From various hospitals, Dr. Livingston gathered samples of human cancers removed during surgery and put the pathological tissues under the microscope. The microbe was indeed present in every one of the samples. When she isolated and cultured the microbe from the cancer tissues and injected it into mice, the mice developed cancer in about 20 percent of cases. Dr. Livingston decided to call this microbe *Progenitor cryptocides*.

PROGENITOR CRYPTOCIDES

After several years of careful research at Newark Presbyterian Hospital, Dr. Livingston published her findings in the *American Journal of Medical Sciences* in 1950, much to the verbally expressed dismay of many members of the cancer establishment. After all, they had long accepted as an article of faith that cancer is caused by a virus. Medical technology has long been able to develop antibiotics to deal with bacteria but has yet to find any consistently effective protection against viruses. The fact that cancer might actually be caused by a bacteria thus should have come as good news, but the medical establishment refused to give creditability to Livingston's findings by setting up testing procedures to verify or disprove her findings. Instead, the traditional researchers simply continued to voice denial of the credibility of the microbe theory.

Both Dr. Livingston and her opponents—including the ACS—cited as evidence in their favor experiments performed by Dr. Peyton Rous in 1910 which demonstrated that roughly 90 percent of the chickens sold in New York City contained cancers caused by a microbial agent small enough to pass through a filter designed to catch bacteria while allowing viruses, which are much smaller, to pass through. Although Dr. Rous did not conclude that this "filterable microbial agent" was a virus, scientists who came after him assumed this to be the case. Dr. Livingston, however, believed her *Progenitor cryptocides* (PC) was in fact the cancer-causing agent discovered by Dr. Rous.

Since PC bacteria are highly pleomorphic (i.e., often assume forms that do not resemble bacteria at all) and have different growth requirements depending on the stage they are in, Dr. Livingston proceeded with extra tests to make certain that she was not dealing with a virus. She discovered that PC would indeed pass through Dr. Rous' filter just as viruses were supposed to do. But then she took samples of the filtered microbes and regrew them in cultures, something impossible to do with viruses, since they are unable to survive outside of living organisms. Dr. Livingston also discovered that unlike viruses, both PC and Dr. Rous' cancer agent could be dried, stored indefinitely, and then reactivated to produce new tumors. For Dr. Livingston, the PC cancer-causing agent was not a virus but was only viruslike. The PC bacteria had to be reincubated and made larger in order to be kept from passing through very fine filters that usually hold back bacteria.

In the course of her research, Dr. Livingston reached another conclusion that put her at odds with the cancer establishment, especially the part of it which believes implicitly in surgery as a first recourse. PC, as Dr. Livingston found out, was present not merely in the cancer but throughout the patient's entire body. In her view, cancer is not a localized disease. Rather, it is a generalized or systemic illness affecting the entire body, not just the particular area manifesting symptoms. Thus, while surgery can be helpful in that by removing cancerous tissue it helps the immune system fight the disease, it is a serious error to think of the tumor or lesions as constituting the disease and of surgery as being the cure. Indeed, from Dr. Livingston's viewpoint, it was no surprise that a patient could develop cancer in a totally different site after a "successful" operation, despite the surgeon's having "gotten it all." Since surgery does nothing by itself to enhance the body's immune system, it may even make another onset of cancer more likely—and more serious.

Dr. Livingston might have concluded that once a drug to combat or at least control PC bacteria was developed, a cure for cancer would be on its way. Careful research on the microbe in laboratory animals, however, convinced her that the solution was far more complex than finding a "magic bullet" to strike down PC. The PC bacteria, she discovered, are normal constituents of every cell in the human body.

"The microbe is present in people from the time of conception," she stated in a WBAI radio interview in 1987. "It is not always harmful. It is useful, for example, in the knitting of wounds. But when it begins rampant proliferation, it produces a hormone called choriogonadotropin, which promotes tumor growth and is present in abnormally large amounts in cancer tissues."

Dr. Livingston went on to explain that PC normally remains dormant in the cell and emerges only to help in healing after injury to the body. Ordinarily the immune system monitors the production of PC, keeping it at the amount needed to cope with the damage. But when immunity is weakened by stress, poor diet, old age, surgery, and/or other debilitating factors, the body may no longer be able to regulate PC production and PC bacteria may begin to proliferate, releasing choriogonadotropin as it multiplies.

TRANSMISSIBILITY THEORIES

Theories about the transmissibility of cancer have alarming implications for public health. Dr. Livingston's experiments convinced her that cancer can be transmitted from human beings to chickens and guinea pigs. This conclusion raises the disquieting implication that the transfer mechanism may work in the other direction as well, allowing cancer to pass from animals to humans.

For obvious reasons, the poultry industry finds such an idea unthinkable. However, Dr. Livingston's chicken vaccine was licensed in California in 1985.

"Cancer is a very serious disease in chickens," Dr. Livingston noted in her radio interview. "Each year many thousands of chickens are lost to cancer. The organism is carried from chicken to chicken, even in the unhatched egg."

If all of these birds were simply "lost," the problem would be confined to the poultry industry, but there is considerable evidence, Dr. Livingston stated, that many infected fowls are finding their way into supermarkets. She believes that the chickens we consume today are just as cancer-ridden as the ones Dr. Rous examined in 1910 when he determined that 90 percent were so afflicted. A March 1987 report on 60 Minutes, while not concerned specifically with cancer, certainly supported her contention that FAA enforcement is both lax and ineffective in keeping questionable poultry off the market.

The question of whether cancer can pass from animals to humans takes on even wider dimensions when one considers that livestock, often living in cramped and unhealthy conditions, are frequently fed chicken manure because of its high protein content, and are thus exposed to the infectious cancers so prevalent on the poultry farm. But avoiding eating beef and pork, while desirable, is not sufficient, according to Dr. Livingston. Even drinking milk is risky, she asserted, since "about 80 to 90 percent of cattle are carrying leukemia," according to the cattle industry's own literature.

The doctor's views on milk are met with as much skepticism in the dairy industry as her views on meat and poultry are in the meat and poultry industries. But Dr. Livingston's legacy is not without support. Her views are accepted in Europe. In Switzerland and Sweden, where dairy is a major industry, milk from leukemic cows is not permitted to reach the market because the authorities consider it a serious risk to the public health. Such strictures have not been imposed in the United States in part because the U.S. dairy industry simply doesn't believe, and no government authorities will test, Dr. Livingston's theories. The doctor never denied that the expense of enforcing strict quality control and rejecting milk or meat from diseased animals would be tremendous. However, it would also alleviate a great amount of human suffering.

THE TREATMENT Dr. Livingston pondered this evidence for many years beginning in the 1940s and 1950s and continued gathering data and doing research until she developed a program of cancer treatment: diet, antibiotics, and a therapy she called autogenous vaccines. Eighty percent of her cancer patients improved. In 1992, while on a vacation in Europe, Dr. Livingston died. We all mourn her loss. But the challenge her work presents to the medical establishment lives on.

THE ANTICANCER DIET

The Anticancer Diet is not in itself a cure for cancer, nor is it intended as such; however, it works with the other aspects of Dr. Livingston's therapy to strengthen the immune system. A healthy immune system not only keeps normally present PC under control but combats any disease-causing PC taken in with food. Meats, especially chicken, beef, and pork, are the most likely sources of dietary PC.

Since the immune system of a cancer patient is already seriously depleted, it is necessary to avoid these kinds of foods in order to minimize the influx of pathogenic, cancer-causing PC. For this reason, Dr. Livingston's diet goes beyond the usual tenets of sound nutrition. It emphasizes raw or very lightly cooked fresh food full of vitamins, minerals, and enzymes for rebuilding the body. Refined or processed foods are eliminated. Most animal products are excluded, both because of their suspected ability to transmit pathogenic PC and because they are often full of toxins, hormones, antibiotics, chemicals, and pesticides that deplete the immune system and may interfere with treatment. In fact, the diet Dr. Livingston developed is basically the one which the ACS is now only beginning to promote: primarily vegetarian, low in fats and cholesterol, low in animal products and protein, and high in fresh fruits, vegetables, whole grains, and legumes.

Dr. Livingston stipulated that her patients do the following:
➤Avoid the obvious carcinogens and immune system depleters, such as cigarettes, alcohol, caffeine, and drugs, both recreational and prescription.
➤Avoid the empty calories of foods that are high in white flour and sugar or that have been deep fried.
➤Cut down on salt and on food high in sodium while increasing consumption of potassium-rich fresh fruits and vegetables.

As patients began to recover, Dr. Livingston allowed them to eat some fish, but chicken, eggs, beef, and milk products remain prohibited, since her research has led her to believe that these foods have a high potential for transmitting cancer to humans. The PC microbes in their pathogenic state are in the animals, and when the animals are eaten, the microbes are transmitted and proliferate in humans.

The most unusual aspect of Dr. Livingston's diet is its focus on abscisic acid, an essential immune nutrient forming part of the vitamin A molecule. As Dr. Livingston stated in her 1984 book, *The Conquest of Cancer: Vaccines and Diet*, "Abscisic acid is the keystone upon which all cancer immunity is built in your body. If you already have cancer, abscisic acid is absolutely critical to your defense, because it actually stops cancer cells from multiplying. If you don't have cancer (or if it is latent in you system), it is imperative that your diet contain high amounts of vitamin A and abscisic acid if you are to immunize yourself against it."

Raw juices, especially carrot juice, and fruits and vegetables high in vitamin A have a prominent role in the Anticancer Diet. However, because many cancer patients have extensive liver damage and therefore are unable to break down vitamin A to obtain abscisic acid, Dr. Livingston's diet also includes a number of foods such as mangos, avocados, tomatoes, and green leafy vegetables that are naturally rich in abscisins. To break down the vitamin A in carrot juice, Dr. Livingston recommended adding a tablespoon of dried liver powder (from organically fed cattle, of course), which contains enzymes that predigest the carrot juice and thus make the abscisic acid available.

AUTOGENOUS VACCINE

Besides the diet, Dr. Livingston developed an autogenous vaccine made from the PC in the individual patient. "We make the vaccine," she reported in the radio interview, "and as the body builds immune bodies to the organisms, the deleterious effects of the *Progenitor cryptocides* are nullified. But each time we make it, we make it for the individual. It cannot be made for your neighbor, and it cannot be sold."

ANTIBIOTICS

Since PC microbes are bacteria, they are vulnerable to antibiotics. Dr. Livingston found that the administration of safe, nontoxic antibiotics such as ampicillin and penicillin G can reduce the excessive amount of PC in the bloodstream and thereby cause cancerous tumors to shrink. The term "excessive" is used here because, as has been noted, normal amounts of PC do not cause a problem in the healthy body and in fact contribute to one's well-being. It is only when they become excessive that they contribute to cancerous growth in the body.

OTHER PARTS OF THE PROGRAM

Other elements of this safe, nontoxic program include the following:

➤Transfusions of fresh whole blood, preferably from a healthy family member, to reduce the risk of contamination, increase oxygenation, and replenish the body's enzymes.

➤Injections of gamma globulin to provide fresh antibodies.

➤Injection of spleen extract derived from immunized animals to increase the patient's white blood cell count. White blood cells play a critical role in arresting foreign substances and toxic intruders into the blood.

➤Injections of nonspecific vaccines, such as one containing numerous mixed bacteria, for use in respiratory infections and to increase general resistance.

➤Supplements and/or injections of vitamins C and B_{12}, plus tablets of vitamins such as A, C, E, B_6, and B_{12}, and minerals to stimulate the immune system.

➤Oral supplementation of hydrochloric acid where needed to correct overly alkaline blood caused by digestive difficulties.

THE PATIENTS Dr. Livingston's ideas about the treatment and prevention of cancer are not purely academic. They have been put to the test in her clinical practice as well as in her laboratory. In *The Conquest of Cancer*, she listed over 60 cases of patients she treated; these were pulled at random from her files. Of course, not every story is a success story, but the sample does show an improvement rate of 82 percent, a statistic that conventional therapists can only dream of.

> *A 66-year old man came to the clinic in 1978, diagnosed with inoperable cancer of the liver. By 1980 the patient reported feeling much better, and tests showed that his tumor had shrunk 50 percent. When Dr. Livingston contacted him in 1983 while writing her book, he said that he was still following the program and was in general good health.*

A 12-year-old boy was diagnosed with Hodgkin's disease. His mother, however, refused to subject him to chemotherapy and brought him to Dr. Livingston's clinic instead. A year later, his lymphoma was in remission. Follow-up testing revealed that he was totally clear and that a lesion on his liver had disappeared. He went back to school, gained weight, and was soon participating in sports.

A 51-year-old woman could no longer endure the side effects of radiation and chemotherapy for cancer of the ovaries which had spread to her colon, causing a tumor about the size of a baseball. Her prognosis was terminal when she started treatment at the clinic. A computed axial tomography (CAT) scan and an ultrasound test taken the following year showed no abnormalities. She went back to work, and 2 years later she was still free of cancer.

None of these case histories, of course, constitutes experimental proof that Dr. Livingston's therapy is effective. Such proof is not likely to be forthcoming, since it is not morally feasible to establish a control group of cancer patients, give them a placebo, and see how many of them die. However, Dr. Livingston always stood ready to put researchers who wished to verify these stories in touch with these patients or any others in her files.

The doctor's work is continued by others in San Diego. Whether her theories will ever find acceptance and be applied in the wider arena of public health in the United States remains to be seen.

Dr. Lawrence Burton's Immuno-Augmentative Therapy

The majority of patients arriving at the Immunology Research Center (IRC) in Freeport in the Grand Bahama Islands have been pronounced terminal by orthodox medicine. Many are crippled and unable to walk, others bloated beyond recognition with ascites, an abdominal fluid buildup that is a common symptom of malignant carcinomas. Some have been bedridden for long periods, others are mentally disoriented, and many are in such constant pain that the simplest outing is unthinkable. They come to receive the Immuno-Augmentative Therapy (IAT) developed by Dr. Lawrence Burton, a Ph.D. in zoology who also had a strong background in cancer research. The IRC in Freeport was opened by Dr. Burton in 1977, where he acted as director until his death in March of 1996. Since then, the center has been headed by Dr. John Clement, a British physician who is an internationally respected cancer specialist and who studied with Dr. Burton.

What is going on at the IRC that makes it a fortress of hope for so many cancer "immigrants," most of them outcasts deemed hopeless by established medicine? On Grand Bahama Island, the IRC has taken in people considered doomed. Many are still alive, long after the terminal prognoses given by their traditional physicians and oncologists have come and gone. Others have died but were enabled to survive longer than anyone had imagined possible. Many now lead happy, fruitful lives with much less pain than they had come to accept as an inevitable accompaniment of illness.

Not everyone can be accepted for treatment, unfortunately. Dr. Clement and his staff must first be reasonably sure the treatment they offer is the right thing for the prospective patient's condition. For those patients who are accepted, however, something new appears: a restoration of hope. The center holds out a small but significant promise to them.In an interview given prior to his death, Dr. Burton was quick to note that IAT "is not by any means a cure for cancer." However, he also relates how "cancer patients who have been treated with IAT... often respond with cessation of tumor growth and, in some instances, with no tumor growth. In many there is actual reversal as well as necrosis [complete stoppage] of the cancer growth."

THE DISCOVERY The man who made such startling progress in the treatment of cancer had a long career in research. Dr. Lawrence Burton decided to go into cancer research after seeing "firsthand the many horrors of cancer" while assigned as a pharmacist's mate to the U.S. Navy's Cancer Center at Brooklyn Naval Hospital in 1944. In those days, he recalled "the accepted procedure for cancer treatment was radical surgery. If you had a cancer of the foot, the leg was removed at the hip."

After World War II, Dr. Burton studied genetics, cancer etiology (the cause of cancer), oncolysis (destruction of cancer cells), and immunology. He received a Ph.D. in experimental zoology from New York University in 1955. Dr. Burton became a research associate at the California Institute of Technology and began to publish the results of his work in leading scientific journals such as *Cancer Research*. He became a research associate at New York University in 1957, moving up to become an associate in oncology in 1966 at St. Vincent's Hospital, a noted teaching hospital. In 1966 he became a senior investigator and oncologist at St. Vincent's.

Immuno-Augmentative Therapy has its roots in this period of Dr. Burton's career. In 1959, he and a team of cancer researchers accidentally discovered a tumor-inhibiting factor that reduced or eliminated cancer in a special breed of leukemic mice. In the November 1962 issue of *Transactions of the New York Academy of Sciences* they reported on certain natural substances that were capable of causing remission in over 50 percent of the leukemic mice treated.

In the fall of 1965, Patrick McGrady, Sr., science editor for the American Cancer Society (ACS), observed Dr. Burton's experiments and was amazed. In a radio interview, McGrady told my audience, "they injected the mice and the lumps went down before your eyes—something I never believed possible."

McGrady had Dr. Burton and his associate, Dr. Friedman, also with a Ph.D. in zoology, repeat the experiment at the ACS's 1966 Science Writers'

Seminar. The two doctors, in the presence of 70 scientists and 200 science writers, injected mice having mammary cancer with the serum they had isolated during their research. An and a half later, the tumors had disappeared almost completely.

The next day, the results of these experiments received front-page coverage throughout the world. The *Los Angeles Herald Examiner's* headline read "Fifteen Minute Cancer Cure for Mice: Humans Next?"

Unfortunately, this enthusiastic publicity backfired. As Dr. Burton recalled, "This caused a misleading specter of 'cure' to which no researcher would ever dare lay claim..." Furthermore, when word about the experiments spread throughout the medical community, many traditionally trained physicians questioned their validity, suggesting that the results had been accomplished by trickery.

In September of the same year, Drs. Burton and Friedman were invited to repeat the experiment before the New York Academy of Medicine. This time, in order to avoid accusations of fraud, they had the mice selected by independent oncologists and pathologists. Again, an or so after injections with the newly isolated tumor-inhibiting factors, the tumors started to disintegrate.

During 1970 and 1971, Drs. Burton and Friedman were assisting Dr. Antonio Rottino, a medical doctor on the cancer research team, in treating his cancer patients at St. Vincent's with their antitumor serums. In 1972, Dr. Rottino announced that the treatment had to cease. The IAT treatments were considered experimental and therefore unproven, and so were not appropriate to use in providing regular medical care.

Also in the early 1970s, Long Island psychologist Martin Goldstone's wife was being treated with the Burton-Friedman technique. She had enjoyed such promising results that when they learned that the treatments had been stopped at St. Vincent's she and her husband and other prominent people in their Great Neck, Long Island, community raised enough funds to establish the Immunology Research Foundation to continue the work of the two doctors.

In 1975 *New York* magazine published an article on the work of Drs. Burton and Friedman entitled "The Politics of Cancer—Why Won't the Medical Establishment Pay Attention to These Two Men?" The article drew considerable public attention and inquiry. Senator Howard Metzenbaum of Ohio, whose wife had just died of cancer, wrote a letter to the National Cancer Institute (NCI) demanding to know why the public was being kept in the dark about this treatment. He was informed that the NCI was of the opinion that the Burton-Friedman work was nothing new, couldn't possibly be effective, and was therefore not worthy of further investigation or testing.

Perhaps the most important result of the article was that after extensively investigating Drs. Burton and Friedman, Champion International, a philanthropic organization interested in alternative medical therapies, decided to fund the two men's work. Champion International's patronage became all-important 3 years later, when Dr. Burton decided to relocate his clinic.

THE THERAPY The Immunology Research Center moved from Great Neck, New York, to Freeport on Grand Bahama Island in 1977. Since then, over 2,500 terminally ill cancer patients have undergone treatment there. About 50 to 60 percent of patients experience tumor reduction. Many resume normal lives; frequently they survive 5 years and more beyond the initial diagnosis of cancer. The 5-year survival period is sufficient for the American Cancer Society and the National Cancer Institute to consider a patient cured.

I have visited the IRC on a number of occasions and have analyzed the records of many of Dr. Burton's and Dr. Clement's patients. This investigation has confirmed the remarkable success that IAT continues to have on a regular basis. In sharp contrast to the depressing environment of most cancer hospitals in this country, the attitude of patients at the IRC is one of optimism and hope. Most patients are off drugs and free of pain and report that they feel well. Perhaps the most telling endorsement comes from the family members of non-surviving patients who have continued to support the clinic with financial contributions and moral backing.

Dr. Burton did not believe that we should use the word "cure" in relation to cancer. "Immuno-Augmentative Therapy," he explained, "augments the immune system and enables it to control and combat cancer." But it does not totally eradicate cancer. No therapy does that. Cancer patients, no matter how long the cancer is under control, must always be watchful of their condition to be sure that the cancer does not begin growing again or growing somewhere else. Cancer is not a localized condition but a systemic disease. While it may clear up in one organ, it may flare up in another.

INJECTING BLOOD PROTEINS

Immuno-Augmentative Therapy consists of injections of four blood proteins that Dr. Burton discovered and was able to isolate. These proteins are essentially responsible for the control and even shrinkage of tumors. When injected in the proper amounts and at proper intervals, they can help the weakened body do what it would do normally: control the growth and proliferation of cancerous cells.

One of the proteins is a tumor antibody that can destroy tumors. Another is an antibody complement that stimulates the tumor antibody. Without the stimulation from the complement, the antibody will remain inactive. The other two proteins have a direct effect on the destruction of tumors: The "blocking" protein inhibits the antibody to give the body a chance to clear away the toxic waste of tumor destruction; otherwise the body would go into toxic shock. The blocking protein is itself then inhibited by an antiblocking protein. When the blocking protein is prevalent, the antibody and tumor complement are prevented from attacking tumors, which therefore may grow; when the antiblocking protein is prevalent, the blocking protein is held in check, enabling the tumor antibody and complement to actively seek and destroy cancerous cells.

AUGMENTING THE IMMUNE MECHANISM

Dr. Burton applied his discovery of blood fractions to create a harmonious balance in the patient's internal chemistry. Once this balance has been established, the patient's body is able to defend itself naturally against the continued proliferation of cancer cells and frequently is able to attack and begin to reduce existing tumors. Dr. Burton's therapy does not attempt to shrink a tumor directly or intervene in the growth of a cancer. It is designed only to "augment an immune mechanism in the patient." The stimulated immune mechanism itself is then responsible for attacking the tumor.

IAT therapy involves two separate stages. The antibody, antibody complement, and antiblocking proteins help the body fight cancer. Every time a tumor cell is destroyed by these three proteins, the fourth one—the blocking protein—is released to inhibit further destruction of the tumor. The role of the protein, as noted above, is not to protect the tumor but to give "the liver a chance to eliminate the waste by-products of cell destruction." The blocking protein actually helps the body recover from the toxic shock caused by killed cancer cells. It plays a vital role not in the actual destruction of cancer but in the body's ability to recover afterward.

IAT involves a careful consideration of the alternating roles of tumor destruction, on the one hand, and the body's recovery from toxic breakdown, on the other hand. The timing of these two processes is all-important. While the blocking protein is eventually deblocked by the antiblocking protein, this process may take too long. During therapy a decision must be made as to when and how aggressively to intervene in this process. The body—especially the liver—must be protected from the toxic waste of the destroyed cancer cells, but it must at the same time be protected from the ravages of the tumor. The attending physician has to decide when the blocking process has given the body enough recovery time. The system is then deblocked by the intravenous introduction of specific amounts of the antiblocking protein, and the cancer destruction continues. The immune mechanism may be bolstered further by the injection of the tumor antibody and tumor complement.

The timing and the quantities of protein introduced are the critical issues. As Dr. Burton explained, "In time, the patient's own body deblocks the system [enabling cancer destruction to be resumed]. But if there is a large amount of tumor, we cannot wait indefinitely while the process is repeated. The patient has a limit. He or she can produce only so much antibody and so much deblocking protein. Thus we have to augment these proteins—once a day, twice a day, as many as six to eight times a day. If the augmentation is done properly, we can produce, to quote the National Cancer Institute, many, many 'spontaneous remissions.'"

THE RESULTS In a recent interview, Dr. John Clement noted that despite the progress that has been made with numerous cancer patients at the center, success rates are still relative at IRC. He says, "The majority of the patients coming here are already pronounced as terminally ill. We can produce almost invariably some slowing down or even stopping of the cancerous process. And we have been lucky, of course, in a number of patients, we've been able to prevent the cancer, cause a regression. We do not like to use the word 'cure' because even though we may stop the process going on you have to realize that if you've got cancer once you're still the same person and you're likely to get cancer again. You still have the same immune system. You still have the same genetic background. And you are likely to get a recurrence."

Dr. Burton had particular success with mesothelioma and metastatic colon cancer, two supposedly "incurable" cancers.

MESOTHELIOMA

Mesothelioma, or "asbestos cancer," typically attacks the lungs (the pleural cavity), sometimes the stomach (peritoneal cavity), and occasionally the heart (pericardial cavity). It is characterized by a number of tiny tumors initially resembling shotgun pellets that spread and grow rapidly. There is no treatment for mesothelioma according to an NCI treatise on the subject, only pain management. The survival rate is 0. The prognosis is only 2 to 10 months' survival.

The use of asbestos in building has decreased sharply because of the associated health risks. Nonetheless, the treatment of mesothelioma will continue to be a major health priority for many years because of the unusually long latency period of asbestos cancer. There are no known survivors of mesothelioma in the traditional medical health care system.

Dr. Burton reported that the average survival rate of his mesothelioma patients was already 47 to 48 months, and a number of survivors are currently residing at the clinic. Some have been released and now live normal lives since, "in contrast to other types of cancer, once you get rid of all tumor cells containing asbestos, the patient is safe," said Dr. Burton. This is due partly to the fact the mesothelioma is strictly an environmental disease and is in no way genetic.

Eleven IRC peritoneal mesothelioma patients were the subjects of a report published in the early 1990s by Drs. Burton and Clement. They had suffered such physical defects as abdominal distention, obstruction, and ascites. The four women and seven men had an immune profile typical of advanced cancer populations: elevated levels of blocking proteins and suppressed levels of deblocking protein and tumor complement. All were "augmented" with injections of immunoglobulin serum antibodies and deblocking protein. The results of the study were as follows:

"Four males and one female are alive, with survival among the five ranging from 22 to 80 months. The mean survival for those living is 43 months, and the median is 52 months. Of the other six cases, mean survival was 23 months and the median was 16 months, with a range of 7 to 50 months. The total subject population represented mean (or average) survival of 35 months and a median survival of 30 months, with a range for all cases from 7 to 80 months."

METASTATIC COLON CANCER

Dr. Burton had equal success in treating metastatic colon cancer. He noted that "Dr. DeVita, director of the NCI, announced on television around December 1984 that the 5-year survival rate for metastatic cancer of the colon is zero. This means that nobody under traditional treatment survived 5 years. But we have over 10 patients who have lived past the five-year mark and are still alive today."

One of those surviving patients is Robert Beasley, who was diagnosed with colon-to-liver cancer (meaning that the cancer metastasized—traveled—from the site of the primary tumor, the colon, to a remote site, the liver). Beasley says that his doctor "not only could tell I had liver trouble, he could hold the tumors in his hand. That's how bad it was. So he sewed me up and he said, "Take him home. I will not offer him chemo. He has 3 months to live." Eleven years later, after being treated for this condition by Dr. Burton, Beasley reported that he was in perfect health.

Dorothy Strait is another survivor of colon-to-liver cancer. When she was diagnosed, her surgeon told her that her case was hopeless. Having seen and biopsied her liver metastases and having viewed her liver scans, he gave her a prognosis of 3 months of survival or less. After being treated by Dr. Burton for a few months, she returned to her surgeon, who was surprised to find no trace of the tumor in her body. Twelve years after the original diagnosis, she was still alive and healthy.

There are many other cases of metastatic colon cancer survivors among IRC patients, with some patients living 7 to 10 years after having received prognoses of less than 12 months' survival. But the traditional physicians who are informed of these drastic turnarounds in their former patients frequently write them off as "spontaneous remissions" rather than giving credit to the "unproven" therapy of immune augmentation. Still, neither the NCI nor the ACS has been able to explain why their "spontaneous remission" rate is zero while that of the IRC is about 1 out of every 10 patients.

IAT UNDER ATTACK

Despite its successful pioneering work in cancer treatment, the Immunology Research Center came under attack from the traditional medical establishment in 1985. The ACS and NCI regard cancer "cure" as their exclusive province, heavily supported by public funding. Many outside efforts were regarded as intrusions and trespasses, and when they departed significantly from traditional treatment approaches, they were suspected of being quackery.

The American cancer establishment finally convinced the Bahamian government that Dr. Burton's Immuno-Augmentative Therapy (IAT) might have involved the use of contaminated blood. The clinic was forced to close on July 17, 1985, but was reopened the following spring after investigation proved that these allegations could not be substantiated.

While the clinic was closed, a group of Dr. Burton's patients formed an association dedicated to reopening the IRC. Since most of these patients were Americans, they sought the assistance of the U.S. Congress. A congressional hearing on the matter was conducted in January 1986 by Representative Guy Molinari for the purpose of fact-finding and to make these complaints public. During the hearing, many members of the patient association had a chance to tell the public about their personal experiences at the IRC. One of the witnesses was Sherry Costaldo. Her story follows.

Patient Story

Sherry Costaldo was diagnosed as having breast cancer at the age of 28 after many doctors had dismissed her, insisting that she wasn't sick. She underwent a radical mastectomy at Memorial Sloan-Kettering Cancer Center in New York and then 5 weeks of daily radiation and 19 months of chemotherapy, which she was told at the time was only experimental. Subsequent radiation treatments continued on a regular basis before she suffered a massive seizure, resulting from the spreading of her cancer into the brain.

Displeased with what she had come to learn was experimental treatment at Sloan-Kettering, she went to Nassau Medical Center. There she underwent surgery to remove a brain tumor and then endured 5 more weeks of radiation treatment while she was on Dilantin (phenytoin) and prednisone. She remembers being "extremely ill from the treatment and medication, and seizures occurred periodically." She was "almost always dizzy, disoriented and nauseous, and very ill." She was told she might go on to chemotherapy administered through a shunt in her skull or through the spine, but she would have to suffer even greater pain, and the results were not guaranteed. She returned to Sloan-Kettering, where her ovaries were surgically removed (oophorectomy) in the hope that once estrogen production was stopped, tumor growth might be halted. But a subsequent brain scan confirmed that four tumors were lodged in her brain. Her oncologist told her that nothing more could be done. Two months later, she headed for Freeport and Dr. Burton's IRC, which she had heard was helping many cancer patients.

Although her husband was vehemently opposed to her being treated by Dr. Burton, she underwent IAT therapy for 14 weeks. During that time she was able to get off prednisone completely and eventually found herself "swimming, walking with confidence, and able to take care of my family and myself." She noted her progress from that point on during the congressional hearings: "The improvement has been almost unbelievable, and I am now living a fairly normal life. I have taken aerobic dancing, organized and directed a children's choir, and seldom need to rest. I run circles around my husband."

40

Cancer Therapy: Rebuilding the Body's Biochemistry

A number of alternative therapies for cancer focus on biochemical imbalances as a cause of disease development and progression. These include 714X, hydrazine sulfate, shark cartilage, and antineoplaston therapy. The latter treatment will be detailed in this chapter.

Antineoplaston Therapy

Thirty years ago a medical student in Poland took a new and different approach to cancer research. He decided to find out why all people don't have cancer. Everyone is exposed to the same known and unknown causative agents of this disease. What is different about the people who never contract it? Is this difference the key to developing a cure?

The Discovery: Dr. Stanislaw Burzynski

Dr. Stanislaw Burzynski believes so. Now working out of a research facility he founded in 1970 in Houston, Texas, Dr. Burzynski has treated about 2,000 patients with advanced cancer with impressive success. Most of these people turned to him as a last resort when conventional treatment with radiation, chemotherapy, and surgery had failed. What they found was a therapy based not on the abuse of the body's built-in defense systems but rather on the transformation of cancerous cells into healthy, normal tissue.

Dr. Burzynski's solution lies in a group of chemical substances, part of a larger group of chemical compounds called peptides, which exist in every human body. His research points to a severe shortage of these substances—called antineoplastons—in cancer patients. Simply stated, antineoplastons are a special class of peptides, found in the body, that combat neoplastons—abnormal cells or cancer cells. Antineoplastons could be the vehicle needed by the body to ward off and even reverse the development of these cancerous cells.

Dr. Burzynski has put this theory into action, treating patients by reintroducing antineoplastons into the bloodstream either intravenously or orally with capsules. In many cases, tumors shrank in size or actually disappeared. Some patients even experienced complete remission of their cancers, and years of follow-up study have revealed no sign of any return.

Such results are almost unbelievable. Dr. Burzynski appears to have tapped the power of antineoplastons to naturally "reprogram" cancer cells. His approach could virtually eliminate the need to destroy these cells or remove the tumors they create. This therapy was not developed overnight. It has taken Dr. Burzynski nearly three decades of research, first in Poland, then at the Baylor College of Medicine in Houston, Texas, and ultimately at the Burzynski Research Institute in Houston. During this time, Dr. Burzynski has zeroed in on the substance he named antineoplaston. But to get back to Dr. Burzynski's original concern, why do tumors develop in the first place?

WHY TUMORS DEVELOP According to his theory, cancer is due primarily to an information-processing error. Good information produces healthy cells; bad information results in cancerous cells. Antineoplastons are important because they carry "good" information to the cells. They can "tell" the cells to develop normally.

All cells start out with specific goals. Some turn into skin, some into blood vessels, some into bone or other body tissues. However, they will never go on to perform these highly specialized functions in the body unless they go through a process called differentiation. Cancer cells, or neoplastons, which everybody produces regularly, never differentiate. They are abnormal cells that the healthy body rejects and destroys because they have not received good information and so have no constructive role to play. When the body is in a weakened state, these neoplastons are not destroyed but rather are left at the mercy of cancer-causing agents that invade the system and "turn them on." They begin to multiply, forming large, constantly growing lumps. They are victims of bad information and assume a destructive role in the body.

This is where antineoplastons come in—as a means of relaying positive messages. Forming various combinations of the substance, Dr. Burzynski sends instructions to the cells that can allow them to differentiate or specialize. He seeks to correct the information-processing error and restore the body's normal defense mechanisms. The beauty of the treatment is that harmful drugs, radiation, and surgery are not required. The body virtually heals itself.

A BIOCHEMICAL DEFENSE SYSTEM According to the research done by Dr. Burzynski and others in this country as well as abroad, antineoplastons are components of a biochemical defense system that parallels our immune system. Unlike the immune system, which protects us by destroying invading agents or defective cells, the biochemical defense system protects us by reprogramming, or normalizing, defective cells. Errors in cell programming may lead to such diverse disorders as cancer, benign tumors, certain skin diseases, AIDS, and Parkinson's disease.

EVOLUTION OF A THERAPY How did Stanislaw Burzynski develop this amazing therapy? The doctor's progress in medical research is characterized by a rare ability to look further, to take that extra step onto an untried path and go beyond the status quo. Considering that the doctor was born into a family with a passion for learning, these traits aren't altogether surprising. His parents had university degrees, his father a total of five before retiring as a university professor. Stanislaw followed suit, becoming at age 25 one of Poland's youngest men ever to earn both an M.D. and a Ph.D. He began his research at one of Poland's finest medical schools, the Lublin Medical Academy. Its prestigious faculty provided the mentors he needed to shape his embryonic theories on anticancer defense mechanisms.

The Polish government eventually granted him leave to emigrate to the United States, and by 1970 Dr. Burzynski had become a staff member at Baylor College of Medicine. Since his research had been interrupted by obligatory military service, nearly a decade had passed since he had fixed on the notion that the human body must possess a built-in system to resist cancer and similar diseases. He believed that without this system, no one could hope to ward off the cancer-creating "sea of carcinogens" that surround us. Of course, believing that a natural defense system exists does not explain what it is made up of and how it works, but mentors from his university days offered some clues.

From a former chemistry professor Dr. Burzynski had learned about the information-carrying peptides, which are related to the antineoplastons he had yet to uncover. Other clues had come from Dr. Marian Mazur, professor at the Polish Academy of Science and a widely acclaimed authority in the cybernetic field of science. Cybernetics looks at how systems work; one of its key elements is feedback, which provides a way to control and communicate within a system. If cancer cells become destructive because they have received only bad information, the task is not to kill them but to get the right information to them to make them normal and healthy. Cybernetics provides insight into the nature of improving communications within a system so that the desired information or feedback is properly transmitted. A household thermostat is an example of a feedback device: a tool used to close the gap between an actual result—say, room temperature of 90 degrees—and a desired result—a more comfortable 70 degrees.

Dr. Burzynski concluded that active ingredient of the body's cancer defense system might be found in the family of peptides—small blood proteins—which were known to communicate with and affect the growth of cells. Within that system, these substances could operate as a feedback device to correct the difference between actual cancer cells and the desired healthy cells or to reprogram cancer cells with good information so that they could become constructive and vital instead of pathogenic.

Peptides are a popular subject of modern medical research. Nearly 50 different types have been found that can stimulate cell growth. One, known as peptide T, is attracting attention for its potential in treating AIDS. Dr. Burzynski is thus by no means the only scientist exploring the potency of peptides, but he has been at it longer than most and has achieved findings unique to cancer therapy.

An early discovery involved the level of peptides in advanced cancer patients. Their blood samples revealed only 2 to 3 percent of the amount typically found in healthy bodies—a drastic difference. If peptides, as Dr. Burzynski assumed, played a role in the body's natural defense system, these cancer patients had at some point been disarmed. They were victims of misinformation, since there were not enough peptides to carry good information to the cancer cells.

The next task was to determine exactly what kind of peptides cancerous bodies lack. Burzynski put his doctorate in biochemistry to good use, studying the makeup and structure of the deficient substances and uncovering an interesting effect. When applied to tissue cultures, the peptides missing from cancer patients actually suppressed the growth of human cancer cells.

But while progress was evident, the puzzle was far from solved. It was not enough to know that antineoplastons could carry appropriate information to cancerous cells; it had to be determined how to get them to do it in order to ameliorate tumor growths. Dr. Burzynski turned to his knowledge of systems, cybernetic science, and information theory. The idea of using feedback to adjust and correct an obvious imbalance seemed appropriate to the possible role of antineoplastons in treating cancer.

The Treatment: "Reprogramming" Cancer Cells

Dr. Burzynski's concept constituted a scientific leap, yet it appears amazingly simple in light of the most basic function peptides perform: they transmit information to the cells. Some aim to spur on, others to inhibit, cellular growth—but they all do it by sending messages the body can obey.

Dr. Burzynski likens the process to the use of the alphabet: "It's like having 26 alphabet letters—you can create an infinite variety of words." Using the right "code" becomes the key to reprogramming cancerous cells. Theoretically, it is possible to stop a peptide messenger carrying dangerous, damaging goods and hand over a more beneficent, favorable package for it to deliver instead.

The best time to change the peptide code is when cells are new and immature. Guided by good information, the cells can successfully pass through all the normal stages of development. They can gradually take on the special traits they need to serve different parts of the body, in other words, differentiate. When cells differentiate, they have reached maturity.

Imagine being stuck in childhood or puberty, never given the means to change and grow into a finally functioning adult. This is the state of a cancer cell. It doesn't know how to differentiate and mature, because its genetic code is garbled. In a healthy body with a sufficient level of peptides and antineoplastons, good information is quickly communicated to the cancer cell, and the cell is rendered harmless. But when these levels are low, the cancer cell continues to be victimized by the wrong information. Dr. Burzynski's treatment is aimed at ending the cancer cell's confusion. He puts antineoplastons into the bloodstream to carry the proper genetic code, halt the growth of useless tumors, and encourage cancer cells to differentiate.

Antineoplastons are not foreign substances. Because they appear naturally in the body—and evidently are found at a much higher level in healthy bodies—they don't pose a toxic threat. This fact alone sets Dr. Burzynski's approach miles apart from traditional cancer therapies. Radiation treatments and chemotherapy destroy cancer cells but also destroy any other cells in their path.

Two significant observations have been made about the side effects of antineoplaston treatment. First, most patients experience virtually no side effects. The few that have appeared have been minor, short-lived, and easily controlled, such as skin rashes, chills, and fever. The second and more remarkable observation is that the treatment can actually create positive side effects in decided contrast to traditional medical treatments. Patients have shown increases in white and red blood cell counts, decreases in blood cholesterol, and stimulated skin growth; these and other effects are known to aid the body's natural healing powers. Antineoplaston therapy has tremendous promise not just in theory but in practice.

However, a new medicine or medical treatment is not accepted overnight. The medical and scientific communities as well as certain governmental bodies set rigid testing standards to ensure the safety and effectiveness of every supposed curative. Antineoplastons are no exception.

TESTS AND RESULTS For several decades Dr. Burzynski has been subjecting his theory to the testing procedure required to "prove" its worth, and it is holding up well under pressure. More than 60 percent of the patients treated during the

Burzynski Research Institute's phase I testing showed considerable improvement, whereas the norm is only 3 percent at best.

Each phase of testing has different goals. Phase I is designed to examine any side effects that may occur and to determine proper dosages of the antineoplaston "medicine." Phase II entails a more specific study of whether and how the medicine acts to reduce or eliminate cancerous growth, and phase III would take an even closer look at these issues, among larger groups of people with the same types of cancer.

When phase I clinical trials began, Dr. Burzynski didn't expect much in the way of an anticancer effect. His aim was to find out how much medicine patients should be given, starting with very small doses that could be increased over time. He had no way of knowing but could only suspect which kinds of cancer would respond best to his treatment. What he expected and what he got were two different things.

The results in the best cases of 20 different phase I trials showed significant anticancer activity. In the most successful trial, not only did more than 60 percent of the patients respond to treatment, more than 20 percent remained cancer-free for over 5 years. These patients suffered from some of the most serious and difficult to treat forms of cancer, including advanced lung and bladder cancer, and malignant mesothelioma, a type of cancer that results from asbestos exposure and is especially resistant to traditional medicine.

In phase II trials, patients are grouped according to their basic type of cancer. Depending on how and where those basic types develop in the body, different phase II treatments are tried. For example, in current trials with breast cancer, treatment varies depending on whether the disease has spread to the lungs or to the liver or bones.

In 1992, 24 patients with malignant lymphoma (cancer of the lymphatic system) had been treated in phase II trials. Chemotherapy had failed to help nearly 70 percent of these patients. Only certain forms of this cancer, such as Hodgkin's disease, have ever shown real success from conventional treatment. But with antineoplaston care, 85 percent showed vast improvement.

The most impressive results have been in brain cancers (astrocytoma stages III and IV and glioblastoma) and metastatic cancer of the prostate. In a small phase II trial of astrocytoma conducted by Dr. Burzynski, 20 patients were enrolled. All diagnoses were biopsy confirmed. All but one patient had received (and failed) one or more prior standard therapies. Four patients achieved complete remission and two others partial remission. The responses of 10 patients were classified as objective stabilization (less than 50 percent decrease of tumor size). Since the end of this study in May 1990, some of these patients have achieved partial and even complete remission. Even if they are only preliminary findings, such results are impressive in this type and stage of cancer.

In another phase II study of stage IV prostate cancer refractory to hormonal treatment begun in 1988, two complete and three partial remissions were reported in a group of 14 patients. Seven patients obtained objective stabilization.

From a 1997 interview, Dr. Burzynski offers us more of the clinic's success stories: "When we started our program, we concentrated on the type of cancers which are uniformly deadly, such terrible types of malignant tumors as primary malignant brain tumors that are known in medical terminology as astrocytoma, glioblastoma, medulla blastoma. These tumors are uniformly deadly. Practically everybody who develops high grade astrocytoma or glioblastoma dies from the disease. There's no cure available, and the death comes quickly, usually within a year.

"We concentrated on the treatment of such highly malignant tumors to prove a point that antineoplastons work. Otherwise, if there are some other treatments available, we could be accused of perhaps using these additional treatments which could make the tumors disappear. But those treatments do not exist. If we are able to eliminate highly malignant brain tumors by the use of antineoplastons, these are the first cases in medical history of this happening. Since we concentrate our efforts on the treatment of such bad malignant brain tumors, of course, most of our statistics concentrate on these tumors. We already finished three clinical trials, phase II trials, in such malignant brain tumors. And we found that the success rate of the patients who are responding to the treatment is between 67 to 80 percent among these trials, which means that only 20 percent to 33 percent of the patients do not have any proper response to the treatment.

"We already have long-term follow-up for some of these patients, including 8-year follow-up when the tumors disappeared and did not come back. We can say that we were able to not only decrease and eliminate these tumors, but also cure a number of patients from these tumors. We continue to have clinical trials in different types of malignant brain tumors. Currently, we have over 20 different clinical trials in the area of malignant brain tumors, and we are accepting the patients through such trials. If somebody is interested we can, of course, offer him the treatment, and then he can go back home and continue the treatment back home under the care of his doctor.

"The other areas where we have success is the treatment of non-Hodgkin's lymphoma. Certain kinds of non-Hodgkin's lymphoma respond well to chemotherapy and radiation. But we usually see the types which do not respond to these other treatment modalities, such as low grade lymphoma or cases of intermediate or high grade lymphoma, which already fail to respond to chemotherapy and radiation, including bone marrow transplantation. We already have a number of successful treatments in this area, and we are conducting a number of different clinical trials. We can accept patients who would like to be treated. We don't yet have statistics because we did not finish any of these clinical trials yet. We hope to have statistics in various lymphomas perhaps within the next 6 months.

"We see encouraging results in the treatment of cancers of gastrointestinal tract. Again, we see optimistic results in the treatment of pancreatic cancer, colon cancer, stomach cancer, and cancer of the esophagus. However, the number of cases is still too small to jump to a conclusion. We have clinical trials in each of these areas. Some of these patients are treated by simply taking capsules of anti-neoplastons. Some other patients are required to take intravenous infusions.

"Another exciting area is the treatment of kidney cancer and cancer of the bladder [although] the success rate is rather small. We have success in certain types of lung cancers, such as large cell type. The other type is non-small types, especially a large cell undifferentiated carcinoma of the lung. But in the other types of lung cancer, it still is hard to tell if you can successfully help these patients.

"In breast cancer, we have few clinical trials, and in certain cases we see successes. In other cases, we see failure. We still have problems when we have extensive liver involvement or lung involvement.

"In other types of cancers, we don't know whether we can have any success or not because the number of patients is too small. There are certain types of malignancies such as sarcomas, for instance, malignant melanoma, where we don't yet have sufficient numbers to come to a conclusion. And there are certain types of cancer where we know that we are not getting good results and we don't accept such patients. For instance, in acute leukemia in children, in Hodgkin's disease, in cancer of the testicles, we usually don't have good results, and we do not accept such patients to our program.

"Of course, there's still a lot to learn, and we hope that as time goes by we accumulate a lot of scientific data which we will prove in which types of cancer antineoplastons work best, and will also prove which types of cancers they don't work at all. It will take some time, but we are committed to continuing our research to have the best results possible."

THE CLINIC Most of Dr. Burzynski's patients, during all phases of testing, are treated without being hospitalized. Checkups are conducted every day or every other day for the first 2 weeks and then less frequently depending on the improvement of the individual patient. The Burzynski Clinic in southwest Houston operates on an outpatient basis, with the average period of care ranging from 6 months to 3 years.

There are certain insurance companies that evaluated Dr. Burzynski's program and decided to cover practically every patient who is coming for the treatment. Conversely, other insurance companies will not pay for the Burzynski treatment. In most cases it depends on the patient's policy. Most of the patients who are coming to the Burzynski Research Institute are in very advanced stages of cancer; they've tried everything possible. Many of them are devastated by chemotherapy or radiation therapy. They may easily catch pneumonia or have bleeding or some other medical complications which require hospital admission. But according to Dr. Burzynski, the great majority of his patients can take treatment at home, and can lead normal lives and go back to work soon after they start treatment.

The antineoplastons that have been responsible for the dramatic results mentioned above are manufactured in Dr. Burzynski's plant in Stafford, Texas. According to Dr. Burzynski they are considered a form of chemotherapy since a chemotherapeutic agent is technically any "organized mixture of chemicals that fight a malignancy." However, they do not have the devastating side effects of the traditional class of chemotherapeutic drugs because they are formulations that are identical to proteins that are present in the body. Natural antineoplastons are small proteins isolated from human urine or blood. Synthetic antineoplastons are chemically identical to the natural proteins but are synthetically derived. Synthetics are easier and cheaper to manufacture and are even more efficacious in treating specific cancers such as brain and prostate cancer. Other cancers, though, respond better to the natural substances.

Dr. Burzynski uses a deliberately coordinated assortment of antineoplastons, both synthetic and natural, as the case requires. When he thinks it is appropriate, he refers patients for other types of treatment (chemotherapy, radiation, or surgery) to augment the antineoplaston injection or capsule therapy. While he has had little success with cancer of the testicles and childhood leukemia, he has had astounding results with brain tumors, malignant lymphomas, and cancer of the bladder and prostate.

Other groups have reproduced and are expanding Dr. Burzynski's preclinical work, including researchers at the Medical College of Georgia, the Imperial College of Science and Technology of London, the University of Kurume Medical School in Japan, the University of Turin Medical School in Italy, the Shandong Medical Academy in the People's Republic of China, and the Uniformed Services University of the Health Sciences in the U.S.

Some of the most exciting preclinical research was reported by Dr. Dvorit Samid from the Uniformed Services University of Health Sciences in Bethesda, Maryland. She reported that "Antineoplaston AS2-1 profoundly inhibits oncogene expression and the proliferation of malignant cells without exhibiting any toxicity toward normal cells." Dr. Samid explained that AS2-1 does not kill cancer cells, rather it reprograms them to behave like normal cells. Clinical results of antineoplastons in patients with cancer refractory to other forms of therapy included reports of complete remissions from Japan and the U.S. in inoperable metastatic ovarian carcinoma and advanced stage prostate cancer, respectively.

ATTACKS FROM THE MEDICAL ESTABLISHMENT During the past several years, there have been efforts made by various medical agencies skeptical of the Burzynski treatment to get Dr. Burzynski's license revoked. In response to these efforts,

Dr. Burzynski says, "The efforts against us are tremendous. And I did not expect, when I started this program, that I would be harassed mercilessly by the FDA [Food and Drug Administration] and by some other agencies. Currently, we enjoy peace at the state level. Whatever battles we fought seem to be over. Our main problem now is with the FDA despite the fact that I am approved by the FDA to conduct so many clinical trials. Every patient seen by us is approved by the FDA. The FDA would like to put us out of business without any concern about what would happen to the patients. They are not really worried that the patients who are receiving treatment now will die if they put me out of business. I don't think that effort will succeed because we think and strongly believe that we are doing the right thing; we are saving the lives of many American people, and we will continue."

Looking to the Future

Prevention is the focus of several studies Dr. Burzynski has undertaken. In one study, two groups of mice were exposed to the main cancer-causing agent from cigarette smoke. One group was given food containing an antineoplaston preparation; 80 percent of these mice avoided lung cancer. Among the group that was not given antineoplastons, 100 percent got the disease.

The next step in this research is to use antineoplastons as part of a preventive treatment among humans. Dr. Burzynski believes that this would best be done with apparently healthy individuals who have low levels of antineoplastons. Smokers may well benefit in this respect since they fit this requirement and are therefore prime candidates for cancer and so are in dire need of a preventive program.

The possibilities of Dr. Burzynski's therapy appear endless. Antineoplastons correct (i.e., stop) cancer development in a way the body understands and easily tolerates. Even with phase I treatments, which aren't intended to produce maximum benefits, some patients have emerged cancer-free.

Of course, successful outcomes result from traditional approaches as well. Careful surgery can aid recovery, and chemotherapy has had particular success with rarer types of cancer such as Hodgkin's disease and childhood leukemia. The regrettable part is that these "answers" to cancer can also cause more harm. Typical and devastating side effects accompany methods to which many patients never respond. Surgery and radiation can lead to serious damage to organs and tissues, and radiation and chemotherapy may drastically undermine the ability of the immune system to fight off even the simplest bacteria and toxins.

What Dr. Burzynski offers is an opportunity to use and strengthen the body's natural defense system. The need to explore and develop antineoplastons and other safe remedies will continue as long as people are exposed to air pollution, radiation, chemicals, ultraviolet rays, and the like.

The Burzynski Research Institute is currently conducting Food and Drug Administration-authorized clinical trials of antineoplastons in the treatment of cancer as well as other diseases. For more information on this therapy, contact:

The Burzynski Research Institute
Suite 200
9432 Old Katy Road
Houston, Texas, 77055-6330
7213-335-5697
E-mail: info@burzynskiclinic.com

41

Cancer Therapy: Whole–Body Approaches

Whole-body therapies involve a combination of approaches to cancer treatment and prevention, including diet and nutrition, herbs, immune enhancement, and detoxification.

Dr. Joseph Issels' Whole-Body ("Ganzheit") Approach

Trained as a traditional surgeon, the late Dr. Joseph Issels became aware of the limitations of orthodox therapy when he began treating cancer patients. He became convinced that the successful treatment of cancer required a return to the whole-body approach to the disease. As he once said, "cancer is not just a local disease confined to the particular place in the body where the tumor manifests itself but is a general disease of the whole body."

Based on this approach to cancer, Dr. Issels developed a broad-spectrum therapy to restore and regenerate the body's natural defense mechanisms that complement the specific measures of traditional medicine directed at the elimination of the localized tumor. With this approach, Dr. Issels achieved a degree of success in treating his cancer patients that is unparalleled in traditional medicine.

THE DISCOVERY How did it all begin? In his early years of medicine, Dr. Issels put some of his theories into practice in what he would later call a "*Ganzheit*" or "whole-body" approach to healing. He required that all his patients have infected teeth or tonsils removed, since he strongly believed that they release poisons into the body which lower natural resistance and trigger disease. Proper diet was also considered critical. The usual foodstuffs had to be replaced by biologically adequate ones adjusted to fit the actual organic conditions of individual patients. Chronically ill patients usually had to receive lactobacillus acidophilus, a cultured milk product which served as a ferment substitute to compensate for a loss of efficiency in their digestive systems. Tobacco, alcohol, coffee, tea, and other substances the doctor considered harmful were banned. Whenever possible, long-standing emotional stress was relieved or eliminated. In the meantime, the doctor went ahead with treatment of the particular diseased organ, confident that he was also addressing the root cause of the patient's sickness.

Dr. Issels was soon getting remarkable results with this combination of *Ganzheit* therapy, homeopathy, dietary control, and other therapeutic techniques. His practice became the largest in town, although it did not make him a rich man, since his fees were low and he treated for free those who were unable to pay.

Yet these successes contrasted grimly with his inability to help cancer patients. He knew that his colleagues were equally baffled by the disease, but that knowledge did not ease his frustration. Surgery and radiation seemed to bring temporary improvement, but it was clear that they did not get at the cause of the cancer and could not protect the patient from further occurrences. Surely, Dr. Issels thought, there had to be a way of applying the principles of *Ganzheit* therapy to the treatment of cancer to produce not just remissions but genuine cures. There had to be an alternative to disfiguring surgery, toxic chemicals, and poisonous radiation.

USING HISTORY AS A GUIDE

The antipathy Dr. Issels had felt toward cancer in his early years became almost an obsession with the disease. He read everything he could find on cancer and in the process became an expert in medical history. He discovered that cancer, contrary to popular opinion, was not a modern affliction but had been observed by Chinese and Sumerian physicians and described in manuscripts dating back 3,000 years before Christ as resulting from a malfunction in the body's regulatory mechanisms that was to be treated with acupuncture and drugs.

Hippocrates (460–377 B.C.), the founder of Western medicine, was the first to use the word "carcinoma" in referring to malignant tumors, which he believed arose from a "separation of the humors" (blood, bile, and phlegm) and was to be treated with surgery and drugs. But what Dr. Issels found especially noteworthy was Hippocrates' recommendation that the entire body be detoxified and that cancer patients be put on a special diet. Further research showed that for the ancient Greeks, *diata*, or "diet," referred to far more than what a patient was to eat or drink. The term was closer in meaning to "way of life" or "lifestyle" and strongly suggested abstinence from anything that might be spiritually as well as physically harmful.

The Roman physician Claudius Galen (131–200 A.D.), the founder of scientific physiology, whose authority had gone unchallenged in Western medicine for over 1,000 years, had also turned his attention to cancer, as Dr. Issels soon discovered. The doctor's interest became more than academic when he read Galen's opinion that cancer is a disease of the entire body, not confined to the site of the tumor.

Moving forward in time, Dr. Issels encountered the world-famous doctor of the Renaissance, Philippus Aureolus Theophrastus Bombast von Hohenheim, better known as Paracelsus, who also felt that the physician's role in treating cancer and other diseases was not to interfere with the body but rather to stimulate the healing processes nature had provided to correct the imbalances in the body that result in illness. Dr. Issels also encountered the pioneer surgeon Ambroise Pare, who shared Paracelsus' view of cancer as a disease of the entire body, and the French thinker Rene Descartes, who thought cancer was caused by abnormalities in the lymph glands. He pored over the work of Percival Potts, the 18th century British physician who was among the first to describe cancer as an "occupational" malignancy when he noticed an abnormally high rate of cancer of the scrotum in young chimney sweeps. In short, no one who might have something useful to say about cancer escaped Issels' scrutiny.

The work of Dr. Edward Jenner, the English physician who had developed a vaccination and checked the scourge of smallpox, seemed to offer special promise in regard to both theory and practice. Although Dr. Jenner had not been successful in treating cancer, he had produced vaccines which had shown promising results against other disorders. Equally important for Dr. Issels, his British predecessor believed that cancer stemmed from inadequacies in the immune mechanisms and that it could have a fatal effect only when the body's natural immunity had broken down completely.

SEARCHING FOR A VACCINE

Following this line of thought, Dr. Issels searched for a vaccine that would bolster the body's immune system to the point where it could fight back successfully against cancer. Neoblastine, a vaccine he developed by culturing cancer tissues in a controlled medium many times over a long period to insure safety, seemed to offer some promise. After testing the vaccine on laboratory animals, he tried it on a terminally ill lung cancer patient, together with his *Ganzheit* therapy involving extraction of infected teeth and tonsils, and strict dietary control. Although the patient lived 3 months longer than expected, the results were ambiguous, since there had been no cure and it was impossible to attribute the patient's improvement to any single factor in the treatment.

Another case, on the surface equally disappointing, occurred when Dr. Issels agreed to treat a woman with an enormous uterine tumor who had already been given up on by her doctors. Heeding her husband's pleas, Dr. Issels agreed to see her but he could do nothing beyond prescribing painkillers and ordering a change in her diet. Nonetheless, the fact that Dr. Issels had undertaken to treat her gave the woman a much better outlook. Until her death two months later, she maintained steadfastly that Dr. Issels' treatments had freed her of pain that drugs had been unable to eliminate.

These patients and others all succumbed to disease and left Dr. Issels little cause for optimism. Yet these cases did serve to convince him that *Ganzheit* therapy had been helpful and to confirm his long-standing belief that cancer is not a mysterious ailment but a chronic systemic illness, to be treated like other diseases of this kind. The tumor, he became convinced, was merely a late-stage symptom, accidentally triggered off but able to grow only in what he described as a "tumor milieu," the result of prior damage to organs and organ systems, especially those involved in maintaining the body's resistance to disease. The disease would never gain a foothold unless the body's defenses were depleted.

Once it had gained a foothold, conventional treatments, Dr. Issels decided, could usually provide only temporary relief. While surgery, by removing large masses of tumor, might stimulate the immune system to regenerate, it was not likely to provide a cure by itself, since the operation could not get at the underlying cause of the cancer. Radiation and chemotherapy, while initially successful, frequently provided only temporary relief. Nonetheless, Dr. Issels did not offer *Ganzheit* therapy as a substitute for the usual treatments but as a supplement which he believed would make the conventional therapies more effective by rehabilitating the entire patient, not just attacking the tumor.

COMBINING TRADITIONAL AND UNCONVENTIONAL METHODS

As the number of his cancer patients continued to grow, Dr. Issels began specializing in that disease. In 1950, he took charge of a 30-bed cancer unit at a small suburban clinic, where he put in 17-hour days, treating patients with a combination of traditional and unconventional methods. Surgery was used to remove large tumors. Drugs were administered to improve the functioning of various organs, especially the liver and kidneys, which usually are severely damaged in advanced cancer patients. The body was detoxified through the use of purifying drugs; mild purgatives; a diet high in fruit, vegetables, and grains; and the consumption of large amounts of water, juice, and herbal teas. Homeopathic remedies were used along with vaccines to stimulate antibody production.

Dr. Issels' cure statistics were not numerically impressive, but there was no lack of patients for treatment. Those who came to him were not in the early stages of the disease but were, for the most part, patients whom the medical establishment had been unable to help. For them, Dr. Issels offered the proverbial "last, best, hope" of staying alive, a hope he was sometimes able to fulfill in ways that bordered on the miraculous.

THE TREATMENT Although about 90 percent of the patients he saw had already been designated as incurable and beyond the help of orthodox medicine, Dr. Issels continued conventional treatment if it was possible and appropriate. He viewed *Ganzheit* therapy as a supplement to make these treatments more effective rather than as a substitute for them.

TONSILLECTOMY AND TOOTH EXTRACTION

As mentioned, in *Ganzheit* therapy, patients part with infected teeth and tonsils, since Dr. Issels viewed these as sites of infection that place an unnecessary burden on the immune system and act to lower the body's general defenses against disease. Dental amalgams also are removed.

DIET AND NUTRITION

Diet is a critical component of *Ganzheit* therapy. Most meats are avoided, since meat is difficult for advanced cancer patients to digest and is usually filled with hormones, antibiotics, and pesticides that place further strain on the body. The recommended diet is primarily vegetarian, focusing on organically grown whole grains, fruits, and vegetables, supplemented by enzymes, minerals, and vitamins, with emphasis on A, B-complex, C, and E. Yogurt and acidophilus supplements are used to eliminate abnormal intestinal flora.Serum activator is administered to bring the metabolism of red blood cells up to normal levels, allowing the release of additional hemoglobin and thus increasing the supply of oxygen to the body's cells.

Organ extracts are supplied to help repair secondary damage to organs and improve their functioning, while a high fluid intake backed up with herbal extracts is used to detoxify the body; improve kidney, lymph, and liver functions; and bolster the excretory systems.

PSYCHOTHERAPY

Since *Ganzheit* therapy entails the treatment of the entire patient, individual and group psychotherapy is an important element. Through this treatment, Dr. Issels hoped not only to help the patient come to terms with the disease, but also to remove, or at least alleviate, the psychic stress which he felt could help bring on cancer and hinder its cure.

IMMUNOTHERAPY

A major component of the treatment is a highly sophisticated form of immunotherapy, geared specifically to fighting cancer and supported, where necessary, by surgery, radiation, and chemotherapy. This immunotherapy involves a twofold approach: specific immunization against the particular type of cancer and a general effort to augment the body's natural immune responses.

"Specific immunization works on a well-tried principle," Dr. Issels wrote in his 1975 book, *Cancer: A Second Opinion*. "Once a particular cancer antigen has been identified, it is administered under conditions most favorable for the induction of an immune response that will destroy cancer cells bearing that antigen. This is really no more than an extension of the standard vaccination technique against any infectious disease."

For specific immunization against the tumor, Dr. Issels often administered a vaccine shown to cause regression of malignant tumors that was developed by Dr. Franz Gerlach, a Viennese scientist. Other tumor-specific immunization was effected with standard non-toxic vaccines such as Centanit for carcinoma, Sarkogen for sarcoma, and Lymphogran for Hodgkin's disease.

General immunotherapy is used to bolster the patient's overall immunity and to destroy the "tumor milieu" that makes it possible for the cancer to sustain itself and grow. Here the primary means of attack consists of autovaccines prepared from extracts from the patient's own teeth and tonsils as well as other nontoxic vaccines designed to boost general resistance to disease.

OZONE THERAPY

Ozone therapy, although not a direct aid to the immune system, is also used as a means of increasing the oxygen supply to the cells and destroying viruses and bacteria in the bloodstream. This method of systematically exposing portions of the patient's blood supply to medically pure ozone is almost unknown in the United States but has been used against blood-borne infectious diseases in Germany for more than 25 years. Dr. Issels found the therapy to be effective in purging the blood of oxidation-resistant pesticides and other toxins.

HYPERPYREXIA (FEVER INDUCTION)

Hyperpyrexia, homeopathy's long-sanctioned induction of fever, is also used in much the same way as ozone therapy to make life uncomfortable for the tumor. Once a month patients get a "fever shot," which can raise the body temperature as high as 105 degrees Fahrenheit, where it stays for 2s or so while the patient is under constant medical supervision. In the evening the body's temperature is lowered again.

While Dr. Issels may not have shared the enthusiasm of the ancient Greek physician who remarked, "Give me a chance to produce fever, and I can cure all illness," he knew that fever was a natural reaction of the body to foreign invaders and that it made these invaders more vulnerable to attack. He also discovered that the number of disease-destroying leukocytes in the patient's bloodstream rose enormously after each fever shot and that the patients uniformly reported feeling much better afterward, as their bodies were detoxified.

Even localized heating of the tumor area, Dr. Issels discovered, can have effects which, while not as spectacular, were clearly beneficial.

THE RESULTS Three independent studies of Dr. Issels' medical records conducted by highly reputed experts have confirmed a 16.6 percent cure rate among the terminal patients treated with *Ganzheit* therapy, a figure that no doctor or hospital anywhere in the world comes close to matching. The other alternative therapies mentioned in this section have success rates (5-year complete remissions) ranging from 5 to 15 percent.

To understand the significance of this figure, it is necessary to recall that all these patients were terminal, already given up on by conventional medicine. In the United States, for example, such a patient has virtually no chance of survival, let alone of cure.

This distinction between survival and cure is also crucial. For conventional medicine, "cure" simply means that the cancer patient has survived 5 years after the initial diagnosis. It says nothing about the state of the patient during that time or at its end. Dr. Issels used a different standard.

While even Dr. Issels did not think of *Ganzheit* therapy as the be-all and end-all, his indisputable successes bring one face-to-face with some uncomfortable facts. The tremendous advances in the development of symptom-oriented treatments, which include surgery, radiation, and chemotherapy, have been of benefit to some cancer patients, but these benefits appear to have peaked in the mid-1950s. Notwithstanding the stunning array of new high-tech surgical procedures and chemotherapeutic drugs, traditional medicine has not been able to obtain more than a slight increase in the survival rates of patients. Despite the expenditure of billions of dollars in the war on cancer, there is growing evidence of the limitations of conventional therapies and evidence that statistical manipulations have inflated the amount of actual progress.

Of course, the shortcomings of conventional therapies do not by themselves constitute proof of the accuracy and efficacy of Dr. Issels' theories and methods. But at the very least these limitations should indicate that it is time to take a long, hard look at conventional therapies and the theories behind them.

Dr. Issels continued his fight against cancer throughout his life. In the years before he died in 1998, when he was well into his 90s, Dr. Issels and colleagues at the Centro Hospitalario Internacional Pacifico, S.A. (CHIPSA) Center for Integrative Medicine refined a program that combined his comprehensive immunotherapy with the similarly holistic approach developed by the late Dr. Max Gerson, another leader in the alternative medicine field. (See the next section for a full discussion of Dr. Gerson's approach to cancer.) The Issels-Gerson Combination Therapy is now being offered at CHIPSA, a modern, full-service 70-bed hospital in Tijuana. Several program plans are available, including supportive therapy, full intensive therapy, advanced therapy, and therapy with hyperbaric oxygen.

Dr. Max Gerson's "Environmental" Approach to Cancer Therapy

With the advance of technology, an ever-increasing number of new substances are introduced into the environment each year. These substances range from chemicals, pesticides, and drugs to the byproducts of nuclear weapons and energy. There are also new agricultural and manufacturing techniques such as genetically engineered microorganisms and food irradiation. Until relatively recently the human body, which has evolved over thousands of years, seemed to do a fairly good job of adapting to the changes within the environment. Within the past century, however, the rate at which people have been exposed to new and toxic substances has accelerated so rapidly that the result has been a breakdown in the body's natural adaptation and defensive processes. Certain physicians view this breakdown as one of the major contributing factors to many of today's most dreaded diseases, especially cancer.

The theory that cancer is triggered by environmental factors that deplete the body's natural immunity and defensive capabilities is not a new one. In fact, the late Dr. Max Gerson took an "environmental" approach to cancer therapy more than 60 years ago. The cornerstone of Dr. Gerson's therapy is detoxification of the body through diet designed to rehabilitate the body's natural immunity and healing processes.

Although Dr. Gerson died in 1959, his work is being carried on by his daughter, Charlotte Gerson, in the Gerson clinic located on the western coast of Mexico about 30 minutes south of San Diego. Dr. Gerson was eulogized by Dr. Albert Schweitzer, whose wife Gerson cured of lung tuberculosis in the 1930s. Schweitzer wrote in a letter to Ms. Gerson, "I see in him one of the most eminent geniuses in the history of medicine. Many of his basic ideas have been adopted without having his name connected with them. Yet he has achieved more than seemed possible under adverse conditions. He leaves a legacy which commands attention and which will assure him his due place. Those whom he cured will now attest to the truth of his ideas."

THE DISCOVERY Dr. Gerson was born in Germany in 1881. The roots of his work date to his early days as a young intern and resident before World War I. At that time he was suffering from severe migraine headaches, which were considered incurable. But Dr. Gerson, after a fruitless search through the medical literature, turned to nutrition to change his body chemistry and gain relief. He was already convinced that contamination of foods by artificial fertilizers and processing had a deleterious effect on body chemistry. He felt that by restoring normal metabolism through a healthy diet, he might be able to improve his migraine condition, and so he started to experiment on himself with certain foods. His first experiment was with milk. He thought that milk, being the first food, was something that even a baby could handle, so that his body should have been able to utilize it properly. But when he drank nothing but milk, his headaches became worse. Then it occurred to him that milk is not normally consumed by adult animals other than humans anywhere in nature and that maybe milk is a foreign substance rather than a natural nutrient in the adult human diet.

Dr. Gerson decided to conduct his next experiments using foods that were more suited for the human type of build and body chemistry, namely, fruits and vegetables. (Contrary to popular belief, human physiology is basically vegetarian and not carnivorous. The human intestinal tract measures 30 feet in length and as such is unsuited to the proper digestion and elimination of meat.) When Dr. Gerson found that he did not experience migraines when he ate nothing but grains, fresh fruits, and vegetables, he began experimenting with single foods to discern their particular effect on his physiology. He found, for instance, that when he ate cooked foods, they often did not agree with him. But it turned out that it wasn't the cooking but the added salt that made the difference. When he ate the same cooked foods without salt, he was able to handle them very well.

Little by little Dr. Gerson began to piece together a menu of foods that he could safely consume, together with a list of foods that would almost invariably give him migraines within a few minutes of his eating them. In the end he arrived at a diet very high in fresh fruits and vegetables and freshly prepared vegetable and fruit juices and very low in fats. Later, in his treatment of tuberculosis patients, Dr. Gerson would use a small amount of raw, fresh unsalted butter because it is a good source of the phospholipids which form an important part of the body's defense mechanism, but otherwise the diet was largely free of animals fats, especially cooked fats, and totally free of meats and cooked animal proteins of any sort.

By the early 1920s, Dr. Gerson had succeeded in completely curing himself of migraines with his special diet. He then started extending his findings to patients who came to him suffering from migraines. They too benefited.

Eventually, although by accident, Dr. Gerson began to use his "Migraine Diet" in the treatment of tuberculosis as well. His daughter, Charlotte, relates how this occurred:"One time, a patient came to him suffering from migraines and was given what he called his 'Migraine Diet.' When the patient came back after 3 or 4 weeks, he told Dr. Gerson that along with his migraines, he also had been suffering from lupus vulgaris, a form of skin tuberculosis, and that with the diet, not only had his migraines disappeared but the lupus had also begun to heal. Dr. Gerson found this almost impossible to believe, because he had learned that lupus was really an incurable condition. But there was the proof before his eyes. He saw that the lesion was healing, and he verified that it had been properly diagnosed and that there had been bacteriological studies showing that, in fact, the man had skin tuberculosis.

"After that, he was able to cure many other patients with skin tuberculosis. This therapy was later verified in large experiments in Munich, involving 450 terminal or incurable cases of skin tuberculosis treated with his Gerson dietary therapy. The treatment was shown to cure 447. From there Dr. Gerson felt that if tuberculosis could be influenced by nutrition, then why only skin tuberculosis —why shouldn't other forms of tuberculosis respond? He applied this same dietary treatment to people with lung tuberculosis, bone tuberculosis, kidney tuberculosis, etc. One of the most famous patients he had at that time was the wife of Albert Schweitzer, who had contracted TB in the tropics. She had been given up because her TB had spread to both lung fields and was quite extensive. Well, among others, she too recovered and lived many, many years, until age 80 or so."

As a result of this healing, Drs. Gerson and Schweitzer became friends and remained so throughout their lives. Dr. Schweitzer followed the progress of the Gerson therapy as it was later applied to a wide variety of diseases, and when he developed adult diabetes, he found relief through Dr. Gerson's treatment. Unfortunately, the American medical establishment has never shared Dr. Schweitzer's high opinion of Dr. Gerson. Instead of being praised, he was persecuted and harassed. Today, more than 40 years after Dr. Gerson's death in 1959, his therapy remains on the American Cancer Society's "Unproven Methods" list.

THE TREATMENT Before discussing Dr. Gerson's therapy, it is important to look at its theoretical basis. Like the other alternative cancer approaches discussed in this chapter, it differs fundamentally from the traditional medical treatment in that it deals with cancer as a generalized disease rather than a localized one. More specifically, Dr. Gerson's therapy aims at rebalancing and revitalizing the cancer patient's entire physiology in order to rectify this systemic disorder. It looks for the cause of the illness and works to correct it, thereby causing the cancer to regress and preventing it from recurring.

According to Dr. Curtis Hesse, former director of the Gerson Therapy Center (in a personal correspondence to Charlotte Gerson), "Ironically, the main problem we actually have in this treatment is not always cancer or disease but the other medications and treatments that the patients have already undergone. In cancer therapy, we do not as a general rule accept any patient who has undergone chemotherapy. From past experience, we know that liver damage and damage to other organs, as well as the immune system, have been such that they do well for a 2- to 3-week period but then go downhill."

The core of Gerson therapy is a regimen consisting primarily of a salt- and fat-free diet of organically grown fresh fruits and vegetables, which are usually served raw or as juices. The primary objective of the diet is to detoxify the body and rebalance the whole metabolism, not simply to eliminate the symptoms of the disease. "The treatment has to penetrate deeply to correct all vital processes," said Dr. Gerson. "When general metabolism is restored, we can again influence the functioning of all organs, tissues, and cells though it."

LIVER THERAPY

Dr. Gerson placed particular importance on the condition of the liver, which is a primary regulator of metabolism. According to Dr. Gerson: "The problem of the liver was and still is partly misunderstood and partly neglected. The metabolism and its concentration in the liver should be put in the foreground, not the cancer as a symptom. There, the outcome of cancer is determined as the clinically favorable results, failures, and autopsies clearly demonstrate. There the sentence will be passed—whether the tumors can be killed, dissolved, absorbed, or eliminated, and finally, whether the body can be restored.

"The progress of the disease depends on whether and to what extent the liver can be restored."

The liver's many functions, coupled with its constant interaction with the other organs of the body, give it a crucial role to play in the maintenance of health. Dr. Gerson and many other scientists have noted that in all degenerative diseases, including cancer, there are varying degrees of liver dysfunction and deterioration. Fortunately, however, while the liver is not easily destroyed and liver damage may not even be detected until liver function has been greatly impaired, the liver is also one of the organs that has the greatest capacity for regeneration. Consequently, the restoration of the liver is a significant objective of Dr. Gerson's diet (se below).

Dr. Gerson's liver therapy is multifaceted. First, animal proteins are eliminated or greatly reduced in the diet because they have been found to interfere with liver therapy and impede the body's detoxification. The ideal diet for patients on liver therapy, as mentioned above, is low in salt and fat, and high in potassium and fresh fruits and vegetables, mostly in juice form. The juice is always prepared freshly and is not mixed with other medications that could alter the pH and thereby decrease its efficacy. Restoration of the liver, which may take from 6 to 18 months, depending on the severity of the illness, allows it to detoxify the body and produce its own oxidative enzymes.

Other aspects of liver therapy include liver injections, and lubile and pancreatin tablets. The liver injections are composed of liver extract and are given daily for 4 to 6 months. They, too, provide important vitamins, minerals, and enzymes that aid in restoring the liver to its proper functioning. These liver injections are usually combined with vitamin B_{12} injections, which Dr. Gerson believed are important for proper protein synthesis. Cancer patients are often unable to combine amino acids properly in order to form proteins within their bodies.

Lubile (defatted bile powder from young calves) was used more frequently in the earlier stages of the therapy; it is not used for most patients today. However, it is beneficial in cases where the liver is extremely damaged and the whole bile duct system is impaired.

Pancreatin tablets are given during and after the detoxification program is completed as a backup source of digestive enzymes, since those are also deficient in most cancer patients.

According to Dr. Gerson, patients on the therapy actually begin to break down, assimilate, and eliminate cancer tumors. This is accomplished when the repaired liver is adequately producing oxidative enzymes, the general detoxification process (of which the liver is a critical part) is active, and potassium levels throughout the body are adequate.

COFFEE ENEMAS

During the period when the body is killing, absorbing, and eliminating the tumor, detoxification is of the utmost importance. Dr. Gerson admitted that in the early stages of development, the therapy did not contain adequate detoxification techniques. "After a tumor was killed," he says, "the patient did not die of cancer but of a serious intoxication with 'coma hepaticum' (liver shock) caused by absorption of necrotic cancer tissue."

Thus, in addition to the other cleansing aspects of the therapy, Dr. Gerson began to prescribe frequent coffee enemas, which at the outset of treatment can be given as often as every 4 hours. This prescription derives from the work of two German researchers who found that caffeine administered rectally causes an opening of the bile ducts, releasing accumulated toxins and causing an increased production of bile, which flushes out these toxins. After these enemas, Dr. Gerson noticed that patients were often relieved of pain such as headaches, fevers, and nausea and could easily discontinue sedation. On the other hand, Dr. Gerson noted that coffee taken orally seemed to have exactly the opposite effect: It caused the stomach to go into spasm and produce a "soaping" over or contraction of the bile ducts. Hence, while regular coffee enemas are an indispensable part of Gerson therapy, drinking coffee is discouraged.

Gar Hildebrand, president of the Gerson Research Organization, tells us more:

"These enemas have been used by thousands of cancer patients, outside the realm of traditional medical care, because they work. Boiled coffee in retention enemas stimulates the liver's enzyme system, which in turn causes great relief from pain in cancer patients. The liver has more than a thousand documented medical functions. When we help it work better and faster, a cancer patient's overall physiological condition changes, sometimes within hours and certainly within the first several weeks of treatment. You have a whole different person. People come off gurneys and out of beds, excruciating chronic pain is eased, and addiction to morphine is broken.

REESTABLISHING POTASSIUM LEVELS

Muscles, the brain, and the liver normally have much higher levels of potassium than of sodium. Early in his research, however, Dr. Gerson noted that in cancer patients this ratio is reversed; that is, he found that sodium is elevated in cancer cells and that in the ailing body, potassium is often inactive and/or improperly utilized. He felt that at the beginning chronic disease is caused by the loss of potassium from the cell system. Accordingly, another primary objective of Gerson therapy is to reestablish proper levels of potassium in the body. Because of the specific relationship between sodium and potassium, in which an increase in one mineral causes a decrease in the other and vice versa, one of the first things Dr. Gerson advocated was the elimination of salt and sodium-rich foods from the diet.

Additionally, all patients on Gerson therapy immediately begin receiving large amounts of a potassium solution which Dr. Gerson developed after 300 experiments. The potassium compound he used, which is still used at the Gerson clinic, is a combination of potassium gluconate, potassium acetate, and potassium phosphate monobasic. This is administered in the form of a 10 percent potassium solution, which is added to juices 10 times daily in 4-teaspoon doses. The potassium solution is never added to the liver juice because Dr. Gerson believed that it can alter the juice's pH, thereby decreasing its efficacy. After a month, the amount is decreased by about half. The fluid retention and edema (caused by a sodium overabundance) is usually the first thing to disappear when patients are given high amounts of potassium in juices.

Dr. Gerson noted that even in a healthy person it is very difficult to restore potassium deficiencies. In seriously ill people, it may take as long as a year or two before normal levels in major organs are reestablished.

In patients suffering from dehydration, potassium is added to the fluids therapeutically administered in the form of a GKI (glucose, potassium, insulin) solution. According to Ms. Gerson, this solution is not specific to Gerson therapy but is recognized and utilized by the American medical establishment in general. "Dr. Demetrio Sodi-Pallares, a world-renowned cardiologist from Mexico City," says Ms. Gerson, "very much recommends this solution." He agreed with Dr. Gerson that disease is systemic or metabolic. His own research in heart disease has shown that it is not a disease of the heart but a metabolic disease that must be treated with a high-potassium, low-sodium diet.

Dr. Sodi-Pallares found that giving GKI to heart patients with fluid retention is also very helpful. Ms. Gerson noted that "This solution helps restore potassium to the cell system. Energy is required in order for potassium to go back into the cell system, and this energy is supplied by the glucose and insulin. We use this solution quite successfully in two ways: first to replenish the patient with fluids, but also to restore potassium to the cells and reduce edema."

DIET

All aspects of Gerson therapy revolve around the diet, which is designed to support all the other efforts to rebalance the internal body chemistry. At the clinic, all meals are prepared with fresh, organically grown produce. Nothing is canned, jarred, pickled, frozen, or preserved in any way. Between the juices and the meals, the total average intake of food for each patient is approximately 20 pounds of fresh raw food a day, mostly via juices.

All refined, processed, and empty-calorie foods are avoided. This includes obviously treated foods such as white sugars and flours, and smoked, sulfured, packaged, or mass-prepared products. Other obvious taboos include cigarettes, alcohol, drugs, and caffeine, which are known to deplete the immune system and act as carcinogens. All animal proteins such as meat, poultry, and dairy products are avoided, since they are difficult to digest and hinder, rather than promote, the restoration of the liver.

Both animal and vegetable fats are also avoided as they too can be difficult to digest and can impede detoxification. Additionally, Dr. Gerson found that dietary fats actually have the effect of promoting tumor growth. This accords with cancer research indicating that the higher the level of cholesterol and fats in the blood of cancer patients, the less chance of their surviving. Dr. Gerson slowly eliminated all fats from the diets of his cancer patients and found that the results improved substantially. On the other hand, whenever he added fats (even oils that are low in cholesterol) to the patients' diets, he observed regrowth of tumor tissue. Consequently, for cancer patients receiving Gerson therapy, fats of animal and vegetable origin are eliminated as much as possible. The only exception is linseed oil, which Dr. Gerson found is particularly well tolerated. (For patients suffering from other illnesses, while the diet is still essentially low in fat, some raw fresh butter, egg yolks, and low-cholesterol vegetable oils such as safflower oil and sunflower oil may be eaten in small quantities.)

Dr. Gerson was a strong believer in the importance of organically grown produce, and as mentioned above, all food used at his clinic must be grown in this manner. Chemical pesticides and fertilizers, he said, essentially poison and denature fruits and vegetables by altering their chemical composition. For instance, he found that many chemical fertilizers cause the sodium content in the affected foods to rise while decreasing potassium levels, which is precisely contrary to what the body requires to restore its healthy metabolic function.

THE "HEALING CRISIS"

A "healing crisis" is an activation of the body's defenses, and often takes the form of fever as the immune system begins to be functional again. Ms. Gerson says that "almost invariably, once the patient begins to produce a fever, this is followed by a tumor reduction. It seems as though the fever helps the body break down and dissolve the tumor tissue. Along with the fever comes flulike symptoms such as aches and pains all over the body.

"This healing crisis can be quite severe in cases where the body is getting rid of accumulated heavy toxic materials. These toxins are removed through the coffee enemas, but sometimes the patient will have a very irritated colon because these materials literally burn as they are being released. In those cases, we alter from the coffee to chamomile tea enemas, which are soothing and help the body release toxic materials which have built up. We see that type of problem with patients who have been medicated a lot with tranquilizers and antidepressants. The latter are especially toxic. When they have been used a fair amount, the patients suffer a lot as they are released from the body. We have to give these patients chamomile tea enemas, peppermint tea and chamomile tea by mouth, and oatmeal gruel—all are soothing."

Usually these reactions last no longer than 3 to 4 days, and when they are over, the patients claim to be much relieved and improved, with a better appetite. Sometimes, if patients have experienced a good deal of weight loss, they become ravenously hungry. This is part of the body's normal healing process. Ms. Gerson tells of a 38-year-old patient with liver and pancreatic cancer who had been told in October 1 that she would not survive past Christmas. She was on 12 morphine tablets a day and had lost 25 pounds. In 2 days she was free of pain and off the morphine, went through a healing crisis with fever, came out of it after about 6 or 7 days, and started to be very hungry. Every time she went to dinner, she took food back to her room so that she could have an extra meal or two in the middle of the night. This patient not only survived past Christmas but told Ms. Gerson years later that she was feeling wonderful and had resumed most of her normal activities.

OZONE THERAPY

Ozone therapy, used in Europe for decades but still considered an unproven method in the United States, is one of the most effective new techniques added to Gerson therapy. In an interview Ms. Gerson explained what is used: "Ozone actually, in chemical formula, O_3. Plain oxygen that we breathe all day in our air is O_2. Now, that little extra oxygen atom that's loosely attached... comes off easily and is highly active.... It circulates very quickly through the bloodstream and attaches very quickly to the red blood corpuscles and is released, among other places, at the tumor site. The ozone molecule [is] extremely active and can directly attack and destroy malignant tissue...."

She continues, "The ozone can be used in many ways. We have used it, for instance, as an insufflation into the rectum. The patients can easily hold it, and it is then absorbed directly into the bloodstream. It is also extremely effective in colon cancers.... It can be put into the vagina for tumors in the cervix or uterus. It can also be given intravenously; ozone gas can be injected into the veins without any adverse effect. This is something that makes people worry a bit, because they still remember the horrible exterminations done on prisoners in concentration camps. By simply injecting air into the vein, you can cause spasms of the heart and death. But this isn't air; it's oxygen and ozone. This has to be done properly, with very, very thin needles so that the bubbles that go into the vein are very, very tiny. And they disperse very quickly in the blood and are picked up very rapidly by the red blood cells. If it's done slowly, there is absolutely no adverse effect. To be quite sure of that, I'm usually the first one to get any of these new techniques done on me. I've had it done a couple of times; I've had as much as 20 cc of ozone gas put into my veins and I'm here to talk to you about it. We also use room ozone generators, so you can breathe air augmented with ozone; it goes through the lungs very quickly and into the bloodstream.

"Ozone has been proven to be very effective at killing viral and bacterial infections.... Besides that, there is a feeling of well-being in the patients who are given ozone because it increases oxygenation and energy. Ozone is also, with its extra single oxygen atom, an excellent scavenger of free radicals, in other words, a very good detoxifying agent. It's altogether a wonderful material, and we feel that since we started using it quite extensively...we have vastly improved our results."

COLEY'S TOXINS

Gar Hildebrand explains this aspect of the program. "Coley was a physician who searched the literature for cancer treatments after a heartbreaking experience of losing a child patient to the disease. Much to his surprise, he found a skin infection called erysipelas. Erysipelas is caused by a streptococcus that causes a skin fever of 105 to 106 degrees Fahrenheit. This fever causes an inflammatory infection which interferes with tumor action.

"Coley constructed a live erysipelas vaccine, which was too toxic at first. Some patients died, but others experienced a tumor regression. He went through a lot of trial and error and eventually settled on something which we now call *Serratia marsecens*. He mixed the *Serratia* and the strep in a ratio of 1,500 cells to 1, and then crushed the mixture through a microfilter to liberate the internal toxins of the bacteria. This liberated antigens, which in turn caused the immune system of the patient to think that there was a chronic infection that had to be fought.

"The effectiveness of Coley's toxins seems to be due to the fact that the immune system, when turned on, can cause a lot of dust to rise. These patients need to be put into an intensive care unit and hooked up to monitors in case there is a problem, although there have never been any heart attacks or kidney failures reported in the 900 cases that have been thoroughly studied. Then a tiny amount of toxins is administered intravenously for 4 hours through a drip. About 2 hours into the process, the immune response begins. The patient will develop chills and shaking that last for about half an hour to 90 minutes, followed by a rise in temperature of about a degree every 10 minutes. Once that temperature hits 105 or 106, the ICU staff lies the patient down or puts in a suppository of Tylenol to stop it.

"The reaction is the immune system's response. This is not a poison. This is not a toxin. It's not like chemotherapy making your hair fall out or causing bone marrow suppression. The Coley's toxins are much more like what happens when your immune system decides to cure you of an infection. So the symptoms are more flulike, without the nausea and vomiting. After the second or third IV application, patients usually get sleepy and actually nod off. The fever lessens progressively. In other words, there's a honeymoon period.

"Coley himself said that if you don't keep these up for at least 3 or 4 months, in booster dosages, you won't get a permanent response. The literature reveals that gains are lost when Coley's toxins are given in lower concentrations or for shorter durations."

THE PATIENTS Cancer patients have been treated with Gerson therapy for more than 50 years, and the results have been amazing, especially in contrast to those reported by conventional cancer specialists and agencies. The therapy was administered at treatment centers in New York and then California before the establishment of the new Gerson Therapy Center in Mexico in 1977. It was at this time that statistical analyses began to be recorded. A 40 to 50 percent improvement rate was recorded in terminal patients, and an 80 percent improvement in early to moderate cancer cases.

The following are examples of the types of improvements patients have experienced using Dr. Gerson's therapy.

A 15-year-old girl had been treated for a tumor in the spinal cord. She had been paralyzed and her father had been told that she would die. When she came to Dr. Gerson, she couldn't walk or feed herself. Approximately 8 months after beginning Dr. Gerson's treatment, she could move her arms and hands, and her tumor had vanished. Decades later, she reported, "I have been tested throughout the years, and there is no sign of any tumors." She concluded by saying, "I truly hope that our government will soon open its eyes to the truth, even if it does hurt the canned food business."

A 30-year-old man was diagnosed with melanosarcoma (a skin cancer) which was spreading over his body. He had undergone surgery once for removal of tumors. New nodules appeared 2 months later, and doctors recommended radical surgery and removal of the left half of the neck and neck muscles as well as removal of glands in the groin. Refusing surgery, the patient started Gerson therapy, and within a few weeks all glandular nodes had disappeared.

Three years later the patient wrote the following to Dr. Gerson, as reported in his book: "I am now more vigorous and stronger than ever. The long 18 months to 2 years which we spent in following your orders have paid off with the very best of health. At present I weigh 187 pounds and am full of pep and health. I have worked harder this year than in any year of my life and I eat a well-balanced diet of all normal, healthy food."

A woman arrived at the clinic with a confirmed diagnosis of breast cancer with bone metastases. She had had a mastectomy but subsequently the cancer had spread. When she arrived at the clinic she had six "hot spots" in the spine and one in the shoulder. Her outlook was extremely poor and she was in considerable pain. Two years after she started on Gerson therapy she reported to Ms. Gerson that not only did she have a clear scan, she was horseback riding three times a week, was in excellent shape, and had plenty of energy.

For more information on Gerson Therapy, contact:
Gerson Institute
P.O. Box 430
Bonita, CA 91908
1-888-4-GERSON
www.gerson.org

Herbal and Nutritional Therapy

Dr. Donald Yance, a practicing clinical herbalist, certified nutritionist, and author of *Dietary, Herbal and Nutritional Strategies for Treating and Preventing Cancer*, describes his plant-based protocol for treating and preventing cancer.

"The foods that I would emphasize in general are first of all the highest quality attainable, as fresh as possible and organic. I always stress quality and balance. I don't care if you think you should be juicing carrots, beets and celery, in my opinion they must be organic and they must be fresh. I tend to base a lot of my specifics on the person's health status, the person's genetic makeup and the type of cancer they have. Of course I am going to emphasize foods that contain a high level of phytochemicals that we know inhibit cancer and possibly can reverse cancer."

"Phytochemicals and phytonutrients are new terms that describe plant constituents that are not vitamins or minerals but various compounds that play an important role in cell protection. They protect against the initiation and promotion of cancer. Of the flavones my favorite is called quercetin which is found abundantly in broccoli and in onions and is a wonderful inhibitor of a number of different cancer cell lines. Isoflavones are found in the soybean food family. Tryterpines, limolines and nomlines are found in citrus fruit, mostly in the rind and the oil of the citrus, which can be made into a tea with orange peel, lemon peel or from the oils. Some of these are in clinical trials for cancer therapy."

Dr. Yance continues, "I am a big believer in omega-3 fatty acids. Not only do they have strong inhibitory effects on cancer growth from many mechanisms but they also help to feed the body nutritionwise, particularly combined with protein. I know there are a lot of different viewpoints on this topic. Do I need to build up this person while at the same time detoxifying them? That is where you play the balance between foods that will build a person and inhibit cancer, and foods that will detoxify the person." So a combination of detoxification and health-restoring diet is essential to Dr. Yance's approach.

DETOXIFICATION Dr. Yance describes his detoxifying program. "I use Epsom salt baths which do a number of things. First, you raise the thermal level of the core body temperature. Most people with cancer have a very subnormal body temperature. It is important to get the body's immune system activated by raising the body temperature. When people are in contact with some sort of pathogen the body's natural response is to secrete pyrogens that raise the body's temperature. We do this artificially because cancer does not provoke the usual immunological reaction so we do things to help that. I mix essential oils, mostly lavender, into the bathtub and give them an herbal compound along with an herbal tea.

"I also put an big emphasis on liver detoxifying, in which I will use a number of different plant compounds along with various supplements. I favor alpha lypoic acid combined with some very concentrated forms of herbs, particularly turmeric. Alpha lypoic acid is a highly absorbable nutrient that is both fat and water soluble. In my opinion it is the first precursor of glutathione, which is part of the phase two liver enzyme detoxifying system. It helps detoxify zenoestrogens, lipid soluble toxins, some other drugs and pollutants and possibly some other things like dead cancer cells. The liver is the main vehicle for breaking these things down and helping the body secrete them. The dosage I use is 300 milligrams of lypoic acid twice a day.

"As far as turmeric goes, I use a compound of standardized curcuminoids, the active constituent in turmeric about 95 to 97 percent. I use 1 gram three or four times a day on an empty stomach combined with bromelain. Bromelain is an enzyme from pineapple that interacts with the turmeric and with corsatin. The dosages of corsatin and bromelain are the same, 1 gram three or four times a day on an empty stomach. These three compounds have a synergistic effect in that they all help each other to be absorbed more efficiently."

OTHER HERBS Dr. Yance tells about some other commonly used herbs. "An interesting plant that I use quite a bit in breast cancer is an herb called pulsatilla, which has no anticancer activity but tends to lift a person's spirit. I think that ability is the first and foremost part of any person's treatment. Then we move on to plants like schisandra, known as a five spice herb in Chinese medicine because it has salt, sweet, bitter, pungent, and sour taste all in one plant. It is a wonderful hepatic protective agent and detoxifier and also is used to treat nervous exhaustion. It helps the body's endocrine system with the stress of having cancer. It balances the pH of the digestive system which may be too alkaline or too acidic and so improves the ability of the body to absorb. It is perhaps the most powerful liver protective agent of all plants.

"Red clover is a wonderful plant particularly with some of the hormonal-type cancers, like breast cancer and prostate cancer. Because of the isoflavones and curcuminoids present in this plant, I use a one-to-one extract of red clover instead of the over-the-counter preparations of one-to-five, which are not as strong. I make a teacoction (a tea you basically cook) of blossoms of red clover which is also very nice."

"Licorice is also a wonderful plant. It has hormonal regulating properties, liver protective properties, it is a demulcent so it soothes mucus membranes and it is a precursor to aldosterone. Aldosterone is the hormone that tells the body to hold onto fluids. If a person has very dry skin and every time they drink liquid they urinate it right out of their bodies, their blood pressure tends to be very low, they may have low levels of aldosterone, so think of using a little licorice."

EMOTIONAL AND SPIRITUAL HEALTH Attitude, love, and spirituality play a part in healing cancer as in many other diseases. As Dr. Yance says, "I believe this is the essence of healing. It is difficult to give any kind of nutritional support until a person has their fear of the cancer removed. When they have fear they have very poor quality of sleep. Sleep is essential for detoxification. The body does most of its detoxifying while it is in the deepest rest. Fear is an obstacle in the way of healing and I believe this is where you tap into a person's spirit. Once a person is comfortable with who they are spiritually, then they no longer have fear. The whole body, mind and spirit are interrelated. When you feel comfortable with who you are spiritually you don't worry about things as much.

"I always explain that we are all going to ultimately die. We need to come to grips with that and not fixate on it. Let's think about the living, let's think about today, let's think about how we can step forward and be healed because you don't want to live miserably anyway. Let's think about how you can enrich yourself on all levels and that everything complements each other. One of my great loves for plant medicine is that plants are here on earth just like we are and they exude a tremendous amount of healing. We have only scraped the iceberg of the ability of plants to heal."

PART NINE

Chronic and Degenerative Conditions

42

Digestive Disorders

In examining digestive disorders, one must realize that there are no special clinics where research and treatment focus exclusively on these disorders and that there are no particular pioneers in the field of digestion. One reason for this is that digestive disorders are not often clearly diagnosed as such. A determination may be made that a person has cancer, arthritis, or renal failure, for example, but not that the condition is related to a chronic digestive disorder that has gone undetected for a long time. While you may be undergoing extensive, costly, and perhaps toxic treatment for a diagnosed disease, it is possible that only the symptoms of your disease are being treated, not the underlying cause.

Furthermore, many people go through life with a chronic digestive problem and assume that it is a normal state of affairs. Any complications that result again are rarely understood as being connected to an underlying problem with the digestive mechanism. Some disturbances that obviously are related to digestion—diarrhea, constipation, and the like—are handled by taking over-the-counter drugs such as laxatives and antacids. Some people think they have a "weak" stomach or that these problems are just a part of getting older, and so end up taking drugs habitually, unaware that they are likely exacerbating the real problem. This chapter will enhance your understanding of the great effect that digestion has on your total health.

Traditional vs. Alternative Approaches

The differences between traditional and alternative medicine are particularly evident in the treatment of digestive disorders. In the traditional paradigm, a person is generally deemed healthy unless he she has a major breakdown in the digestive apparatus or a major disease. In essence, the paradigm says that health is the absence of disease.

Traditional physicians are more used to treating symptoms than correcting causes. For this reason, one of the most common problems in digestion—a "cause" rather than a "symptom"—is one that is rarely considered in traditional medical practice. This is the *malabsorption syndrome*, or the failure of the body to absorb the nutrients that have been ingested. The problem here is that even though a food is eaten and goes through the digestive system, the nutrients, minerals, and vitamins do not get into the blood and hence do not penetrate the body at the cellular level.

Traditionally trained physicians are skilled at identifying and treating conditions when they have reached a disease state. Their approach to diagnosis and treatment is anatomical in nature. They use sophisticated technologies to evaluate the anatomy of the digestive tract—the stomach, pancreas, small intestine, colon, and liver—and look for evidence of tumors, polyps, ulcers, and other problems. They are less likely to search out or treat conditions such as underactivity, sluggishness, or suboptimal function. Even when such conditions are detected, they often are not considered significant.

The digestive process, like all body systems, produces a wide spectrum of symptoms when it is not functioning properly. Complementary physicians, who combine traditional medicine with alternative practices, consider mild or moderate symptoms to be signs of suboptimal functioning that should be addressed as such. These symptoms include burping, indigestion, and constipation. Complementary physicians often analyze the body biochemistry using sophisticated blood laboratory testing that goes beyond traditional medicine's use of the standard SMA-24 profile to identify major digestive disorders. They are very interested in the foods a person eats, and whether any specific foods cause irritation or other reactions. Thus they tend to test for food sensitivity as part of a complete analysis of body function.

In terms of treatment, complementary physicians tend to use natural substances such as foods, herbs, and homeopathic preparations. Supplements that contain concentrated forms of vitamins and minerals are fundamental elements of body rebalancing. Complementary physicians tend to be attuned to the concept of even the mildest malabsorption since they frequently see the end product of this condition, namely, deficiencies of nutrients.

Symptoms

Digestive system disorders can be placed into two main categories: those that are clearly and directly related to digestion, and those that are a step or two removed from the digestive process, and therefore more difficult to connect with digestion.

Symptoms of disorders in the first category are more easily recognized. The most common include burping, belching, flatulence, a feeling of indigestion, undigested food in the stool, or a feeling of food "just sitting there." When such symptoms are present, it is relatively easy to connect the problem to some malfunction in the digestive process.

Problems that occur over time and are related to the long-term inefficient absorption of nutrients and/or an insufficiency of nutrients in the food to begin with are often not directly connected to digestive difficulties. Insufficient stomach acid production can result in malabsorption of calcium, leading to osteoporosis and osteoarthritis, for example. Periodontal problems may be caused by a deficiency of calcium and other nutrients. Anemia may be linked to low stomach acid levels, because iron is not absorbed efficiently. Poorly nourished skin is another common result of malabsorption due to digestive problems. The skin may show minor symptoms, such as blemishes, dryness, scaling, or a tendency toward irritation. These are often due to dietary deficiencies and/or poor absorption of calcium, zinc, vitamins A and E, and essential fatty acids.

Why Digestive Problems Occur

MALABSORPTION OF NUTRIENTS If any of the systems involved in digestion are faulty in any way, the efficiency of the absorptive process will diminish and the body will not be receiving the nutrients it needs.

INSUFFICIENT PRODUCTION OF STOMACH ACID Insufficient or suboptimal production of stomach acid, which is not an illness but a sluggish stomach, is the most common digestive problem, especially in people over 40. In the presence of low stomach acid, food digestion in the stomach is impaired and thus protein and minerals are not digested efficiently. Many people with this problem burp and belch after meals.

PROBLEMS WITH THE PANCREAS AND DIGESTIVE ENZYME PRODUCTION The pancreas is a gland that produces enzymes for digesting protein, carbohydrates, and fats. The enzymes neutralize the acidity of partially digested food (chyme). If the enzymes are inefficient, difficulties will result. Very often, when a patient complains of digestive problems two to three hours after eating, the pancreas is the culprit.

PROBLEMS WITH BILE The liver produces bile, which is stored in the gallbladder and sent into the small intestine through the bile duct. This alkaline fluid is partly responsible for fat absorption, as it emulsifies or breaks down fats into smaller particles. The liver is a major workhorse of both digestion and the detoxification of the body, and it can be overtaxed by a poor diet or by any inefficiencies in the digestive process. If production of stomach acid or pancreatic enzymes is sluggish, this sub-par functioning can be a major stressor on the liver.

PROBLEMS WITH THE SMALL INTESTINE The pancreatic enzymes described above come into play when partially digested food moves from the stomach to the duodenum, which is the first part of the small intestine, The digested food then moves farther down the small intestine into the jejunum, where food absorption takes place. The nutrients are then carried through the bloodstream to various parts of the body. A malfunction in this part of the process, or anything leading up to it, can impair nutrient absorption.

MALFUNCTIONS OF THE ILEOCECAL VALVE The ileocecal valve is located between the small and large intestines. Diarrhea and constipation are often associated with malfunctions of this valve. The valve's job is to open when the contents of the small intestines are ready to pass through, to let a certain amount through, and then to close. However, if the valve stays open too long, or is too tight or closed, problems can occur.

If the ileocecal valve remains in the open position, it can enhance diarrhea, because everything is flushing through too quickly. Food passes through the digestive apparatus so rapidly that the absorptive process is impaired. In addition to the rapid transit due to the open valve, the movement of food may reverse, as the contents of the colon backflush. The colon is the "garbage disposal" area, whereas the small intestine is the "kitchen" area. Therefore, a backflush of waste material puts biochemical stress on the small intestine and irritates the liver as well. In short, the waste material makes a mess in the kitchen. The material may be absorbed into the bloodstream, causing various toxic reactions.

If the ileocecal valve is too tight or too closed, this can cause constipation. The tight valve, by not facilitating the passage of the small intestine contents into the colon, retards the entire digestive flow, which leads to infrequent bowel movements, or constipation.Unfortunately, most people are unaware of this valve and its importance in the regulation of proper digestion.

IRRITATION OF THE COLON When the stomach acid and pancreatic enzyme systems do not work properly, undigested particles of food or actual pieces of food may reach the colon, also called the large intestine. This not only irritates the colon, but also leads to flatulence because the undigested food will be fermented by the friendly and not-so-friendly bacteria residing in the colon.

The colon may be irritated throughout its entire length or in any of its anatomical parts: the ascending colon, the transverse colon, or the descending colon. Often, the most common pattern is that all three parts are out of balance. In this case, the patient should consider how he or she handles stress because the colon may be the organ in which various stress elements are manifesting themselves.

There has been found to be a high correlation between food intolerances or allergies and irritation in the descending colon (see below). It's always a good idea to keep a careful food diary to identify frequently eaten foods and those you may suspect are culprits in allergic reactions. Foods that commonly prompt allergic reactions include gluten foods (wheat, barley, oats, and rye), sugar, peanuts, citrus fruits, dairy products, soybeans, corn, and caffeine.

Irritation of the ascending colon alone means that its ecology is off balance. For example, there may be an overgrowth of yeast because the ascending colon becomes a fermentation factory of sorts when undigested food particles reach it. The unfriendly bacteria that live in the small and large intestines may be especially likely to overgrow if the production of stomach acid is so low that the digestive system becomes under-acidified or excessively alkaline. A highly alkaline environment favors the growth of yeast, which may then exceed the usual niche it maintains within the ecological population of the colon.

Food Allergy and Digestion

Foods to which a person is allergic or sensitive are considered invaders by the body's immune system. Thus, they irritate and weaken the digestive apparatus. It is quite common to find that people consume large amounts of foods to which they are allergic. Reading food labels and choosing food correctly is a critical part of treatment.

Digestive malfunctioning can cause complications when allergens are present. If there is a deficiency of the gastric juices or pancreatic enzymes, for instance, a food will be in the system for a much longer time than it would if there were adequate amounts of acids and enzymes to break it down. If the food is one to which the body is sensitive, that sensitivity will be heightened by the delayed action of the digestive mechanism. Furthermore, if protein molecules are not broken down into small enough particles because of faulty digestive processes, the larger units entering the bloodstream will be treated like foreign invaders by the body's immune system, and an allergic reaction will ensue.

Children have less developed gastrointestinal systems than adults do, and so they often suffer from obvious food allergies. Later in life, though, as the digestive system becomes more sophisticated, these allergies are manifested in less obvious ways. Even if the symptoms are not the same, the underlying allergy may be. A child who has suffered milk-associated asthma, for instance, may have severe acne as a teenager. The milk allergy is still there, but its symptoms have moved to a different organ system, often misleading the patient and physician into thinking that the original allergy has been outgrown.

HIGH-PROTEIN DIETS High-protein diets pose a special problem with respect to food allergies. People who consume a lot of protein usually tend to have it in their systems around the clock. This is because it takes at least 4 to 7 hours for proteins to be digested, and if the protein is fried, deep-fried, or charcoal-broiled, it can take even longer. Consider the person who starts the day with bacon and eggs, has a sandwich of cold cuts and cheese at lunch, eats more meat and drinks milk at dinner, and tops it off with a late night snack of ice cream. This person will have protein in his or her system all the time.

If any substance—in this case, protein—sits in the digestive system virtually all the time, two things will occur. First, the person will almost certainly develop an allergy to it because of overexposure. Second, the person will probably not be aware of the allergy because his system will never be without the substance long enough for him to notice changes due to its presence or absence. The negative symptoms then become cumulative and chronic, and are manifested as disease states. Digestion is usually strained, and the disorders that appear are generally regarded as signs of poor health, which becomes tolerated as unavoidable or is attributed to genetics or age.

FOOD ROTATION Food rotation is one way to help alleviate this problem. It can be combined with medical care. Don't eat the same foods day after day, because no matter how healthy and nutritious they are, you will not benefit from them if your body rejects or reacts negatively to them. Wheat, for example, is nutritious, but because it is found in practically every processed food, it is also a very common allergen. Therefore, it must be rotated in the diet with other grains. Eat it no more frequently than every fourth day and in no more than a 4-ounce portion at each meal. Then there is a good chance it can be eaten without causing an allergic reaction.

All foods should be rotated in this manner. Even if your body is not responding negatively in an overt way, you may be having hidden reactions to many different foods. Even if you are not, by overusing a food—eating it too frequently and in oversized portions—you may eventually develop an allergy to it. Try to make a routine of rotating all foods and avoid eating processed foods as much as possible because certain foods, such as corn and wheat, are ingredients in many of them. (See chapters 11 and 12 for further discussion of rotation diets).

LACTOSE INTOLERANCE Lactose intolerance is a common digestive disorder. Probably two-thirds of the world's adults cannot tolerate lactose, which is found in milk and all milk products. When lactose-sensitive people continue to eat dairy products, they begin to suffer from a wide range of symptoms, which include abdominal cramping and bloating, chronic nasal discharge or postnasal drip, puffiness under the eyes, gas, and diarrhea.

Lactose intolerance is a malabsorption of lactose caused by a deficiency of lactase, the enzyme responsible for milk digestion. Lactase breaks lactose down into the readily digestible forms glucose and galactose. If it is absent or deficient, lactose remains undigested in the system. Some passes through the blood and is excreted in the urine, but most ends up in the large intestine. The lactose molecules draw water out of the tissues and into the intestinal cavity, while the undigested glucose is fermented by intestinal bacteria. Carbon dioxide is given off during this process, and diarrhea, bloating, flatulence, and belching may result.

The lactase deficiency can be caused by damage to the intestinal mucosa; this damage may be brought on by acute infectious diarrhea in infants. Malnutrition, cystic fibrosis, and colitis also have been known to cause lactase deficiency. Even in the absence of these traumas, lactose deficiency is very common.

The most obvious remedy for lactose intolerance is to stay away from milk and all milk products. Also, keep in mind that lactose is found in many vitamins and most processed foods, and so it is best to avoid processed foods and request from vitamin manufacturers a full disclosure of their exact ingredients. It is important to eliminate lactose from the system completely in order to recover from its ravages. Another option may be to purchase a commercially prepared lactase supplement that boosts your supply of lactase and enables you to better digest the lactose. Some lactase-deficient people, however, can still eat a few fermented milk and dairy products without negative consequences. These items—primarily yogurt, buttermilk, and cottage cheese—must be tested on an individual basis to determine one's reaction to them.

GASTRITIS Gastritis, another common digestive disorder, involves an inflammation of the mucosa lining the inner wall of the stomach. The inflammation is accompanied by symptoms such as nausea, vomiting, and loss of appetite. In the acute form, gastritis can be caused by infections and/or the ingestion of corrosive agents such as alcohol and aspirin. In the chronic form, gastritis is a serious condition that may be the cornerstone of degenerative diseases such as ulcers.

The treatment of gastritis should include the elimination of any substance (an allergen or anything else that is difficult to digest) known to be causing or aggravating the condition. The diet should include lots of liquids. Vegetables should be steamed to maximize their digestibility and reduce their acidity. A blood chemistry test should be performed to determine what, if any, vitamin deficiencies exist, since they often play an important role in this disorder. Vitamin deficiency related to gastritis is responsible for many complications, among which are a prickly sensation in the skin, loss of memory, depression, and general weakness.

PRESSURE DISEASES Another group of disorders associated with the digestive system have been termed "pressure diseases" because they are caused by a pressure buildup that results from failure to eliminate waste efficiently. They include diverticulitis, hemorrhoids, hiatus hernia, and appendicitis, among others.

DIVERTICULITIS Diverticular disease is the most troublesome and widespread of the pressure conditions. It occurs when the muscle rings encircling the colon, which move along bulk matter, become clogged. Try clenching your fist and then imagine that mud is stuck in the creases of your hand. The creases can be thought of as diverticula, and the mud in them is food being trapped in the digestive organs. When bulk and fiber are lacking in the diet, the colon must deal with a mass of food too dry to be pushed along with ease, and so it becomes overworked, overstressed, and overstrained. Its membranes eventually herniate, or rupture, and it is these ruptures that are called diverticula. When there are many diverticula—and there can be hundreds—they tend to become inflamed and cause more acute symptoms. This condition is known as diverticulitis. Approximately one in four people with diverticular disease develop these acute symptoms.

Diverticulitis barely existed before the 20th century, but now is said to affect one-third of all adults middle-aged or older, half the population over 50, and two-thirds of the population over 80. It is the most common digestive disorder of senior citizens.

Research on the genesis and development of diverticular disease has shown that it results from a gross lack of fiber in the diet. The refining of carbohydrates seems to be the main culprit here, since this condition is almost wholly absent in cultures where whole grains, legumes, vegetables, and such are the mainstays of the diet and where processed foods are not used.

The traditional treatment for diverticular disease has been to give the patient stool softeners to help the stool pass through the system and expanders to force it out. Antibiotics also are used. The patient is placed on a fibrous diet that helps the colon begin processing waste more efficiently and with less strain. Bran is usually prescribed, and patients are often told to avoid milk products and spicy foods since these tend to produce abdominal pain, pressure, and gas.

Alternative treatments for diverticular disease may include the above suggestions, but will add to the patient's diet other abdominal and intestinal cleansers taken orally. These include cellulose, hemicellulose, pectin, and noncarbohydrate lignin. Celery, brussels sprouts, broccoli, and especially beet juice will also help the condition. Bran should be unprocessed because this type has a shorter intestinal transit time and helps increase stool weight. The diverticula pockets may be cleansed with dietary supplements of chlorophyll, chamomile, garlic, vitamin C, zinc, nondairy acidophilus, pectin, and psyllium. Instead of medicinal antibiotics, natural antibiotics such as garlic may be used.

HEMORRHOIDS Constantly straining to push dry, compacted stools out of the system causes the veins in the rectal and anal passages to become distended and engorged with blood. The veins become weakened, lose their elasticity, and can no longer carry blood properly. This causes the blood to pool instead, creating a ballooning effect known as a hemorrhoid.

When the hemorrhoids are internal, they can become obstructive to stool passage. With constant pressure being exerted against them, they may rupture and bleed and, in severe cases, hemorrhage. External hemorrhoids, also called piles, are very sensitive and may grow to the size of golf balls.

It is estimated that half of all Americans over 50 years of age have hemorrhoids and that hemorrhoidal treatment is a $50 million a year industry. Most of the profit comes from sales of suppositories. Suppositories are given to shrink and lubricate hemorrhoids to prevent them from rupturing. Alternative treatments for hemorrhoids center on hygiene, diet, and exercise. Warm tub or sitz baths and ice packs may help. If you increase your intake of water, vitamin C, and fiber, and exercise regularly, the blood trapped in the hemorrhoidal veins will be reabsorbed into the body and the problem will be cleared up. However, it will recur unless you integrate these changes into a new, more healthful lifestyle.

Prevention of the recurrence of hemorrhoid is aimed at changing conditions associated with the pressure and straining of constipation. Doctors will often recommend increasing fiber and fluids in the diet. Eating the right amount of fiber and drinking six to eight glasses of fluid (not alcohol) result in softer, bulkier stools. A softer stool makes emptying the bowels easier and lessens the pressure on hemorrhoids caused by straining.

Eliminating straining also helps prevent the hemorrhoids from protruding.

Good sources of fiber are fruits, vegetables, and whole grains. In addition, doctors may suggest a bulk stool softener or a fiber supplement such as psyllium (Metamucil) or methylcellulose (Citrucel).

In some cases, hemorrhoids must be treated surgically. These methods are used to shrink and destroy the hemorrhoidal tissue and are performed under anesthesia. The doctor will perform the surgery during an office or hospital visit.

HIATUS HERNIA Hiatus hernia is another condition related to constipation and low-fiber dietary regimens. Like the other pressure diseases, it is essentially a modern-day Western disorder affecting primarily middle-aged and older people. There are no warning symptoms until it causes a sharp pain just below the breastbone. It is a condition in which part of the stomach wall becomes extended and pushes up against the diaphragm and the skeletal system. Obesity may contribute to the condition, which also sometimes develops during pregnancy.

The traditional treatment of hiatus hernia usually includes antacids, a bland diet, and sometimes surgery. These steps are adequate to relieve the pain, and you certainly should follow the suggestions of your physician. The alternative (or even complementary) approach is aimed at going beyond alleviation of the painful symptoms by establishing a dietary regimen that can reverse the condition while ameliorating the source of discomfort. Since constipation due to a low-fiber diet is frequently the cause of this condition, make sure to get plenty of high-fiber bulk foods. Losing weight may also help.

APPENDICITIS Appendicitis is an inflammation of the appendix, a small pouch that extends from the first part of the large intestine. The appendix has no known function. It can become diseased as a result of infection or obstructed from contents moving through intestinal tract.

Appendicitis caused mainly by troublesome elimination. The most common abdominal emergency in the Western world, it is often brought on by continuous constipation, straining during stool elimination, and anal retention—failing to evacuate solid waste when the body tells you to. By delaying your bowel movements, perhaps because you are too busy to be inconvenienced, you confuse your body. The water from fecal matter begins to be reabsorbed, and the dry, hard stool that is left will pass only with great pain and difficulty. In the meantime, you strain the muscles that must retain this mass and eventually train them to delay normal elimination.

Some people learn to have a bowel movement only once a day or even once every 2 or 3 days. You should have two or three bowel movements a day, depending, of course, on what and how often you eat. When there is not enough dietary fiber to move food and waste readily through the digestive system, pressure builds up and blocks the passage of stool. Bacteria accumulates and backs up into the 3 to 6 inch long appendix which is attached to the large intestine. The appendix becomes inflamed and infected, and an appendectomy must be performed.

To see how critical the issue of fiber is here, consider the 6,000 appendectomies performed in the United States each week compared with only a handful per year in rural Africa, where processed fiber-depleted food is virtually nonexistent. This again is a pressure disease that can be avoided or even treated with a high-fiber diet consisting of complex carbohydrates.

ULCERS Ulcers of the digestive tract afflict as many as 14 million Americans. About 1 in 10 men and 1 in 20 women suffer from ulcers. Digestive system ulcers occur most often in the duodenum, which is the upper portion of the small intestine. The duodenal ulcer is usually found in the first few inches of the duodenum. The second most common type is the peptic or gastric ulcer, which affects the stomach.

Some ulcers are slight abrasions of the internal mucosal lining; others advance to the stage where they totally perforate the stomach or intestinal wall. Their three stages of development are known as perforation, penetration, and obstruction. In acute perforation, the ulcer eats through the wall of the abdomen. This is the most serious state and causes the greatest number of deaths. Surgery to close the perforation is virtually unavoidable.Penetration is the stage where the patient usually awakens at night with severe pain in adjacent areas of the body—the back, liver, and so forth—not just the stomach. This transfer of effect to other organs makes the ulcer hard to diagnose. Obstruction is the stage in which swelling caused by inflammation affects the stomach and the opening to the small intestine.

The vast majority of ulcers are caused by the helicobacter pylori bacteria. These bacteria take up residence in the lining of the digestive tract and then contribute to the breakdown of that lining, resulting in a lesion or crater. Doctors used to think that ulcers were caused by stress or the production of too much hydrochloric acid.

TRADITIONAL TREATMENT Traditional physicians generally limit their treatment to the use of antibiotics to combat the bacteria and acid-production blockers such as Tagamet and Zantac to prevent the stomach acid from irritating the broken-down tissues in the mucosal lining. The heavy reliance on acid-production blockers is troublesome for two reasons: the drugs do not address the real issue, which is why the bacteria have proliferated in the digestive wall; and since the natural stomach acid opposes the bacteria, the blockers may reduce the body's ammunition against the infection. In the process, these drugs also may lessen the effectiveness of the overall digestive process. The stomach's role in digestion is to produce acids that help to digest foods. When that mechanism is suppressed by acid-production blockers, the body may not digest foods efficiently and absorb nutrients. Thus, a patient may suffer from malabsorption.

ALTERNATIVE APPROACH As a complementary physician, Dr. Martin Feldman advocates a much more comprehensive approach to the treatment of ulcers. In addition to eliminating the bacteria, he says, the treatment should accomplish three goals: helping the stomach to heal the erosion; rebalancing the stomach acid production so that it works properly; and optimizing the immune system so that the body can protect against reinfection.

DIAGNOSIS

The mainstream medical community uses endoscopes and upper GI x-rays to determine if an ulcer actually exists. Dr. Feldman may call on these diagnostic techniques as well to obtain as much scientific data as possible on the status of an ulcer. He also uses tests performed by specialty laboratories to identify the presence of *Helicobacter pylori*. Dr. Feldman also draws on his clinical judgment in the diagnostic process. If the blood laboratory test is negative but his clinical experience suggests the presence of *Helicobacter pylori*, he may conduct a therapeutic trial by having the patient take some natural substances that combat the bacteria. He can use this technique because the substances are safe and well tolerated, producing very few side effects. Dr. Feldman then monitors the patient to determine if the therapy reduces the symptoms.

OPPOSING THE BACTERIA

Both antibiotics and natural substances can be used to fight the *Helicobacter pylori* infection. For antibiotic treatments, Dr. Feldman favors the use of amoxicillin because it is usually effective and well tolerated by most patients.

In addition, he may combat the bacteria at a second level with natural therapies. These include goldenseal, an herb that has antibacterial properties, the mineral bismuth in a citrate form, and various combinations of homeopathic solutions. Because homeopathic solutions function primarily as transmitters of energy, Dr. Feldman can test the effect of specific homeopathic products on the body's acupuncture-meridian energy fields.

HEALING THE ULCER

In addition to removing the bacteria, it's important to help the body heal the ulcer irritation or erosion. Dr. Feldman uses a variety of natural treatments to heal the digestive lining. These include cabbage juice, aloe vera, licorice herb, and n-acetyl-glucosamine, a nutrient complex. Other substances that soothe the irritation and thus promote the healing process are marshmallow, ginger, cayenne, and an herbal combination called Robert's Formula.

TESTING FOR FOOD ALLERGIES

Food allergens tend to irritate the stomach, making it harder to heal an ulcer or any other irritation of the stomach or intestines. Therefore, any foods to which a patient is allergic should be eliminated from the diet. To identify such offenders, Dr. Feldman will test a patient's reaction to various food substances by placing them upon the taste portion of the tongue. The brain-taste mechanism, which is very highly developed, has the ability to ascertain if a given food substance is a danger to the body.

REBALANCING THE ACID-PRODUCTION MECHANISM

Paradoxically, many patients with ulcers have a low production of stomach acid. As Dr. Feldman notes, the low-acid environment allows the *Helicobacter pylori* bacteria to get a foothold in the mucosal lining, while a normal acid level would tend to provide some antibacterial protection.

In addition to allowing the bacteria to grow, a low acid production can cause other problems. One is that food will sit in the stomach for a long period of time and ferment abnormally due to the lack of sufficient stomach acid. This fermentation then produces abnormal acids that irritate the stomach and the ulcer. The result: people with low stomach acid experience the symptoms of a high acid production. They may take antacids to suppress the symptoms, but that remedy doesn't correct the true problem. The stomach must work efficiently so that food does not ferment abnormally.

Dr. Feldman has found that many patients suffer from this problem, so he puts a strong emphasis on reoptimizing the stomach's acid mechanism. Again, he uses a variety of natural therapies to get the acid-production system back on track. These remedies include zinc, folic acid, intrinsic factor, and duodenal substance. In some cases, he also prescribes oral acid supplements, which may assist the acid mechanism in strengthening itself. This latter treatment requires careful supervision to ensure that a patient takes the proper form of acid in the proper doses.

REPAIRING THE IMMUNE SYSTEM

As a final phase in his treatment of ulcers, Dr. Feldman focuses on rebuilding the immune system. The logic here, of course, is that the immune system must be working at its maximum level to fight the bacteria that causes most ulcers to begin with. This part of the treatment consists of nutrients that serve as the building blocks of the immune system. They include vitamins A, E and C, bioflavonoids, gamma linolenic acid (GLA), essential fatty acids, zinc, and selenium.

FOODS TO AVOID

As a final note, people who suffer from ulcers should avoid ingesting substances that exacerbate the condition. These include alcohol, nicotine, aspirin, coffee, soft drinks, salt, high-oil nuts, and even raw fruit (except bananas). Foods that are excessively spicy and difficult to digest should be avoided as well.

You don't want to eat a lot of high-protein foods, especially those that are high in fat. Animal foods require more gastric involvement and should be avoided if possible. If you do eat meat, at least trim the fat; also, avoid overcooking, deep frying, and charcoal broiling since these processes make the molecules bond more tightly so that more digestive effort is required to break them down.

Carbohydrate foods have their own protective buffer in the natural state (brown rice and whole grain and vegetables), but once they are refined (white flour and white rice, cakes and pastries) the buffer is stripped away. Therefore, avoid denatured, processed carbohydrates. Vegetables are usually quite acidic, so avoid those causing gas (turnips, cucumbers, brussels sprouts, broccoli, radishes, and cauliflower), especially in the raw state. Vegetables will be less acidic if you cook them, preferably by steaming since it does not destroy their fibrous structure.

Dr. Martin Feldman's Approach to Digestive Wellness

Dr. Martin Feldman, whose ulcer protocol is described above, is a traditionally trained physician who practices complementary medicine. Over many years of practice, he has found that a surprisingly large number of health disorders are related to suboptimal digestion, which as mentioned earlier reduces the body's ability to absorb the vital nutrients needed for proper functioning. Rather than taking the traditional approach of waiting for symptoms to develop into full-blown disease states, Dr. Feldman strongly believes in treating sluggish conditions before they progress. By identifying and treating digestive system disorders when they first begin, he believes that many degenerative diseases can be avoided.

DIAGNOSIS This approach makes use of standard medical procedures and tests. A complete medical history is taken, and comprehensive blood and laboratory analyses are conducted. Dr. Feldman looks for indicators of suboptimal functioning in the digestive system, such as a slight elevation of SGOT enzymes on an SMA-24 blood test. The SGOT, an enzyme found in liver cells, can double or triple in the presence of hepatitis. Traditional physicians will generally look for such extremely elevated levels and tend to disregard slightly elevated levels. Dr. Feldman, however, considers that even a small increase in the level of this enzyme can indicate that the liver, while not diseased, is off balance and in need of attention. As he explains, "I'm looking for the early evaluation of an imbalanced or a suboptimal liver, not a very diseased liver."

Lab tests can also disclose other indicators of malabsorption. These include low levels of minerals such as calcium, magnesium, zinc, manganese, chromium, and selenium, and deficiencies of fat soluble vitamins such as vitamins A, D, and E. The water-soluble vitamins, including B complex and C, are generally less affected because they are more easily absorbed. Dr. Feldman also may test for bacteria and parasites.

In addition, Dr. Feldman uses a noninvasive technique, based on acupuncture pressure points, to test the strength of various internal organs and mechanisms. This technique can determine which components of a patient's digestion are sluggish by testing the level of electrical activity in their specific meridians. If the flow of energy in a given meridian field is deficient, that aspect of digestion is often suboptimal.

Dr. Feldman explains, "Acupuncture theory has taught us that there are many energy flows throughout the body. The energy flow is quite specific along anatomical pathways. A deficient electrical flow often reflects an organ weakness. Traditional acupuncture intervenes by inserting needles into specific acupuncture points to either improve the flow of electrical energy through that flow channel or meridian, or to reduce the flow." Because he uses acupuncture theory only for diagnosis and not for treatment, Dr. Feldman has no need for needles. Instead, he uses meridians to profile the component parts of the digestive apparatus and pinpoint areas that are underactive or suboptimal in strength. In this way, he can determine the energy flow or lack of flow and thus assess the body's function.

"Without needles, without any invasion of the body, we can profile the liver's energy, the stomach's energy, the pancreas's energy, the small intestine's energy, and the colon's energy," Dr. Feldman says. "We can see which areas are the weakest, where imbalances are occurring, and where the problems are most severe."

Once the areas of weakness are identified, Dr. Feldman may consult with a gastroenterologist to see if additional testing is needed, such as x-rays or colonoscopy.

TREATMENT Dr. Feldman then begins to formulate a plan to soothe, replace, repair, and rebuild faulty mechanisms. Treatment decisions are based on area of dysfunction, whether and where irritation is present, and whether any pathogens are present, such as parasites or unfriendly, harmful bacteria. To correct any of these problems, Dr. Feldman's treatment relies heavily on natural substances, including vitamins, minerals, herbs, and occasional homeopathic preparations.

The first step in this process is to soothe any parts of the digestive system that are irritated, whether the stomach, the small intestine, or the colon. Various herbal preparations, such as marshmallow, slippery elm, and aloe vera, may be used for this purpose. Aloe vera, in particular, can help soothe the ileo-cecal valve, the ascending or descending colon, or the entire digestive tract when it is irritated.

Next, it is important to replace whatever is insufficient or suboptimal. When deficiencies of stomach acid are determined, oral acid tablets (such as betaine hydrochloride or glutamic acid) may be prescribed in order to optimize the stomach acid phase of digestion. Dr. Feldman warns that this therapy must be supervised by a knowledgeable practitioner. Other natural substances, including zinc, folic acid, intrinsic factor, and duodenal substance, can help get the stomach back on track to produce its own acid.

The most crucial step in Dr. Feldman's treatment is repair. The focus is on (1) eliminating negative influences on the organ in question, including foods that provoke allergic reactions, irritants such as caffeine, and poor food choices (such as fatty and denatured foods) that stress the digestive system; and (2) using natural therapies to rebuild the suboptimal or sluggish components of digestion. For example, the following substances may be used:

STOMACH: Cabbage juice, licorice, zinc, vitamin A, n-acetyl-glucosamine, marshmallow, ginger, and cayenne. Natural therapies such as goldenseal and a citrate bismuth can help to combat an infection of helicobacter pylori, although an antibiotic may be needed as well to eliminate the bacteria.

ILEOCECAL VALVE: Lipid soluble chlorophyll, aloe vera, slippery elm bark, and echinacea. Increased consumption of water can also help in the case of a closed valve.

COLON: For an imbalance of the ascending colon: bifido bacteria (which can help rebalance the ecology of the colon), fructooligosaccharides (FOS), insoluble fiber, and calendula. For a parasitic infection of the descending colon: grapefruit seed extract, black walnut herb, artemesia, and homeopathic antiparasite remedies. For a general irritation of the colon: aloe vera, lipid soluble chlorophyll, butyric acid, Jerusalem artichoke flour, 1-glutamine, a mix of soluble and insoluble fiber, calcium, and magnesium.

LIVER: Choline, methionine, inositol, milk thistle, combination herbal formulas, and homeopathic solutions.

43

Chronic Fatigue Syndrome

Chronic fatigue syndrome poses a major problem for traditional medicine. The medical establishment has fumbled in its treatment to the point of sometimes claiming that the illness does not exist, but chronic fatigue is a major problem in the United States. Millions lack the energy they once had, ranging from people who have just a little bit of energy to those who are maximally depleted, in bed and unable to function.

"Chronic fatigue syndrome" is the term used to describe a state of constant exhaustion. A syndrome is a disorder that includes a collection of symptoms but is not necessarily a disease entity. Although not labeled as such until the late 1980s, chronic fatigue syndrome is quite similar to other disorders that have been known for centuries. In the 19th century, for example, a common complaint of middle-class women was neurasthenia, which was characterized by chronic exhaustion and a variety of other physical symptoms.

Why is it that for years Americans with a debilitating illness were not recognized as having a disease? They were simply told that chronic fatigue syndrome does not exist. Dr. Dean Black says, "If you go back to the last century, you can read about women suffering from nervous disorders—so many of them that clinics had to be set up to care for them. There was always the search for a cause, but one couldn't be found, and so, without a cause, doctors wouldn't say it was a disease. It had to be in the patient's mind. This is not a new way of sweeping things under the carpet."

Dr. Black brings up another historical example to explain traditional medicine's current difficulties in coming to grips with chronic fatigue syndrome. He says we need to go back to the origin of the current paradigm in the 17th century, when René Descartes promulgated his doctrine of universal doubt. This doctrine held that one could know nothing without using the scientific method: "People would say things to Descartes, but he would explain them away, saying, 'I can see this, this, or this equally plausible alternative.' He felt we could know things for certain only if we had a scientific method whereby we could define truth in a rational cause-and-effect manner. Now, that method had a certain number of rules, one being that there had to be a straight line between a single cause and a single effect. Deviate from that and you introduce so much complexity that the idea of certainty is lost.

"Medicine's power base is the idea of its basis in certainty, which hinges on the concept of a single linear cause-and-effect relationship. That's why medicine is always looking for a single causal factor. This is called the theory of specific etiology."

Dr. Black compares the situation of chronic fatigue syndrome to that of the Epstein-Barr (EB) virus, which was initially thought to cause chronic fatigue syndrome, although later this theory was challenged. "That is why they were so happy to discover this EB virus," he explains. "It seemed marvelous to them because it served to justify the single-cause idea. Yet, as has been frequently pointed out, everyone may have Epstein-Barr [it is so widely distributed]. Chronic fatigue syndrome is caused by many factors operating together. But this idea has been excluded by traditional medicine, which refuses to come to grips with multifactorially generated disease. Medicine is reluctant to accept this multifactorial explanation because it holds to this idea of absolute truth, which requires simplicity and must have one cause and one effect."

Dr. Andrew Gentile stresses that we need to be able to differentiate between chronic fatigue syndrome and other health problems: "Since chronic fatigue syndrome has no known cause, we need to rule out other disorders whose cause we do know. The working definition provided by the government for this disease says there is no other illness at the root of it. Differentiating it calls for great care, since fatigue is ubiquitous as a symptom of many diseases, such as anemia, low thyroid, hypoglycemia, and a variety of other illnesses. These other illnesses must be clearly ruled out."

Symptoms

Chronic fatigue syndrome causes fatigue and usually begins after the onset of flu-like symptoms. The fatigue is not a simple tiredness; it is an exhaustion accompanied by feelings of being unwell. Many people have difficulty getting out of bed and may become weakened to the point of needing to lie down all the time. Often patients are bedridden for months; extreme tiredness can last for years.

Chronic fatigue syndrome may be accompanied by depression, irritability, headaches, low-grade fever, infection, confusion, focusing difficulties, spaciness, diarrhea, sharp muscle pain and weakness, swollen glands, and sleep disorders. The patient is not able to fall asleep or stay asleep and does not feel refreshed or restored even after much sleep.

"Patients will go from one room to another, and when they get to the new space, they cannot remember why they are there," Dr. Gentile says. "They cannot remember the name of a colleague they worked with for years. There are difficulties with concentration and an inability to read complex texts. So there are cognitive symptoms, sleep disorder, flulike symptoms, frequent sore throats, tender lymph nodes, and often fevers and chills."

Dr. Martin Feldman adds that "immune system difficulty somehow pulls down hormonal function. Almost all patients with this syndrome have low adrenal function, and many have low thyroid function. So we have a hormonal mix-up causing fatigue, but behind this is the viral disease pulling down the immune system."

Potential Causes

VIRAL INFECTION Dr. Gentile explains that a number of studies have looked at viruses in connection with this syndrome. One theory posits a single viral agent. In fact, he states, "I have heard chronic fatigue syndrome being called a number of things from Epstein-Barr to mononucleosis.

"Epstein-Barr was brought into the discussion by way of a lab in Philadelphia that exclusively studies this virus. One of the lab assistants was negative for current and acute Epstein-Barr virus, but during the course of the study developed the symptoms of chronic fatigue syndrome. He was treated and found to be positive for Epstein-Barr virus. So we had the first studied case in which a person went from Epstein-Barr-negative to Epstein-Barr-positive at the same time that he had all the symptomatology for chronic fatigue syndrome. That began a flurry of studies investigating the Epstein-Barr connection. We now know there is not a high degree of correlation between the symptoms of chronic fatigue syndrome and Epstein-Barr serological titers. So Epstein-Barr is probably not the cause of chronic fatigue syndrome."

Dr. Gentile goes on to note that the Epstein-Barr virus is widely distributed in the populace. Most people have it by age 8. Thus, there is no clear distinction between those who have it and those who do not. We would expect many more people to be ill with chronic fatigue if it were indeed Epstein-Barr that was causing it.

Several other candidates have presented themselves, including human herpes virus 6 (HHV-6), a B-lymphocyte virus that was studied by the National Institutes of Health. "But again," Dr. Gentile says, "studies showed that this virus is very widely distributed and thus could not be the distinguishing agent responsible for the syndrome. Other studies are proceeding. Wistar, a renowned laboratory in Philadelphia, is looking at a retrovirus, HTLV-2 [human T-cell lymphotropic virus] as a possible cause."

Dr. Neenyah Ostrom, author of *America's Biggest Cover-Up* believes that HHV-6 may be involved. "What is interesting is that there are two types of this virus. One form is found very widely in the general population, and the other is found in people with cancer, AIDS, chronic fatigue syndrome, and other immunological problems. That virus can attack the immune system very effectively, and I believe it will eventually be found to be instrumental in causing chronic fatigue syndrome, AIDS, and some forms of cancer."

Other viruses that have been thought to contribute to chronic fatigue syndrome are coxsackie virus, adenovirus, enterovirus and the hepatitis virus, among others. Dr. Gentile states, "The consensus among practitioners is that a single virus probably does not cause this illness. We have to carefully distinguish between cause and trigger. Clearly, a virus may trigger a cascading set of events in various body systems: neural, endocrine, cognitive, hormonal. A variety of abnormalities may be found in these systems, but if viruses do trigger these imbalances, then they quickly hide within the normal cells—which is usually how viruses behave—while their effects wreak havoc in the body system."

It is as if the virus triggered something in the immune system that makes the system unable to self-regulate and find its way back to homeostasis. Thus, each time the immune system is stressed by a toxic load from the environment or food allergies, or when infections are reactivated, there is a breakdown. The flare-ups and relapses occur and recur frequently, reproducing all the symptoms. These relapses then compound themselves. If a patient is not sleeping every night, symptoms such as exhaustion and lowered immune crop up.

"We know, by the way," Dr. Gentile adds, "that the rhythms of this illness dovetail nicely with 90-minute circadian rhythms. In sleep, we have a REM [rapid eye movement] cycle that occurs every 90 minutes, and this is the cycle by which our immune system is synthesizing proteins. The immune system works lock and key with this cycle. But if one has a sleep disturbance caused by a virus or a set of viruses from this disorder, one's sleep will be off and so the immune system will be off."

ENVIRONMENTAL FACTORS, NUTRITION, AND ALLERGIES Dr. Majid Ali sees the surrounding environment and lifestyle as playing causal roles. He says that the immune system becomes injured by environmental pollutants such as mold, formaldehyde, and pesticides as well as by allergenic foods, poor nutrition, stress, and lack of physical fitness.

Dr. Shari Lieberman, a professor of nutrition, expands on this point. She has published articles and several books, including *The Real Vitamin and Mineral Book*. "We as a country are not healthy. We have all these discussions, lectures, books, and so on, concerning a healthy lifestyle. We have the information, but we are not actualizing it. I don't think people understand how all of the body's circumstances are impacted by the immune system."

Dr. Michele Galante also believes that allergies are important: "The patients I have seen have been very allergic not only to pollens and airborne agents but especially to foods and chemicals. These people are so sensitive and so debilitated that a short exposure to perfume, nail polish, gas fumes, carbon monoxide, or even just paint, such as from a freshly painted room, will give them headaches, make them weak, even make them emotionally upset. Chronic fatigue syndrome is closely connected to allergy."

Unfortunately, Dr. Ostrom adds, "some of these allergy-causing substances are unavoidable. Chemicals in our environment, aside from those in our foods (coloring, preservatives, and so on), are everywhere. There is chlorine in our water; the air is filled with pollutants—things that were not in our ecological system 50 or 60 years ago. Recent phenomena that accompany technological advances, such as the mercury in silver amalgam dental work, are weakening our systems. Each of these chemicals in itself does not necessarily have so strong an impact, but exposure to all of them together, day after day, for many years, overloads the liver and immune system. Electromagnetic influences, previously ignored, are now also under discussion. Many believe the cathode rays from computers affect the electromagnetic fields of the body, for instance, as does the electromagnetism of cellular phones, radio waves, and television waves—things relatively new to our environment."

METABOLIC REGULATION Chronic fatigue syndrome can also be explained in terms of immune system depression related to a failure in metabolic regulation. When glucose production is up, it brings on hypoglycemia, with a high degree of glucose in the blood causing an increased level of insulin, which lowers the glucose level excessively. Because of poor utilization of glucose, fatty acids increase in the blood to provide a sufficient level of energy. A high level of triglycerides will occur, and the immune system will be depressed because it needs a new army of T lymphocytes, which are not being produced because of derangement in lipid metabolism.

VITAMIN, MINERAL, AND HORMONAL DEFICIENCY Dr. Neil Block explains that lack of necessary vitamins, including C, E, and beta carotene, can also affect your immune system, as can a lack of minerals, particularly calcium, vanadium, copper, magnesium, potassium, molybdenum, boron, iodine, selenium, and chromium. The trace minerals are especially important for organ function.

Dr. Block also points to hormonal imbalances, particularly thyroid imbalance (especially hypothyroidism), which affects women six times as often as men. It tends to develop spontaneously between the ages of 20 and 50, although it can come at any time, often from unknown causes. The rare causes, which are the ones known for this disease, involve either a superabundance or a deficiency of iodine in the body, although the latter is unlikely in our society, where we have iodized salt and other sources. Another rare cause is consuming too many of certain vegetables, such as cauliflower, broccoli, and brussels sprouts, which tend to bind the active ingredient and inhibit thyroxin production.

Other hormones frequently out of the normal range include the adrenal hormones. "There are a number of tests we can run for this, none of which is perfect," Dr. Block continues, "for we have to remember that the adrenal gland is really two glands in one. On the inside, the adrenal medulla is making adrenaline and noradrenaline, and the outer coating, the adrenal cortex, is making cortisonelike substances that are related to our immune system and blood sugar control as well as corticoid steroids. The last thing the adrenal cortex is important for is modulating the male and female hormones that are in conversation with the pituitary gland and primary sexual organs. And, lastly, some chronic fatigue syndrome patients have imbalances in gender hormones. It is not unusual to have imbalances in the estrogen that governs the ovarian function or in other governors, such as LH [luteinizing hormone] from the pituitary gland or progesterone." In fact, women frequently come to Dr. Block with lack of menstruation, milky discharge from the breast, breast tenderness, or more menstrual cramps than usual. And every month one or two men come who are low in blood testosterone.

DRUG USE Dr. Galante remarks, "The allopathic drugs, conventional drugs, antibiotics, and steroids are major influences. The use and abuse of these drugs in childhood, for example, sets up chronically weakened conditions that will extend into adulthood and contribute to a predisposition for chronic fatigue. These drugs are suppressive in nature, not curative. They themselves impose an illness on the system. This may be one of the largest of the causal factors."

Dr. Ali talks about a young person suffering from chronic fatigue syndrome who went to a medical clinic and was given a prescription for steroids. We know steroids suppress the immune system, so why would anyone give these drugs to someone with this disorder? Steroids can create a sense of well-being and euphoria for a couple of days, but it is false.

PSYCHOLOGICAL FACTORS Dr. Gentile tells us that chronic fatigue seems to reduce a person's tolerance to stress. He has had patients who were marathoners before contracting the illness. They report that they had been working hard and then got sick with fever and chills. The illness waxed and waned. They would feel better at times and go back to running but then quickly relapse. These patients cannot tolerate stress in either the physical or the psychological form. Stress will exacerbate the illness again and again.

According to Dr. Paul Epstein, a key tenet of naturopathic medicine is to treat the underlying cause: "A person diagnosed with chronic fatigue syndrome has a suppressed immune system, which can be documented by blood tests and other measures. But what caused this? It may be improper diet; then the patient will need to eat properly. But we also need to ask why he adopted that diet in the first place. If the answer is stress, we can then ask what caused the person to follow certain patterns of reaction to stress. As we treat the patient, going through all the different problems layered one on top of the other, we eventually get in contact with the person's core self.

"One way to make this contact is through the inner child. Many people have been influenced by John Bradshaw's work on recovering and healing the inner child and on seeing how the wounds and scars of childhood may have led us to create lifestyles that are addictive. Thus, even as I help the person medically by giving advise on diet, stress reduction, and so on, I remember this. If we do not touch deeper problems, healing may not occur."

Diagnosis

Dr. Michael Vesselago uses laboratory tests to diagnose his patients and then treats them accordingly. He looks for viruses as well as allergies and stress: "I test the person for allergies with an IgE RAST [radioallergosorbent test] and get back a report showing how the body responds to over 100 tested foods. We adjust the diet so that the person is no longer eating allergy-causing foods, and that alone brings about a significant improvement in over 70 percent of individuals.

"If someone collapses unduly fast or wakes up tired and requires several cups of coffee to get going, then I will focus on the adrenals first. I do a test for adrenal function that involves checking cortisol, which is one of the main adrenal hormones. From that I get a picture of how well the adrenal glands are coping with stress during the day."

Dr. Martin Feldman says that the first step in the analysis of any patient who comes to him with fatigue, whether mild, moderate, or severe, is to profile the patient to see how she or he fits with the five major problems associated with the syndrome. Almost all people with chronic fatigue syndrome have at least one of these problems:

➤an immune viral breakdown, leading to low adrenal function
➤thyroid imbalance
➤vitamin B deficiency
➤hypoglycemia
➤cerebral allergies

Dr. Feldman also tests the thymus, spleen, and lymphatic system. "You could test the T- and B-cell counts. That's easy to do, but it's very expensive, so in daily practice it's easier to test thymus electrical energy. You can also do this for the spleen. When we find a weak thymus circuit, we can try any aspect of therapy within the weakened circuit to obtain a resonance that will help strengthen that circuit."

Dr. Gentile is more concerned with self diagnosis: "If you feel you have chronic fatigue syndrome, ask yourself these questions: Have I had debilitating fatigue for 6 months? Do I have flulike symptoms? Have I not found any physiological cause? Do I have pronounced sleeplessness? Do I have low stress tolerance so that if I take a short walk or try any sport, I feel vaguely ill and tired?"

Dr. Majid Ali states that most physicians have a tendency to focus narrowly on a problem. But, he says, "I don't think trying to find a diagnosis for one or two symptoms is terribly important. What is important is how the patient describes his or her suffering. We need to think of what we can do at a molecular and energetic level to relieve his or her suffering and restore his or her health.

"I've seen patients whose lives have been devastated by chronic fatigue syndrome. They've gone through all these drugs, antivirals, steroids. With each drug, they get better initially and then nose-dive. What do we do?

Alternative Therapies

The key to finding treatment for chronic fatigue syndrome, according to Dr. Gentile, is choosing the right expert. "It has reached the level of scientific respectability, and most practitioners and medical examiners believe it exists. It is important to have someone who is up to date on the literature and who has seen at a minimum 50 to 100 patients, someone who understands the ups and downs of the disease and is aware of the number of different treatments that have developed."

He points out several ways to locate a credible expert. For one thing, there are chronic fatigue syndrome support groups in every major town in our country and now worldwide that have lists of physicians who have tended to specialize in the disorder. There are national groups such as the Chronic Fatigue Syndrome Association. They maintain a list of doctors who understand the disease and have treated it and are sympathetic and believing.

"This last trait is so important," Dr. Galante explains, "because many sufferers have gone through scores of doctors. We're treating a woman now who has already seen 75 physicians all over the world. She was ready to give up because she feels people do not believe her. So a critical part of treating this illness is belief. A second thing to bear in mind is that because this is a chronic illness with a wide range of symptoms, it will tend to fall between the cracks of all the medical subspecializations. With this disease, it will not be adequate to go to a single physician. It would be worth considering putting together a team, which would include a GP/internist, one who works both with traditional and alternative therapies; an allergist/infectious disease specialist; and a psychologist/psychiatrist. This team could coordinate to work out a treatment plan, working so that the client understands what is coming next. And if these treatments don't work, they could determine why that might be and what would be worth trying next."

THE SPIRITUAL ELEMENT Dr. Ali tells us that in dealing with a chronic, devastating illness like this, hope and the spiritual element are essential for long-term success. He has had case histories that truly stretch the bounds of credulity: "Creating hope is very easy to do; sustaining hope is difficult, but it is central to healing. Before I see a patient, he or she has seen at least seven specialists. They've had biopsies, CAT [computed tomography] scans. When they come to me, it's not that easy to simply reassure them that they'll get better after they've seen the previous failures. But fortunately, by the time they get to me, they've listened to some of our tapes, read our books, and, most important, talked to some of the other patients who have gotten better. So when they come in, and they've seen our nursing staff, our ancillary staff, they see we are all serious. If they ask how my program differs, we say this: They do not have the option to remain sick."

VITAMIN SUPPLEMENTS Another component of treatment is supplements. The hope, according to Dr. Shari Lieberman, is not only to repair damage and stabilize the weakened immune system but also to overboost the system:

At Dr. Ali's clinic I watched a nurse making up an intravenous (IV) chronic fatigue syndrome protocol with vitamin C, magnesium sulfate, pantethine, calcium, pyridoxine, and a multivitamin formula. She says that patients who come in are very tired and have joint pains, headaches, and memory loss. These IVs help repair cell membranes and boost the immune system, which will then hopefully function better. About 90 percent of the patients have responded well. Dr. Ali will usually order a set of five to begin with, she says, and after that he can measure the patient's response, see how deep the problem is, and whether she requires further treatment.

"I see these drips as jump-starting the cellular enzymes," Dr. Ali says. "The enzymes, which are detoxification enzymes, are dependent on minerals and vitamins. If I feel there is enough time, when the patient is not acutely ill or has been chronically ill for a number of years, I will try to use a more conservative approach. But when I see people with severe, incapacitating fatigue, I use the IV. In fact, in one of our studies where we compared one group that had the IV and one group that didn't, we saw that the IV speeds up the recovery process."

Dr. Ali continues, "We have 14 different formulations or protocols to manage different clinical problems in our IV drips. For chronic fatigue syndrome, we use vitamin C, magnesium, calcium, pyridoxine, pantethine, zinc, B vitamins, molybdenum, potassium, copper, and selenium. Most of our protocols have 15 to 18 items, and we change their quantities depending on the individual's state."

Dr. Feldman has found that "people suffering from chronic fatigue syndrome are deficient in such nutrients as vitamins A, B_5, B_{12}, and E;

bioflavonoids; the essential fatty acids; zinc; selenium; and GLA (gamma-linoleic acid). All those must be put into order before we can proceed further."

Dr. Neil Block discusses his treatment: "If proteins or amino acids are low, we can try to individually supplement the amino acids. If minerals are lacking, they can be given individually or in tandem, trying to operate by an economy of scale so that a patient doesn't have to take from more than 10 to 15 bottles at a time.

"As for hormonal imbalance, I have 20 to 25 percent of my chronic fatigue syndrome patients on thyroid hormone. I prefer to use the more natural brands of thyroid hormone. Again, I believe in giving both the male and female hormones. We also have to try to adjust the pancreas and adrenals. For the pancreas I use chromium or chromium picolinate. For adrenals, the glandulars or homeopathics, and sometimes things such as licorice tend to help multiple hormones. If we are working on the pituitary, we use glandulars, the homeopathics, and on rare occasions I use a lot of the amino acids to try to build neurotransmitter activity. The amino acids to be used are arginine, tyrosine, and phenylalanine. Tryptophan was also once useful to me until they took it off the market. I'm also not afraid to use, correctly and in small doses, items obtained from the pharmacy. What I tend to shy away from are the tranquilizers, such as Valium and Librium. I do make use of antidepressants on occasion."

Often his patients have seen other physicians and holistic healers and may need only one or two things to turn the body around on multiple levels: "With neurotransmitters being easily adjusted nowadays, with items like the newer antidepressants such as Paxil and Zoloft, which lack drastic side effects and have a response beginning in 2 to 4 weeks, they're worthwhile. It's nice for a patient who has suffered 2, 4, or 6 years to take these new agents and within 2 to 4 weeks get at least some indication of the direction in which he or she is going."

ENZYMES Dr. Steven Whiting, author of *The Complete Guide to Optimal Wellness*, tells us about enzyme supplementation. There are two forms of supplementation, he says, and it is important to understand the difference between them. One type of product you can get at health food stores consists of whole enzymes and actually contains such things as pepsin, rennin, and trypsin, the real enzymes. They have their place, and they have their drawbacks. Their primary use is for chronic disease and for people who are very debilitated. The big problem with using them is that the body can grow to be dependent on them quite rapidly. When they are taken orally in the form of supplements, the body is not always encouraged to make them on its own.

"The second group of supplements," Dr. Whiting says, "is called enzyme precursors. These are substances that not only contain the raw materials for the body to build its own enzymes but frequently contain the vital stomach acid hydrochloric acid, which helps the body build many of the protein digestants. Remember, proteins are digested in the stomach, and carbohydrates and starches are digested in the intestinal tract. This is why a very unique enzyme system has been created and needs to be maintained."

He continues: "For the average person looking for a good enzyme product, I recommend one that would contain at least the following things. First, hydrochloric acid. After years of eating junk foods and dead, lifeless foods, we need it to help with stomach digestion. According to a recent survey by the University of California at Berkeley, only 9 percent of the population eats the recommended number of fresh fruits and vegetables per day. This product should also contain protein digestants, which should include papain and pepsin. There should be fat digestants, ox bile and pancreatin. Also a starch digestant, which would be bromelain."

"The bulk of the five years of research I have done for my book is about what I call whole-spectrum nutrition. We have been able to isolate about 102 nutrients that the body needs every day. These include the 16 vitamins, the three fatty acids, 8 to 12 amino acids, and about 72 minerals.

"What we found out in working with patients, such as those with chronic fatigue syndrome, in a clinical environment is that the concept that has developed in the last 20 years of using potency to address chronic diseases may have been only part of the picture. In reality, we are finding that the ratio of nutrients to each other is as important as if not more important than potency alone."

He illustrates by talking about calcium absorption. Calcium is one of the more difficult minerals for most people to absorb. As they age, people's overall pH increases, and they lose the natural acids in the body, making calcium absorption even less efficient. Dr. Whiting describes a study he conducted with Paul Saltman, head chemist at the University of California at San Diego, in 1991 on the use of calcium. They divided 59 postmenopausal women into several groups: "One got a placebo, one got calcium, one got a mixture of trace minerals, and the fourth group got calcium with the trace minerals. Essentially, at the end of two years all the women had experienced substantial bone loss, which would be expected because of osteoporosis in that time period—all, that is, except the last group, who got the calcium and the trace minerals together. They actually had a 2 percent increase in bone density.

"This is very indicative of what has been found in many recent studies, which is that it is the combination of nutrients that is extremely important." Thus, when Dr. Whiting sees a patient with chronic fatigue syndrome, "The first thing I recommend is that she take a full spectrum of supplements that provide all the needed vitamins and minerals. Once they are on a full program, we will be in a much better position to address various health challenges."

HERBAL THERAPIES Many herbs can help to heal the immune system, and thus play a role in chronic fatigue syndrome. Herbologist Letha Hadady offers some recommendations. Strengthening agents include Chinese ginseng, dandelion, false ginseng, *Andrographis*, *Eclipta alba*, and honeysuckle. Honeysuckle flower,

Andrographis, and dandelion may also help to destroy germs. Chinese blood tonics, include *han lien tsao*, which is called *Eclipta alba* in Latin and grows wild in the American southwest. It builds blood without any side effects, such as inflammation. You can take it every day in powdered form. Hadady also mentions *fo ti*, which builds blood while it keeps us cool.

There are three types of ginseng: American, Chinese, and false. The American type provides more moisture and more saliva and is good after a fever. Chinese ginseng, called *ren shen*, gives us energy. *Dang shen*, or false ginseng, makes us feel stronger without feeling hotter. All can be used in soups. When *dang shen* and astragalus are used together, the first lifts our energy and the second sends our defenses to the surface. Cayenne pepper increases circulation and makes us feel stronger.

There are also herbs for relaxing the nervous system. Siberian ginseng can be taken as an extract or in capsule form. Valerian, taken in capsules, can quiet the nervous system: "For people who are depressed," Hadady says, "we need to bring them to their center as a way to be grounded and to feel more whole. Use ginger and mint. Mint helps bring the worries out of the head, and ginger helps burn them away, because it is digestive and heating and so it brings us warmly to our centers. They make a good combination."

High Energy preparation is an herb mixture that uses western and Oriental ingredients: *gotu kola*, American ginseng, damiana, red clover, peppermint, and cloves. It strengthens the adrenals and lungs.

Hadady adds that cloves and hot water will increase your energy and make you breathe more deeply.

Dr. Lieberman has looked at American plants to find ones that can strengthen the debilitated immune system that accompanies chronic fatigue syndrome. "I'd say hands down that about the most important herb in this area is licorice root," she says. "A specific valuable compound found in this root is glycyrrhizin, available at health food stores as a supplement. It's not the easiest thing to find, but a few companies make it. Glycyrrhizin is just remarkable at boosting the lymphatic and immune systems, the white blood cells, and the thymus gland."

Glycyrrhizin can actually be therapeutic in relation to some of the viruses implicated in chronic fatigue syndrome. Glycyrrhizin stimulates the production of interferon naturally. It supports the thyroid gland and boosts natural killer cells and other aspects of immune functioning. A therapeutic dose ranges from 75 to 300 milligrams per day. It's important to monitor your blood pressure while taking this supplement. "I haven't seen many patients' blood pressure go up when taking this, but it will occasionally happen," Dr. Lieberman notes.

Another antiviral is echinacea. Dr. Lieberman believes that it is not used nearly enough for chronic disease and immune dysfunction. Many people use it for influenza, but it can be useful for other viruses as well. Echinacea has a remarkable ability to naturally stimulate interferon, natural killer cells, and phagocytes.

The liquid extracts of echinacea work best, Dr. Lieberman says. Use 50 drops once or twice a day, depending on the severity of your symptoms. "It's been recommended that you use echinacea four days on, four days off. There is some concern that if you use it all the time, you may adapt to it and it may stop boosting certain aspects of immune function. We don't know that for sure, but to be on the safe side, that's my recommendation. But I keep my patients on glycyrrhizin long term, though I gradually cut the dose down and maybe eventually have them on 75 milligrams per day as a prophylactic."

DIETARY CHANGES Gracia Perlstein, an alternative health care practitioner with a private practice in New York says that for chronic fatigue, food is the best medicine: "We really don't have any existing drugs on the market to help this condition. In fact, most drugs will weaken immunity and delay recovery further. It is best to approach this with natural supports to inherent healing processes." While there are no quick cure-alls, she makes the following recommendations to speed up recovery.

A diet of pure, dense, nutrient-rich whole foods is imperative for this condition: "You want to include plenty of fresh organic vegetables. Cruciferous vegetables such as broccoli, cauliflower, and brussels sprouts are very important for their immune-enhancing properties. You want onions and garlic, the poor man's cure-all.

"Choose from a wide assortment of whole foods. Don't eat the same few over and over again. In this weakened state you can develop allergic responses to foods consumed repeatedly in large amounts. Eating different foods will ensure that you get a variety of nutrients and will keep you from developing allergic responses. Amaranth, quinoa, and other grains not commonly eaten by Americans are good to include.

"Really emphasize the green foods. Have a dark green salad daily. Super green powders are very helpful as well. Add them to juices, but do not emphasize sweet fruit and carrot juice.

"Eat an adequate amount of high-quality proteins. The best sources are vegetarian because of the low toxicity and ease of digestion. Good vegetarian proteins are tofu, tempeh, fortified soy milk, and legumes. You can benefit from small amounts of fresh fish because fish is high in omega-3 fatty acids. But there are some precautions you must take. Be sure to find a market that gets fish from clean, unpolluted waters and make sure they do not dip it in chlorine, which is a common practice. If you eat farm-raised fish, it should be organically raised. If you eat poultry, it should be naturally raised as well, free of hormones and pesticide residues. Consume only small amounts of animal protein, no more than 3 to 4 oz a day.

"The best way to have protein is in a soup. An excellent old Chinese recipe for an immune-enhancing soup combines a whole astragalus root with onions, garlic, ginger, and free-range chicken, fish, tofu, or tempeh. Some fresh green vegetables and a handful of brown rice are added to that. The soup is brought to a boil and then simmered. Some miso is added for flavor. This is highly nourishing, easy to digest, and excellent for helping a weakened individual regain strength.

"Drink plenty of pure water daily. In colder seasons unsweetened herb tea, such as immune-supportive echinacea tea, is a very good source of liquid. Cold water is a little shocking to the digestive system for people with chronic fatigue syndrome, so you want warm liquids and plenty of them."

HOMEOPATHY Homeopathy is Dr. Galante's specialty; it has been very effective against chronic fatigue syndrome. Homeopathic remedies, all made from natural substances, are given in microdoses. The essence of homeopathy is to select for each individual a remedy based on her or his unique physical constitution and manifestation of symptoms.

ACUPUNCTURE Registered nurse and acupuncturist Abigail Rist-Podrecca points out that the *chi*, or bioelectrical energy, flows through pathways called meridians in the body. Disease, she says, is associated with an energy blockage. Acupuncture needles inserted in some of the 365 points that can be used open the blockages so that the energy can flow smoothly through the meridians. In addition, the needles dilate the blood vessels so that more blood flows through the area, bringing more oxygen and nutrients, which aid all aspects of health.

TAI CHI A benefit of tai chi is that it increases one's awareness both internally and environmentally. "Then you can choose which to work on, whether there is something physically wrong or something in the environment that needs to be corrected," says Eric Schneider of the Northeastern Tai Chi Chuan Association.

According to Schneider, you have to cultivate a part of your body that can observe phenomena dispassionately without having to grab on to every experience and run with it, so that when you find yourself in stressful situations you can say quietly, "Oh, so this is what is happening now. What can I do about it? What are my options, and how am I feeling?"

However, it takes 10 years to achieve what is called the *gung chi*, which means that the body is able to contain energy. This is not a quick fix.

IMAGERY AND HEALING Dr. Paul Epstein says imagery is a therapeutic technique that helps people explore through words and symbols so they can understand the language of the subconscious.

According to Dr. Epstein, "Usually what comes up is the issue that is at the core of what will be the healing. People may get in touch with childhood wounds or abuse from the past that needs healing. Perhaps they'll get in touch with the fact that the work they are doing is not real work.

"In one such case, with a person suffering from chronic fatigue syndrome, we found that the illness was a case of a person trying to get love. She had not let go of trying to get love from her mom and dad. She was still stuck at that place. And the pain and the grief of not having that love were not only weakening her immune system but keeping her stuck in the unhealthy way she was living her life."

Dr. Majid Ali reiterates some of Dr. Epstein's message: "What I demonstrate to my patients is that the way you look at the world around you determines the biology under your skin. If you can be in a self-regulatory, healing mode, your brain activity, heart activity, muscle energy, skin energy will all be functioning positively. Or you can be trying to figure things out, think everything through in an overly intellectual way, and your biology will be as up and down as the New York skyline. This is the stress mode, and it causes disease. Another mode is an even, steady-state mode, a resting mode.

"Our goal is to perceive the energy in these modes and understand how the energy profoundly affects the electrophysiological profile. Can we allow this energy to guide us into the healing mode? We want a transition from an ordinary, thinking, nervous stressful mode that causes disease to a nonthinking, meditative, deep-breathing mode that makes us well. That is our goal."

AYURVEDA Dr. Nancy Lonsdorf, medical director of the Maharishi Ayurveda Health Center in Washington, D.C., and coauthor of *A Woman's Best Medicine*, defines fatigue as an imbalance in the body's rest-activity cycle. According to Ayurvedic principles, the natural structures of rest cycles allow the body to recover from activity cycles: "A state of chronic fatigue means that the body has not fully rejuvenated itself."

Dr. Lonsdorf reports that many of her clients overcome fatigue by adhering to the basic rules of Maharishi Ayurveda, which address rest, activity, digestion, cleansing, and meditation.

THE NOTION OF SELF-HEALING Dr. Epstein wants to help patients listen, explore, and understand the message of their disease, which is the key that unlocks the door to recovery: "After the diagnosis and medications, natural or other, there still has to be an exploration of healing for this person. We might have conditioned immune-suppressant responses built into our attitudes, beliefs, the way we live our life, the way we think, and the way we eat. An illness cannot be fixed from the outside; there is no magic bullet for chronic fatigue syndrome.

"People heal themselves by engaging in a self-healing process, by looking at their life and its meaning. It may seem rather complicated, but it is not. It is based on the knowledge that we do not get sick overnight. The condition may manifest suddenly in certain symptoms, but it took years and years to arrive. And it was not from one virus, not just from Epstein-Barr or herpes or parasites, low blood sugar, or electromagnetic pulsations. It was a combination of all of them.

"What is needed in treating chronic fatigue syndrome or AIDS and similar problems is a new approach. We should be looking not for the quick fix or what will work for everybody but for an approach that is individualized and holistic and empowers the patient to get involved in the cure and gives that patient belief and hope that healing is possible.

"There are two points in my treatment that I've been told by patients have helped them most: that I have given them hope and belief that healing is possible and that I have shown them that there are things they could do to help themselves. I don't heal anybody. Doctors don't heal anybody. They support people as they heal themselves."

44

Diabetes

Diabetes mellitus is a serious condition that affects nearly 16 million Americans a year. It is the third leading cause of death in the United States and a primary cause of new cases of blindness, renal disease, and nontraumatic amputations. Dr. Robert Atkins, a complementary physician from New York City, says, "Diabetes has tripled in the last 35 years. In addition, certain subsegments of the population are more often affected; African-Americans, for example, are disproportionately affected."

Causes

Diabetes is closely associated with heart disease, and the incidence of both conditions increased when Americans began to change their dietary patterns. "There is a wonderful book written about 25 years ago," Dr. Atkins continues, "called *The Saccharine Disease*, by Dr. Cleave. He made observations, one of which was 'the law of 20 years,' which says that after you introduce refined carbohydrates into a culture, two illnesses emerge two decades later, diabetes and heart disease. We know that a Third World diet without refined carbohydrates leads to no heart disease and no diabetes. When one illness emerges, so does the other. Studies of this sort have linked diabetes with heart disease. We know that a woman who is diabetic is three times more likely than women in the general population to get heart disease."

Under normal circumstances, insulin is released by the pancreas in response to elevated levels of sugar in the blood. It promotes the transport and entry of glucose to muscle cells and various tissues, thus lowering blood sugar levels. In a diabetic, part of the process is interrupted as a result of a deficiency in, resistance to, or insensitivity to insulin.

INSULIN DEFICIENCY For many years, it was thought that diabetes is purely and simply a deficiency syndrome in which the body does not produce sufficient quantities of insulin for proper glucose metabolism and assimilation. More recently, it has been learned that many diabetics do produce enough insulin, but their cells do not take it in. The problem is, then, due to insulin insensitivity or resistance.

INSULIN INSENSITIVITY Insulin enters cells at points known as receptor sites. When the receptor sites are plugged because of fat, cholesterol, inactivity, and obesity, insulin cannot enter. As a result, glucose stays in the blood and creates hyperglycemia, or high blood sugar. This excess sugar is diagnosed as diabetes. In such cases, there is no need to increase insulin production but rather a need to enhance insulin sensitivity. A person with diabetes needs to work at making his or her own insulin more efficient, and simply increasing the amount of insulin will not do that.

INSULIN RESISTANCE Insulin resistance is a phenomenon that is closely related to insulin insensitivity. With insulin resistance, there is also a sufficient or even overabundant supply of insulin, but allergic responses prevent insulin from doing its job. Usually allergies to specific foods suppress the activity and efficiency of insulin. Different factors may be responsible for a disordered carbohydrate metabolism in different people. Wheat, for instance, may create symptoms of high blood sugar in one woman and corn may affect another. Offending substances can be determined on an individual basis with food allergy tests.

Types of Diabetes

Type I diabetes is the most serious form of the disease. Type I diabetes used to be called juvenile diabetes, because for many years it was believed that this type of diabetes only occurred in the childhood or teenage years. This form of diabetes is characterized by a true insulin deficiency. It results when the pancreas is damaged from some exotic viral infection or even a highly toxic state. The disease may also be a genetic condition. In type I diabetes the beta cells in the pancreas that produce insulin are destroyed. Since type I diabetics have an insulin deficiency, they have to take insulin by injection daily, and generally for life.

Maturity-onset or type II diabetes is more of an acquired disease. It is often precipitated by chronic excess weight from poor diet and/or lack of exercise. It may also be brought on by overconsumption of stressor foods or other allergens that are insulin resistors.

Type II diabetes accounts for some 90 percent of all diabetes in the U.S. It occurs most frequently in adults over age 40. In type II diabetes, the beta cells in the pancreas still produce insulin, but for a variety of reasons there may be insufficient insulin production or the body may not be adequately using the insulin that is produced. Thus this form of the disease is characterized by complications of insulin resistance and insulin sensitivity rather than, in most cases, a true deficiency of insulin. For this reason, maturity onset diabetes can frequently be non-insulin-dependent.

Some nondiabetic women develop a type of diabetes called gestational diabetes during pregnancy, usually in the last trimester.

Symptoms

Often there are no symptoms present, especially in the beginning stages of type II diabetes. Obesity is sometimes a sign of a prediabetic state, especially when the excess weight is concentrated at the waistline and just above the waistline. Classic diabetic symptoms are more often experienced by type I diabetics and include frequent urination, especially at night, great thirst and hunger, fatigue, weight loss, irritability, and restlessness. Progressively, the eyes, kidneys, nervous system, and skin become affected. Infections and hardening of the arteries commonly develop. In type I diabetes, coma from a lack of insulin is a constant danger.

Traditional Approaches to Treatment

MEDICATIONS Before the development of insulin in the 1920s, diabetic patients had a bleak prognosis. Sufferers saw the condition rapidly go from bad to worse as complications such as blindness, gout, and gangrene developed. Overall life span was drastically shortened.

In the beginning, insulin appeared to be a miraculous drug, and it probably was. The life span of diabetic children was extended from months to decades. Today, many of these children live normal, productive lives.

Insulin is still the primary therapy for type I diabetes. Type I diabetics generally take insulin at least once a day, frequently several times a day.

While some type II diabetics require injections of insulin, many are given oral hypoglycemic medications. Many type II diabetics incorrectly believe that these pills are simply a form of insulin, but that is not the case. None of the oral medications used to treat type II diabetes contain insulin. They are designed to help your body use the insulin that is in your pancreas more effectively, or to stimulate better insulin production. Consequently, oral medications can only be used by diabetics whose pancreas still makes some insulin. In addition, some type II diabetics can control their diabetes entirely through diet and exercise.

In recent years, a number of new drugs have been introduced to treat type II diabetes. Some of these drugs are being rushed through the approval process without adequate review of their safety. One drug, Rezulin, was pulled from the market in early 2000. Some 500,000 Americans had been using the medication, which was approved for use by the Food and Drug Administration (FDA) in 1997. The FDA asked the manufacturer to withdraw Rezulin after it was linked to 89 confirmed reports of liver failure, including 61 deaths.

COMPLICATIONS AND BLOOD SUGAR CONTROL Although diabetes can cause a wide variety of complications, from kidney and eye problems to nerve damage, some of these complications can be reduced considerably by carefully controlling blood sugar. For many years doctors assumed that diabetics whose blood glucose levels were as close to normal ranges as possible reduced their risk of serious complications. In 1993, the Diabetes Control and Complications Trial (DCCT), one of the largest studies ever conducted, confirmed that diabetics in the intensive control group, with glycohumaglobin rates that averaged 7.1, reduced their risk of eye disease by 76 percent compared with the less aggressively managed group, with glycohumaglobin rates of 8.9 percent. Across the board, diabetics in the intensive control group had a 50 percent reduction in all serious diabetic complications. Although the trial was conducted only on type I diabetics, experts believe that the findings of the study apply to all diabetics.

CURRENT DIETARY RECOMMENDATIONS The findings of the DCCT study make diet and eating habits even more important for diabetics than previously. Eating the right foods can help maintain proper blood sugar levels, as well as helping to boost your immune system. In 1994 the American Diabetes Association changed the dietary guidelines for diabetics.

In the past there was one standard diabetic diet, prescribed for all diabetics. Now the ADA recommends that diabetics work with experts in diet and nutrition to individualize their diets. In the past, complex carbohydrates, like potatoes and bread, were restricted because it was believed that they caused moderate increases in blood sugar. The new dietary recommendations recognize that complex carbohydrates are not the problem they were once thought to be. Emphasis is now put on the total amount of carbohydrates in a meal, rather than the source. Diabetics are frequently taught to count carbohydrates, and match medication requirements to carbohydrate intake. This is especially true for insulin-dependent diabetics.

Unlike simple sugars, complex carbohydrates are beneficial. Although both are broken down into glucose, the latter do not go directly into the bloodstream. While simple sugars immediately enter the blood, complex carbohydrates go through a long process of digestion and only very gradually release sugar into the blood. Therefore, they do not then contribute to the high blood sugar levels, as do simple carbohydrates. Instead, they stabilize and improve health.

In addition, fat and protein are more carefully monitored than in the past. Diabetics who are overweight are told to keep fat intake to no more than 20 to 25 percent of total calories. Large amounts of protein may be related to accelerated kidney damage. This is because protein must be immediately processed by the body; it cannot be stored. This puts a great stress on the nephron cells, which filter the body's toxins. Many diabetics suffer from kidney deterioration as a result and must receive dialysis or a kidney transplant. Studies show that the elimination of meat from the diet is often enough to reverse kidney damage.

The Natural Approach

Despite its severity, diabetes need not be as debilitating as it usually is. While there is currently no cure, there are ways of enhancing the body's natural defenses through nutrition, avoidance of allergy-producing substances, and exercise. A healthy lifestyle and alternative approaches to treatment can decrease the amount of insulin or oral medications needed by some persons, although type I diabetics will need to continue taking insulin for life.

The goal of treatment can and should be to build up the body's ability to function as independently as possible. When changing to a more holistic approach to treatment, it is important not to immediately discontinue any of your diabetic medication. Instead, a preventive medicine physician should assist in the gradual transition. With a doctor's guidance, medication may be reduced or completely eliminated with time. Complete elimination, however, is not always possible.

Physicians who practice alternative approaches to treating diabetes for the most part employ a program combining exercise and dietary modification aimed both at better nutrition and at weight loss, where indicated. Medications are used only as second- and third-line approaches. This sort of program usually controls the disease and its ancillary complications in a less invasive, more efficacious manner, in a short period of time.

While type II diabetics respond most dramatically, even type I diabetics may be able to reduce their insulin dependency. More important, they are able to alleviate many of the insidious complications that have come to be thought of as intrinsic to diabetes.

DIET Since diabetes and heart disease are so closely related, Dr. Atkins recommends that some people with diabetes follow a Dean Ornish program, in which they drastically cut down on dietary fats. The best diet consists of organic vegetarian foods, eaten raw, sprouted, steamed, baked, or stir-fried with little or no oil. Those who have a true insulin disorder will not fare well on a high-carbo-hydrate diet, since diabetes is a carbohydrate metabolism disorder.

"It is important to know who needs carbohydrate restriction versus who needs fat restriction," Dr. Atkins says. "To determine that, there are a variety of tests, including a cholesterol profile in which we look at the ratio between the triglycerides and the HDL [high-density lipoprotein]. When a person has a blood sugar disorder leading to a lipid disorder, the ratio is extremely high. To be really safe, the number should be approximately the same or the HDL should be higher than the triglycerides. It is perfectly appropriate to spend five or six weeks on one diet and then get all of your parameters checked again, and then spend five or six weeks on the other diet and get them checked again. In that way, you can make an intelligent decision."

EXERCISE An exercise regimen is crucial for burning calories and normalizing metabolism, and is especially important for overweight adults, who are often inactive.

Exercise also heightens the body's sensitivity to insulin. By lowering cho-lesterol, it lowers triglyceride levels in the blood, making cells more available for glucose assimilation. This is why the insulin requirements of diabetic ath-letes always drop while they're engaged in swimming, soccer, and other sports. Athletes also notice an increase in their insulin requirements when they cease doing their physical activities for an extended period of time.

Athletes are not the only ones who benefit from exercise. Ten to twenty minutes of light exercise after each meal helps reduce the amount of insulin necessary to keep blood sugar levels under control. A brisk walk gets the body's metabolism working a little faster so that food is more easily absorbed. That prevents blood sugar from rising too high.

An exception to the rule involves diabetics with heart disease. In these patients, exercising after eating may precipitate an angina attack because of the transfer of blood from the intestines to the legs and other parts of the body.

ALLERGY TESTING Testing for food allergies can determine which foods are responsible for insulin resistance. Clinical experience has shown that this approach to treatment is the most useful way to get to the root of adult-onset diabetes and reverse the condition. Patients can usually be weaned from insulin, since an insulin deficiency is not the cause of the problem. Eliminating allergy-producing foods may also foster weight loss. This occurs because people crave foods when they are allergic to them. When these foods are taken out of the diet, the desire for them eventually stops.

To determine whether a specific food is causing hyperglycemia, a doctor can monitor a patient's blood sugar before and after that food is eaten. Foods that raise the blood sugar cause allergic reactions and should be eliminated.

SUPPLEMENTS In addition to diet and exercise, the following supplements are important to know about:

CHROMIUM PICOLINATE. Chromium helps normalize glucose levels in insulin-dependent diabetics.

MAGNESIUM AND POTASSIUM. These minerals also help to maintain a glucose tolerance level.

ZINC. Zinc is essential for normal insulin production.

ENZYMES. Enzymes useful in controlling insulin-dependent diabetes are digestive protylase, amylase, and lipase.

VANADYL SULFATE. Vanadyl sulfate may be the most important mineral for diabetes. It was discovered in France in the late 1800s and used to help diabetics before insulin appeared on the market. It works at the cellular level and is most effective when taken three times a day.

HERBS Plants containing phytochemicals with antidiabetic properties, in order of potency, are as follows:

Cichorium intybus (chicory)
Rauwolfia serpentina (Indian snakeroot)
Thymus vulgaris (common thyme)
Arctium lappa (gobo)
Carthamus tinctorius (safflower)
Passiflora edulis (maracuya)
Opuntia ficus-indica (Indian fig)
Taraxacum officinale (dandelion)
Tetrapanax papyriferus (rice paper plant)
Canavalia ensiformis (jack bean)
Linum usitatissimum (flax)
Pueraria lobata (kudzu)
Hordeum vulgare (barley)
Inula helenium (elecampane)
Althaea officinalis (marsh mallow)
Oenothera biennis (evening primrose)
Avena sativa (oats)
Triticum aestivum (wheat)
Medicago sativa (alfalfa)
Panicum maximum (guinea grass)

Plants containing phytochemicals with insulin-sparing properties, in order of potency, are as follows:

Cocos nucifera (coconut)
Plantago major (common plantain)

TOPICAL TREATMENT FOR DIABETIC ULCERS Ulceration at various locations plagues many patients with diabetes and causes a condition that is often serious enough to warrant amputation. This tragedy may be averted with a simple solution. According to clinical studies, raw, unprocessed honey is an ideal dressing agent for almost every type of wound or ulcer. It sterilizes the ulcerated area, and often works even after antibiotics fail.

OTHER APPROACHES Mucokehl (made from the fungus *Mucor recemosus*), which was originally developed in Germany, may actually reverse diabetic neuropathy. People using this remedy get feeling back in their extremities, and their eyesight improves. Many practitioners also recommend chelation therapy for reducing diabetic retinopathy and healing foot ulcers.

Monitoring and Preventing Diabetes

Diabetics and those who wish to prevent diabetes can do a great deal to monitor themselves. It's important to look for the presence of antibodies that attack some of the body to defend against an ingested allergen. This is easy to see if the symptoms are blatant, but not if they are subtle. The thing to look for is a general lowering of the body's immune response.

The best way to see this is to go 5 days without eating the food (or any of its relatives) you wish to test. If you want to test milk, abstain from cheese, ice cream, and all other dairy items or processed foods that contain milk as an ingredient. After 5 days, eat a meal consisting of just milk and eat generous amounts of it. Then tune in to your body's response. If you experience headaches, stomachaches, pulse rate changes, increased heartbeat or blood sugar, depression, lethargy, dizziness, or even delusions, you can see that your body has reacted negatively to this substance. In other words, you have an allergic response to it. You will have to back off from it. Leave it alone for 12 weeks initially. When it is reintroduced into the diet, it must be rotated with other foods. Eat it in modest amount no more often than once every 4 days.

"Of course, there are a lot of good things about that 4-day basis," says Dr. William Philpott, a prominent diabetes researcher and clinician. "You will eat... 30 or 40 kinds of foods instead of the half dozen you've been eating. This is a very wholesome thing. To have the necessary nutrition you will have a wide range of foods." It is a good idea to try introducing new foods into your diet, ones that you have never thought to eat. Try not to eat any foods more frequently than twice a week.

Dr. Philpott recommends that you invest in some diabetic equipment so that you can monitor your blood sugar an hour after each meal. "At least 110 is optimum," he says, "and 160 or beyond is high blood sugar. Before the next meal, test your blood sugar again to make sure it is at least 120 before starting your next meal. If it is not, wait and exercise. Get it down before your next meal. Monitor your pH from saliva; it should be 6.4. If it is below 6.4, you are having a reaction to the food. Measure your pulse; if it varies drastically, you are reacting to the food. Blood pressure is more significant. Physical symptoms, mental symptoms, and blood sugar are the most important. They are absolutely essential. It will take about 30 days to do this."

Gestational Diabetes

About 3 percent of nondiabetic women develop a type of diabetes called gestational diabetes during pregnancy, usually in the last trimester. Gestational diabetes is diagnosed with an oral glucose tolerance test. In many cases this type of diabetes can be controlled with diet and exercise. Although gestational diabetes disappears after delivery, as many as 50 percent of women with gestational diabetes will develop diabetes later.

Dr. Susanna Reid, a naturopathic physician at the Center for Natural Medicine in Connecticut, says that diet and exercise are the key to controlling gestational diabetes.

DIET Dr. Reid advises women with gestational diabetes to learn how to eat on the low end of the glycemic index. The glycemic index was developed around 1982 by Dr. Sullivan, who gave people glucose and then measured how high the sugar level in their blood rose. He then established that level as 100 percent of the glycemic index. He repeated the experiment by giving people various foods and measuring how high their blood sugar would go just as he had with glucose, and assigned then each food a percentage.

Dr. Reid says that foods we don't normally associate with sugar may still be high on the glycemic index. "A baked potato and puffed rice are both 100 percent on the glycemic index, which means that they raise your blood sugar significantly. This is bad for your body; it goes into a state of alarm when your blood sugar rises so quickly and significantly, and it produces more insulin. Since the rate of rise is so rapid, the body tends to overproduce insulin and people get what is called reactive hypoglycemia (low blood sugar). Then they have to eat sugar to get their blood sugars back up again. Therefore you need to eat foods low on the glycemic index to avoid either hypoglycemia or reactive hypoglycemia."

She explains that the position of some foods on the glycemic index may seem counterintuitive. These include fruits, nuts, and legumes. For example, peaches, plums, grapefruit, and cherries are between 20 and 29 percent on the glycemic index. But potatoes and even carrots and parsnips and rice are at the top level. She says, "When you eat foods that are high on the glycemic index, you need to have a healthy fat with them. Doing this seems to prevent the rapid rise in blood sugar. If you had a baked potato, for example, you'd want to have olive oil in it."

Foods that you may think would be low on the glycemic index, such as vegetables, are often among the highest. "Peas are between 50 and 59 percent on the index and corn is between 60 and 69 percent. Yams are very high, but sweet potatoes are much lower on the index than yams. Brown rice and all the grains tend to be very high."

EXERCISE Dr. Reid also tells her patients about the importance of exercise for gestational diabetics. She says that by exercising regularly, we can often keep our blood sugar levels within the normal range. "When a person exercises, it improves insulin's ability to remove glucose from the blood and also decreases insulin resistance. If you exercise 60 minutes a day at 60 to 70 percent of the maximum heart rate, then usually after just one week of exercise you'll see an improvement in the glucose tolerance test. But be careful not to overdo it and cause your blood sugars to drop too low."

Dr. Reid warns that a woman should not attempt to become a world-class athlete while pregnant. "But she should continue and enhance her current exercise program. There are some things that she needs to be careful about. She should not lie supine and attempt to lift weights, she shouldn't get too warm, she should maintain adequate hydration, and she probably shouldn't take up a new sport in which balance is a main requirement because she is having to adjust daily to changes in the shape of her body and her orientation in space. She wouldn't want to do anything where she might fall, such as inline skating at top speed."

Dr. Reid's favored exercises are running and walking. "Women need to feel free to move when they are pregnant. It is not a pathological state. They are not ill."

NUTRITIONAL SUPPLEMENTS Dr. Reid cautions against using some herbal supplements during pregnancy. "Most of the herbs are contraindicated in pregnancy, so one has to be cautious in treating gestational diabetes. For example, traditional herbs we would use to treat non-insulin-dependent diabetes, which gestational diabetes usually is, are bitter melon (*Mamordica charantia*), fenugreek, elecampane (*Inula helenium*), and garlic and onion supplements. All those are contraindicated in a pregnant woman. Ginkgo and Jerusalem artichoke are not contraindicated, and in all of the research that I've done I can't find a contraindication for *Gymnema sylvestre*, which is an herb that seems to increase the pancreas's ability to produce insulin, which would be advantageous in patients with gestational diabetes."

Patient Stories

Dr. Julian Whitaker, who has worked with many diabetic patients, has had considerable success with a program that emphasizes diet, vitamin and mineral supplements, exercise, and practical education. Here he describes two cases. The first was a 27-year-old patient who was taught to use these essential tools.

He was on insulin for about 6 months and was also having hypoglycemic reactions. When we saw him, he was taking only 10 to 12 units of insulin per day and his blood sugar levels were very low. Whenever you have a situation like this, you can cut down on the insulin and then eventually get off it completely. We measured in his blood a protein called C-peptide which measures the body's production of insulin. If his pancreas was not producing insulin, his C peptide would be about 0. This patient had a close to normal C-peptide, meaning that his pancreas was producing insulin. We put him on a program to sensitize his body to the lower levels of insulin his pancreas was producing. This included exercise, a low-fat diet, and vitamin and mineral supplements.... It has now been about 9 months, and he has been without insulin. His blood sugar level would go to about 140 or so after breakfast, but then he was told to exercise, and when he keeps up his program, his blood sugar level stays under control. I think this indicates that you have a very powerful tool in diet, exercise, and minerals which is patently ignored by most physicians treating diabetes as they systematically utilize insulin and oral drugs for their diabetic patients.

Another case of Dr. Whitaker's illustrates the shortcomings of traditional diabetic treatment and shows how an alternative approach may be more appropriate and efficacious.

Five years before I first saw this patient, he had had mild high blood pressure for which he was started on diuretics. He used hydrochlorothiazide, a thiazide diuretic. This drug has a tendency to lower potassium and elevate blood sugar, findings that are well known and are listed in the Physicians' Desk Reference, *but it is still the most commonly used prescription medication worldwide. The patient's potassium level dropped, he developed some cardiac arrhythmias, his blood sugar level began to go up, and his problem was diagnosed as high blood pressure plus diabetes. He was placed on oral medications that failed to lower his blood sugar, so he was placed on insulin. When a patient like this gentleman, who did not have any diabetes to speak of but had a drug-induced form of diabetes, is placed on insulin, his blood sugar drops to a very low level. The body responds to this low level by generating glucose from the liver and shooting the blood glucose up very high so that when the highs and lows are checked, the physician feels the patient is out of control and increases the insulin level; this, of course, only increases the rebound, or the up and down characteristics, of the blood sugar. This is what happened. Not only was he having much higher and much lower blood sugar levels, he was having one or two hypoglycemic attacks a day. He kept going back to the hospital with this problem, and when he arrived there, his blood sugar would be high, so they increased his insulin. He was taking 130 units of insulin daily and was also taking additional medication for cardiac arrhythmias and high blood pressure, which he didn't have, and 17 prescription pills daily.*

When we saw him, we realized that he had not had any dietary advice at all. This, I think, is in some way systematic malpractice. We very rapidly took him off of all of his medications. When we instituted a low-fat, high-carbohydrate diet plus an exercise program under close monitoring, we were able to test his blood sugars two to three times a day. We cut his insulin in half in 2 days and then eliminated it after another 2 days. For 9 days he went without insulin, and his blood sugar never went back up again. We stopped the diuretics and gave him additional potassium. His blood sugar never went back up again, and he was able to lose some weight in the short time he was with us. When he went home and continued the low-fat, high-carbohydrate diet plus exercise, his weight continued to drop; he lost, I think, an additional 20 pounds. Over this period of time, he never required medications again. Here he had been treated by two board-certified, highly specialized, highly respected physicians in his community, who had been doing—and I went over his chart very carefully—everything appropriately, according to standard methods of practice. In other words, it is currently acceptable that some kind of drug is given for mild elevations of blood sugar. The practice isn't even frowned upon. It's also currently acceptable to prescribe a diuretic for mild blood pressure elevations, even though the diuretic may cause problems down the line.

As a result of following these currently acceptable methods of therapy, the patient was rapidly deteriorating not from any diseases he had but from the treatments he was given. We were able to use diet and exercise to cut through the requirement for medications, and he is still, a year and a half later, not taking any medications. Now he's quite a bit healthier. I think a diabetic patient is prone to excessive drug use not only in the treatment of the initial condition but also in the treatment of conditions associated with diabetes. But when you use a diet and exercise program to cut through that, you can eliminate a tremendous amount of prescription medication, as was done in this patient.

Dr. William Philpott's treatment is based on the detection of insulin resistance factors in specific food and chemical allergies as they affect the individual patient's ability to utilize available insulin supplies efficiently. He describes what happened in his treatment of a 60-year-old man who was a diagnosed type II (maturity-onset) diabetic.

He was placed on an oral medication which he took twice a day. However, I saw him 11 years after that diagnosis at his present age. His fasting blood sugar was usually around 300. The doctors said, "We are going to have to go to insulin." He was very weak—just terribly fatigued—and depressed too. He had read my book Victory over Diabetes *and wanted to give it a try before he went on insulin. When he came to me he was not on insulin yet; he was just ready to be put on insulin. I simply put him on foods that he just never would be addicted or allergic to and put him on intravenous vitamin C, B_6, calcium, and magnesium for about 4 days in a row.*

By the time we reached the fourth day his fasting blood sugar was normal. On the sixth day, we started feeding him foods that he more commonly used. One of those foods was wheat, and within an hour his blood sugar was 270. At about 3 or 4 hours it had normalized and we were able to give him another meal. With rye it was 275. On garbanzo beans it was 206, millet was 189, and even milk was 176. Oatmeal was 206. So we had at least a dozen foods that gave him high blood sugar. Actually the most important was the wheat, which he ate religiously every day.

We find the cereal grains containing gluten—wheat, rye, oats, barley, buckwheat—to be the most serious reactors. Through the years, only sugar and glucose have been used as the criteria for response, but we found much higher reaction to wheat.

As we studied him, we grew a fungus from his mouth and from his stool and rectal area called Candida albicans. He also had rather high antibodies. A lot of diabetics are made toxic by this organism.

We spotted that and found that he was deficient in magnesium and folic acid. We found that he was taking in 400 milligrams of caffeine, in coffee, every day. This was an important factor that was helping to disorder his functions. Now, knowing the foods he reacted to and leaving them out of the diet for at least 12 weeks while treating his infection and making his nutrition optimum, we were able to very quickly leave him with good energy, good control, and no high blood sugar at all.

Instead of going on insulin, here we have him strong with no high blood sugar at all and without infections. If we had just given him insulin and paid no attention to this fungus infection, he'd still be toxic. If you monitor him from any standpoint you wish, this man doesn't have diabetes. That's the difference between the types of symptom management: just giving insulin to cover this insulin resistance that he had. We measured his insulin, and actually he had a normal amount of insulin.

His problem was insulin resistance. Now he knows that the disease process is not deteriorating him any more. The consequences of this deterioration are depression, weakness, infection by fungi and viruses, and soon the whole degenerating disease process. Now we have him on a high-fiber diet, which will feed the right kind of bacteria. There will be good bowel function, moving the toxins out of the body, which is necessary.

But this is a very small part of what you need to do. People should lose weight and should use this kind of diet, but there is something much more central to this disease process, which is the insulin resistance to the food and your ability to isolate which foods prevent your body from using insulin properly.

45

AIDS

Probably the most popular new musical on Broadway in the 1990s was *Rent*. Although it suffered from a saccharine quality, it was a crowd pleaser because it mirrored something in the times. The central characters were a pair of couples—one straight, one gay—and all four members of the group were HIV positive. One dies of AIDS in the course of the drama but even more important for the theme of this chapter is the fate of the straight male's former girlfriend. When she finds out she is positive, she commits suicide.

In some ways this death may be more tragic than the AIDS death, insofar as it's partly driven by an establishment-induced myopia. The plain fact is: It has not yet been proven that HIV (human immunodeficiency virus) causes AIDS, though there is clearly an association between the two. Moreover, the woman's despair may have been so overwhelming partly because she only knew about AZT and the other drastic treatments touted by conventional doctors. She was probably unaware of the less toxic, more natural treatments we will explore in this chapter.

In 1984 at a conference in Maryland, Dr. Robert Gallo claimed to have isolated the HIV retrovirus, which he conjectured was the active agent causing AIDS. The press front-paged the story, not only lauding Dr. Gallo and his fellow researchers, but also predicting a cure was just a short distance down the road.

Well, more than 15 years have passed and we find that in relation to AIDS, we are not on the high road of hope but slogging through a quagmire of failed studies that provide little sense or information about how the disease progresses; confusing, unworkable, and expensive treatments; and toxic drugs that often do more harm than good. That's the bad news coming from the medical establishment. The good news is where the establishment failed, that is, in the accuracy of their doomsday predictions about the inevitable, plaguelike spread of AIDS. AIDS has not spread with either the speed or decimating broadness that was foreseen. On the other hand, if there is to be any good news on the treatment front, it will have to come from the alternative doctors who concentrate on such healing remedies as the use of nutritional and lifestyle changes as well as oxygen and ozone therapies.

In this chapter, we will comment briefly on some of the problems with the conventional understanding and treatment of AIDS. We will devote the bulk of the chapter to the alternative and complementary treatments for AIDS that seem to be working.

Does HIV = AIDS?

In 1984, Dr. Robert Gallo found the presence of human immunodeficiency virus (HIV) in the majority of the AIDS sufferers whose blood he tested. From this he concluded that HIV causes AIDS. So far this is still the best evidence that HIV equals AIDS, but it relies on a peculiarly strained logic.

Even if HIV were found in every AIDS patient, this alone does not settle the question of what causes the syndrome. HIV could simply be a cofactor, an agent which is necessary but not sufficient to create AIDS. Prominent AIDS researcher Dr. Root-Bernstein writes in *The Scientist*, "We also thought we knew that HIV alone is sufficient to cause AIDS. But such researchers as Luc Montagnier... and many others... now believe that cofactors are necessary and, therefore, that HIV by itself cannot cause AIDS."

The case for labeling HIV as partially, not wholly, the cause of AIDS is summed up well by Dr. Root-Bernstein. He notes, "All AIDS patients do have multiple, well established causes of immunosuppression prior to, concomitant with, subsequent to, and sometimes in the absence of, HIV infection." If HIV infection in AIDS patients is always found with other debilitating conditions— "chronic or repeated infectious diseases caused by immunosuppressive microorganisms; recreational and addictive drugs; anesthetics; antibiotics; semen components; blood; and malnutrition"—then it seems reasonable to conclude that these factors are as necessary as the presence of HIV to bring on the disease.

THE NATURE OF THE RETROVIRUS HIV is a retrovirus and part of the debate around it is whether a retrovirus could be powerful enough to play a determinative role in creating the AIDS disease.

First, we need to describe a virus. A virus is an extremely simple organism that contains genes (strands of DNA or RNA holding the information needed by the virus to copy itself) within a shell with, possibly, an outer membrane around that. The virus is so absolutely simple it cannot reproduce, feed itself, or carry out any other functions on its own. To survive, it has to get into a living cell and use that cell's machinery. It can only survive as a parasite, though; perhaps surprisingly, these viruses are not always detrimental to their host. A virus may move from cell to cell, leaving its own genetic material behind as it travels. In the best of cases, this new material may be valuable, and, if nothing else, will account for increased genetic diversity.

A retrovirus is a particular, only recently discovered, subtype of virus. To understand its action we need to step back a minute and look at how genes operate. Until 1970, it was believed the DNA in a cell's nucleus was the sole possessor of the genetic code. When it was necessary to direct cell operation, RNA (a messenger version of the code, created on the DNA template) would be manufactured and sent out to carry the DNA's orders. This seemed to be an adequate explanation, except for viruses. They were so simple they could only contain either RNA or DNA, not both. However, while a DNA-carrying virus could be easily understood—it entered a host cell and used its DNA to form RNA out of materials from the host cell—the operation of RNA-carrying viruses seemed inexplicable.

In 1970, biochemists Howard Temin and David Baltimore overthrew accepted thinking by showing that certain types of RNA could themselves manufacture DNA. They deservedly won a Nobel Prize for their findings. This is relevant to our study because it led to an explanation of how RNA-carrying virus operated successfully. Once it entered a likely host, it used the host's machinery to manufacture its own DNA, which then took over operation of the host cell. A virus that functions in this manner, as does HIV, is called a retrovirus.

Where this causes a problem for AIDS researchers is that it adds yet another puzzling element to the disease, since the retrovirus, in general, is not actually threatening and tends to leave its host unaffected by its presence.

Harvey Bialy, editor of the science journal *Bio/Technology*, rounds out this point by mentioning, "HIV is an ordinary retrovirus. There is nothing about this virus that is unique. It does not differ substantially from all the benign retroviruses.... It contains no gene different enough from the genes of other retroviruses to be a possible AIDS gene."

He also remarks that HIV uses all of its genetic information when it first infects a cell. "It doesn't hoard any for later use, so there is no conceivable reason HIV should cause AIDS 10 years after infection, rather than early on when it is unchecked by the immune system."

Why AIDS Hasn't Spread As Predicted

For the moment we can leave these problems to be sorted out by the scientists, since we want to turn to the less speculative question of what inroads AIDS has made into the world's populations.

Predictions based on the HIV theory have failed spectacularly. Here are the bare facts. AIDS in the United States and Europe has not spread through the general population. Rather, it remains almost entirely confined to the original risk groups, mainly sexually promiscuous gay men and drug abusers. The number of HIV-infected Americans has remained constant for years instead of increasing rapidly as predicted.

These statements may seem bold to the point of being outrageous to anyone who keeps up with the AIDS story by following it in the mass media. However, there is one thing that escalating predictions of the ravages of AIDS conveniently tend to leave out of their reports. That, in many cases, when a report of a sudden increase of AIDS patients is made, it is accompanied by a redefinition of what the disease is.

Recall that people only die indirectly of AIDS. AIDS weakens the immune system and then they die of another disease, such as tuberculosis. Now suppose—and this is not a theoretical case—a fatal disease that was not classified as AIDS-related is reclassified as AIDS-related. Obviously, you would be adding the people who had died of that disease previously to the AIDS death list and driving up the figures.

As I said, this is not hypothetical. In January 1993, the Centers for Disease Control (CDC) changed the definition of AIDS so that anyone who had a low CD4 blood cell count was defined as an AIDS statistic. According to the previous definition, a person did not have AIDS until he or she came down with an AIDS-related disease. Is it any surprise then, after this redefinition, that the CDC's 1993 report said the disease was exploding? The reported cases had doubled from about 48,000 to about 107,000. However, a task force for the Society of Actuaries didn't fall for this explosion. Robert Maver, speaking for the task force, said the increase was artificially produced, created by widening the net of people who were considered to be suffering from the disease. He commented, "Under this new category [low CD4 level] alone, more than 50,000 cases were added to the 1993 total."

Although there is not the time in this chapter to deal with the similar numbers game being played with the statistics of African AIDS victims, a similar situation is occurring. At this point, the reader might wonder why projections have been and continue to be so flawed. In the book *Rethinking AIDS*, P. Plumley lists three reasons why public health officials tend to vastly exaggerate the number of people that will get AIDS in the future. "(1) no one wants to appear complacent; (2) the worse the epidemic is projected to be, the more money will be available for public health work; and (3) when the numbers turn out to be lower, the officials can take credit for having done a good job of AIDS education."

Of course the downside of this is that the money the public health officials have accrued by pumping up the number is largely wasted, because it is not properly targeted. David Mertz points out, "Only 5 percent of all U.S. AIDS educational materials are directed at gay men. Instead, a sizable majority of safe-sex material is targeted to young, white heterosexuals. Injecting drug use receives similar short shift in these materials." This results in a dangerous squandering of resources.

Problems with Conventional Treatments

Among the difficulties I have with conventional programs is that they are restricted in purview almost exclusively to drugs. If one brings up measures to help the AIDS patient that go beyond ingesting pharmaceuticals, according to Dr. Dean Black, "This opens up the door to all the lifestyle measures that medicine has so long discounted, the idea that it could be in the behavior of the AIDS victim, in the diet, in the lifestyle in some fashion."

Researcher Bill McCreary points to the absurdity of doctors who ignore their own intuitions about the people they are treating to await orders from on high: "Doctors say it's not approved by the FDA so we can't touch it…. Doctors usually do a better job because they're there, they know the patient…. Today, the doctor works from a cookbook that is issued out of federal government. They have to abide by that cookbook or they may be found guilty of malpractice."

AZT The major recipe in that cookbook now is AZT, widely prescribed as the "approved" AIDS treatment. AZT was developed as a chemotherapy agent in the late 1960s for the treatment of leukemia, but was never patented by its creator, Dr. Richard Beltz, after he established that his chemotherapy compound was "too toxic for even short term use" and "caused cancer at any dose." Because of this, AZT was never used for its intended purpose as a cancer chemotherapy. Laboratory studies revealed some of its side effects to be hair loss, weight loss, muscle loss, anemia, and the very same pneumonia associated with AIDS. The drug was then shelved.

The drug's antileukemic mechanism of action is to kill growing lymphocytes by termination of DNA synthesis. The rationale of AZT therapy is simple, if not naive: the retrovirus HIV depends on DNA synthesis for multiplication, and AZT terminates DNA synthesis. Thus AZT should stop AIDS.

It should—but there's one catch. As Huw Christie explains, "Cancer cells, which AZT was designed to kill, grow faster than normal tissue cells, the idea therefore being that, when incorporating AZT, they die more quickly than normally replicating cells too. When the treatment is finished and the chemotherapy stopped, the normal tissue cells can set about making up for their own lower rate of loss." Studies show, on the other hand, that no more than 1 in 1,000 lymphocytes are ever infected by HIV—even in people dying from AIDS. Since AZT cannot distinguish between an infected and an uninfected cell, 999 uninfected cells must be killed to kill just one HIV-infected cell.

In 1984, the U.S. Department of Health granted a contract for AZT to Burroughs-Wellcome which remarketed AZT to AIDS doctors as an "antiviral." AZT was first given to human beings in the initial AIDS treatment trials.

A campaign was then waged to get every HIV-positive person on AZT. Researcher John Lauritsen explains, HIV-positive patients "were told that they should go for what was called early medical intervention. There were slogans put out, 'Put time on your side.' The early intervention meant purely and simply AZT. And rather than putting time on the side of these people, what the drug did and is doing is to terminate their lives."

Here's another difference from cancer treatment. In cancer, you begin to take chemotherapy after you contract the disease. AZT, as we saw, originally developed for chemotherapy, would be the first "chemotherapy" prescribed as a preventative before a person shows any symptoms.

Activist G. Hazlehurst put it like this: AIDS "is the only disease I know of where treatment with powerful drugs is begun several to many years prior to the actual onset of any illness, when there is still the possibility it may not even develop."

HOW AZT AFFECTS THE IMMUNE SYSTEM Dr. Martin Feldman told me, "The current drugs on the market, primarily AZT, tend to severely weaken the immunity and make the body have to work harder to have immune strength. The body uses up its basic nutrients in the process. Really, the body is fighting against the AZT."

Another commentator notes that if you give AZT indefinitely, so that every 6 hours the patients take 250 milligrams of AZT, they are going to "lose weight, they become anemic, they lose their white cells, they have nausea, they lose their muscles…. That is what you call AIDS by prescription."

AZT challengers agree that it can only weaken the immune system further. Dr. Dean Black castigates the developers of the drug for the whole rationale of the treatment. "By virtue of determining to substitute for the immune system, by attacking this alien agent with a drug, medicine has literally replaced the body's immune system. What can it do but become weak?"

A number of advocates of alternative treatment tell us that we need to change the focus of treatment toward "stimulating, activating, and increasing" the body's antibody system. "Since it is the evolutionary responsibility of the cytotoxic T-lymphocytes to destroy infected and abnormal self-cells, increasing their numbers would be beneficial." The best direction of treatment, according to this perspective, would be to help the body to use the immune system it already has instead of forcing it to tolerate an artificial one.Since we've brought up the subject of better treatments, let's move on to three doctors who have already developed alternative treatments.

Alternative Treatments

A number of alternative treatments are having some success with AIDS. In this chapter we will highlight three of the newer approaches, pairing each description with a brief mention of a doctor who has pioneered the approach as well as the histories of some of the patients he has worked with. It is important to discuss with a medical professional any alternative therapies you are considering or already using. The three approaches are (1) supporting the body's own methods of healing and defense by bringing nutrient levels up to optimal levels; (2) working on improving the body's metabolism using a special fatty acid preparation; and (3) elevating the level of oxygen in the blood to boost the immune system and cell activity.

Optimizing Nutrient Levels: Dr. Christopher Calapai

In an article published in a scientific journal, Cohen and Kutler note that in evaluating the health conditions of HIV-infected persons, before they showed any disease symptoms, most had poor nutrition. They had decreased body mass, fat, and protein, resulting from malabsorption. They would be eating but their bodies were not adequately breaking down the food and assimilating its nutrients. A further study, "Influence of HIV Infection on Vitamin Status and Requirement," points out that a vicious circle will result from this malabsorption. "Once occurring, malnutrition leads to immunosuppression, infection, and mucosal damage… resulting in further malnutrition."

Dr. Christopher Calapai sees the body's inability to profit from food nutrients as stemming not only from absorption problems, but from anorexia and high resting energy expenditure (REE). REE means that the body is overstimulated. While it should have slowed during rest, the metabolism is still using up nutrients at an accelerated pace. In any case, the HIV-infected person is either not getting or using too quickly the nutrients he or she needs to support bodily functions.

It is no question that certain vitamins are needed to maintain immune response. These include E, B_6, C, and beta carotene. Studies of the elderly, who generally have impaired immune systems, have long shown that these vitamins, taken as supplements, will improve immune response.

In fact, there is evidence that certain vitamins as well as herbs can counter the progress of AIDS as they bolster the immune system. Let's highlight some of the more notable successes that have been seen with these types of therapies, many of which are used by Dr. Calapai.

VITAMINS AND OTHER NUTRIENTS In my forthcoming book *AIDS: A Second Opinion*, I detail the vitamins and herbs that have been used for treating people with AIDS with positive results. In this briefer space, I will touch upon some of the substances that have recorded good results.

GLUTATHIONE

Glutathione is an antioxidant that protects against cellular damage. It stimulates lymphocytes that help defend the body against viral illnesses, such as AIDS. When N-acetyl-cysteine (NAC) is given to a patient, the body will convert it to glutathione. A study in *Nutrition Review* indicates that HIV-positive individuals are deficient in glutathione. On the other hand, results have been reported from a number of studies that indicate HIV activity is reduced by glutathione's presence.

Dr. Joan Priestley gives her HIV-infected and AIDS patients intravenous glutathione, because, she says, "Glutathione specifically attacks the AIDS virus in about four different steps."

At an AIDS symposium, Dr. Calapi stated: "When we add glutathione intravenously with vitamin C, we see a significant turnaround in the patient's comfort, attitude, and well being... NAC taken intravenously can inhibit reverse transcriptase [HIV replication] activity better than 90 percent. There is no drug available for any treatment or disease that can do better than 90 percent with minimal or no side effects."

BETA CAROTENE

Beta carotene is a safe form of vitamin A, which stops damage from bodily pollution, bolsters the immune system, inhibits viruses, and prevents premature aging.

A study done by Dr. Semba of Johns Hopkins showed that a vitamin A deficiency found in HIV-positive and AIDS patients was a serious risk factor for the disease. In a different study, Dr. Semba's team found that a lack of vitamin A was positively correlated with death from AIDS.

On the other hand, a number of studies chart improvements when beta carotene is administered. In one, 11 HIV-positive patients received 60 milligrams of the vitamin per day for 4 months. They recorded an increase in natural killer cells and other vital parts of the immune system, which HIV infection tends to diminish. Another study was done on 10 patients who had just gotten off AZT and began taking 120 milligrams a day of beta carotene. Although one died a few months into the treatment, the other nine experienced an HIV burden diminution, clinically measured improvements in health, and evaluated themselves as having a better quality of life.

VITAMIN C

Vitamin C is one of the stars among the vitamins in treating AIDS. Basing his opinion on numerous clinical studies, Dr. Robert Cathcart confidently states, "Vitamin C can double the life expectancy of AIDS patients." He says that his treatment, which involves using massive doses of buffered ascorbate of 50 to 200 grams every 24 hours (in combination with other treatments for secondary infections), will produce a clinical remission of the disease that shows every evidence of being prolonged if the treatment goes on.

Other doctors report similar results. Dr. Raxit Jariwalla, a virologist from the Linus Pauling Institute, says, "In laboratory cultures of HIV-infected cells... vitamin C can significantly suppress both the activity and replication of the AIDS virus."

Joy DeVincenxo, who is HIV positive and has used massive doses of vitamin C, explains, "A lot of doctors... do not believe in giving me vitamin C... [but] without it, I know I wouldn't have stayed stable for so long."

These statements are supported by a host of studies, such as the one that appeared in the volume *Nutrition and AIDS*, which summarized the results of various examinations of C's value. The authors point out, "A striking property of ascorbic acid is its ability to inactivate viruses and inhibit viral growth in their host cells." Experimental studies reported in the same volume show that vitamin C will directly interfere with HIV replication, carrying the assault on the disease into the enemy's camp.

VITAMIN E

Vitamin E is an antioxidant that seems to prevent many diseases caused by environmental stressors. It is found in fish and vegetable oil, nuts, and whole grains. However, the majority of Americans do not get enough of this vitamin in their foods and need supplementation. Studies are piling up showing that vitamin E is a warrior against AIDS. One study showed that the administration of 50 milligrams per kilogram per day over 5 days already began to inhibit the replication of HIV. Another study showed that if the dosage of E was increased 15-fold (to 160 IU/liter), immune system functions that had been suppressed by HIV presence were restored.

HERBAL TREATMENTS Again, we can only skim the surface in mentioning some herbal treatments that have shown themselves as powerful agents in working against AIDS.

The Institute for Traditional Medicine in Portland, Oregon, has done some vital work in looking at how Chinese herbs can be used in treating AIDS. The founder of the institute has developed a specific herbal combination, which combines strong tonic herbs with those that fight inflammation and infection. Of 150 patients who have undergone therapy with this herbal formula over 3 months, 76 percent experienced an increase of energy, and 62 percent of the patients who suffered from diarrhea saw a cessation of the problem. Other symptoms were similarly improved.

Dr. Chang of the Sun Yat Sen Medical Center also found a mix of Chinese herbs to work strenuously against AIDS. He found that extracts from 11 different herbs inhibit the activity of HIV. Dr. Quingcai Zhang notes these Chinese herb treatments are effective because they work with the body to fight infection, rather than, as do such drugs as AZT, by trying to override the body's own creative functioning.

Following are some of the herbs that have a good reputation for working against HIV.

ASTRAGALUS

Astragalus root has been used for centuries in China because it was thought to strengthen the immune system. Current research shows the truth of this belief since astragalus is now known to correct T cell (part of the immune system) deficiency and promote antiviral action.

A study at the University of Texas showed that taking astragalus extract stimulates T cell production in healthy animals and restores it in cancer patients who have seen their T cell production impaired. In another study involving 19 cancer patients with weakened immune systems, an extract of astragalus induced such a complete recovery that it was noted, "People whose immune systems were devastated by cancer experienced full restoration of immune function."

Of course, studies need to be conducted on AIDS sufferers, but astralagus's aid to the immune system is evident.

GARLIC

Garlic has a number of antitumor and antiviral mechanisms. It stimulates the immune system's productions of phagocytosis, which eliminates abnormal cells from the body. It is toxic to some abnormal cells and inhibits the implantation of others. It has even proven effective against some bacteria that do not respond to antibiotics.

In fighting AIDS, it is especially good in eliminating the opportunistic infections that set in once immune systems have been weakened. A German study of seven AIDS patients who were given 5 grams of garlic daily found that five showed significant improvements in their T cells, along with other improvements in health and fewer outbreaks of opportunistic infections.

GINSENG

Numerous studies of ginseng's benefits were conducted in Russia in the 1960s and 1970s. Norman Farnsworth collected and translated many of these studies, which indicated that various types of ginseng acted to normalize body temperature, enhance the body's ability to resist infection, improve cells' ability to dispose of the byproducts of metabolism, and counter the effects of environmental pollution.

Its effects in treating AIDS patients have also been shown. In a study by Y. K. Cho and others, Korean red ginseng improved weakened immune response in subjects infected with HIV.

LICORICE ROOT

Licorice root has also been effective in stopping the HIV virus from replicating, according to a scientific study. The study, done at the World Life Research Institute, recorded no toxicity to normal cells.

The plant is known to strengthen the immune system by increasing macrophage activity and that of interferon-gamma, both vital actors in combating infections and viruses. Licorice is a detoxifying agent and has anti-inflammatory, antiallergic, and antispasmodic properties.

ST. JOHN'S WORT

Studies at New York University have shown that St. John's wort contains two potent chemicals that are highly effective in preventing the spread of retro-viruses, like HIV, both in laboratory samples and in patients.

One of the researchers found that one of these chemicals would stop the spread of AIDS, even crossing the barrier into the brain, which serves as a reservoir of HIV cells, to combat the disease there. This researcher comments that St. John's wort's "antiviral activity is remarkable both in its mechanism... and the potency of one administration of a relatively small dose of the compounds."

PHYTOCHEMICALS Before moving on to the lifestyle components that form part of Dr. Calapai's program, I want to call your attention to a newer area of research in supplementation that I believe will have a lot to offer toward helping AIDS patients in years to come. This is the area of phytochemicals.

Phytochemicals are disease-preventing or healing substances found in edible plants, such as those found in licorice root, which are believed to account for the plant's valuable immune-system strengthening qualities that have already been outlined. These chemicals are found in frequently consumed foods such as fruits, vegetables, grains, legumes, and seeds as well as in less common foods such as soy and green tea. They have already been associated with the prevention and treatment of four of the leading causes of death in this country: cancer, diabetes, cardiovascular disease, and hypertension. Although not enough studies have been done on these substances, those that have been done hint that quite large benefits are to be expected.

Research on limonene, found in citrus fruits, shows that it increases the body's production of enzymes that help it dispose of potentially carcinogenic substances. It is well known that people whose diets are heavy in fruits have lower rates of most cancers than those who don't have such diets. Many are attributing this low cancer rate to the effect of the phytochemicals.

LIFESTYLE CHANGES

DIETARY MODIFICATION

Dr. Calapai's treatment program involves both building up the body with proper nutrients and calling on his patients to make lifestyle changes. Research supports the long-term efficacy of dietary counseling and use of nutritional supplementation for people with AIDS to increase or maintain weight, restore lean tissues, and lessen the effects of the disease. These factors could help decrease mortality as well as improve bowel function.

Patrick Donnelly, program coordinator for the Whole Foods Project, says AIDS patients must be made aware of the need to eat nutritious foods. He advises working with what are being called "the new four food groups, which are grains, legumes, fruits, and vegetables." These foods are high in antioxidants. and have nutrients like beta carotene, vitamin C, zinc, and selenium. Such nutrients are not found in the high-fat, high-protein standard American diet. Donnelly says, "We're trying to get people to look at a new way of eating that is not about providing calories so much as supporting the immune system."Another member of the project staff, Richard Pierce, comments, "You only have to look at this food [we provide] to see that it's full of life.... The vitality of the food is what nurtures us."

Along with eating healthy foods, one must learn to avoid the foods that contribute to the growth or virulence of disease, counterproductive foods, particularly yeast and sugar. Yeast is a natural part of our makeup but it can wreak havoc on the body when it gets out of control. Sugar is an immune suppressant. If one takes 100 grams of sugar, it will cut antibody production by 50 percent for 24 hours.

EXERCISE

Studies have shown that regular exercise has long-term benefits on the biological condition of HIV and AIDS patients as well as on the course of the illness. Researchers have found that exercise will improve a patient's health at all stages of the disease. Moreover, it seems that complications of the disease will be delayed by exercise.

ACUPUNCTURE Acupuncture has proven to be one of the most popular treatments that HIV-positive people turn to. One study followed the development of acupuncture for AIDS treatment in the United States and found that people with HIV who use the treatment have extended survival rates. In addition they regularly report a substantial reduction in symptoms and side effects from HIV-related drugs. Acupuncture frequently provides relief from AIDS-related diseases, and most patients report a reduction in fatigue, abnormal sweating, diarrhea, and acute skin reactions after four to five treatments. Some patients have a 15- to 20-pound weight gain and return to long hours of work.

Abigail Rist-Podrecca, a registered nurse, notes that acupuncture works by "dilating the blood vessels, so that the vessels can open. You get more circulation, more of the nutrients, more oxygen flowing through those meridians [the places where the acupuncture needles are stuck]."

She believes one of the reasons people with AIDS weaken is that they lose the ability to take up nutrition through the intestines. Acupuncture acts to reverse this digestive problem as well as working on the lungs and other bodily centers.

Studies conducted at the Lincoln Hospital Acupuncture Clinic in the New York the AIDS Alternative Health Project in Chicago, and the Quan Yin Herbal support program in San Francisco have reported symptomatic relief and overall physical improvement following acupuncture.

REFLEXOLOGY AND AROMATHERAPY Reflexology is a form of relaxation treatment. It was used in an AIDS program in Uganda in 1993. Four months after the program began, 85 percent of those treated noted pain relief, better relaxation, and better sleep following the reflexology sessions.

Aromatherapy is the use of plant essences in healing. Pure oils are used, some of which have already proven to have antifungal and antiviral effects.

One study looked at the effect of aromatherapy when used in conjunction with other therapies to see if it would lessen the need for toxic drugs. Using 80 randomly selected AIDS patients, the study concluded that the group that utilized aromatherapy, in contrast to the control group, reported fewer aches and pains, faster healing of wounds, greater physical strength, and a better ability to cope.

HOW DR. CALAPAI'S PROGRAM WORKS As mentioned, Dr. Calapai's program centers on nutrition and lifestyle changes. When he first sees a patient, he asks him or her to bring in a week's worth of diet history, which he goes over very carefully. He immediately tells the patient how important it is to institute lifestyles changes that will provide strong benefits. These changes include immediately stopping smoking and drinking alcohol.

He orders a detailed diagnostic protocol that includes blood evaluations of cellular, mineral, vitamin, hormone, and viral and antigen levels. He also does aggressive testing for common infections, such as herpes and tuberculosis (TB), which can contribute to the progression of the disease. He allows a patient to take the antiretroviral drugs if that patient so desires. He also lets the patient consult other doctors.

Once Dr. Calapai has the test results, he uses them along with the patient's history to devise dietary recommendations.

RESULTS Dr. Calapai reports good results with his program. "Many of the patients that I have put on the protocol after 2 weeks or so say they're feeling very good." He continues, "They have a lot of energy; they're sleeping better…. The overwhelming majority say they feel better in a number of ways."

He has had patients who have followed his nutritional and lifestyle alteration program and, though they have very low T cell counts, have been free of coughs, colds, and other opportunistic infections for a year.

Improving Metabolism: Dr. Emmanuel Revici

Dr. Emmanuel Revici's program is similar to Dr. Calapai's insofar as it also affirms that AIDS must be managed by addressing nutritional deficiencies. However, it is much narrower in locating the deficiency only in certain fats. At the same time, it is broader in that it is based on a well worked out philosophy.

This philosophy, though not based on Chinese medicine, does resemble the Asian system in seeing the body as driven by two crosscurrents. Elsewhere in this book, I make mention of Chinese thought on yin and yang. Traditional Chinese medicine sees these two energies as creating the body's vitality. The body's health depends on their balance.

Similarly, Dr. Revici sees two basic processes in the body: the anabolic, which builds up, and the catabolic, which breaks down. He writes, "The two antagonistic intervening factors... act alternately, each being predominant for a period of time. The result is... an oscillatory movement with successive passages from one side to the other of the average value." When an organism is working normally, it maintains its characteristic rhythms and intensities by means of this oscillation. However, when there is a breakdown, it will be because the alternations are lopsided and either catabolic or anabolic influences are unduly dominating. It is as if a pendulum's swing were being artificially pulled to one side.

In the case of AIDS, as Dr. Revici sees it, there is a deficiency in certain of the body's phospholipids (a type of fat), which normally play a role in disease prevention. He traces the course of the disease: A primary viral infection occurs, which brings about the weakening of the body's line of lipidic defense. This is followed by secondary, opportunistic infections which are allowed to run wild due to the body's lowered defense threshold. Then comes an exaggerated catabolic imbalance whereby the body's breakdown of substances is outrunning its construction of others.

The treatment called for in such a case is a four-pronged one. To deal with the viral infections, antiviral agents should be introduced into the system. To deal with the lipid deficiency, these lipids have to be reintroduced by injection. For the secondary opportunistic infections, proper antibiotics are applied. And for the catabolic imbalance, balancing agents are prescribed. I examined ten of Dr. Revici's cases and about them I can make these generalizations. Of these patients, only three seem not to have improved during therapy. Yet, of these three, one, though worsening in immunologic markers, nevertheless felt "well" at the end of ten years of treatment. Another, though his T4 count also declined considerably over 4 years of treatment, was still "feeling fine" at the end of that period. Thus, of the ten patients, eight currently (or recently) report feeling well after an average period of 5.2 years of therapy. Five of the eight also report no remaining symptomatic complaints; and two of those have had a marked improvement in immune markers. All are currently continuing in therapy.

Oxygen and Ozone: Dr. John Pittman

Dr. John Pittman's treatment is based on the use of ozone and oxygen. Before describing his treatment in more detail, it will be helpful to give some background on medical applications of ozone with viral infections.

Oxygen is an essential nutrient. It is, in fact, the most essential, as it is the only one which must be continuously available, at pain of quick death. As we all know, life ceases if the supply of oxygen is cut off for more than a few minutes.

Those observations are so taken for granted that we hardly think about them further. Specifically, have we thought in any depth about how ubiquitous "hidden" hypoxias (lack of oxygen) may be? A number of studies, such as ones by M. Carpendale and colleagues and another by Wagner and others, indicate that ozone inactivates HIV at low and safe concentrations. Carpendale reports, "Ozone... has been shown to inactivate human immunodeficiency virus (HIV) in serum at noncytotoxic concentrations."

It has been conjectured that ozone kills HIV cells. Ozone is also able to strengthen immune responses.

TREATMENT PROTOCOL Ozone therapy is a prime component in Dr. John Pittman's Carolina Center for Bio-oxidative Medicine where he and his staff treat and study patients with AIDS, HIV, and other immune-compromising conditions. Dr. Pittman believes that ozone can arrest the progression of AIDS' diseases and turn the syndrome into a manageable condition. He values ozone's ability to help alleviate chronic problems that plague patients, including dermatological conditions and low level infections. He also notes a relationship between ozone and improved T cell and CD4 counts. Best results occur when an intensive series of treatments are taken every 4 to 6 months.

Dr. Pittman uses ozone as an integral part of a wider treatment protocol: "The first 10 days of their program entails a modified juice fast. Everyone drinks fresh pressed vegetable juices and no solid food." Patients are then put on an intensive detoxification program. Nutritional supplements are given. The patient begins autohemotherapy. This involves the removal of blood from the body, so it can be filled with ozone, then reinfused.

After 5 days of autohemotherapy, Dr. Pittman says, "if the patient has tolerated that... we begin with the direct intravenous infusion of ozone gas... on a daily basis, gradually increasing concentrations and volume until we observe a healing crisis in the patient." The patient will experience fevers, chills, and sometimes flu symptoms. When the healing crisis passes, the doctor tapers off dosage and concentration, and goes into lower doses, "which have a more immune stimulating effect."

Concurrent with ozone therapy are other intravenous therapies, which include intravenous vitamin C and mineral infusions as well as EDTA chelation therapy. The doctor also employs acupuncture and other dietary therapies throughout the program.Although I was not able to obtain the same detailed case histories from Dr. Pittman that I had from the other practitioners mentioned here, I did gather very positive anecdotal evidence, including the story of a man who came to the clinic with a CD4 count of 42. In 2 weeks of intensive therapy, his count soared to 285.

As you can see, Dr. Pittman believes in a nontoxic multifactorial approach in the treatment of AIDS. He says, "I think the approach for AIDS has got to be one from a multimodality standpoint. There is no one single approach. It is only through the combination of appropriate antiviral therapy, immune stimulating therapy, diet, and detoxification programs that a patient is really going to be maintained and have any hope of improvement."

Alternative Health Therapy Concepts

Theories and methods that seem very different can have broadly similar results. All three of the treatment approaches mentioned have, at the very least, reversed some of the symptoms of HIV infection in some patients, and have improved the quality of life, according to the patients themselves, in many.

The three approaches are not mutually exclusive. Is there any reason why they should not be used together, complementing each other? For example, it was noteworthy that some of the reported actions of the vitamin C infusions used by Dr. Calapai were very similar to those of the ozone infusions used by Dr. Pittman. Both were found to be highly effective in inactivating many viruses, and HIV in particular; and both seemed to augment the effectiveness of the immune system. Perhaps if they were used together, the effects of each would potentiate each other, with results better than either alone.

One of the very important advantages of many of these "nonconventional" methods is that, whether or not they are effective (and there is evidence that some are), they are generally safe. Most nutritional and herbal methods cause far fewer side effects than the pharmaceutical and surgical methods now in favor. This is a major argument for permitting them to be used at the discretion of the individual.

That is a reason for not bringing these modalities under the regulatory authority of the state or organized medicine. It is a matter of constitutional freedoms. But there are also strong economic arguments. The costs of these alternative techniques are almost always far lower than the treatments now approved by organized medicine for the same disorders. Thus, encouraging the use of these other approaches can save the American public, both as taxpayer and as health-care consumer, vast amounts of money.

Yes, the physicians whose work with HIV infection we have examined approach health and illness from different perspectives. But they do share a basic world view that separates them from the practitioners of conventional medicine.

According to the conventional view, my body consists of congeries of mechanisms, with subsystems that can be adequately understood separately, with little regard to the status of all the myriad other subsystems. The view of the body found in alternative healthcare is one which sees its level of interconnectedness as far higher. In a healthy organism all the subsystems are supporting each other in myriad ways (most of which are not yet observable or understood). In the first (allopathic) world view, most disease originates through the breakdown of some one mechanism, or a few discrete mechanisms; disease then is to be treated by fixing (or bypassing) the defective mechanism(s). In the second (holistic) world view, however, disease has to do not only with individual mechanisms, but with weakenings of many kinds of couplings between mechanisms, and with overstressing supporting systems through excessive demands for support. In this view, the total system can be strengthened by adding inputs that may rouse relatively quiescent supporting subsystems to become more active, as well as by giving additional resources to many different supporting systems—therapeutic strategies that are emphasized in the work of the three doctors we have used as examples.

SURVIVOR PORTRAITS Literature on long-term survivors with AIDS is replete with anecdotal evidence linking survival to such things as holding a positive attitude toward the illness, taking control of one's health, participating in health-promoting behaviors, engaging in spiritual activities, and taking part in AIDS-related events.

Survivors are very pragmatic problem-solvers who educate themselves about alternative treatments, nutrition, and exercise. If something isn't working for them, they change it.

While AIDS survivors generally do not follow mainstream treatments, they are not loners. They maintain good relationships with their friends, families and doctors, and often belong to support groups. Bill Thompson, an AIDS survivor and activist says, "It was through... the help of my friends, I learned about carrot and beet juice and I went out and got a Champion juicing machine. That's how I've been maintaining good health."

Another feature of long-term survivors is that they are passionately committed to life, believe in the possibility of survival, and surround themselves with people who will love and support them. They make major lifestyle changes. They have also dabbled with dietary changes. A writer who studied the lives of survivors says:

> They all talked about what they called "emotional house cleaning." Usually after they had survived their first major opportunistic infection, it represented a crisis to them and they did some soul-searching. They either repaired relationships, or ended them. And all but two talked about a rebirth of spirituality.

Half had returned to the religions of their childhood—although none in a fundamentalist, ,judgmental way—and half spoke more generally of there being a meaning to suffering…. This gave them a sense of purpose in the here and now. They were not done with life yet. They had a reason to stick around.

46

Migraines

Twenty-three million Americans suffer from migraines. One in five women is affected, compared to only one in twenty men, making women four times more susceptible to this widespread health problem.

Causes

It is now believed that migraine headaches occur when a sudden dilation of the blood vessels creates pressure on the brain. There are numerous triggers for migraines. Dr. Mary Olsen, a chiropractor from Huntington, New York, who specializes in craniosacral adjustments and applied kinesiology, tells about the eight most common reasons for their occurrence.

ALLERGIC REACTIONS Dr. Olsen states, "Allergies can be dietary or environmental. Dietary triggers can be foods, food combinations, or additives in foods. Alcoholic beverages, particularly red wine and beer, are among the most common causes of migraines. Tyramine, a chemical found in cheese, smoked fish, yogurt, and yeast extracts, may be involved. Monosodium glutamate (MSG), which is found in Chinese cuisine and most processed foods, is often implicated, as is sodium nitrate, which found in cold cuts and hot dogs. Aspartame, a commonly used artificial sweetener, may lower serotonin levels in the body. Some researchers believe that this contributes to severe headaches. Chocolate and other foods containing caffeine can also be dietary triggers. In addition, people can have allergies to such common foods as wheat, dairy products, corn, and eggs. A person can have environmental allergies to toxic fumes emitted from modern products found in the home."

HORMONAL FLUCTUATIONS Dr. Olsen explains, "Women suffer from migraines to a much greater extent than do men. Among women who suffer from migraines, approximately 60 percent correlate headaches to their menstrual cycle. The major contributing factor is the hormone estrogen. We know that women who take oral contraceptives are more susceptible to severe migraines and that women experience a lower frequency and severity of headaches after menopause, when there is a sharp reduction of estrogen. Unfortunately, the widespread use of estrogen replacement therapy has resulted in many women having a return of these headaches. Although the exact relationship between migraines and estrogen is unknown at this time, we do know that estrogen affects the central nervous system, including the systems involving serotonin, which can be involved in the development of migraines."

CRANIAL FAULTS "Malposition in cranial bones or cranial faults is another factor contributing to migraines. Trauma to the head, such as striking the head on a car door or birth trauma, may be enough to lock a bone into a particular position. A whiplash injury may also result in cranial faults."

MERIDIAN IMBALANCE "Applied kinesiologists and acupuncturists check for a meridian imbalance. Meridians are 12 bilateral electromagnetic channels of energy in the body identified within the Chinese science of acupuncture. Blocked energy, or *chi* within a meridian causes dysfunction, including migraine headaches."

UPPER CERVICAL SUBLUXATION "Another common cause of migraine is cervical subluxation in the upper part of the neck. This is especially prevalent among people who use the telephone as a regular part of their work. The tendency to hold the phone between the neck and the shoulder forces the vertebrae in the opposite direction. You also see this with people who tend to read in bed. Propping the head up in one direction causes the vertebrae to shift, which puts stress on the nerves and contributes to the migraine."

LOW MAGNESIUM LEVELS "A number of studies have noted that many people suffering from migraines have low levels of magnesium in their blood. This is also true of people who suffer from fibromyalgia, a myofascial condition that can cause severe pain to the head, mimicking a migraine."

DRUGS "If you use aspirin, acetaminophen, mixed analgesics, or other acute care medications to get rid of your headaches, you actually may be causing them. The use of these painkillers is the single most common reason for migraines. They are called rebound headaches, and this is why they occur. When you take a painkiller often, the body gets used to having a certain amount of that drug in the bloodstream. When the level falls below that threshold, the body begins to experience withdrawal symptoms. One of these symptoms is a headache. If this situation exists, any preventive treatment for migraine will be undermined."

STRESS Finally, Dr. Olsen cites stress as a factor in migraines: "Although stress is not a cause in itself, it can exacerbate the effects of a headache or cause an increase in the frequency of headaches."

SYMPTOMS Migraines differ from regular headaches in that they usually occur on one side of the head. They can be accompanied by nausea, vomiting, sensitivity to light and sound, fatigue, weakness, irritability, and vision problems. An aura sometimes precedes a migraine. Usually, this is a visual phenomenon that may appear as flashes of light or visual distortions. However, other sensory systems can be disturbed, causing the aura to manifest as numbness, tingling, odor hallucinations, language difficulties, confusion, or disorientation.

Alternative Treatment Approaches

Although the exact treatment depends on a patient's individual needs, Dr. Olsen suggests general guidelines for treating migraines brought on by different factors. Of course, combination approaches are often indicated as well.

Addressing the Causes of Migraine

FOOD ALLERGIES As Dr. Olsen explains, "Since migraines don't necessarily follow immediately after ingesting a food, it may be difficult to make a connection between a particular food and the resultant headache. We often have patients keep a food diary to record what is eaten and their physical reactions. That makes it easier to correlate foods with delayed reactions. If we suspect that a particular food is troublesome, the patient is asked to place a sample of that food under the tongue. If there is a sensitivity, a muscle that tested strong previously will weaken. Pulse is also evaluated for such changes as increases in intensity or frequency. Treatment can be as simple as removing the offending food from the diet."

ENVIRONMENTAL ALLERGIES Dr. Olsen states, "If the migraines appear to be caused by environmental allergies, the British Migraine Association recommends keeping houseplants. Different plants have the ability to absorb different toxins. For example, spider plants absorb the formaldehyde released from particleboard, plywood, synthetic carpeting, and new upholstery, while chrysanthemum protects against the toxic effects of lacquers, varnishes, and glues. If you don't feel like keeping a lot of chrysanthemums around the house, the same effect comes from drinking an herbal tea made with this flower."

HORMONAL IMBALANCE Dr. Olsen suggests that supplementing the diet with vitamin B$_6$ and evening primrose oil around the time of a woman's menstrual period may help restore hormonal balance enough to forestall migraine attacks.

CRANIAL FAULTS Dr. Olsen says, "Since migraines involve the cranial nerves, patients suffering from migraines should always be examined for cranial faults. These faults are extremely difficult to evaluate, due to the subtle movement of bones, but correcting them can be key to healing.

"One of my patients responded only partially to treatment after we corrected other findings that contributed to her headaches. Although the frequency decreased, she still reported migraines. At first, she had a general examination for cranial faults; there were no positive findings. Finally, after examining every single sutral point (or area of articulation) along the frontal bone in the forehead, we found the problem and corrected it. Her headaches stopped. In this case, the patient had an internally rotated frontal bone. Applied kinesiologists find this to be the most common cause of migraines from a cranial fault. This is particularly true if the patient reports eye pain with the migraine.

"The correction for this is done in three steps. First, pressure is applied to the posterior aspect of the palate on the side of internal rotation. Then light pressure is applied on the lateral pterygoid muscle, located behind the upper molar in the mouth. Next, pressure is applied to the medial pterygoid on the opposite side. That completes the treatment."

MERIDIAN IMBALANCE Dr. Olsen states, "The task of the practitioner is to balance the energy by stimulating the meridians. There are various ways of accomplishing this. Acupuncturists use needles, while applied kinesiologists prefer to stimulate the meridians with a finger.

"Three acupressure or acupuncture points are helpful in treating migraines. Lung 7 is located about two finger widths from the crease in the wrist, on the thumb side of the anterior part of the arm. Bladder 67 is found at the nail point of the little toe, and gallbladder 20 is located between the mastoid and the occipital protuberance in the skull. These points are stimulated in a circular or tapping motion until there is an effective change."

UPPER CERVICAL SUBLUXATION Dr. Olsen suggests that migraines caused by upper cervical subluxation will cease with chiropractic adjustment to the proper area.

LOW MAGNESIUM Dr. Olsen says that for migraines caused by low magnesium, "I have found a combination of magnesium and malic acid to be helpful. A health care practitioner should be consulted because the dose varies with each patient."

MEDICATIONS Dr. Olsen says that people whose migraines are triggered by medications "must gradually wean themselves away from drugs, with the help of their doctor. When they are no longer dependent on these medications, treatment can begin."

STRESS According to Dr. Olsen, "Studies in England suggest that the herbal remedy feverfew can reduce the frequency of migraines. Feverfew has sedative qualities and can be taken as a tea. One cup per day is usually effective. In addition, relaxation techniques such as meditation, progressive muscle relaxation, and yoga can help to reduce stress. Regular moderate exercise, such as swimming or walking, also lowers tension and creates a psychological sense of well-being."

Dr. Jennifer Brett, of Stratford, Connecticut, also comments on the benefits of feverfew: "An important study reported by the *British Medical Journal* back in 1983 found that 1 to 2 capsules of a freeze-dried extract of feverfew would prevent most migraines from occurring."

Supplements

In addition to feverfew, Dr. Brett makes the following recommendations: "When feverfew is taken with magnesium in doses of 250 to 500 milligrams daily and Ginkgo biloba, most people notice a significant reduction in the number of migraines, even to the point of disappearance. This includes people who suffer daily migraines. Many people come to me who have had no success with more conventional treatments. After I start them on feverfew and magnesium, they get a significant reduction in the number of headaches and the severity of pain. Even when they have headaches, they tend to be less frequent and less painful. In my experience, this combination will work for more than 70 percent of migraine sufferers.

"Some people find that they need to add the nutrient niacin. Niacin causes flushing in many people, and it is exactly this flushing that stops the migraine headache. When the blood moves out of the head and into the skin in the form of a flush, the migraine can be aborted before it even starts."

Biofeedback

The July 14, 1998, issue of the *Canadian Medical Association Journal* reported that people using thermal control, a biofeedback technique, were able to control migraines by learning to raise their finger temperatures with a digital-temperature device. They learned the technique in the practitioner's office and from manuals and audiotapes at home. Generally people need about two months to learn the technique. It appears to work by increasing blood flow, which is decreased by nervous tension.

Another biofeedback technique places sensors on the temples, over the temporal arteries. People learn to change their pulse rates in order to diminish their migraines.

Other Therapies

A variety of therapies can help relieve or prevent migraines, says naturopath Dr. Emily Kane, in an article on the website of the American Association of Naturopathic Physicians (www.naturopathic.org). She cautions, however, that people with severe or frequent migraines should first have a physician rule out serious conditions that may be causing their headaches, including diseases that cause seizures, brain tumor, aneurysm of a carotid artery, Meniere's disease (which affects the inner ear), and hemangioma (a tumor composed of new blood vessels).

PHYSICAL MEDICINE Aerobic exercise, says Dr. Kane, can lessen the frequency of migraines if it is performed regularly, three times a week for a minimum of 20 minutes.

There are many inventive forms of hydrotherapy which involve applying cold to the head and heat to the feet. For example, cold wet packs on the forehead, back of the neck, and head will constrict the blood vessels so that less blood flows into the head. Soaking the feet in a hot footbath in which peppermint and apple cider vinegar are added to the water will bring the blood away from the head and into the feet, and also cool and cleanse the blood. A hot hip bath will also bring the blood away from the head. When the headache is severe, try alternating hot and cold, using towels that are soaked and then wrung out and applied to the face and head. The last application should be cold. You can also alternate hot and cold hip baths. An enema with cool water may give relief, since migraines are frequently related to wastes remaining in the colon.

HERBS If you are interested in taking herbs, Dr. Kane recommends that you consult a qualified professional, especially since different herbs are effective for migraines with different causes. Some nontoxic recommendations are as follows. For migraines associated with poor digestion or depression, lavender, which calms the nervous system, can be added to your bath water or rubbed into your temples. Feverfew works for the kind of migraine that is relieved by applications of heat. Eating three leaves a day has been known to prevent migraines. Willow relieves pain and reduces inflammation.

Dr. Kane suggests that this herbal tea, by cleansing the system, can prevent or decrease migraines:

1 part hops
1 part chamomile

1/2 part oatstraw
1/2 part catnip
1/2 part skullcap
1/4 part peppermint leaf

You can make this formula yourself or order it from Frontier Herbs (1-800-669-3275). Add a heaping tablespoon to a cup of water that has just boiled and steep for 3 to 5 minutes. You can add honey to sweeten. Drink this tea two to three times a day.

DIET One strategy is to fast for a few days to detoxify the body. A glass of water to which lemon juice and a half teaspoon of baking soda have been added can help eliminate waste in the digestive tract.

Certain foods, says Dr. Kane, tend to promote migraines and should be avoided. These include spicy foods; stimulating foods such as chocolate, tea, and coffee; alcohol; and fried food. Obviously, any food to which you personally have a bad reaction should be avoided.

HOMEOPATHY Many homeopathic remedies can help relieve migraines; the remedy must be matched to the particular symptoms. Some of those mentioned by Dr. Zane include the following:

ARNICA MONTANA. Arnica montana is for treating migraines that feel as though the head is burning but the rest of the body is cool. There is aching above the eyes that radiates to the temples. Sneezing and coughing cause shooting pains. Arnica is also used for migraines caused by head injuries such as concussion.

LACHESIS. Lachesis is for a severe congestive migraine, usually on the left side, that involves vomiting and loss of sight. There is throbbing and a sense of bursting. The headache is induced by sun (chronic). It is relieved by pressure on the top of the head and gets worse if discharges are suppressed (e.g., with antihistamines).

NATRUM MURIATICUM. Natrum muriaticum (table salt) is particularly effective for chronic headaches that involve intense pain accompanied by a feeling of bursting or of compression, as if in a vice.

NUX VOMICA. Nux vomica relieves migraines associated with stomach, liver, abdominal, and hemorrhoidal conditions. The migraine comes on when the person awakes or gets up, after eating, in the open air, or when the eyes are moved.

PHOSPHORUS. Phosphorus is used to treat congestive migraines in which the head throbs. These headaches are made worse by motion, light, noise, lying down, hunger, and heat; they improve with rest. The person feels cold but likes cold applied to the head.

PULSATILLA. Pulsatilla is used for congestive migraines in which the head throbs and is hot. The headache improves with applications of cold or walking slowly outside. It may be associated with overeating and menstruation.

RHUS TOXICODENDRON. Rhus toxicodendron is used in cases where the person feels intoxicated or stupefied, as though the head were being weighted down. When the person wakes and opens her eyes a violent migraine comes on. Children may get this type of migraine when they get cold or damp or have wet the bed.

SEPIA. Sepia is used for migraines, especially in women, that are related to nervousness, indigestion, or heartburn, and may be violent or periodic and improve when the person lies quietly. This type is often cured by sleep, by strenuous activity such as dancing, or by long walks outdoors.

SILICA. Silica relieves chronic migraines involving nausea and vomiting that begin at the nape of the neck and move over the crown of the head to the eyes. The headache improves with pressure, lying down, heat, and urination.

THUJA OCCIDENTALIS. Thuja occidentalis is used for the person who feels as though a nail were being driven into the top of the head and who has severe stitches in the area of the left temple and pulsation in both temples. Thuja is effective for severe headaches that follow vaccination.

ACUPRESSURE Dr. Kane describes acupressure points that can be used to relieve different types of migraines. A point known as Wind Gate is effective for migraines related to the change of seasons. It is actually two points located at the highest point of the neck just below the hairline on either side of the muscles that run up the spine. You can press these points or put two tennis balls in a sock and lie on your back so that the balls press into these two points.

Another point is in the fleshy area between the thumb and forefinger. Squeezing it can reduce migraine pain and also stimulate a bowel movement, which itself often relieves the headache. A point below the bottom of the big toe can relieve migraines that affect the upper part of the face and the eyes.

A PSYCHOLOGICAL APPROACH Dr. Kane suggests pondering some themes that make connections between migraines and a person's emotional or mental condition. Insight into hidden stresses that manifest physically as migraines may help you release the tensions that lead to the migraine. For example, Dr. Zane explains, some experts believe that migraines represent an attempt to live out one's sexuality through the head. On a physiological level, the pattern of tension manifested as constricted blood vessels releasing into relaxation when the vessels finally dilate and the pain is relieved can be compared to an orgasm. This type of migraine can frequently be relieved by masturbation, although it may require more than one orgasm to bring relief. Dr. Kane notes further that constipation and problems with digestion are often associated with migraines. This indicates a "closed-up" condition in the lower body.

COLORS Dr. Kane describes the use of color to relieve migraines as well as other ills. You can wear certain colors or use gels placed over lamps or other light sources. The colors most effective during a migraine, she says, are purple and scarlet. Purple increases the ability to tolerate pain and makes a person drowsy when a purple light is shined on the chest, throat, and face. Scarlet can be shined on the face to raise blood pressure, though only for migraines caused by decreased blood flow. For migraines that affect the right side of the head, shine blue on the face or the liver for five minutes.

In between migraine attacks, use lemon (said to dissolve blood clots) and yellow (which works on the lymphatic system and motor nerves) for two weeks. Then use lemon and orange, which act as decongestants, for four weeks. Repeat this pattern for as long a period as required.

REFLEXOLOGY Applying pressure to the feet can alleviate migraines because specific reflex points correspond to the head area. Reflexologist Gerri Brill says that the greatest benefit comes from a routine that encompasses all body systems. Here she gives a detailed description of her program.

CREATING A COMFORTABLE ENVIRONMENT. "I start off by getting you to feel relaxed. Sometimes I use a foot basin to soften and warm up the feet. Then I have you lie down on my massage table while I explain the anatomy of the foot and the idea that each part corresponds to an area of the body. The big toe relates to the head, and the little toes relate to the head and sinuses. Under the toes is a ridge that corresponds to the neck and shoulders. The chest-lung area corresponds to the ball of the foot. The narrow part is the waist area, and at the heel you have the small and large intestines, the sciatic nerves, and the lower back."

RELAXING BREATHING. "There is a special place on the foot that corresponds to the solar plexus. This is a little notch just below the ball of the foot. The solar plexus is the seat of the emotions. By placing my thumb in this little notch as you inhale and releasing as you exhale, I help you to let go of a lot of stuck feelings held inside. It helps promote relaxation and is good to do at the end of the session as well."

WRINGING THE FOOT. "As you lie down, I wring out your foot three times or so, as if I were wringing out a washcloth. That helps the foot relax." Lung press. "This is where I press the fist of my right hand into your chest-lung reflex while holding your foot with my left hand. This area is on the pad of your foot, directly beneath the ridge of the toes. As I press, I slowly bring the flat of my fist down to the heel. I repeat this action three times. It is another relaxation technique."

FOOT-AND-TOE BOOGIE. "Next I do what is called the foot boogie. That means rocking your foot back and forth to loosen it up. Then I do the same with your toes. I place my hands around each toe as I shake your toes back and forth. It sounds silly but it feels great."

ZONE WALKING. "Zone walking is performed with the outer aspect of the thumb. If you place your thumb on your lap, it is the area that rests on your lap. It's important to keep the fingernails short to avoid digging into anyone. Using the outer aspect of my thumb, I start way down at the heel. I mentally divide the foot into five zones, with each zone leading to a different toe. Starting at the outside portion of the foot, the fleshier part, I bend the working thumb at a 45-degree angle and apply pressure as I creep up the foot ever so slightly. Each move is no more than a sixteenth of an inch. There are a lot of nerve endings in the feet, and I want to hit all of them. Applying steady pressure, I work my thumb upward all the way to the tip of the toe. When I reach the top of the toes, I go back down to the heel again to repeat the process. These steps are repeated for all five zones. By covering the whole body in this way, I help to create an equilibrium."

SPINE REFLEX. "Now I am at the inside aspect of the foot. That's the spine reflex, and it is very important because the spine supports you and holds you erect. I start at the bottom by your heel with my thumb. Again, I work with the outside corner of my thumb held at a 45-degree angle and walk up your spine. I go all the way up to the big toe. Then I turn around and thumb-walk down, using little steps and steady pressure. I don't want to hurt you, but I do want to exert a good amount of pressure since this is pressure therapy."

SHOULDER AND NECK REFLEX. "Now I move to the ridge underneath the toes. This corresponds to the neck and shoulder line, and it is important for headache relief because when people have tension and headaches, their neck and shoulders are usually tense. Again, I use the thumb-walk. I start at the outside of the big toe and thumb-walk to the ridge. I bend the toes back slightly to get inside. This is repeated until I get to the little toe. Then I turn around and thumb-walk back."

HEAD AREA. "The big toe relates to the head, so of course I want to work this area. I place the fingers of my right hand over my left hand and thumb-walk down the fleshy part of the big toe. I divide the big toe into five zones and work down each area using very, very tiny bites or steps. My aim is for 25 bites on that big toe. That covers the whole area. I do that five times. This is very important."

BRAIN REFLEX. "Rolling my index finger over the top of the big toe stimulates the brain and relieves aches caused by migraines. Often this area feels sensitive because of crystal deposits that accumulate. These deposits need to be broken up."

HEAD AND SINUSES. "After finishing the big toe, I move to the little toes. Again, using my thumb, I divide each toe into three zones and thumb-walk, using little bites. This is repeated three times on each toe. This is another place where I feel tiny grains of sand.

"Breaking them up is the main way to relieve migraines."

CLOSING THE SESSION. "Just to make the session complete, I go back to the top of the foot while supporting the heel with the fist. I finger-walk with the right hand between the little bones on the top of the feet. This area helps the lymphatics, chest, breast, and part of the back. Massaging here helps you to achieve a state of balance. Then I work around the ankle areas. The ankles relate to the reproductive organs and alleviate headaches caused by PMS. That's just one foot. Now I wrap up the foot that was worked on and start over on the other side. Afterward, I massage both feet at the same time, which is very sooth-ing. At this point, you know that the session is coming to an end. Once again, I massage your solar plexus area and have you take a deep breath. Finally, I do a nerve stroke to soothe the feet. This is where I ask you to imagine taking in peace and balance with each breath. This promotes a profound sense of relax-ation. At this point the session is over, but you should rest a few moments instead of getting up quickly. Just relax and acknowledge how great you feel. Be sure to drink some water after the session to flush out the deposits."

47

Multiple Sclerosis

ultiple sclerosis (MS) is a progressive and deteriorating muscular disability
in which there is a loss of the protective covering of nerves in the brain and
spinal cord. Some 350,000 Americans have this debilitating disease.

Dr. Michael Wald, who holds degrees in nutrition and chiropractic, and has
authored five books about health, explains. "Multiple sclerosis is a syndrome of
progressive nerve disturbances. What we have is a gradual loss in myelin, which
is part of the outer covering of the nervous system. The nervous system breaks
down."

MS is a condition that can present itself quite suddenly, Dr. Wald says. A
young adult could be quite healthy and then one day have problems moving the
limbs. Muscle weakness, dizziness, and problems with perception and touch
may appear. Vision may be blurred.

"Generally the person will go to a neurologist and the neurologist will take
an MRI," Dr. Wald continues. "Maybe he will take some of the patient's cere-
brospinal fluid and look for things. Then the doctor says, 'You've got the disease.' Then the person is put on one of several steroids and that is the end of
that.."That's really not enough. There is enough nutritional and medical literature to support the use of a whole host of dietary and nutritional changes in the
lives of these people. What we want to do in natural medicine is slow down and
reverse the degeneration of myelin. When myelin breaks down, it's called
demyelinization. In about two-thirds of the cases of MS, the onset is between
20 and 40. We are talking about the most fit people in the prime of their lives,
being struck with this condition."

Possible Causes

No one pretends to know the causes of MS. Some postulate that it is due to a virus. Often, a person will have a viral problem and will get MS shortly thereafter. So that may be a cause or a trigger. Yet, Dr. Wald cautions, "Human beings are complicated, as we well know, so even if we knew the cause, we would still want to approach it from a natural medicine perspective by giving the body whatever it needs to help whatever it wants to correct. Whether it's MS or a headache or some other problem, the natural healer strives to give the body what it needs."

The theory that MS is caused by a virus is based on animal studies. "Certain viruses can be given to certain animals, for example, which will cause every single symptom of MS," Dr. Wald says. "So it's not unreasonable. The common viruses they think might be involved in causing MS are the rabies virus, herpes simplex virus, and the parainfluenza virus. So natural approaches should be antiviral in nature. We want to think of echinacea, astragalus, goldenseal."

Multiple sclerosis is classified as an autoimmune disease. An autoimmune disease is one in which the immune system fails to recognize a component of the body's systems as "self" and mounts an attack on that component. For example, says Dr. Wald, "The body may be breaking down the myelin, causing symptoms of MS. So anything we do to slow that down or reverse it should theoretically help." He adds, "In autoimmunity, the problem with immune breakdown occurs eventually to everyone as aging happens, so we are really talking about a situation that will affect everyone."

Natural Treatments

DIET In terms of diet, the first thing is to identify and eliminate food allergies. Dr. Wald remarks that allergies also indicate problems with the immune system. "An allergy means that the immune system becomes hyper-responsive. We already have that going on in MS, so we don't want to create any other hyper-responsiveness with foods."

A number of foods commonly cause allergies, including gluten-containing foods such as barley, rye, oats, and wheat. "These are common offenders. Also milk products fit this category. In fact, the intake of milk in adolescents is correlated with a far higher MS incidence. That much has been proven."

How would a person determine if he or she were allergic? Dr. Wald says, "You can do what is called an IgG4/IgG1 combination test for allergy, which is a blood test. Ninety foods can be checked, and you can determine quite quickly how your immune system hyper-responds to some of them. Then you eliminate the foods and use substitutes. Another way to approach this would be to look at your diet for the top 10 or 15 foods that you eat most often or that are your favorite and eliminate them, because those best-loved foods tend to be the allergy foods. Even allergists recognize this."

Dr. Wald adds, "Most people find it strange that their favorite foods are what are getting them into trouble. A person will say, "But I eat the food all the time." Yes, but you are also causing some disruption of the immune function by doing that, particularly if you have a weak immune system to begin with." By eliminating these foods, "you will reduce overall stress on the immune system. That means healing has a chance to take place."

Aside from allergens, other foods to be avoided in relation to this disease are animal fats. "A high intake of saturated fats in the diet, animal fats, is definitely linked to MS."

Dr. Wald notes that some studies have supported vegetarianism as a positive path for MS sufferers. "Dr. Roy Swank, professor of neurology at the University of Oregon Medical School, did one of the longest studies of MS ever done, which was about 26 years in duration. People who had MS symptoms were put on essentially a vegan diet, cod liver oil, and several other similar things. Over time he noticed that those on this diet who initially had symptoms had fewer exacerbations and less worsening of their condition over the years or had no exacerbations, and did very well or better in comparison to those who had an initial MS diagnosis and were given the standard drugs."

SUPPLEMENTS Another important avenue to explore is supplementation. Dr. Wald told me about an unusual new supplementation therapy developed at Harvard. "One practical suggestion is something called myelin basic protein. This is something that you or anyone can buy in the health food store. Harvard has investigated reactions with MS patients, using oral myelin from a cow, actually. Basically, if you eat myelin, the stuff in the nervous system will attack the myelin you are eating, leaving your nervous system alone and giving it a chance to repair. The technical term for that is molecular mimicry. You are mimicking your myelin, so it's a distraction technique. That's very important."

Less experimentally, there are certain supplements of proven effectiveness, particularly the omega-3 and omega-6 fatty acids. Dr. Wald notes, "Most of the readers probably know something about these. Evening primrose oil is an example of an omega-6. We get that from grains and seeds. The omega-3s can be obtained from such things as flaxseed oil and fish oil. There are dozens of other types of fats that are important. I do recommend that those with MS have what is called an essential fatty acid blood test done, so you can find out exactly what oils you need and then simply put them back."

These oils control inflammation in the body and immune function. They also are needed for vascular function—in other words, all the things we need for healing MS. Dr. Wald says that even if you don't have these special tests done, you certainly would want to at least purchase a supplement that contains a reasonable balance of omega-3 and omega-6 oils. Probably, you should look for one that is heavier on the omega-3 oils, the flax and fish oils.

"I myself find that MS patients have difficulty metabolically breaking flaxseed oil down into what they need. So, rather than flax, I tend to recommend what is called ephedra, a supplement. For dosage, you should follow the directions on the bottle unless you are seeing a health care practitioner who can individually tailor the dose."

Another very important nutrient for MS is glutathione. This amino acid is the major immune booster in the body. If you are going to help your health, regardless of what the concern is, you have to somehow raise glutathione levels. Dr. Wald recommends anywhere from 250 to 500 milligrams orally.

Selenium helps the body utilize the glutathione. The recommended dose would be in the 200 to 400 microgram range.

Vitamin B_{12} is also extremely important. Dr. Wald says, "Alcoholics, for example, can have the shakes, which are caused by degeneration of their myelin, due to a B_{12} deficiency. This seems very similar to the problems of MS. So, though a B_{12} deficiency is probably not the cause of MS, many MS sufferers have a B_{12} imbalance, one that doesn't necessarily show up on a blood test. So every MS patient we see gets a B_{12} shot. Oral supplements might do it, but it really depends on the level of disability."

Enzymes are also extremely important. As Dr. Wald puts it, "Any conversation about autoimmune disease would not be complete without speaking about them. Bromelain and papain are plant-derived enzymes. They are pancreatic enzyme supports."

Dr. Wald notes that these enzymes are key to defending the body against autoimmune chemicals in the blood which irritate and break down tissues. Enzymes that you eat like bromelain, papain, and others found in fresh fruits or vegetables, as well as pancreatic enzymes, get into the blood and literally digest some of these irritating chemicals. It's a must to include lots of those enzymes.

"Lastly," Dr. Wald says, "some other supplements should be mentioned. One is N-acetyl-cysteine (NAC). Cysteine and methionine are sulfur-containing amino acids that help liver detoxification and overall body detoxification. So any anti-autoimmune approach should contain generous amounts of NAC, between 250 to 1,000 milligrams orally. It works really well orally. The NAC increases glutathione levels. As we said earlier, glutathione is the single most important immune-boosting chemical in the body."

HERBS, OXYGEN, EXERCISE Dr. Wald also uses extracts of herbs that are standardized, meaning they have been assayed for the active ingredient. "In other words," he says, "what the bottle says is in there, is in there." The herbs goldenseal, astragalus, and echinacea are the ones most often recommended for autoimmune disorders.

He mentions a common criticism of herb use. "I do want to recall a question I often field about herbs. A person will ask, 'If MS is a case of the ultra-sensitization of the immune system, would you want to take herbs that would bolster the immune system?'

"Well, the wonderful thing about how nature has worked this out is that these supplements will not enhance immunity. They are what are called biologic response modifiers. They work to balance what is wrong. If your immunity is too high, they will work to bring it low. If your immunity is low, they will bring it up. Of course, you can abuse these things to a certain point. But almost no one, if she follows the general directions on the bottles, will be caused any harm. The most the person will experience is a little gastrointestinal upset, and once she experiences that she will naturally decrease the dose." In taking herbs, no matter which ones, Dr. Wald recommends a 4-day on, 4-day off cycle, so the body doesn't become insensitive to the herbs, which could result in the herbs losing some of their effectiveness.

He also notes that work has been done with oxygen in aiding sufferers from this illness. "Something not commonly talked about in MS is hyperbaric oxygen. It is possible—and there are many studies on this with MS—for a person to get into a chamber and be exposed to clean, purified oxygen under pressure for health reasons. The purpose of the pressure is to increase oxygen levels in the blood so that healing can take place. As we age—and you can think of MS as accelerated aging of the immune and nervous system—we do not use oxygen well and so tissues break down, producing lots of free radicals. Anything that helps prevent or reverse that has to be healthy just in general. So for those with less severe cases of MS, hyperbaric oxygen will be quite valuable."

In his experience, the effectiveness of exercise for those with MS depends very much on the individual. "Sometimes exercise worsens MS and sometimes it helps it. I think the reason is that if someone's nutritional status is lousy, and the person is exercising, she is only increasing her stress. So, you want to have a complete holistic program where supplements, diet, exercise, and stress reduction are all combined intelligently."

48

Parkinson's Disease

Michael J. Fox, the television and film actor, has had his career cut short by Parkinson's disease. He seemed to be a young, healthy, happy, and active person. How could this have happened to him? It raises all kinds of questions as to what is Parkinson's disease and how we can prevent it. He is devoting his life now to raising awareness of Parkinson's disease. It could happen to any of us.

What is Parkinson's Disease?

Dr. Michael Wald, who holds degrees in nutrition and chiropractic, and is the author of *BioEmotional Healing*, has had experience with Parkinson's patients. He describes the condition, also known as PD: "It is characterized by tremors and muscular tightness and problems with posture and reflexes. It is one of the most frequently encountered disorders and is a predominant cause of disability in those greater than 50 years of age. Its prevalence is estimated at 1 to 2 million cases in the United States and the incidence increases with age. There are different types of Parkinson's, primary and secondary.

"Particular to PD is a loss of cells in the area of the brain known as the substantia nigra, locus cerleus, and substantia innominata, and a formation of abnormal bodies called Lewy bodies. Basically we don't know the cause but the most likely mechanism of the cellular damage is oxidation by toxic free radicals. In particular, this oxidation might break down a certain amino acid we need for normal health and normal motor function that leads to dopamine depletion.

"Someone with PD has what is called a 'resting' tremor or 'pill-rolling' tremor, as if they were rolling something between their thumb and their first finger and their hands are moving. During sleep it fades away. If you try to move their arms and legs, the muscles are very rigid, called 'lead pipe' rigidity, and the muscles move with a 'cogwheel phenomenon'. These individuals walk very slowly and often shoot forward and fall down and hurt themselves because their motor function is skewed. Infrequency of blinking is one of the early signs and a loss of overall facial expression, a loss of voice volume, with a poverty of body movement. Reflexes are diminished."

This lack of movement is called bradykinesia and the shuffling gait with poor arm swing is very characteristic of Parkinson's patients. One key is that the incessant tremor disappears with intentional movement and then returns as soon as the arm is at rest. There is also a very strong association with depression and eventual dementia with PD.

These clinical signs are because the nerves in the brain start to degenerate and are a strong clue in the diagnosis. MRIs sometimes show atrophy, or wasting, in advanced cases but mostly the CT scan and MRIs of the brain do not show anything. The diagnosis is usually made based on the clinical picture.

Parkinson's is mostly a disease of the elderly but it is seen in younger people like Michael J. Fox. Younger people tend to develop the motor and muscle problems first. In the older population there is a much higher incidence of dementia. Other kinds of dementias can also have features that look like Parkinson's disease and many times there is an overlap of different causes for the dementia.

Potential Causes

The cause is unknown but there is a lot of speculation. A current theory is that PD may be caused by a toxic environmental agent or chemical compound. This is because there were reports of greater prevalence in rural areas. The herbicide Parquat is a likely culprit. Dieldrin and DDT have also been implicated. Another study by Scheider and colleagues in 1997 found that the antioxidant lycopene (found primarily in tomatoes and related products) was not associated with higher PD risk but intake of sweet foods, including fruit, was. They theorized that pesticide residues in the fruits and vegetables may have contributed to the development of PD.

"There have been a number studies of pesticides and insecticides," Dr. Wald says. "If you are genetically susceptible and are exposed to toxins in the soil or air, they can breakdown or oxidize the dopamine. In the *Journal of Neurology* they reported causing PD with pesticides that they were able to reverse. It is our liver that detoxifies toxins. Manganese and copper were studied and they say that ongoing exposure to manganese and copper of greater than 20 years will cause PD. A diet higher in mono and disaccharides, the simple sugars, is associated with a higher risk of PD."

Dr. Jay Lombard is chief of neurology at Westchester Square Medical Center and assistant professor at Cornell University Medical College. He has seen and treated many Parkinson's patients. He has this to add about the causes of Parkinson's:

"Environmental toxins have been implicated in the etiology of Parkinson's disease, particularly pesticides. It appears that patients who have Parkinson's disease have an inability to detoxify these very common pesticides found in the environment because they lack a particular enzyme."

It is also known that certain drugs can cause a reversible form of PD. These drugs are the phenothiazines and butyrophenones, drugs that affect the central nervous system. Carbon monoxide poisoning has been known to induce a parkinsonism.

Conventional Treatment

Medical doctors usually prescribe a drug called selegline (Eldepryl) at first. It may help by delaying the amount of time before the patient gets L-dopa, the standard treatment. It interacts with SSRIs and TCAs, drugs often given for the part of PD that results in severe depression. As the disease gets worse and interferes with any kind of reasonable life or falls start because of the postural instability, then the doctors start L-dopa. None of these drugs can cure the disease and it keeps progressing.

Alternative Approaches to Treatment and Prevention

Dr. Jay Lombard is also the author of *Brain Wellness Plan*. He talks about some of the things we can do to prevent PD. "It is known that glutathione is diminished in the brains of Parkinson's patients. One of the major strategies in preventing the progression of Parkinson's disease is to boost up the natural glutathione levels in the brain. There are various compounds that do that, for instance, antioxidants like lypoic acid.... It is worth further study to see if indeed giving dihydrolypoic acid prevents progression of the disease.

"Gangliosides are a type of lipid or fat membrane that is found in high degrees in our nervous system. Gangliosides have also been studied to help prevent progression in Parkinson's. Administering medications that increase dopamine production are beneficial for symptomatic improvement but the underlying process in Parkinson's patients has to do with our antioxidant defense systems being deficient. Anything we can do to raise those defense systems certainly would help with the underlying disease.

"What I tell patients with Parkinson's disease is that the medication they have been given will help them feel better and the natural products or antioxidants that I prescribe may not really make them feel much different but are addressing the underlying cause of Parkinson's disease. It is possible that those two things don't always match."

Dr. Lombard follows three general strategies in attempting to prevent progression of the disease. He remarks, "These strategies are useful for other neurodegenerative conditions as well. We know the immune system is overactive in particular ways that is destructive to the brains of Parkinson's patients. We know that patients with Parkinson's have an inability to handle a particular metal found in our diets called iron and we know that Parkinson's patients may have a deficiency of a part of the cell called the mitochondria that is responsible for the manufacture of ATP [adenosine triphosphate, which is involved in the storage and transfer of cellular energy]. Using these three evidences a comprehensive program can be drawn up that addresses each of these issues separately.

"In regard to excessive inflammation, certain types of white blood cells make a compound called nitrous oxide, which is a free radical. It is very destructive to areas of the brain in Parkinson's disease. There are certain antioxidants that are effective in quenching or inhibiting the effects of this free radical. These include an extract of green tea that has profound antioxidant properties. Dihydrolypoic acid, which is a glutathione precursor, increases brain glutathione levels and is very effective as an antioxidant. Lycopenol is another antioxidant that crosses the blood-brain barrier and inhibits excessive free radical activity.

"Second, we know Parkinson's patients have too much iron in their brains and iron acts as a free radical inducer. The idea of buffering the effects of increased iron with a protein called lactoferrin. This prevents excessive iron absorption from the intestinal tract into the bloodstream.

"Finally the mitochondria, the energy producing units of the cell that make ATP, are also deficient in Parkinson's patients. Ways of increasing the mitochondria include coenzyme Q10, serotonin and two other compounds, NADH, which is also called ignatia, and ubiquinone, which is a coenzyme Q10 analog. They dramatically increase brain ATP levels. These three things are a very worthwhile strategy to treat a Parkinson's patient."

Dr. Wald has devised a detoxification program that he feels is worthwhile for PD. "Beta carotene has been fairly well studied in PD. It is an antioxidant and I use about 50,000 units. It helps protect the liver and other cells and the nervous system from premature degeneration. Vitamin C helps protect dopamine, an important neurotransmitter that is low in those with PD."

"Essential fatty acids, like omega-3 and omega-6, are important for protecting the nervous system. Toxins in our environment known as zenobiotics are fat soluble, meaning they love to hang out in the nervous system. We need to take all the antioxidants I already spoke of with essential fatty acids like omega-3 and omega-6. So we want to get vitamin E, 400 to 800 IU a day and vitamin C to balance tolerance. Some of the studies show PD patients have low levels of vitamin B$_3$, niacin. There is a nonflushing form called hexaniacinite, 250 milligrams a day. Melatonin is a very important hormone not just for sleep and repair but also as an important antioxidant in the nervous system. It slows down the breakdown of dopamine. Another important amino acid is N-acetyl cysteine or NAC. It is used by the liver to convert fat-soluble toxins into water-soluble toxins so we can excrete them in the urine. The body must be able to eliminate toxins once they are mobilized. Any detoxification program needs to focus on the liver and intestine and the lymphatic system and so on to get these things out."

Dr. Wald adds, "Glutathione has been found to be low in PD. The most effective way to increase it is with vitamin C. Glutathione is not only an immune booster but helps fight degenerative changes. It tends to become lower as we age."

49

Alzheimer's Disease

lzheimer's disease is the leading cause of senile dementia in this country. It is a degenerative disease of the nervous system, meaning that the nerve cells in the brain start to malfunction and then degenerate and die. Alzheimer's disease is slow but progressive and wipes out many functions of the brain, especially memory. The heartbreaking tragedy of Alzheimer's disease is that it steals the person by taking away who they are. Over time, they do not know themselves or remember anything familiar from their past—not their family, their homes, their careers, or their life histories.

In the last 10 years, there has been an explosion of Alzheimer's disease in this country—up to a 10-fold increase. We know Alzheimer's dementia is a disease of old age, as many as 30 percent of those over the age of 85 are suffering from this dementia. And we can anticipate Alzheimer's disease to reach epidemic proportions in the 21st century as more and more people reach their 70s, 80s, and 90s, and even their100s.

Signs and Symptoms

How can you know if someone is starting to suffer from Alzheimer's dementia?

It can be tricky because there is such a *gradual* decline. The decline in cognitive function usually starts with memory loss. First, the ability to learn new material and recent, short-term memory starts to go. There may be some language paucity, mild impairment in drawing or puzzles, and difficulty with higher functions like planning and problem solving. The personality starts to change with occasional irritable outbursts and sometimes apathy. But you can think to yourself that grandma or grandpa is just getting on in years and getting more forgetful or crankier.

As the disease progresses, memory becomes worse and the personality more flat. Constant restlessness and wandering without direction can start. If the doctor orders a CT scan of the brain at this later stage, there is 50-50 chance that it will start to show brain atrophy.

In the end, there is no memory, no trace of former personality, difficulty talking—in fact, difficulty making any sense with language. Intelligence is gone. Limb become rigid. People at this stage develop poor sphincter control and become incontinent of urine and stool.

Diagnosis is made on clinical grounds. There is a short test doctors give called the Mini-Mental Status Exam (MMSE) that can provide some clues. It tests things like short-term memory, language skills, and perception. It is useful information for the doctor but cannot be used to make a firm diagnosis of Alzheimer's. The head CT scan shows more definite atrophy but only at the late stages of the disease. The definitive diagnosis is only by brain biopsy after death, although there is a lot of research now underway to find some way to make the diagnosis before death.

There is another disease that looks just like Alzheimer's disease on clinical grounds. It is called Lewy body disease and researchers are finding that this disease is much more common than previously thought. The differences from Alzheimer's disease—and these are subtle distinctions—are that Lewy body disease patients are more psychotic with visual hallucinations and severe depression, and also have some features of Parkinson's disease.

At autopsy what the doctors see when they examine the brains are neurofibrillary tangles, senile plaques, cell loss and impaired synaptic function. They find that cholinergic, noradrenergic, and dopaminergic cells in the brain are lost. It is believed that oxidative stress and the accumulation of free radicals leads to this nerve cell degeneration. Excessive lipid peroxidation seen in the brain is the cause of the nerve cell death.

Causes

Dr. Michael Wald, who holds degrees in nutrition and chiropractic, and is the author of *Bio-Emotional Healing*, has studied Alzheimer's disease and other degenerative diseases of the nervous system.

"There have been extensive studies of this condition and certainly genetics plays some role," Dr. Wald says. However, he remarks, "even though genetics plays a significant role in determining susceptibility to the condition, like most chronic degenerative diseases, environmental factors also play an extremely significant role."

In talking about causes of dementia, Dr. Wald mentions metabolic disorders such as vitamin B_{12} deficiency, folate deficiency, hypoglycemia (low blood sugar), and thyroid disease. He also enumerates environmental causes such as trauma, aluminum or silicon ingestion, and exposure to known neurotoxins such as pesticides, insecticides, and other chemicals from the environment in water, food, and air. All of these things cause free radical damage. Free radicals are highly reactive molecules that interfere with normal function of the body. Dr. Wald says, "As we age normally, free radicals increase that actually cause the aging but in certain susceptible individuals, either genetically or environmentally, they've got too much aging in specific areas that result in these kinds of symptoms [of dementia]. In medicine they call it Alzheimer's or Parkinson's."

Dr. Wald explains his concern with aluminum ingestion. "With Alzheimer's disease, we really must focus on aluminum and metals in general. Aluminum specifically concentrates in an area of the brainstem causing neurofibrillary tangles. This is a type of defect that is characterized by Alzheimer's disease. Whether aluminum causes it or results from the formation of these neurofibrillary tangles no one quite knows, but in either case we want to make sure aluminum is removed. Basically this aluminum has a very strong affinity for the nervous system…. The fact is that as we grow older blood levels of aluminum increase and studies of Alzheimer's patients show that they have higher aluminum levels than normal people without dementia or symptoms. It doesn't have to be high doses of aluminum. It could be very low, trace doses over a long period of time that cause oxidation in the brain which causes neurofibrillary tangles and all the symptoms."

So what are sources of aluminum that we want to eliminate? "Antacids commonly have aluminum. Drinking water has trace amounts of aluminum. Researchers have shown that trace amounts of aluminum from water—just that single source—immediately enter brain tissue. The frightening news is really that aluminum in water not only occurs naturally but is added to some water supplies. There is aluminum in deodorants, cooking pots and pans, aluminum foil. Certain nondairy creamers have aluminum, as does baking powder to help the powder from becoming very lumpy when you mix it with fluid."

Dr. Wald explains that there are ways to decrease the body's aluminum absorption. "It can be chelated or removed with either intravenous chelation or oral chelating supplements," he says. "Calcium citrate prevents the absorption of aluminum. Aluminum absorption can be decreased not just with calcium but with its partner magnesium. Magnesium, like calcium, competes with the aluminum for absorption. Probably people with Alzheimer's disease need much higher levels of calcium and magnesium. It's very important to supplement these on a daily basis. So if we are juicing every day, if we are taking our natural antioxidants and our natural chelaters, we will offset this accumulation over a lifetime."

Conventional Treatment

There is currently very little that can be done by Western medicine to stop the progression of Alzheimer's disease. One drug given regularly is Aricept (donepezil). It has been shown to slow the rate of decline in early Alzheimer's disease. It is an acetylcholinesterase inhibitor. Its side effects are nausea, vomiting, and diarrhea, all because it increases cholinergic activity. A study published in 1997 in the *New England Journal of Medicine* showed that megadoses of vitamin E together with the drug Segeline slowed the progression of moderate Alzheimer's disease. A decade ago they gave a drug called Tacrine but it caused so much liver toxicity that they had to stop.

Alternative Therapies

Dr. Jay Lombard is a practicing neurologist in New York City and has published several papers in medical journals. He has studied many neurological diseases and is the author of *The Brain Wellness Plan*.

He outlines a four-pronged approach for the treatment of Alzheimer's disease. "The broad headings for treating Alzheimer's have to do [number one] with reducing excessive inflammation. Number two is raising a neurotransmitter called acetylcholine, which is very vital to memory. Number three is reducing antioxidant activity. Free radicals appear to be very involved in Alzheimer's disease. Fourth is boosting the mitochondria. The mitochondria are the energy-producing units of the cell that make ATP [adenosine triphosphate, which is involved in the storage and transfer of cellular energy]." Dr. Lombard feels the mitochondria play an important role in neurological diseases such as Alzheimer's disease and Parkinson's disease, and that "increasing mitochondrial activity is a common theme in treating these diseases."

So what specifically does Dr. Lombard suggest? He says, "In regard to raising brain acetylcholine levels, there is a natural product that is currently available called hypericin A, which acts to block the enzyme that breaks down acetylcholine and therefore raises our brain acetylcholine levels. [It is] very effective in improving memory and preliminary data in Alzheimer's hopefully will be available soon." Dr. Lombard also recommends ginkgo biloba, vitamin E, and melatonin. In addition, there is an analog of coenzyme Q10 and the amino acid acetyl-l-carnitine. Ignatia has also been shown in preliminary studies to be effective in raising brain ATP levels in Alzheimer's.

"Finally the last thing in Alzheimer's is looking at hormones, particularly estrogen and DHEA," Dr. Lombard says. "Estrogen is very effective in inhibiting an enzyme that is detrimental to Alzheimer's patients…. Estrogen blocks that enzyme and therefore inhibits the production of these pathological proteins found in the brains of Alzheimer's patients. DHEA, a natural adrenal steroid, again may be effective in Alzheimer's disease."

Dr. Wald offers the following additional nutritional advice for Alzheimer's disease and dementia in general. Start by avoiding processed foods, milk and dairy products, and increasing consumption of vegetables, grains, nuts and seeds from organic sources. Avoid aluminum and the metals. Then, he says, "Take a high potency mulitvitamin. Supplement that with vitamin C, between 500 and 3,000 milligrams three or more times a day, vitamin E, between 400 and 1,000 IU, and flaxseed oil. Flaxseed oil is needed in terms of overall cell membrane health and nervous system repair, about a tablespoon per day. Also I recommend thiamine (vitamin B_1) 3 to 8 grams per day, phosphatidyl serine, about 100 milligrams three times a day, acetyl-L-carnitine, about 500 milligrams three times a day, vitamin B_{12}, about 1,000 micrograms twice daily, and ginkgo biloba."

"The importance of thiamine or vitamin B_1 in Alzheimer's disease,' Dr. Wald says, "is that it has a profound effects on the brain. It actually mimics an important transmitter in the brain known as acetylcholine, which tends to be low in Alzheimer's patients."

He continues, "B_{12} deficiency is one of the more common deficiencies in the elderly to begin with. Up to 42 percent of people over age 65 are absolutely deficient of B_{12}. A deficiency of that will cause every symptom of Alzheimer's disease—neurological and motor or muscular symptoms, plus impairing mental function."

Zinc deficiency is another common deficiency seen in the elderly. Dr. Wald suggests "it could be a major factor in the development of Alzheimer's disease. There are many zinc-containing enzymes involved in cellular repair and DNA repair. Ineffective DNA and error-prone DNA can cause mental diseases.... Zinc supplementation has been used with as little as 27 milligrams in a study of 10 Alzheimer's patients and only two failed to show remarkable improvements. I think that is pretty good."

Dr. Wald also recommends phosphatidyl choline. "To date there have been 11 double-blind, published studies that all reported success using phosphatidyl choline in Alzheimer's disease. People with anywhere from mild to moderate dementia using a very high quality phosphatidyl choline can expect some improvement. The doses are between 15 and 25 grams. If you don't see improvements within 2 weeks, it probably isn't going to work."

What role do hormones play? Dr. Wald remarks, "There have been 12 population-based studies indicating that women on hormone replacement therapy have a lower rate of Alzheimer's disease. If we need to do hormone balancing, we want to use natural hormones whenever possible and see what happens. Even these studies admit that these people were much healthier to begin with."

Dr. Wald has used DHEA, an adrenal hormone. "DHEA has been found to be low in the blood and brain of Alzheimer's patients. I have used between 25 and 50 milligrams per day in men and 15 to 25 in women with benefit."

In the October 1997 issue of the *Journal of American Medical Association*, a study concluded that ginkgo biloba stabilized and in some cases improved cognitive performance and social function for 6 months to a year. LeBars and colleagues, the authors of the study, stated that ginkgo may be as effective as any drug, hormone, or vitamin used to treat Alzheimer's. It is safe and inexpensive.

PART TEN

Women's Health

Although this is beginning to change, there has in the past been little research on women's health issues. And in many cases the research done on health concerns affecting men and women equally has emphasized the men's side and understated the differences pertaining to women.

The natural healing tradition, however, has always emphasized women's health. At many points in modern history, the natural healer was the only person to whom women could turn to have their problems taken seriously and managed appropriately. And natural healing techniques were often nearly exclusively a woman's domain. Just as doctors have traditionally been men, and midwifes and nurses traditionally women, women are still often excluded from the highest levels of the medical establishment, where the decisions are made as to which types of treatments to favor and which to ignore.

As mentioned throughout this book, we are at a moment in history when alternative approaches have, in theory, finally been accorded a newfound legitimacy in the eyes of the medical establishment. It is only now that more and more people, especially women, will turn to the long, strong, and wonderful natural healing tradition. International in scope, it spans many cultures and synthesizes ancient folkloric remedies together with cutting-edge technologies. If doctors practicing Western medicine in the conventional way are going to ignore women's issues, let's see if the alternative medicine community can take up the slack. Let's see if we can help women keep themselves healthy by emphasizing good nutrition and all the individual alternative therapies that address their specific health concerns.

50

Menstrual and Hormonal Concerns

Menstrual Cramps and Irregular Menstruation

Painful and difficult periods are so commonplace in our society that some women have come to think of them as normal. However, they are not normal at all. Many experts feel that the symptoms of menstrual cramps (dysmenorrhea) are related to dietary practices as well as to unresolved emotional difficulties.

What factors may contribute to menstrual cramps? Dr. Pat Gorman, an acupuncturist and educator from New York City, explains, "In addition to toxins found in foods with preservatives, additives, and caffeine, they are due to putrid proteins found in dairy and red meat. These foods contain a lot of hormones that upset the system. In addition, foods fried in heavy oils cause problems and should be cut out immediately by any woman interested in getting rid of dysmenorrhea."

Dr. Gorman adds that the Chinese attribute this condition in part to pent-up anger and frustration: "If you are not happy with your life, if you are angry with people, you must work this out. The liver, which stores blood and prepares it for the period, is also responsible for anger. That's not a Western concept, but with my patients I find that working out anger helps the liver relax. As a result, there is far less of a problem with dysmenorrhea."

Dr. Marjorie Ordene, a gynecologist in Brooklyn, New York, agrees that hormonal and psychological factors cause painful periods and explains the underlying factors: "What causes dysmenorrhea is exaggerated uterine contractions. These contractions are mediated by receptors in the uterine lining that are stimulated by hormonal and psychological factors. Hormonal factors that stimulate the uterine receptors have actually been isolated. They are chemical messengers called prostaglandins. Two things are clear: People with menstrual cramps have an excess of prostaglandins, and there is an imbalance in the types of prostaglandins they produce." She adds that eating foods we are allergic to can increase prostaglandin production: "For example, many women are sensitive to yeast, and eating baked foods, breads, pastries, and processed fruit juices can cause an increase in prostaglandin production."

CONVENTIONAL TREATMENT Medical doctors often prescribe medications such as ibuprofen to inhibit prostaglandins. While these agents work to relieve menstrual cramps and the accompanying symptoms, problems occur when drugs are taken month after month. The side effects can include gastrointestinal bleeding, decreased blood flow to the kidneys, and leaky gut syndrome, a condition that allows undigested food particles to enter the blood.

NATUROPATHIC TREATMENT

DIET

Changes in diet can decrease overproduction of prostaglandins and restore normal balance. Cool green foods help reduce hot stabbing pains and inflammation. It is good to eat foods such as organic grains, legumes, oatmeal, and steamed green vegetables. Deep-sea fish such as salmon, tuna, and mackerel can be included, as well as flaxseed oil. Hot spices should be avoided, along with fried greasy foods, sugar, salt, alcohol, and stimulating foods such as garlic and onions. Foods that produce allergies should be eliminated as well.

Women who have nerve-related menstrual pain can benefit from tofu but should stay away from too many cold raw salads, hot spicy foods, and even white potatoes. The herbalist Letha Hadady suggests this soothing recipe: warm tofu cooked with sweet spices such as pumpkin pie spices and nutmeg. This quiets the nerves and helps a woman feel nurtured and relaxed.

Dr. Anthony Penepent, a physician who practices natural hygiene, helps patients with painful menses by placing them on a strict hygienic regimen: "I put them on a fast a day before the onset of their period. In serious conditions, I might have them fast one day and then prescribe juices or juice blended with salad and fruit for the following days until they complete their menses."

SUPPLEMENTS

Taken throughout the month as a daily supplement, evening primrose oil prevents headaches and blemishes that occur just before the period. Magnesium deficiencies are common and result in the release of prostaglandins that cause spasm and pain. Magnesium citrate is antispasmodic and helps relieve the problem. You can take 300 to 500 milligrams daily and work up to bowel tolerance.

HERBS

The following herbs may help alleviate menstrual problems.

Gardenia and philodendron. These are popular in Chinese medicine and can be obtained by prescription from an herbalist.

Corn silk tea. This tea helps get rid of the bloating that comes from too many hormones stored in the blood. Women's Rhythm also eliminates bloating.

Xiao yao wan. This a wonderful remedy that can be purchased at pharmacies in Chinatowns in major cities. It helps digestive processes. Not only does this formula relieve painful periods, it also alleviates anger.

Green tea. Green tea is cooling and satisfying and has very little caffeine. A pinch of tea can be added to a pot of boiled water, steeped for 5 minutes, and sipped throughout the day. People experience an energy pickup from the digestion being activated, not from the nerves being stimulated. Green tea helps soothe sharp, stabbing pains.

Aloe vera juice or gel. Aloe can eliminate headache, irritability, fever, stabbing pain, blemishes, and bad breath associated with menstrual cramps. Aloe also reduces acid from the stomach and liver and is slightly laxative. Just add to juice, tea, or water.

Dandelion. Dandelion helps break apart impurities in the system. It can be bought as capsules or tea.

Sarsaparilla. Sarsaparilla helps hot, stabbing pains brought on by inflammation. It is anti-inflammatory, antiseptic, diuretic, and soothing.

Valerian. Valerian is a sedative herb that makes a woman feel quieter, more relaxed, and grounded. It is especially good for nervous women who experience insomnia, anxiety, crying jags and emotional upsets, and other nervous problems. Valerian quiets the nerves that go to the uterus.

Yunnan pai yao. This combination of herbs helps reduce heavy bleeding and stabbing pain. Because it increases the circulation, internal bleeding is healed and swelling and pain are reduced.

HOMEOPATHY

Homeopathy was developed in Germany over 200 years ago by Dr. Samuel Hahnemann. The word "homeopathy" means "like cures like." The same substances that cause a disease in a healthy individual can heal an ailment in a sick person when they are diluted and given in minute proportions.

Homeopathic physician Dr. Ken Korins explains that the dilution process is what makes homeopathic remedies so safe: "Homeopathy is a vibrational medicine. We are dealing with very subtle energies. Substances are given in extremely small dilutions that cannot possibly have any toxic effects. In fact, if you were to analyze these substances, you would not find a trace of the original material in the final dilution."

The correct homeopathic remedy is the one that most closely matches the symptoms that manifest themselves. Dr. Korins recommends that dysmenorrhea sufferers choose from among the following:

Colocynthis. Colocynthis is a frequently indicated remedy that is useful when you have a severe onset of sudden cramps, particularly on the first day of menstruation. Emotionally, intense irritability and anger are associated with the menstrual cramps. A key indication is that you feel better when your knees are pulled up toward the stomach and held with firm pressure.

Magnesia phosphorica. Magnesium phoshorica helps spasmodic cramps with bloating. The key indication for this remedy is that you feel better from warmth. Magnesia phosphorica and colocynthis help alleviate the symptoms in 85 percent of cases.

Pulsatilla. A key indication for pulsatilla is variation; the cramps and the flow of bleeding are changeable. The pains themselves are typically cutting and tearing and may be felt in the lower back or kidney region. Generally, you feel worse in warm stuffy rooms and better in the open fresh air. Emotionally, you tend to be mild, gentle, and weepy when entering the menstrual state and prefer the company of other people to being alone.

Viburnum. Viburnum is indicated when the menses are very scanty and often late. In fact, they may last only a few hours. When you get cramps, the flow of blood stops. Cramps tend to radiate to the sacrum and the thighs. You may feel faint or feel like passing out.

Cimicifuga. Cimicifuga is indicated for spasmodic, cramping pains. The pain radiates across the pelvis from one thigh to the other. It is often associated with a premenstrual headache. Increased flow results in more pain. Emotionally, you may feel nervous to the point of being scattered and often are somewhat depressed.

Chamomilla. Chamomilla is helpful if you are either hypersensitive or insensitive to pain. Emotionally, you tend to be irritable and contrary. Someone brings you something that you ask for, and then you don't want it. During intense periods, you may become dependent on coffee and other stimulants and sedatives. Another symptom is anger. When you become angry, your symptoms become worse.

AROMATHERAPY

Marjoram, clary sage, and lavender are wonderful analgesics. Eighteen to 20 drops of oil added to a lotion or oil and massaged into the abdomen and lower back will help relieve menstrual pain. Breathing in the cooling fragrances of rose, lavender, or sandalwood can alleviate sharp, stabbing pain.

STRESS MANAGEMENT

Deep abdominal breathing, meditation, tai chi, and other mind-body disciplines eliminate frustrations and anger that bring on pain. Additionally, it is helpful to slow down the pace of life from the time of ovulation to the period.

Amenorrhea and Menorrhagia

Amenorrhea and menorrhagia are medical terms for abnormal blood flow. Amenorrhea refers to the cessation of bleeding or very light and infrequent periods, most often caused by an abnormally functioning hypothalamus, pituitary gland, ovary, or uterus as a result of drugs or surgery that removes the ovaries or uterus. "Bulimics and anorectics also exhibit this pattern," notes Dr. Pat Gorman. "Sometimes this is caused by excessive dieting and overexercise. Not accepting who she is, a woman thinks, I've got to make myself thin, beautiful, and perfect. If this is going on at the end of the cycle, when toxins are being released into the system, the woman is aggravating her body to the point of saying, We're not going to give up this blood. We desperately need it. Forget ovulation, forget periods."

Dr. Ruth Bar-Shalom and Dr. John Soileau, naturopaths from Alaska, in an article on the website of the American Association of Naturopathic Physicians (www.naturopathic.org), list several other causes of amenorrhea. First, it happens normally after a woman stops using birth control pills, during pregnancy, and during all or most of the breast-feeding period. It is important to establish that pregnancy is not the reason for amenorrhea, since some of the remedies for this condition may harm the woman and her child while she is pregnant or nursing.

Malnutrition, crash diets, obesity, stress, intensive exercising, extreme obesity, abuse of antidepressants and amphetamines, and mental illness are other causes of amenorrhea, say Drs. Bar-Shalom and Soileau. When a young woman of 16 has not yet begun to develop sexually, when weight fluctuates dramatically, and when amenorrhea is accompanied by severe depression, drug use, or pain, consult a qualified health-care professional.

With menorrhagia the opposite scenario occurs, and there is profuse bleeding. The condition can be debilitating, sometimes bad enough to warrant immediate attention in a hospital's emergency ward. "The Chinese say menorrhagia is caused by excess toxins and heat in the blood from foods containing preservatives, additives, and caffeine, especially coffee. It's like water in your car radiator becoming low," Dr. Gorman says. "The engine will overheat and explode. Alcohol adds more toxicity because it constantly removes water from the blood. As water diminishes, it heats up the blood. When the blood is what we call 'hot,' or fast-moving, it's very hard for the body to hold it in. It can't stop the bleeding."

The emotional profile of a menorrhagic individual is someone who sees herself as a victim. Dr. Gorman explains: "This person feels the need to serve everybody. She does not know how to set boundaries. Whatever anybody wants, they get. She keeps pouring out her energy and pouring out her blood."

Dr. Vicki Hufnagel, a gynecological surgeon and activist for women's health rights, adds that heavy bleeding is often a sign of an underlying problem in the female system, especially when it is accompanied by pain. The problem frequently is due to a hormonal imbalance. "Anything can throw off a cycle," she says, "including emotional stress, insomnia, too much estrogen in the system, or too little light, as in the winter. Other physical problems that can cause menorrhagia are fibroids, polyps, and a malfunctioning thyroid gland."

Before you can restore the blood flow in patients with amenorrhea or menorrhagia, you must discover the reason for the problem. Once the cause is addressed, periods should return to normal.

SYMPTOMS Asian medicine can diagnose amenorrhea and menorrhagia by examining the skin. Amenorrhea manifests as pale, sallow, slightly yellowish skin from a deep lack of blood and nutrients. Often this is accompanied by a great deal of emotional anxiety. With menorrhagia, the tongue has a red tip and tiny red dots. When the condition is long term, a woman can become anemic.

HORMONAL BALANCING FOR MENORRHAGIA Dr. Hufnagel says that hormonal dysfunctions in women with menorrhagia can be corrected with oral doses of natural progesterone. "Often the creams women use are not adequate because they don't cause a rise in the blood level. We often have to give what we call oral physiological levels of progesterone. I give women natural hormones in a cyclic manner, the way the body should be getting them." Hormone balancing also can be accomplished through the diet. Fatty diets cause higher levels of estrogen in the system, which in turn can cause menorrhagia. Lean diets and exercising with weights produce more testosterone, which in turn helps balance hormones and put an end to menorrhagia.

DIETARY REMEDIES Dr. Anthony Penepent, a natural hygienist from New York, says that amenorrhea is one of the easiest conditions to correct. He recommends a diet that includes two green salads daily, using romaine lettuce, fresh lemon juice, olive oil, and some brewer's yeast. You should also include two pieces of fresh fruit and two soft-boiled eggs in the daily menu. When amenorrhea is caused by a thyroid condition, a thyroid supplement is needed. Additionally, if stress is in the picture, the stressful situation must be remedied. For more serious cases, additional dietary intervention is necessary.

Usually, small changes in diet are all that are needed. Dr. Penepent says, "Even if the woman doesn't follow a completely natural hygienic regimen and is not vegetarian, she still can get tremendous results simply by increasing the amount of green leafy vegetables in the diet and providing concentrated nutritional sources, such as eggs and unsalted raw-milk cheese."

Drs. Bar-Shalom and Soileau add that women with amenorrhea need adequate protein, which means eating a number of grams per day equal to half your weight in pounds. They advocate fish and chicken instead of red meat, as well as nuts, seeds, and beans. Second, they advocate eating seaweed of all kinds.

SUPPLEMENTS Drs. Bar-Shalom and Soileau recommend the following supplements: 400 international units (IU) of vitamin E a day; 25 milligrams of B-complex vitamins a day, 1,000 milligrams of vitamin C twice a day, and 1,200 milligrams of calcium a day.

HERBS Several herbs are good for amenorrhea, say Drs. Bar-Shalom and Soileau.

GINGER TEA. Drink one to four cups of ginger tea each day (made from powder or grated fresh ginger).

BLAZING STAR, FALSE UNICORN, BLUE COHOSH, CHASTE TREE, AND ANGELICA. Mix together equal parts of these herbs and steep 1 tablespoon of the mixture in a cup of boiling water for 20 minutes. Drink three cups a day. You can also combine tinctures of these herbs. Drink 1 teaspoon of the mixed tinctures added to 1/4 cup of water three times a day.

The following Chinese herbs have specific effects on the blood and are needed at different times of the monthly cycle. Dr. Gorman recommends working with a health practitioner to create an individual protocol and monitor progress but offers these general guidelines.

At the beginning of the cycle:

DONG QUAI. High in vitamins A, E, and B_{12}, this blood-builder can be taken most days of the month, up to the point of menstruation, or just before it begins if there are strong premenstrual symptoms. "You don't want to be building blood if you are having trouble moving that blood," Dr. Gorman warns.

WOMEN'S PRECIOUS. This formula is a tremendous blood builder that is taken for about 3 weeks after the period ends. Women's Rhythm is then used the following week.

At the end of the cycle:

GARDENIA. Gardenia is taken when the symptoms of premenstrual syndrome (PMS) arise. By moving blood that is stuck, gardenia helps relieve that heavy, bloated feeling.

WOMEN'S RHYTHM. Women's Rhythm helps release a woman's blood. It is usually taken a week before the period to help move toxins out of the organs. (Women's Precious and Women's Rhythm are Ted Kapchik formulas that can be found in some health food stores and ordered directly from Kahn Herbs.)

Can be taken every day:

FLORADIX WITH IRON. This wonderful product is available in most health care stores. Liquid Floradix is superior to the dry form because it contains more live nutrients.

PHYSICAL MEASURES Drs. Bar-Shalom and Soileau stress the importance of focusing on deep breathing, consciously giving yourself periods of relaxation, and getting sufficient exercise to reduce stress as much as possible. Other suggestions include:

SITZ BATH. Make an infusion of a pound of oatstraw boiled for a half hour in 2 quarts of water and add it to warm bathwater. Sit in the water, which should reach your navel, with your feet propped on a chair outside the tub. Cover your top so that you stay warm. Soak like this for 10 to 15 minutes once or twice a week.

CLAY COMPRESS. Sterilize clay by heating it in a low oven for an hour and then grind it and make a paste with water. Apply the paste to your abdomen, cover with a cloth, and leave until the paste dries.

CASTOR OIL PACK. Put a cloth soaked in castor oil on your abdomen and then cover with plastic and then a dry cloth. Rest for an hour.

HOMEOPATHY Two homeopathic remedies are good for amenorrhea, according to Drs. Bar-Shalom and Soileau.

NATRUM MURIATICUM is for amenorrhea that occurs after extreme mental strain in women who have trouble expressing emotion. Use the 12c potency.

PULSATILLA is for a woman who misses her periods after stressful and emotional situations. Take it in the 6c potency three times a day for 3 weeks or until the period begins.

Toxic Shock Syndrome

Toxic shock syndrome (TSS) is a rare but serious and sometimes fatal disease.

The victims tend to be tampon users under the age of 30, especially those between 15 and 19. This sudden and serious disease affects persons with severely compromised immune systems who are poisoned by a strain of bacteria called Staphylococcus aureus, phage group I. This type of staph produces a substance called enterotoxin F, which can overpower and destroy a weak body.

Toxic shock syndrome is linked to the introduction of tampons with four new ingredients in the early 1980s. Before then tampons were made primarily of cotton. In the 1980s, though, highly absorbent polyester cellulose, carboxymethyl cellulose, polyacrylate rayon, and viscose rayon came into use. Three of these new ingredients were soon taken off the market; today only one of the new ingredients, viscose rayon, is in use. Today's tampons are either entirely viscose rayon or a blend of cotton and viscose rayon. In addition, the tampons on the market today may contain an assortment of chemicals, including pesticides used in growing cotton, chemicals used in the manufacture of viscose rayon (lye, sodium sulfate, and sodium hydroxide), and dyes (some of which have been considered carcinogenic since the 1950s).

One theory about the cause of TSS is that the vagina is normally an oxygen-free environment that limits the growth of dangerous bacteria. However, air is trapped between the fibers that make up tampons. When that air is inserted in the vagina along with the tampon, the possibility of toxin production increases. Even after the tampon is removed, some of its fibers may remain.

TSS was originally thought to affect only women who wore high-absorbency tampons, but now it is known to affect newborns, children, and men as well. The initial indications can include a high fever, headache, sore throat, diarrhea, nausea, and red skin blotches. These signs can be followed by confusion, low blood pressure, acute kidney failure, abnormal liver function, and even death.

A severe case of TSS is a medical emergency that may necessitate hospitalization. However, there are many natural ways to support the system once a crisis is over for quick recovery and prevention of recurrence.

NATUROPATHIC PROTOCOL Dr. Linda Page, the author of *Healthy Healing: An Alternative Healing Reference*, developed a protocol for healing from TSS out of necessity: "I actually came close to death on an operating table from TSS. I had to bring my body back, and I did it herbally. It took a couple of years, and now I can speak from experience."

HERBS

Dr. Page's personal ordeal gave her a great deal of confidence in the power of natural remedies. The following herbs helped her overcome toxicity, restore immunity, and return to health.

Ginseng. Both Panax ginseng and Panax quinquefolius (American ginseng) varieties are general tonics that balance and tone all body systems as well as improving the circulation. Ginseng should not be used when there is a high fever.

Cayenne and ginger. These nervous system stimulants can help the body recover from shock. They can be taken internally or applied to the skin in compresses.

Hawthorn extract. Hawthorn speeds up and normalizes the circulation and restores a sense of well-being.

DIET

In addition to herbs, Dr. Page ate supernutritious foods that could be easily digested and quickly utilized by her failing system. These foods included high-potency royal jelly, bee pollen, wheat germ, brewer's yeast, and unsulfured molasses. The addition of green drinks, including chlorella, barley grass, spirulina, and wheatgrass, supplied her with high potencies of vital minerals. "All these go into the body very quickly and help it recover even from a death situation," explains Dr. Page. "By going on a program of concentrated nutrients, I was eventually able to create a state of health that was better than before."

PREVENTION

Alternatives to tampons have included sea sponges. However, sea sponges are no longer sold as menstrual products. A 1981 report alleged risks from embedded sand, chemical pollutants, bacteria, and fungi. No additional studies were done, but the U.S. Food and Drug Administration (FDA) halted menstrual sponge sales. Another alternative is called the Keeper, a rubber cup that sits in the lower vagina. The Keeper may hold an ounce of menstrual blood and should be emptied several times a day. This device does not promote the growth of bacteria in the vagina. However, the Keeper is not widely available. Tampons that are 100 percent cotton and thus present less risk than do modern superabsorbent tampons that may also contain added chemicals are available in many health food and natural goods stores.

Premenstrual Syndrome (PMS)

Premenstrual Syndrome (PMS) refers to the symptoms that begin during or after ovulation and end with the conclusion of the menstrual flow. Because of diet and lifestyle, PMS is more widespread in Western societies than in Asian societies and in less developed countries. Dr. Jeese Hanley, in an article in *Alternative Medicine* magazine, says that PMS is an indication of imbalance in the body, which can be psychological, nutritional, or hormonal. Dr. Hanley sees PMS as "a wake-up call" signaling us to pay attention to these imbalances and fix them before they turn into a more serious condition.

Dr. Hanley points out that menstruation does not create pain and discomfort when a woman is healthy. However, we live in an environment full of synthetic chemicals, including herbicides and pesticides, that mimic estrogen once they get inside the body, enhancing the effects of natural estrogen and disturbing the hormonal balance. Further, an excess of estrogen in relation to progesterone causes problems of hormonal imbalance.

The effects of PMS range from mild to severe, and they vary from person to person. They may include bloating, cramps, headaches, swelling, fluid retention, low back pain, depression, abdominal pressure, insomnia, sugar cravings, anxiety, irritability, breast tenderness, mood swings, and acne.

DIETARY REMEDIES Dr. Michael Janson, an orthomolecular physician and author of *The Vitamin Revolution*, says, "Sugar, caffeine, and alcohol precipitate or worsen symptoms and should be avoided. This is because a lot of patients with PMS have overt hypoglycemia. Their sugar levels fluctuate up and down. Eating sugar sends blood sugar levels way up, and the body responds by dropping sugar levels way down. Additionally, caffeine, even when taken in small amounts in the morning, can aggravate symptoms such as breast tenderness and sleep disturbances."

According to Dr. Janson, the best diet for lessening the symptoms of PMS is high in fiber and complex carbohydrates; meals should be small, with snacks in between. This helps to regulate blood sugar, and in many cases is enough to reduce or eliminate PMS symptoms. Herbalist Letha Hadady recommends eating a lot of cool green foods such as salads; avoiding hot, spicy, and acidic foods; and eliminating coffee from the diet. Some people, however, need more help and can benefit from vitamin therapy, exercise, and a stress management program.

Dr. Hanley recommends that a woman who suffers from PMS should completely avoid milk and milk products, for milk has a high concentration of pesticides and other estrogen-mimicking chemicals.

NUTRITIONAL SUPPLEMENTS When symptoms are severe, diet alone may not be enough. The following nutrients may prove useful.

VITAMIN B6 (PYRIDOXINE). Pyridoxine has a number of helpful properties for alleviating PMS. As a smooth muscle relaxant, it can decrease cramps. As a diuretic, it reduces fluid retention, swelling, and breast tenderness. Between 200 and 400 milligrams should be taken daily, and vitamin B_6 can be taken throughout the month, rather than just premenstrually. For the first 2 weeks of the cycle, take 100 milligrams a day in a B-complex vitamin; take an additional 250 milligrams the last 2 weeks of the cycle. Note that the more B_6 you take, the more magnesium you need.

MAGNESIUM. Magnesium calms the nervous system and relieves anxiety, depression, irritability, nervousness, and insomnia. As an antispasmodic, it alleviates cramps and back pain. Magnesium also helps reduce cravings for sweets. Between 500 and 1,000 milligrams may be needed.

GAMMA-LINOLENIC ACID (GLA). GLA is a precursor of prostaglandin-E1, a hormonelike substance that helps to regulate neurological and hormonal functions. Prostaglandin-E1 helps reduce muscle spasms, cramping, sugar cravings, mood swings, depression, anxiety, irritability, acne, and to some extent breast tenderness. It also reduces inflammation and decreases the stickiness of the platelets, which prevents blood clotting. One 1,000 milligram capsule of borage oil provides a daily dose of 240 milligrams of GLA.

EICOSAPENTAENOIC ACID (EPA). EPA, which is found in fish oil and flaxseed oil, produces prostaglandin-E3, which helps to alleviate breast tenderness. Flaxseed oil is fragile and should not be used for frying. It can be used in salad dressings or over cooked foods.

VITAMIN E. Vitamin E, 400 to 800 units, can reduce cramps, breast tenderness, and fibrocystic breasts, which often swell up before a woman's menstrual period.

EXERCISE Exercise helps to improve mood, reduce cramps, eliminate excess fluid, and control sugar cravings. Aerobic exercises should be performed three to four times per week.

HERBS Naturopathic physician Dr. Janet Zand, in an article on the HealthWorld Online website (www.healthy.net), suggests the following herbal program, which builds blood and balances hormones during the first 2 weeks, then decongests the liver during the second 2 weeks.

For the first and second weeks, or until ovulation occurs take a combination of red raspberry leaf and *dong quai*, taken as tablets, capsules, tinctures, or tea, three times a day. For the third and fourth weeks (starting when ovulation occurs, until the menstrual flow begins), take the following: magnesium and vitamin B6, two to three times a day; choline, methionine, and inositol, two to three times a day; bupleurum and dandelion, taken as tablets, capsules, tinctures, or tea, two or three times a day.

Herbalist Letha Hadady finds the following Chinese herbs useful for alleviating symptoms of PMS:

LUNG TAN XIE GAN WAN. This Chinese remedy alleviates anger associated with PMS.

XIAO YAO WAN. This helps relieve PMS symptoms of depression, poor circulation, indigestion, and bloating.

WOMEN'S HARMONY. This herb increases circulation.

HOMEOPATHY The homeopathic remedy chosen should correspond to the symptoms described; only one should be used for best results. Sometimes it's a matter of trial and error; if one does not work, try another.

Dr. Ken Korins, a classically trained homeopathic physician in New York City, recommends these remedies for PMS and lists the type of PMS symptom for which they are most useful.

LACHESIS. Lachesis helps most physical and emotional symptoms that accompany PMS, such as headaches, right ovarian pain, and breast tenderness. It may be indicated if PMS symptoms stop once menstrual flow stops. It is also indicated when symptoms get worse with heat and with constricted clothing around the abdomen. Emotional indications are restlessness, paranoia, and a tendency to be talkative.

LACCANINUM. Think of laccaninum when the only symptom is a painful, swollen breast, the pain leaves once the menstrual flow begins, and there is a tendency to be irritable.

BOVISTA. Bovista is indicated when gastrointestinal symptoms, such as diarrhea, occur before the period begins. There may also be traces of blood before the actual flow begins. Subjective and objective feelings of swelling occur throughout the body, even through the hands, resulting in a tendency for the women to feel clumsy.

PULSATILLA. Pulsatilla is good for emotional symptoms of PMS involving a weepy disposition and a need for consolation from others. It helps curb a strong craving for sweets.

NATMUR. Natmur is good when the woman's emotional state is melancholy and sad and worsens when others attempt to console her. Headaches occur before, during, or after the period, and there is a craving for salty foods and an aversion toward sex at the time of the period.

SEPIA. Sepia is indicated in the presence of symptoms such as sadness, depression, indifference, and feelings of discontent and discouragement about life. Often a colicky pain is felt before the menses. There may also be a sensation of the uterus dropping, as if it would fall through the vagina due to congestion in that area.

FOLLICULINUM. This is a new French remedy that can be given on the seventh day of the cycle in a 30 to 200c potency.

Homeopath Dana Ullman, in an article on the HealthWorld Online website (www.healthy.net), suggests some additional remedies. Take each one in the 6c, 12c, or 30c potency every 2 hours while symptoms are strong, then every 4 hours after symptoms diminish. When symptoms become mild, stop the remedy. If you experience no clear improvement within 12 hours, try another remedy.

BELLADONNA. Use belladonna when the major symptom is "bearing down" pains or cramps that appear and disappear suddenly. It is also useful when cramps are made worse by motion, a draft, or being jarred, and when they are associated with a headache.

MAGNESIA PHOS. Magnesia phos is recommended for cramps made better by warmth, by simply bending over, or by bending over and at the same time firmly massaging the abdomen, and made worse by cold and by being uncovered.

COLOCYNTHIS. Colocynthis is indicated for cramps like those just described when those cramps are accompanied by feelings of extreme restlessness and irritability.

IGNATIA. Ignatia is good for bloating accompanied by strong emotional downs, such as hysteria and grief, and when the woman experiences conflicting feelings.

CIMICIFUGA. Cimicifuga is used for bloating accompanied by sharp, laborlike pains shooting across the body, perhaps accompanied by sciatica or back pain, difficulty tolerating pain, hysteria, talkativeness, and a sense of everything being "just too much to bear."

NUX VOMICA. Nux vomica is used for Type A personalities who are often highly stressed, who experience bloating and nausea along with irritability, and who become quarrelsome and critical.

PROGESTERONE To restore hormonal balance, Dr. Hanley advocates natural progesterone, preferably in the form of cream made from wild yam, which is rubbed into the skin. This is because only 10 percent of hormones taken by mouth actually reach the bloodstream; the liver filters out the rest, which stresses the liver and gallbladder and increases the risk of gallstones, gallbladder disease, and liver cancer. Progesterone cream is used between ovulation and the day before the menstrual flow starts.

Progesterone promotes youthfulness, and is beneficial against cancer and fibrocystic breast disease. Dr. Michael Janson says additional progesterone is especially important for women exposed to estrogens from pesticides, food additives, drugs, and other chemicals in the environment. These lead to an overload of estrogen and a deficiency of progesterone. Progesterone is extremely helpful for treating PMS symptoms when such an imbalance exists.

Dr. Hanley also cautions that women taking herbs to relieve PMS symptoms should be sure to include herbs that promote progesterone production. Dong quai, alfalfa, licorice root, ginseng, anise seed, garlic, fennel, papaya, red clover, and sage are all estrogenic herbs. They may relieve symptoms, but they may also lead to fibroids, tumors, and cancers. They should be balanced with progesterone-precursor herbs, including wild yam, sarsaparilla, and chaste berry.

LIVER DETOXIFICATION According to Dr. Hanley, detoxifying the liver can relieve many female health problems. The first step is to reduce fat in the diet; and the second is to use a detoxifying formula that contains herbs and plant enzymes that work to remove toxins from the liver. The herbs and enzymes must be used together; neither should be used by themselves. Dr. Hanley recommends a liver detoxification program 2 or 3 months out of each year; women who suffer from severe PMS is severe can do the program for longer time periods and more frequently.

REFLEXOLOGY Reflexology is a science and an art based on the principle that we have reflex areas in our feet that correspond to every part of the body. Massaging specific reflex areas in the feet helps to improve the functioning of specific organs and glands.

Laura Norman, a certified reflexologist from New York City, describes three reflexology techniques.

"Thumb walking can be used on the bottom, tops, and sides of the feet, although it is most often used on the bottom. The procedure entails bending the thumb at the first joint and inching along the bottom of the foot like a caterpillar, pressing from the heel up to the toe. The right hand is used on the right foot. Taking little tiny bites, press, press, press the whole bottom of the foot.

"Finger walking is similar to thumb walking, but is done by bending the finger at the first joint and using the tip of the finger on the outside edge.

"Finger rotation is where you rotate the finger into the foot."

Massaging the feet with thumb walking, finger walking, and finger rotation using a nongreasy, absorbent cream warms the feet and helps promote overall relaxation. For addressing specific problems, reflexology must be applied to specific areas.

Reflexology for PMS helps most when performed 3 or 4 days before and then during menstruation. First the right foot is worked on, while resting on the left leg. Then the same actions are repeated on the left side.

Hormonal Imbalance

Disturbance of a woman's hormonal cycle can play a major role in the development of various medical conditions. Women are affected both by their monthly hormonal cycle and by the hormonal phases associated with the life cycle of adolescence, maturity, pregnancy and childbirth, and menopause, so an understanding of these natural cycles is invaluable in understanding and treating a multitude of symptoms.

Sherrill Sellman, a psychotherapist and writer on women's health, author of the best-selling book *Hormone Heresy*, tells us that for the body to function properly, estrogen and progesterone have to be in balance. Progesterone and estrogen stimulate each other and help balance each other. One function of estrogen is to stimulate estrogen-sensitive tissues, which include cells in the breast, ovaries, and uterus. Estrogen helps develop the curviness of women. It produces their secondary sex characteristics. It is a very powerful stimulant of these tissues. Progesterone, on the other hand, helps slow down the growth of cells and stabilizes mature cells so their growth doesn't get out of hand. The proper relationship, as Nature designed it, is one of checks and balances.

"We are seeing a predominance of estrogen in relation to just a little progesterone," Sellman says. "That's caused by the drugs and food we eat and the disharmony in our own bodies. It's been noted that 50 percent of women over the age of 35 are not ovulating each month. Now only if women are ovulating, releasing an egg, can a little endocrine gland called the corpus luteum, which is the primary source of progesterone, be formed on the surface of the ovary. If a woman doesn't ovulate due to stress or bad diet, she can go a whole month without producing the progesterone to balance the estrogen. As a result, women are progesterone-deficient."

Dolores Perri, a nutritionist from New York City, sys that many factors can interfere with normal hormonal production and balance, including alcohol, animal proteins, caffeine, sugar, phosphates and polyphosphates (found in many food products, such as soft drinks, processed meats, and cheese), smoking, stress, weight problems, excessive exercise.

SYMPTOMS Dr. Elizabeth Vleit is founder and medical director of the Women's Center for Health Enhancement and Renewal in Texas, and author of *Screaming to Be Heard: Hormonal Connections Women Suspect and Doctors Ignore*. She describes some of the conditions that hormonal imbalance can trigger and tells when they are likely to occur: "Women's bodies are cyclic in their response to hormones. They have a monthly rhythm of hormonal changes from puberty to menopause, which have a critical bearing on many dimensions of health. Men's bodies, on the other hand, have a tonic pattern of secretion, which means that the same amounts of key hormones are produced every day. They vary within 24 hours in terms of their hormone production. But basically each day is similar to the day before and the day after.

"For women, the first half of the menstrual cycle is dominated by a rise in ovarian estradiol. This is the primary estrogen that is active at receptor sites on all the cells in the brain and body, from puberty to menopause. This rise in estrogen allows the ovary to prepare the follicle that will become the egg released at ovulation.

"At ovulation, when the egg is released, the estradiol level drops briefly. The egg then takes over and produces progesterone for the second half of the cycle. Progesterone levels rise, and estrogen levels rise again, though not as high as in the first half of the menstrual cycle. Progesterone and estrogen drop prior to bleeding, when the egg is not fertilized. The body sheds the lining of the uterus and starts over.

"When hormones fall, right before bleeding, a drop in certain critical brain neurotransmitters, such as serotonin and endorphins, is triggered. This is associated with mood changes women describe—feelings of irritability, insomnia, depression, or anxiety. This may be a time in the cycle when women get migraines. The drop in estrogen that triggers changes in serotonin, norepinephrine, and endorphins sets off a cascade of blood vessel spasms that are involved in migraine headaches. That also affects chemical messengers involved in regulating the immune system, the gastrointestinal tract, the heart, heart rate, blood vessels, and as many as 400 other functions.

"We also see hormonal connections in women who have the diffuse muscle aches of fibromyalgia. These women often develop aches and pains and tender points after some type of hormonal change, such as postpartum or post–tubal ligation, or following a hysterectomy, even if the ovaries are left in place. We see this in menopause too. If we look at the patterns of this type of pain in women, we see that 80 percent of fibromyalgia patients are female, and that the average age when fibromyalgia appears is about 44 or 45."

Sherrill Sellman notes that infertility and miscarriage are both directly related to hormonal imbalance: an excess of estrogen and a deficiency of progesterone.

Dr. Vleit says women need to be aware of the relationship between hormonal cycles and medical conditions: "One of the ways to do that is to track patterns relative to cycles, and to test the blood for various hormones that women's bodies produce. I've developed an approach to doing that by measuring the hormonal levels at the right time of the menstrual cycle. This helps women know what is happening to their hormone levels at the time that they are having symptoms. I become frustrated when doctors tell me that we don't need to measure the female hormones because they vary. I respond that that's the whole point. They do vary, and how they vary, relative to women experiencing problems, is what we must find out in order to offer them the most constructive options."..It is also important to check thyroid function. Thyroid hormone controls progesterone, cholesterol, and the ovaries. It acts as a cascading system. When not functioning properly, other hormones get out of balance.

NUTRITIONAL REMEDIES The typical American diet interferes with optimal hormonal balance. Perri advises us not to reach for a prescription drug for hormonal problems. It is better to eat high-quality organic foods and avoid foods that throw the system off balance. Beans and legumes are better sources of protein than meats, which are loaded with hormones. In addition, Perri recommends cold-processed oils, nuts, seeds, fatty fish, and beans. "These foods are all very high in GLAs," she notes. "The GLAs help us make natural estrogen in our own bodies."

Wild yam and DHEA promote production of natural estrogens in the body, if the body needs them. If estrogen is not needed, these supplements are eliminated by the body, making them completely safe to use. Magnesium and calcium may also be beneficial, since most women do not get enough of these nutrients.

HERBS Blue cohosh, black cohosh, yarrow, and chaste tree help balance hormone production. Other balance-promoting herbs include raspberry leaf, dong quai, wild yam, and passion flower.

Dr. Janet Zand uses programs that rotate the herbs being used in accordance with the 4 weeks of the menstrual cycle. Herbs used during the first 2 weeks nourish blood and balance hormones; those used during the second 2 weeks clear the liver, which tends to become congested during these last 2 weeks.

In an article on the HealthWorld Online website (www.healthy.net), Dr. Zand recommends the following general herbal program for balancing the hormonal system and building general resistance. For the first 2 weeks, take a combination of red raspberry leaf and *dong quai*, as a tablet, capsule, tea, or tincture, three times a day. For the third week, take astragalus, American ginseng, or Chinese ginseng. These adaptogenic herbs tone the deep immune system. Take a tablet, capsule, tea, or tincture, three times a day. For the fourth week, take a combination of goldenseal and echinacea. These herbs have antiviral, antibacterial, and anti-inflammatory properties. Take as a tablet, capsule, tincture, or tea, three times a day.

51

Sexual Dysfunction in Women

Psychologist Dr. Janice Stefanacci says that sexual dysfunction stems largely from a society that offers people no models of normal, healthy sexuality: "If we look to the media, we see things that are totally aberrant in terms of frequency and potency. We see relationships portrayed between males and females where there is power and domination, or submission and seduction. Role models of healthy sexual communication and actualization are virtually nonexistent. People need a sense of what is normal.

"They also need time to think about sexuality as an integrated part of their personality. Our culture is very fragmented in this regard. Many, many people, men and women, never spend time thinking about their sexuality. In fact, if you were to take an informal survey and ask people, 'What is sexuality?' a good proportion of them would say, 'It's sex. It's something you do, maybe in the bedroom, maybe at night.' Nobody is really sure how often you are supposed to have it or how long it is supposed to last. Most people don't realize that sexuality is a completely integrated part of their personality as much as actualizing in education or interpersonal relationships. Sexuality is very much a part of who we are, how we present ourselves in the world, what we do, and how we think of ourselves. Our adequacy and our self-esteem are tied up in our sexuality."

Causes

Some sex researchers are beginning to question the whole concept of sexual dysfunction, promoting broader and less rigid definitions of sexual response and pleasure. "The Masters and Johnson model of sexual response—excitement, plateau, orgasm, and resolution—is very performance-oriented," says Rebecca Chalker, a women's health activist whose book *The Clitoral Truth* explores ways in which feminists are redefining male standards. "After desire and willingness, the only other compulsory element is pleasure," Chalker points out. "Pleasure and intimacy are the real goals of sexual activity, and if you look at it that way, the concept of sexual dysfunction simply collapses."

Nevertheless, women may worry when they have difficulty achieving orgasm, especially with a partner, and men become concerned if they have difficulty controlling ejaculations and getting or maintaining erections. Both women and men are also distressed when they don't feel sexual attraction. In fact, most people who seek out counseling do so for difficulties with sexual communication and the lack of sexual desire.

Early on, through regular masturbation, boys learn what feels good and how to reliably get orgasms. Girls often wait to begin sexual exploration until they engage in sexual activity with a partner; they miss out on the benefits of self-exploration. "Learning about sex from boys or men isn't the best thing for women," Chalker says.

Many sex therapists recommend that women explore their sexual response through masturbation, using a vibrator, sex toys, and sexy videos to stimulate sexual fantasies. You may also want to experiment with things like aromatherapy, oils, and herbs. After sufficient homework, you can try integrating these changes into sex with your partner. Another important change heterosexual couples can make is to try rewriting the "intercourse script." That is, plan to have sexual sessions where intercourse will not take place.

Chalker points out that there are two powerful aspects of our sexuality—the physiological and the psychological—and that "neither can live without the other." Unfortunately, it is the psychological problems which are the more difficult to deal with. Psychological problems manifest themselves in various ways. "Today, we have enormous resources available to help with sexual problems that we didn't have a few years ago," Chalker notes. "I've reviewed some of the herbal aids and remedies here, and I encourage the reader to explore the wide range of resources available in book stores or by mail order.".Of course, sexual dysfunction can also have physical causes. One, Dr. Vicki Hufnagel reminds us, is "improperly performed episiotomies." In *Prevention* magazine, Dr. Tori Hudson lists a number of other factors that can affect the sex drive. She says that sexual problems can be related to menopause, non-menopause-related hormonal changes (often following pregnancy), medications (Prozac, Zoloft, Sertraline, and others), depression, relationship issues, a chronic health problem, fatigue," and others. "In order to diagnose the cause correctly, your health professional would have to ask you many specific questions." Hormonal factors may involve low levels of testosterone or DHEA, although it is not known precisely what effect these hormones have on the libido. If blood tests show that levels are low, supplementation may be in order.

Nutrients, Hormones, and Supplements

Studies show that a heightened libido and orgasmic intensity are related to blood levels of histamine. Women who have low histamine levels tend to experience low sexual excitement, while those with a high level are more able to sustain orgasms. Nutrients that increase histamine levels include vitamin B_5 and the bioflavonoid rutin. Broccoli, parsley, cherries, grapes, peppers, melons, and citrus fruits are good food sources of vitamin B_5 and rutin.

Dr. Tori Hudson says that oral testosterone (available only by prescription), and/or a testosterone cream applied two to three times a week or rubbed into the external genital area before sex have been used to stimulate sexual responsiveness. DHEA, the B-complex vitamins, adrenal extracts, and the herbs ginseng and damiana may also help improve sexual response. Dr. Hudson notes, however, that remedies that focus on sexual drive without addressing general health and emotional issues will not have a consistent effect.

Dr. Janson offers an example of a general supplement program that can be an initial step in treating sexual dysfunction:

Multivitamin, three capsules twice a day.

Vitamin C, two 1,000-mg capsules twice a day.

Vitamin E, 400 IU mixed natural, twice a day.

Ginkgo biloba tincture, 60 mg twice a day.

Gamma-linoleic acid, 240 mg in the form of borage oil, once a day.

Magnesium aspartate, 200 mg, twice a day.

Coenzyme Q10, 100 mg, once a day.

Aromatherapy

"Aromatherapy is fantastic for helping women regain their sense of sensuality," declares aromatherapist Ann Berwick. These are some of the oils she recommends:

"Rose is wonderful for enhancing feminine qualities. It bring out the loving, tender side of us that wants to surrender. Clary sage heightens sensation. It takes you out of your body and into a different realm, allowing you to relax and enjoy the romance. Sandalwood is a wonderful oil for people not in touch with their physical side. It is very earthy and very deep. Jasmine restores self-confidence in people who have been through traumatic sexual experiences. It can help women who have been abused or who are emotionally closed off from damaging relationships.

"By blending different oils, you can create a formula that enhances the sensual side of your nature," says Berwick. She suggests adding them to the bath or using them while massaging a partner or in self-massage. A personal perfume can be made and used daily. "Surrounding yourself with these glorious scents is a wonderful help."

Chinese Medicine

Registered nurse and acupuncturist Abigail Rist-Podrecca explains sexual dysfunction from an Eastern point of view: "Chinese medicine looks to the root of the cause, rather than just the symptoms, and the root seems to be the kidney. The kidneys are called the roots of life. Everything stems from the kidney, they say."

Weak kidney function can be diagnosed in Eastern medicine in multiple ways, including facial diagnosis: "Under the eye is the thinnest tissue in the entire body," explains Rist-Podrecca. "You can see through the skin there. If the blood is not being cleared by the kidneys and detoxified, you will see a darkness under the eyes. People will say, 'I haven't had enough sleep,' but it goes beyond that. In Chinese medicine, that darkness signals that the kidneys are not functioning optimally, so the blood isn't being cleansed."

She goes on describe various factors that can drain the kidneys. "Cold can deplete the kidneys. Many people can't tolerate cold. This is so because in the winter, the kidney's function becomes suppressed, much the same way as the sap in a tree runs to the core and into the roots. When people have a compromised kidney situation, where it isn't functioning optimally, they can't stand the cold weather.

"Overwork and tension can also weaken kidney function because the kidneys and the adrenal glands (the adrenal sits on top of the kidney) are considered one and the same in Chinese medicine. So too much stress, and too many chemical toxins, deplete kidney functioning." Hundreds of Chinese herbs nourish kidney function. Here Rist-Podrecca names a few:

HAR SHAR WOO. This is an essential herbal formula for nourishing kidney function. It is also said to darken the hair. Hair, bone, teeth, joints, and sexual functions are tied up with the kidney energies. When you energize the kidneys, you affect all these different areas. When combined with *dong quai, har shar woo* helps the type of kidney dysfunction that causes low back pain.

ROMANIA. *Romania* is a dark black herb that is high in iron and helps to nourish the blood and improve kidney function.

DONG QUAI. *Dong quai* resembles a cross section of the uterus, and has an affinity for this area of the body.

52

Pregnancy

What we in the United States accept as the safest, most acceptable way to give birth is a historical anomaly—something that has existed for only 75 to 100 years and is not practiced in the rest of the world. Suzanne Arms, an independent researcher and activist who has published seven books on pregnancy and women's health, including *Immaculate Deception*, *Breast Feeding*, and *Seasons of Change*, explains.

"In other parts of the world," she says, "childbirth is seen as a natural process. The only exceptions are areas where American obstetrics and neonatal approaches have been aggressively promoted and marketed. Many European countries and a growing number of Third World countries are gradually adopting these practices as they buy our wares, such as neonatal monitoring devices."

In the United States, the vast preponderance of women give birth in hospitals. They are led to believe, Arms explains, that the larger the hospital, the better the care. They are told that the more narrow the subspecialization training of their doctors, the safer the birth will be. So women don't want to go to a general practitioner (GP), but instead go to a perinatologist with a subspecialty in obstetrics. Says Arms, "Our home birth rate in 1998 was 2.5 percent, the lowest in our history. Although we do have midwives in hospitals and birthing centers outside hospitals, and we do legally permit home births, fewer than 5 percent of births are done with these resources, even if we count births done with midwives in hospitals."

Most of the world—the United States being a large exception—sees the natural way of giving birth as the sanest and healthiest way to bring a child into the world. After examining the issue of natural childbirth and American attitudes toward it, this chapter will turn the stages of pregnancy, certain things you must avoid to have a safe pregnancy, and the many things you can do to make pregnancy as healthy and uncomplicated as possible.

Natural Childbirth

One reason for the greater American preference for hospital births as compared to the rest of the world is that Americans have been led to believe you are risking the baby and the mother if you choose not to have a hospital birth. But, Arms points out, "If we look at the facts, we see this is not true." In the United States, there has been very little comparative study of the benefits of home delivery versus hospital births. "Therefore, to actually compare the safety of hospital and home births, she says, "We have to go to a place like England where they have very good national statistics on births and they have commissioned studies to see which are the safer methods."

Back in the 1970s, a controversial study appeared called the Peel Report. It was used to support a belief among politicians that home birth should be outlawed. At the time, Marjorie Tew, a statistician who was not involved in the controversy but happened to be analyzing statistics in a number of epidemiological areas, noted flaws in the report. She restudied the statistics on home births and found these births were as safe as hospital births. This was true not only for low-risk women—those who enter the process in a healthy state—but even for those with problems.

As a result of these findings, England has reversed its policy, which had been focused on eliminating home births and getting rid of midwifery. The country has gone back to supporting midwives, birthing centers and local home births. They are finding that hospitals are not the best place to give birth. "In fact," Arms concludes, "there is no study that shows a hospital is a safer place than alternative venues for giving birth."

One aspect of women's fear of birth is that they think it will be unendurably painful. So, in many cases, they fill themselves with painkillers before the process even begins.

Arms recognizes this tendency. She says, "Those who advocate natural childbirth are often asked: 'Why should modern women experience painful childbirth rather than benefit from the painkillers modern medicine provides?'

The issue of pain is a complex one, in her view. "Our media tell us that we should be free of any pain and discomfort in our lives. If you look at TV advertising, billboards, and so on, you see there are a tremendous number of products geared to the elimination of the pain that occurs in pathological conditions. We are taught we shouldn't have to experience pain. Since we are used to taking drugs for everything else, why not for labor? But childbirth is not a pathology and the cause of pain during birth is not a disease."

IS CIRCUMCISION NECESSARY?

Sixty percent of babies born in hospitals in the United States are circumcised. Suzanne Arms, an independent researcher and activist who has published seven books on pregnancy and women's health, including *Immaculate Deception*, *Breast Feeding*, and *Seasons of Change*, sees this as a wasteful and counterproductive practice. "The difficulty with circumcision," she believes, "is that it touches some of the most sensitive tissue on the human male body and takes a large amount of material from the penis. You are taking away all the natural protection of the penis, the tissue which keeps it from getting infected and getting diseases and which makes sexuality more exquisite."

She also says that in Europe, circumcision has never been routinely performed on infants, as it is in the United States. She believes that the U.S. practice of routine circumcision is one aspect of a cultural attitude that grew, in part, out of 17th-century Puritanism, which viewed sexual pleasure, including masturbation, as sinful, and advocated tying babies' hands to their cribs to keep them from touching their genitals, which might provide pleasure. (In the 1920s and 1930s, for the same purpose, clitoridectomies were performed on little girls in some parts of the country.) She regards circumcision as an outgrowth of such attitudes: it was done to prevent male babies from using their penises as organs of pleasure.

Arms says, "We can contrast this with the reason for circumcision under Judaic law. In that tradition, circumcision was done on the eighth day as part of a convenant with God. Many Jews now believe that circumcision can be done without cutting the boy."

She also argues that the medical reasons once given for this operation —for example that it prevents cancer—have turned out to be false. Circumcision has no medical value at all and has a lot of risks associated with it, including bleeding and other effects of surgery.

She continues, "It exposes newborn babies to what is for them excruciating pain. Some babies feel it less than others, but, by and large, it puts the baby into shock and trauma."

Many advocates of circumcision apparently feel it is a way to harden the boy. In the past, children to be circumcised were tied down on boards, six in a row. A baby would lie there unable to move, listening to the screams of the little boys next to him. This was considered a way to prepare boys to be ready as adults to give up their bodies in war.

Arms concludes, "I think it's very important that we begin to understand the shock and trauma from this process that we have called normal in the United States. And we don't even acknowledge this trauma, so how can we heal it? People are running around with the long-term effects in their nervous system of an unresolved trauma. Believe me, that is what we are seeing in this culture."

In addition, the potential problems caused by drugs and anesthesia need to be addressed. Drugs and anesthesia can distort and warp the birth process and make it harder for the baby to do the work he or she is supposed to do. They can complicate labor and make birth a pathological problem, something that we do, in fact, need to treat in the hospital.

What is Midwifery?

The most important difference between midwifery and traditional medicine is that medicine treats disease, whereas midwifery is about preventing complications while going through a natural process. Obstetrics, a subspecialty of medicine, seems to consider birth "too unwieldy." Doctors need to get in and out of the hospital quickly, so they want to control the length of time a woman is in labor and how long it takes to give birth. However, the natural variability of giving birth does not conform to their standard. Each human body is unique, as is each human psyche. A 4-hour labor may be normal. A 36-hour labor may also be normal. But under a physician's management, a day and a half is too long.

Medicine focuses on giving drugs and doing surgery. Midwifery concentrates on following through the process normally, spotting problems as they arise and treating them as simply as possible before they become complications, while teaching people how to handle contingencies.

Midwife Jeannette Breen is a great enthusiast for using water during labor: "It has a wonderful analgesic quality, which is much better than an epidural. Being immersed in water provides tremendous relaxation. It does not take the pain away, but women do report feeling less pain in the water. They feel less effect from the pull of gravity. Their movements are very easy, and there is much better tissue relaxation, which means there is almost no tearing in a water birth. It is also easier for the baby because the mother is more relaxed and moving freely. She is not stuck in one position. It is easier for the baby to negotiate the pelvis and to slip out in a warm, moist environment that is quite familiar."

"Two keys to a normal healthy pregnancy and birth are a healthy diet and good social support," says Breen. "Those seem to be overlooked, especially in traditional maternity care in this country. The focus is on diagnostic testing, but not a lot of emphasis is placed on healthy diets, other than prescribing women prenatal vitamins and iron. There is no question that a high-quality diet rich in all the nutrients can make a woman's whole body work more efficiently and effectively.

"Social support creates an environment of love that is all-important but too often overlooked in hospital birthing environments that focus solely on technology. No one can have the baby for the pregnant woman; she has to do it herself. But if she is surrounded by love and support, rather than fear and technology, she is able to give birth in a very intuitive, instinctual way which is satisfying and safe."

Stages of Pregnancy

A woman's body undergoes numerous changes during each stage of pregnancy. These physiological changes are described by nurse practitioner and massage therapist Susan Lacina.

FIRST TRIMESTER "The fetus grows rapidly, and the mother's body changes to support this swift development. Hormonal balance changes. Human chorionic gonadotropin hormone (HCG) is needed for development. As it is released, it causes many discomforts, such as breast tenderness, digestive problems, nausea, and vomiting. Progesterone levels increase and may cause mild hyperventilation, heartburn, indigestion, and constipation. Increased blood flow and its change in composition contribute to fatigue, overheating, and sinus congestion."

SECOND TRIMESTER "The placenta takes over the hormone production, and the levels of HCG drop. Along with that, the discomforts of nausea and vomiting ease up. Physical growth of the fetus crowds the abdomen, and a woman's body expands to accommodate the growth. Fetal production of thyroid stimulating hormone (TSH) begins in the fourteenth week and causes the mother's thyroid level to increase. This can lead to irritability, mood swings, mild depression, increased pulse rate, and hot flashes. Adrenal hormones become elevated and remain that way until delivery. This may cause impaired glucose tolerance and swelling.

"Skeletal structure becomes softer and more flexible to allow for expansion. If a woman doesn't have enough muscle flexibility, she will have some pain, for tight muscles do not allow for these adjustments. She may experience sciatic nerve pain from the lower back down the back of her legs due to the extension of the pelvis, especially at the joint of the sacrum and the pelvic bone. The growing baby puts pressure on the inferior vena cava, which can cause lightheadedness, nausea, drowsiness, and clamminess. Prolonged reduction of blood flow can cause backaches and hemorrhoids. Lying on the side decreases this problem.

"From the twentieth week on, the uterus expands by stretching muscle fibers. Abdominal muscles and ligaments stretch to support the uterus, and there may be abdominal pain. There is an increase in melanin production, causing darkening of the nipples and a line called the linea nigra down the abdomen. If the lymph drainage system is not functioning well, an excess of melanin in the skin can cause brown spots. A well-functioning lymph drainage system is believed to keep melanin levels down so that brown spots do not occur. Increased progesterone causes sinus congestion, postnasal drip, and bleeding gums. Increased capillary permeability may cause the hands and feet to swell."

WHAT TO AVOID DURING PREGNANCY

Before describing the positive steps you can take to make your pregnancy, labor, and time after delivery as healthy as possible, I want to note some things, a few of which are normally benign, that you should avoid during pregnancy.

Susun Weed is an herbalist and teacher with over 30 years of experience. She has written four books on herbal medicine, including *Wise Woman Herbal for the Childbearing Year*. According to Weed, it is well known that the health of a baby's parents affects the health of the baby. If the mother has an overgrowth of *Candida*, so may the child. If the father is a heavy drinker, this may cause liver problems for the child. During the first 2 months after conception, women and their fetuses are the most sensitive to toxins, hair dyes, aspirin, and so on. Thus it is of paramount importance that a woman be aware of what things can have a detrimental effect on her growing fetus.

HIGH HEAT Drawing from her store of knowledge of American Indian lore, Weed tells us, "First of all, we need to be very aware of something that may come up before a woman is even aware that she is pregnant—because, of course, we are pregnant for 2 weeks before we miss that first period—something many women are not aware of, which is that high heat during these first few weeks can permanently damage the fetus." This heat may come from a hot bath, a sauna, or even a sweat lodge. This is one reason why, she elaborates, "in many native American traditions, women in their fertile years do not go into the sweat lodge due to the possible adverse effect to the fetus."

VITAMIN SUPPLEMENTS Women must also be careful about taking vitamin supplements. Women who take 10,000 units of vitamin A during the first 6 weeks of pregnancy are five times more likely to have a child with birth defects than women who don't take the vitamin. "I believe that during her fertile years a woman should be quite cautious in taking supplements," Weed says. "Of course, we want to get those good vitamins, but we want to try and get them from our fruits, our vegetables, our beans, and so on."

It is not only vitamin A that can lead to birth defects; vitamins D and E are also potentially dangerous. "Those three are oil-soluble vitamins," says Weed, "and they tend to be quite detrimental to fetal development when taken in pill form."

MEDICATIONS AND HERBAL THERAPIES Avoid aspirin and certainly antihistamines. This last is a hard one, especially for women who are dealing with hay fever. Antihistamines have a fairly tarnished record when it comes to causing birth defects, Weed says. "I don't just mean drug antihistamines but herbal ones as well, such as ma huang or ephedra."

Laxatives are not the way to go. Unfortunately many people use them and, even worse, many misguided herbalists even suggest women use them to clean out. Of course, there's nothing to clean out. All laxatives, Weed believes, should be avoided by all people, but especially by women during their fertile years, or at least if they are having a baby or trying to get pregnant. This includes herbal laxatives like senna, aloe, castor oil, rhubarb root, buckthorn, and cascara sagrada. Even a bulk-producing laxative like flaxseed should be taken with some caution. To use it, buy the whole flaxseed, grind it up, and sprinkle a small amount into foods.

Generally, you should stay away from diuretics. A woman in her fertile years usually doesn't take them anyway, but anyone inclined to take diuretics should be aware that they could cause problems. Herbal diuretics such as juniper berries and buchu can also cause problems. Avoid hair dyes, all kinds of chemical stimulants and depressants, antinausea drugs, sulfa drugs, vaccines, and anesthetics, especially at the dentist's office.

Weed notes, "There is some question about what happens if we take steroid-like herbs. The more we look into steroids, the more widely we find them spread across the herbal kingdom. As a matter of fact, carrots, the regular carrots you find in the supermarket, contain so many phytohormones that generous use of carrots may prevent conception. We know that wild carrot seed, in fact all parts of the carrot plant, act to prevent contact between the egg and the sperm and prevent that egg from attaching to the uterine wall. So we often advise pregnant women to avoid drinking any carrot juice at all and to cut back on the amount of carrots they are eating."

There are a few other herbs that you need to avoid only if you have miscarried frequently. "Some women get very concerned about miscarriage," Weed states. "If you are concerned, there are some herbs normally used in cooking that you would do well to avoid during the first trimester of pregnancy. Don't go overboard in worrying about them; they will not harm the fetus, but they might, in a highly susceptible woman, cause uterine contractions." They include many herbs in the mint family, such as basil, thyme, sage, rosemary, marjoram, savory, and peppermint itself. The entire family of herbs in the carrot family, such as celery seed, parsley, cumin, coriander seeds, aniseeds, and fennel seeds may cause problems for the sensitive woman. Ginger, nutmeg, and saffron have been used to cause a fetus to leave the uterus. Of course, to achieve that effect, they must be taken in enormous quantities, but for a very sensitive woman, it is best to avoid even small amounts in foods for the first trimester.

One other herb that Weed thinks is especially important for pregnant women to avoid completely is goldenseal. She tells us, "I've been a herbalist for 35 years, and I've never once had the opportunity to use goldenseal. Where I live the native people used to give it to their enemies in order to torture them."

OTHER THINGS TO AVOID It won't surprise you to learn that smoking and drinking are not good for your fetus. Radiation is not good, so even a mammogram should be avoided during pregnancy or if you think you are going to get pregnant. Caffeine in any form should be avoided. Coffee and latte, tea (black, green, or twig tea), and many soft drinks contain generous amounts of caffeine and all can cause birth defects. Nutritionist Gracia Perlstein also says to avoid chemical exposure to toxic household cleansers, and fumes from paints, thinners, solvents, wood preservatives, varnishes, glues, spray adhesives, benzene, dry cleaning fluid, anything chemically based and questionable.

Perlstein also counsels women to avoid a toxic psychological environment. "As much as possible, avoid stress, negative people, and aggravating situations. Instead, try to spend quality time alone and with loved ones, people who are supportive. Spend time in nature. Read inspiring literature. Listen to beautiful music. This has a beneficial effect on your mental and emotional state. That, in turn, affects your baby's biochemistry."

THIRD TRIMESTER "As the baby continues to grow, the expectant mother changes her posture to shift her center of gravity. Heavier breasts can cause shoulders to slump forward. The spine is pulled out of alignment, and this commonly causes backaches. The growing fetus also compresses the veins and the lymphatic system. That can cause ankle edema and varicose veins. There is increased pressure on the intestines and bladder, causing frequent urination and constipation. Pressure on the sciatic nerve can cause more lower back and leg pain. As the diaphragm starts to rise, breathing becomes more difficult. Insomnia is common."

MISCARRIAGE Surprisingly, two-thirds of all pregnancies end up as miscarriages. One reason is that many women miscarry before they even know they are pregnant. Most commonly, genetic abnormalities precipitate the problem. The embryo develops wrongly, and the woman's body naturally aborts the fetus. Endocrine system imbalances are also associated with miscarriages. Women in their late forties have an especially difficult time carrying to term, due to hormonal changes that accompany aging. Poor thyroid gland functioning can also interfere with pregnancy, as can intercourse during pregnancy.

Another cause of miscarriages is low-grade infections, which are often the result of sexually transmitted diseases. The woman is not conscious that a problem exists, but the body knows, and rejects the fetus. Bladder infections are also common; as the uterus enlarges, it places great pressure on this organ. Miscarriages may also occur when women are too hard on their bodies. Women who push themselves to the limit by overexercising and undereating to the point of anorexia are risking miscarriage. They are not getting enough nutrition for their own bodies, much less for the fetus.

When a miscarriage occurs more than once, a woman needs to have a thorough medical workup. Once the problem is understood, it is often correctable. If a woman is having intercourse during pregnancy, for example, she may simply need to take precautions. Using a condom during intercourse can prevent a miscarriage because it keeps male prostaglandins out of the female system, which, in turn, prevents premature uterine contractions. Low-grade infections must be cleared up, and increasing the intake of liquids and vitamin C can sometimes do the trick. Mixing 4 ounces of strawberry juice with 4 ounces of water is an especially good source of vitamin C, which acidifies the urine and helps prevent bladder infections. More serious infections should be cultured and treated appropriately. Sometimes, this means taking antibiotics. Older women who are having a difficult time holding on to a pregnancy due to hormonal changes may need low doses of progesterone, about 25 milligrams, in suppository form.

Some herbs seem to prevent miscarriage. Midwife Jeanine Parvati Baker uses this formula. She mixes together 1 ounce of wild yam root, 1 ounce of Mitchella repens (also called partridgeberry, twinberry, squawvine or partridge root). Baker also adds 1/2 ounce of false unicorn root and 1/2 ounce cramp bark. She puts them together in a half-gallon jar, fills it to the top with boiling water, and lets it sit for about 4 hours. You can sip this brew slowly until you are over the symptoms of miscarriage or, if you are just worried about your pregnancy, drink a half cup each day. The half gallon will keep very well in the refrigerator.

Healthy Pregnancy the Natural Way

DIET The best insurance for a well baby is to follow a highly nutritious whole-foods diet. What you eat now will impact the health of your child later, according to nutritionist Gracia Perlstein: "When a woman is considering pregnancy, it is important that she address her diet to see how healthful it is, as many difficulties have their root in prenatal deficiencies. Scientific studies reveal that birth defects, and even problems that develop much later in life, can be prevented when the mother has excellent nutrition. I would like to include the father there too, because the quality of the sperm is also very important." Since the most crucial stage of embryonic development occurs in the first few weeks, before a woman realizes that she is pregnant, good-quality foods should be eaten all the time.

Eating properly means selecting unprocessed or minimally processed foods. A wide assortment of whole grains, legumes, vegetables, fruits, nuts, and seeds supplies multiple nutrients. "So many people eat the same 10 or 20 foods over and over again," Perlstein says. "In traditional cultures, people have much more variety. I would like to emphasize that supplements should only enhance an excellent diet. Make the effort to eat high-quality, nutrient-dense foods. That means whole foods, the way nature produced them."..The body intuitively knows what it needs to support new life, and paying attention to its messages can be a helpful guide. "A woman's body is very wise when she is pregnant. Many women can't stand the look or smell of coffee or cigarettes, even when they used to smoke or drink coffee several times a day," states Perlstein. She adds that worrying about eating the right foods all the time is stressful and can produce more harm than good. But nutrition education can benefit women with highly processed diets, who need to learn about better food choices. "Vegetarian women may crave animal foods or be drawn to dairy when they are pregnant. Usually it is good to pay attention to these cravings, but to respond in the most wholesome way possible."

Wholesome means organically grown. Pesticide-free fare is better for everyone, of course, but vitally important for young children and developing fetuses, according to recent research. Dairy and other animal products should be from creatures naturally raised. One reason for this is that pesticides and other contaminants tend to concentrate in an animal's tissues. The higher up the food chain, the higher the concentration of toxins. Fortunately, many health food stores, and more and more supermarkets, sell the healthful varieties.

Animal products, when a part of the diet, should be eaten in moderation. Although protein needs increase during pregnancy, they can be easily met from vegetarian sources, which are less toxic than their animal counterparts. Excellent vegetarian protein sources include fortified soy milk, tofu, tempeh, beans, nuts, and seeds, for example.

The increased need for calcium is similarly fulfilled in such a diet: "Many women do not realize that there are excellent sources of calcium other than milk and dairy. There are green leafy vegetables, fortified soy milk, tofu, almonds, and many other calcium-containing foods. If you eat a diet rich in fresh vegetables and fruits, you tend to get quite a bit of calcium. If you want a supplement, calcium citrate is easiest on the stomach. Other forms sometimes cause digestive upsets or constipation. Definitely avoid calcium-depleting foods: coffee, chocolate, and sodium."

Perlstein adds that eating several small meals throughout the day offsets common complications: "Hunger, not calorie counting, is the most reliable guide to eating during pregnancy. Five to six small, nutrient-dense meals per day is a sensible ideal. This is a good habit to develop in the last trimester of pregnancy, when the organs in your stomach are somewhat constricted, and good in the early stages to prevent nausea. It keeps the blood sugar from falling, and nausea has a lot to do with low blood sugar."

Water should be pure and taken in adequate amounts. Eight to twelve glasses are recommended to help flush out toxins from the liver and kidneys: "Many people do not drink enough fluids," notes Perlstein. "This is especially important during pregnancy because the woman is filtering the waste for two bodies."

VITAMIN SUPPLEMENTS Nutritionist Gracia recommends the following daily nutrients for pregnant women: multiple vitamin and mineral supplement, vitamin C, B_{12}, zinc, vitamin E, and folic acid. Folic acid, which is also contained in green leafy vegetable and whole grains, is especially important in pregnancy because science has shown it to prevent neural tube defects. Even when included in the diet, extra folic acid should be taken in supplement form, since it is fragile and easily damaged by heat. Additionally, acidophilus helps prevent constipation and other types of colon problems.

Extra iron may be needed, but a woman should have her hemoglobin tested first, just to be sure it is really needed. Research shows that excess iron in the system can have damaging effects.

HERBS Susun Weed has a number of herbal recommendations for pregnant women.

RED RASPBERRY TONIC

Tonics are herbal preparations that keep your body in good trim, up and running for optimum performance and healthy living. Weed's recommendations for tonics start with red raspberry, Rubus idaeus. "It is probably the best known, the most widely used, and the safest of all pregnancy tonics."

To prepare red raspberry tonic buy dried red raspberry leaves in bulk. Weigh 1 ounce in a quart jar, preferably a canning jar. If you don't have a scale, fill your jar about one-third full. Pour boiling water right to the top of the jar, set it aside, and let it steep for 4 hours or longer. Weed says: "Actually what I do is put up a nice infusion before I go to sleep at night. Then the next morning, it's ready for me. I strain the plant material, squeezing it to get the last of the good stuff out. Give that plant material back to the earth. The liquid is what I drink. I can heat it up, drink it at room temperature, or pour it over ice. Whatever I don't drink right then, I refrigerate and drink up within the next 36 to 48 hours." A quart a day of red raspberry tonic is usually not too much.

This tonic increases fertility in both men and women. It helps prevent miscarriage and hemorrhaging during the birth. It's one of the best herbs to ease morning sickness, and it helps provide a safe, fast birth, reducing pain during labor. It reduces afterbirth pains, helps bring down undelivered placenta, and increases the amount and quality of breast milk. The rich concentration of vitamin C, vitamin E, carotenes, vitamin A, calcium, iron, the B-vitamin complex, and the large amounts of phosphorus and potassium make taking red raspberry well worth it.

STINGING NETTLE TONIC

Another tonic for early pregnancy is stinging nettle, which is one of the most nutrient-rich substances available. It is loaded with carotenes, from which we make vitamin A; vitamins C, E, and D; the B vitamins; vitamin K; and calcium, potassium, phosphorous, and immune-strengthening sulfur.

Make a tonic the same way as for raspberry. Weigh out 1 ounce of the dried herb, put it in a jar, fill the jar with boiling water, then tightly lid it and steep overnight. You can drink it warm, cold or in between, up to four cups a day. The chlorophyll in this brew is so high that the infusion will actually look black rather than green. .Nettle is tremendously nourishing. It eases leg cramps and any other muscle spasms during pregnancy. Because of nettle's high calcium content, it diminishes labor pains and birth pains. It is such a superb source of vitamin C that it is one of the world's most highly favored herbs for preventing hemorrhaging after birth. It's a wonderful way to reduce hemorrhoids. It can increase the amount and richness of your breast milk. Stinging nettle tonic also can help pregnant women who have fatigue, moodiness, and preeclampsia.

DANDELION AND OTHER HERBS

Dandelion is also good for mood swings. You can take it in any form. You'll probably find dandelion root tincture in any health food store. The usual dosage is 10 to 20 drops, taken before meals, in the morning, and just before you go to bed—a total of five times a day.

Dandelion leaves, especially when eaten as a cooked green, provide tremendous amounts of potassium, calcium, and good-quality vegetable salt. They can even be used as a remedy for a woman who already has preeclampsia.

Here are a few more suggestions about herbs. Ginger is one of the best natural remedies for nausea. Ginger works best when the person taking it eats small, frequent meals and gets plenty of fresh air and rest. Ginger can be taken as a capsule or tea. A washcloth soaked in ginger or comfrey tea and applied to the area where an episiotomy has been performed promotes healing. Rosemary added to bath water relieves tension and back pain. Finally, adding jasmine and clary sage to a bath has an uplifting effect and prevents postpartum depression.

MASSAGE Susan Lacina tells why a pregnant woman and her unborn child benefit greatly from massage. "We tend to think of a baby in utero as being cut off from the world," she says. "In reality, the child within is a conscious being that responds to sounds, emotions, and the inner environment that its mother creates, either through her sense of well-being or her lack of it." Here Lacina describes how maternity massage promotes a comfortable and healthy pregnancy:

"Research shows that prolonged stress builds up abnormal levels of toxins and chemicals in the bloodstream. These are passed through the placenta to the baby. Minimizing the buildup of toxins can be achieved by periodic deep relaxation. Relaxation increases the absorption of oxygen and nutrients by the cells of the muscles. When oxygen and nutrition increase, the woman has more energy. Some doctors also believe morning sickness and nausea are eliminated by lowering stress levels.

"Massage assists the lymphatic system in eliminating excessive toxins and hormones. Unlike the heart, the lymphatic system has no pump. It moves freely until muscles tighten up, but when muscles become too tense, either from the fetus or from stress, lymph movement decreases and the concentration of toxins rises. In the lower extremities, the growing uterus can inhibit lymph drainage, leading to swelling, varicose veins, hemorrhoids, and fluid retention. By relaxing the muscles, massage helps stimulate lymphatic drainage of toxins. It decreases the development of varicose veins by its draining effect and helps reduce swelling in the legs."

Massage also helps with overall muscle tone and elasticity. "A woman's body must expand to accommodate the growing fetus," Lacina says. "Hips widen and abdominal, lower back, and shoulder muscles stretch. Legs must accommodate increased weight. Massage promotes flexible muscles, joints, ligaments, and tendons. It also helps decrease muscle spasms and leg cramps by getting rid of lactic acid buildup, and can alleviate the pain caused by sciatic nerve pressure. Added flexibility helps the muscles that are needed for labor."

In addition, massage assists in hormonal balance. "Massage balances the entire glandular system. An overactive thyroid gland becomes less active, thereby decreasing irritability, mood swings, and hot flashes. An underactive thymus gland is stimulated, which increases its ability to fight infection. The alternating relaxation and stimulation that massage provides helps a woman's body function in a more balanced manner."

Lacina describes the benefits of a peroneal massage. "This is a gentle stretch of tissues in the area between the vagina and rectum. Learning peroneal massage increases the mother's awareness of the muscles she needs to relax during the actual delivery and decreases her chances of having an episiotomy, an incision made to enlarge the vaginal opening at the time of birth.

"The actual procedure is as follows: Using warm vitamin E or vegetable oil, the mother places clean, oiled thumbs or index fingers an inch to an inch and a half inside the vagina and applies firm, gentle pressure downward and outward. Stretching continues until a burning sensation is felt. This is held for a few minutes. Performing this once or twice a day, up until the time of delivery, can result in an easier birth."

What about during labor and the postpartum period? "Massage during labor helps to reduce pain and anxiety by offering relief from muscle contractions." Lacina says. "The stimulation of certain acupressure points can speed up labor.

"Postpartum is the name given to the 6-week recovery period after birth. During this time, hormones readjust and the uterus involutes (returns to its prepregnancy size). Massaging the abdomen in a circular motion helps the uterus to contract and helps to expel blood. Massage also helps to stimulate milk flow. The following techniques can be applied for this purpose: (1) The pressure point at the base of the sacrum can be held for about 15 seconds, and then released. (2) Breast massage is another technique that can be used. Using some light oil, a woman circles her breasts with her fingertips. She places the hands flat on the breasts, starting at the nipple, and moves outward and up. That helps the glands to release milk. (3) Additionally, there is an acupressure point at the top and middle of the shoulder. Holding it for 15 seconds helps milk production. (4) Pressing the point between the sixth and seventh ribs (at the nipple level on the breast bone) helps to release milk."

ACUPRESSURE POINTS Thumbs can be applied to the sacrum, at the bottom of the spine, and walked up the spine to the waist. Each point is held for about 5 seconds.

The point in the center of the buttocks is pressed in as the mother exhales and released as she inhales.

Thumbs can be pressed along the shoulder blades between the spine and the scapula.

On the legs, pressure can be applied to spleen 6, an acupressure point located approximately 3 inches above the ankle, on the inside of the leg right below the tibia bone. Holding this spot for 10 seconds and then releasing it helps to stimulate uterine contractions and speeds up labor.

The uterus point is on the inside of the foot, just under the ankle bone. The ovary point is on the outside of the foot, under the ankles, near the heel. Squeezing these points at the same time for about 10 seconds and then releasing them helps to speed up labor.

Breast and nipple stimulation helps create oxytocin, the hormone that helps the uterus to contract.

ALEXANDER TECHNIQUE The Alexander technique differs from massage in that the pregnant woman is actively engaged. Kim Jessor, an Alexander teacher, makes an analogy to a piano lesson: "We talk about being Alexander teachers, the people who come to us are students, and the context is a lesson. So while the results are very therapeutic, I don't think of the work as a therapy but rather as a learning process. This is significant in that it empowers students to take charge in changing their movement habits."

The Alexander technique is based on the concept that all of us know how to move comfortably as children, but lose that natural flexibility over time. The method teaches people how to move freely again, which is especially valuable for women undergoing the stresses of pregnancy.

Jessor describes some of the ways the Alexander technique helps women during and after pregnancy: lower back pressure is relieved, breathing improves, rest is enhanced, labor is eased, stamina increases after delivery, and breast-feeding is easier. In addition, there are less tangible, but equally valuable, benefits from working with the Alexander technique during pregnancy. "Women begin to realize that they can make different kinds of choices about the kind of birth they want to have, where they want to have it, and who they want to use for labor support. In the same way that they begin to find freedom in movement, they find greater options in terms of the choices they make about their pregnancy."

EXERCISE The American College of Gynecologists and Obstetricians (ACOG) endorses physical activity during pregnancy and has created specific guidelines for the dos and don'ts of exercise:

Pregnant women derive health benefits from a mild to moderate exercise routine. Exercising 60 minutes, three times per week, is preferable to intermittent activity, but some benefit can be derived from shorter durations as well. Sometimes little oxygen is available for aerobic exercise due to the body's increased oxygen demands. Therefore, a woman should begin an aerobic activity slowly, and gradually build to capacity. She should not push too hard, and certainly not to the point of breathlessness. Pregnant women should not exercise in the face-up position after the first trimester. This position limits blood supply to the baby.

Avoid standing for prolonged periods of time, doing heavy work in the standing position, and exercising at high intensities. These activities are associated with diminished birthweight in newborns. It's better for women to engage in non-weight-bearing activities such as cycling and swimming, rather than exercises like running. Non-weight-bearing exercise minimizes the risk of injury and allows activity levels to remain closer to prepregnancy levels, right up to delivery. A woman should be aware that her center of gravity is different, and that she might lose her balance when exercising. Anything that could involve falling over, or even mild abdominal trauma, should be avoided. Pregnant women require an extra 300 calories per day in order to maintain their normal metabolic rate. Exercise increases the need for more calories.

A pregnant woman must be careful not to raise body temperature with vigorous workouts, especially in the first trimester. Excessive body heat in the mother can adversely affect the development of brain tissue in the baby. The threshold for this is a body temperature of about 39.2 degrees Celsius, which is 100 or 101 degrees Fahrenheit.

When should a pregnant woman not exercise? "Basically, every pregnant woman can benefit from starting an exercise program at any point in pregnancy. However, there are certain exceptions to this rule. When any one of the following conditions is present, a pregnant woman should limit or avoid exercise: pregnancy-induced hypertension, premature rupture of membranes, incompetent cervix, persistent second- or third-trimester bleeding, premature labor during the prior or current pregnancy, and intrauterine growth retardation.

Other medical contraindications include thyroid, heart, vascular, or pulmonary conditions. Women with medical problems need a physician's evaluation to determine whether an exercise program is appropriate.

AROMATHERAPY Ann Berwick reports that in Europe, where aromatherapy is scientifically studied and widely prescribed, hospital maternity wings utilize essential oils for their soothing and uplifting mind-body effects: "There is a report of one woman who had severe anxiety throughout her pregnancy. They gave her neroli oil, which helped to keep her blood pressure down and allowed her to go into delivery in a more relaxed state. During delivery, she was given lavender and clary sage to relax her uterus. Clary sage is also slightly euphoric, so it helped her to cope mentally with the birth." Here are some formulas to try before, during, and after birth:

As an antidote for nausea and vomiting, peppermint is effective when a very dilute amount is rubbed into the stomach or inhaled.

For relaxation, 8 ounces vegetable oil, 13 drops lavender, 2 drops geranium, and 10 drops sandalwood can be massaged into the skin or used as a compress.

To clear nasal congestion, a teaspoon of eucalyptus oil can be added to a cold-air humidifier or pan of hot water. The steam inhaled reduces congestion.

To help heartburn, place 2 to 3 drops of diluted peppermint oil on the back of the tongue.

A good massage oil to use during labor consists of 5 drops rose oil, 12 drops clary sage, and 5 drops ylang-ylang in 2 to 3 ounces of vegetable oil.

To prevent stretch marks, massage 2 ounces wheat germ oil, 20 drops lavender, and 5 drops neroli oil into the thighs.

To soothe sore nipples, mix 1 pint cold water, 1 drop geranium oil, 1 drop lavender oil, and 1 drop rose oil.

After an episiotomy, a sitz (shallow) bath is helpful, especially when 2 drops of cyprus oil and 4 drops of lavender oil are added. Soak for 15 to 20 minutes.

To promote milk production, take 2 drops fennel oil with some honey water, every 2 hours.

Hemorrhoids will be helped by 5 drops of cyprus oil added to the bath.

The astringent action of cyprus and lemon oil constricts varicose veins. A few drops can be added to a body lotion and applied to the veins morning and evening.

HOMEOPATHY Homeopathic physician Stephanie Odinov Pukit lists a variety of remedies for all stages of pregnancy. She begins with treatments for morning sickness.

SEPIA. Ambivalence is the key word here. There is a conflict between self-preservation and the urge to procreate, which makes wanting a child questionable. The woman becomes angry and irritable and feels as if a black cloud hovers over her. Although her appetite is insatiable, heavy pains worsen with smells or thoughts of food.

PULSATILLA. This is the opposite scenario. Pulsatilla is an excellent remedy for the woman who is cheerful, sweet, and somewhat helpless. The person is warm and may throw the covers off at night. She becomes worse with emotional excitement. Nausea comes and goes and is characteristically worse in early evening.

NUX VOMICA. This is a wonderful remedy for soothing the nerves after a woman has abused her body with alcohol, drugs, or coffee. She tends to be constipated. She tends to wake up at night to think about business because she is ambitious and driven.

ARSENICUM. The picture here is a person constantly anxious about her state of health. She always runs to the doctor fearing that something is wrong. The woman tends to have burning pains. She has great thirst and takes little sips. Symptoms are usually exacerbated at midnight.

COCCULUS INDICUS. This remedy specifically helps motion sickness. The woman tends to lose sleep and to be constantly exhausted. She may be nursing children or caring for someone. The woman feels dizzy standing and better when lying down. She feels worse in fresh air.

PETROLEUM. Petroleum may be indicated if there is a voracious appetite followed by persistent vomiting.

BRYONIA. The person has strong sensitivity to smells and may have connective tissue and arthritic problems. Nausea becomes worse with motion.

Dr. Odinov Pukit suggests these remedies for problems that occur in the latter stages of pregnancy.

SEPIA OR PULSATILLA. In the third to sixth month, the fetus presses high up in the abdomen, causing heartburn, shortness of breath, and indigestion. These remedies also help hemorrhoid problems. The one chosen depends on the other symptoms manifested. Sepia is for a gloomy disposition, while pulsatilla is for a sweet nature.

CARBO VEGETABILIS (CARBO VEG). The woman is slightly heavy and tends to have indigestion and shortness of breath due to poor oxygenation. Although she tends to be chilly, she prefers open windows with the air directly on her.

BELLIS PERENNIS. As the baby drops into the pelvis, pressure is felt on the organs in the lower part of the bladder. Pain and arthritis may occur as a result. Bellis perennis is specific for pain in the uterine area or groin. The woman might be walking when all of a sudden her legs weaken from a sharp nerve pain. After childbirth, when arnica has done its job (see below) and there are still some lumps remaining in the tissues, Bellis perennis is also excellent.

KALI CARBONICUM. Kali carbonicum is for women with back pain, especially those who tend to wake up between 2 and 4 o'clock in the morning. This individual's personality is somewhat crabby and closed. She is vague and evasive about answering questions. Pains are better with pressure and rubbing. The person tends to be anxious and chilly.

ACONITE. High-potency aconite is wonderful to use at any point in pregnancy when there has been shock or fright. Arnica and calendula may be useful for this purpose as well.

Midwife Jeannette Breen finds homeopathy useful during labor and after birth.

ARNICA. Starting a month before delivery, regular application of arnica directly to the nipples prevents later tearing and cracking with breast-feeding. After birth, arnica quickens recuperation. CALENDULA can be used in the same way.

CALIFILUM. Califilum may help a stalled labor. This is specific for a weak uterus or a uterus running out of steam. The woman often experiences weakness, exhaustion, trembling, and shivering. Sharp, brief, unstable, and painful lower uterine contractions fail to completely dilate the cervix and push the baby.

GELSEMIUM. Gelsemium may be indicated as a follow-up to califilum. It is also good for neuralgia, rheumatic discomfort, and pains in the bladder and vaginal area. The person tends to be thirsty and chilly.

CIMICIFUGA. Cimicifuga is good for stalled labor, especially when the woman is becoming fearful, hysterical, and exhausted, and the pains are becoming erratic. This tones the uterus, calms it down, and helps it to become more coordinated.

Corrective Vaginal Surgery

In the United States, about 80 percent of women who give birth have an episiotomy performed. This is an incision that is made during birth when the vaginal opening does not stretch adequately. Of those operations, approximately 90 percent are improperly performed. "Doctors are just not instructed in how to do this surgery," says Dr. Vicki Hufnagel. "All you have to do is go to your local medical school, get out the textbook on obstetrics, and look at what an episiotomy is. It will have a drawing and a discussion that says to put one or two sutures here, and one or two there. They are teaching physicians to close an entire organ system in just one or two layers. If you were to close a laceration on your face in one or two layers, your muscles wouldn't work, your face wouldn't work. You'd be a real mess. We are teaching students how to close the vaginal vault area in a manner that is not allowable in other places. That is the standard of care that we have, and it is completely unacceptable."

Incorrectly performed episiotomies result in problems down the road. Without the support of the vaginal muscles, the cervix pushes through the vagina. It appears that the uterus is being forced out, when really it is not. Doctors mistakenly diagnose a prolapsed uterus and commonly recommend a hysterectomy. Tragically, 100,000 to 200,000 women with this misdiagnosis receive this operation each year.

Corrective surgery easily ameliorates the problem. Repairing the vagina is a simple procedure that can be performed in a doctor's office. It takes all of 45 minutes, and patients can go home the same day.

Postpartum Depression

Depression after childbirth affects thousands of women each year. Although the exact cause is unknown, hormonal shifts after birth, particularly drops in progesterone, may play a large role. Research also links the condition to low levels of the neurotransmitter serotonin. Emotionally, it is often connected to difficult labor and disappointments after birth.

Symptoms range in degree, but are generally worse than a temporary feeling of the blues immediately following childbirth, according to Dr. Marjorie Ordene, a complementary gynecologist from New York: "Postpartum depression is defined as a gradually increasingly sullen mood and a loss of interest and enthusiasm starting around the third postpartum week. This is different from the 'baby blues,' which is a common occurrence in the normal population. The blues happens the first week postpartum, and basically goes away by itself. We are talking about something much more severe." In the worst-case scenario, women can become sick for years and lose touch with reality.

HOMEOPATHIC REMEDIES Homeopathic physician Dr. Jane Cicchetti recommends that women try the 30c potency of the remedy that best addresses their symptoms. If this does not help, a visit to a homeopathic physician can provide more individual support.

SEPIA. Sepia may be needed after an exhausting delivery, after giving birth to two or more children at once, or after having several children. The woman feels completely worn out and depressed. Physically, she feels as if her uterus might fall out, and finds herself crossing her legs a lot. Often there is an actual prolapse of the uterus. Emotionally, a woman who loves her husband and children suddenly has an aversion to them. In fact, she has an aversion to everyone and wants to be alone. She becomes irritable and angry if anyone bothers her, and has an aversion to sex. The woman cries often but cannot understand what is wrong; in fact this problem is caused by a hormonal disturbance rather than an emotional one.

NATMUR. Natmur is for chronic grief. The woman is introverted and dwells on past, unpleasant memories but keeps them to herself. She tries to put on the appearance that everything is fine, and becomes aggravated if someone tries to comfort her.

IGNATIA. Ignatia is for postpartum depression brought on by emotions. It is needed when disappointment follows childbirth. A woman imagines an ideal pregnancy and birthing situation. When that does not work out, she feels extremely let down and depressed. These feelings may occur after a stillbirth or a miscarriage. There is uncontrollable sobbing and sighing, and a rapid change of emotions, which are often contradictory.

ARNICA. This commonly needed remedy is useful for depression, upset, and malaise brought on by bruising, soreness, and pain that lasts a long time. Arnica helps heal the physical trauma and improves the mother's energy and emotional state.

PULSATILLA. Pulsatilla is given when a woman cries a lot and wants to be taken care of. She needs to attend to her newborn baby, but feels as if someone should be attending to her. This individual will eat sweets and other goodies to alleviate overwhelming feelings of sadness and loneliness. The woman often is warm-blooded and enjoys the fresh air. She is happier walking around outside, and much happier if she can be with people.

CIMICIFUGA. This remedy is used less often, but is very important for those who need it. Cimicifuga is derived from black cohosh, a powerful herb for treating hysteria and female complaints. It is needed when a woman feels as if a dark cloud of gloom has settled over her. She fears losing her mind. Often this stems from a very difficult delivery. She may have had a mini-nervous breakdown, feeling at one point as if she was going insane. This leaves her with a great fear of ever having a baby again. Often she alternates between different emotional states. When she is not under this dark cloud of gloom, she becomes excitable and talkative, jumping from one subject to another in an almost hysterical fashion. Cimicifuga heals the nervous system.

KALI CARBONICUM. This deep mineral remedy is indicated for women who become anxious and irritable after a delivery that leaves them feeling weak. Easily startled, they want to be left alone and have an aversion to being touched. They tend to be chilly and to have insomnia from 2 to 4 a.m. Further, they are regimented and have trouble going with the flow of caring for a new baby. Often these symptoms follow a delivery that primarily consists of back labor. Sciatica develops to some degree, which can lead to an emotional state like this.

PHOSPHORIC ACID. Phosphoric acid is helpful when a woman is extremely disappointed from physical or emotional shock. She may have lost the baby, or something might be wrong with the baby. A loved one may have died at the time of birth, or she may be affected from the loss of much bodily fluid during delivery. Indifferent to everything, the woman lies in bed with her face to the wall. It is as if her emotions have completely disappeared. She doesn't want to talk, think, or answer questions.

COCCULUS. This is a remedy for fatigue and emotional depression brought on by loss of sleep. The woman feels drunk and may go through the day feeling dizzy and staggering. These feelings are brought on by sleep deprivation.

AURUM METALLICUM. Arum metallicum is for profound depression characterized by total hopelessness, self-destructive behavior, and a longing for death.

NATURAL PROGESTERONE "Studies show that postpartum depression can be prevented by treating women with progesterone," reports Dr. Ordene. "Companies that make natural progesterone cream recommend using a half teaspoon twice daily, starting a month after delivery. Since postpartum depression is supposed to start 3 weeks after giving birth, it makes sense to begin using natural progesterone at that time."

VITAMIN B$_6$ According to research, this vitamin raises serotonin levels. Patients given B$_6$ for 28 days after delivery did not have a recurrence of postpartum depression.

Abortion Aftercare

Although most women who have abortions do not have any serious medical complications from the procedure, the period after an abortion is a time for a woman to focus on herself; she may have a variety of physical and emotional needs that require attention.

It's particularly important to remember that after an abortion your body's hormone levels have to readjust to the sudden change from a pregnant to a non-pregnant state. Dr. Susanna Reid, a naturopathic physician, describes the physical changes in a woman's body after an abortion.

"Hormone levels are elevated dramatically during pregnancy, and so the body has to readjust itself to its prepregnancy state," Dr. Reid explains. "One way to help the body to do that is by focusing on dietary factors that would be beneficial in regulating hormone levels. As well, you want to increase the circulation in the lower abdomen so that the body can heal itself. The more circulation in an area and the more nutrients that are in that area, the easier it is for the body to remove the toxic waste products. You'd also want to strengthen liver function, since the liver is essential to the balancing of hormones in the body; it functions to promote excretion of hormones. So if the liver isn't functioning correctly, you can have an imbalance of hormones."

To strengthen liver function she suggests eating foods that contain fiber, particularly fruits, vegetables, and whole grains. The gut needs fiber to prevent the reabsorption of hormones. "If there isn't enough fiber in the diet, the hormones are reabsorbed through the intrahepatic circulation. So fiber is very important. In the springtime, one can strengthen liver function by eating large amounts of fresh dandelions and other greens like cleaver. In other seasons, use yellow dock, nettle, dandelion, and cleaver with some red raspberry to make a tea. Red raspberry is a uterine tonic, so it helps to heal the uterus. You can put some peppermint in the tea to make it taste better and aid in digestion."

About 2 weeks after the abortion, she suggests using cold friction on the lower abdomen for 10 minutes at a time before going to bed or first thing in the morning.

PREVENTING INFECTION One of the more common complications from an abortion is infection. It's important not to put anything into the vagina for several weeks after the abortion and to refrain from intercourse. Dr. Reid suggests several natural remedies to help prevent infections.

"If we enhance the immune function, we prevent infection. You can use an immune-enhancing diet that focuses a lot on fruits and vegetables. Fruits in particular are immune-enhancing." She also recommends echinacea, goldenseal, astragalus, and ligustrum to help immune function.

Dr. Allan Warshowsky, a board-certified obstetrician and gynecologist who practices holistic gynecology, recommends taking vitamins C, A, and E and other antioxidants to enhance immune function.

Dr. Reid also emphasizes fluid intake. She explains that an abortion creates many byproducts, and one way the body can help eliminate them is through the exchange of fluids, so you should drink a lot of fluids.

Although each woman experiences abortion in her own way, it can sometimes create a strong emotional response, either positive or negative.

"If it is a desired pregnancy and it's a spontaneous abortion," Dr. Reid says, "then people are dealing with grief. Even if it is a therapeutic abortion, there can be many reasons for the abortion. It may be because the pregnancy isn't viable or wouldn't be viable or maybe it isn't the right time. So there are just a lot of grief issues for some women around abortion."

Dr. Warshowsky believes it is very important to deal with any negative feelings. He suggests that women who experience grief and other emotional and psychological consequences after an abortion may be helped by using meditation or visualization techniques.

Breast-feeding

For many of today's working mothers, breast-feeding is difficult because they can't be at home enough to be with their infants. However, women are further encouraged to neglect breast-feeding by the growth of fallacies about it, as well as a lack of full knowledge of its benefits.

The first major benefit of breast-feeding is the mother's milk itself: it gives the baby the appropriate nutrients. For the first 9 months, Arms notes, the baby doesn't need any other food at all other than from breast milk, which helps establish and nourish the baby's immune system. Feeding the baby from the breast creates in the mother a feeling of calm, relaxation, and deepening love for her child. For the baby, just being there, skin to skin, with the mother, affords immune protection.

The components of breast milk actually change from feed to feed, and, for a mother who has more than one child, the milk changes from child to child. This is why formula can never mimic breast milk. Nor can the container that breast milk comes in ever be duplicated. There's a real difference between providing pumping stations at work and giving working mothers access on their job time to daycare where mother and baby can be together when the baby wakes up—not to mention allowing mothers to be home with their babies until the babies are old enough to be without milk for more than 4 hours at a time.

Breast-feeding does many things for the baby and the mother. It causes the mother's gut to secrete 23 hormones (that we know of), which bottle feeding does not do. These hormones cause a woman to lose weight as well as help her sleep better and feel calmer. If a mother is malnourished and underweight, breast-feeding helps her to get as much nutrient value out of her food as possible.

More nutrient value is absorbed in her gut than would be if she were not breast-feeding.

Arms tells us, "All babies need to be breast-fed and almost all mothers, even those who have had breast surgery, can breast-feed, if we give them 3 months to get settled before we even think of having them go back to work. And then we need to create work situations where they can breast-feed during the day."

The following corrections to common fallacies about lactation and breast-feeding are from K. G. Auerbach, "Breast-Feeding Fallacies: Their Relationship to Understanding Lactation," *Birth* 17, no. 1 (March 1990): 44–49.

➤Nipple soreness is not related to skin color.

➤The lactating breast is never empty.

➤All women do not experience pain during each breast-feeding.

➤Nipples do not get tougher with nursing.

➤Creams and oils on the breast are not encouraged for nipple soreness; vitamin E toxicity could be a concern because of liberal applications, and pesticide residues are a concern in sheep-fat-derived lanolin.

➤Engorgement may be experienced by newly breast-feeding mothers but is almost always indicative of inappropriate or infrequent suckling.

➤The let-down process is not a singular event, but occurs continually during suckling.

➤Noninfectious mastitis rarely requires antibiotic therapy; infectious mastitis includes temperature elevation and flulike systems as well.

➤Extra fluid intake is not needed for breast-feeding; drinking to quench one's thirst is sufficient.

➤The lactating mother's breasts become full usually between 1 and 3 days after the infant starts suckling.

➤Colostrum, which is a highly concentrated source of protein and antibodies, is produced as early as the third month of pregnancy.

➤Women with inverted nipples can breast-feed.

➤Healthy babies do not need supplemental feedings before the mother's milk comes in.

➤Breast milk helps reduce bilirubin concentrations by coating the small intestines, reducing bilirubin recirculation.

➤Additional water or glucose given to the infant reduces total caloric intake and diminishes the coating action of milk feedings.

➤Human milk is far superior in all aspects to artificial formula.

53

Female Infertility

pproximately 2.5 million American couples are unable to conceive. The question of what can and should be done to conquer infertility is not only a complex medical issue but, with the advent of more and more advanced techniques for getting around nature's roadblocks to conception, at times a thorny ethical dilemma as well, with high emotional stakes.

After 10 years of fertility tests and treatments, Carla Harkness, frustrated by the lack of consumer-oriented literature on the subject, consulted over a hundred medical specialists and put together *The Fertility Book*. Harkness sees infertility as an emotional life crisis that is largely unacknowledged by society: "Reactions include grief and mourning, loss of self-esteem, and impaired self-image. Couples often have difficulties communicating with one another. Their sexual relationship is tested and damaged. All in all, it is a traumatic experience." She adds that an early end to pregnancy, due to miscarriage, produces the same frustrations: "The failure of a fertilized egg to implant is amazingly common. Often up to 50 percent of fertilized eggs do not make it past the initial 2-week period to implantation. Up to 20 percent of confirmed pregnancies are miscarried in the first trimester in women under 35 years old. As a woman approaches 40, that number can exceed 25 percent, and by the age of 45, the miscarriage rate is almost 50 percent. The emotional impact of miscarriage is similar to the emotional impact of infertility. There is often grief and mourning that are not accepted as genuine mourning in our society. Couples often hear things like, 'I guess it was meant to be,' 'Something was wrong,' or 'You'll have another.' That is often of little solace to someone feeling this kind of loss."

Causes

Reasons for infertility in women include endometriosis, a condition in which the glands and tissues that line the inside of the uterus grow outside the uterine wall (see chapter 54); poor diet; deficiencies in folic acid, vitamin B_6, vitamin B_{12}, and iron; heavy metal toxicity; obesity; immature sex organs; abnormalities of the reproductive system; hormonal imbalances; and genetic damage from electromagnetic radiation.

It may surprise you to learn that the birth control pill and other sources of estrogen can add to the problem. Barbara Seaman, an advocate for women's health issues and author of *The Doctors' Case Against the Pill*, concludes that the chemicals in the pill may increase infertility in three ways: by suppressing the natural productions of hormones; increasing the risk of sexually transmitted diseases (STDs), especially chlamydia; and upsetting the assimilation of nutrients.

ABNORMAL MENSTRUAL CYCLES As Seaman reports, "Fertility experts confirm that many women who have been on the pill for a long time have problems reestablishing their monthly cycles." Robin Wald, a nutritionist and health-care writer who specializes in infertility, explains further how birth control pills can cause hormonal imbalances that affect fertility.

"The hypothalamus is the gland that produces gonadotropin-releasing hormone, the hormone that triggers the pituitary gland to secrete other hormones that are important for fertility. These hormones, follicle-stimulating hormone, which tells the ovaries to start producing and maturing an egg each month, and luteinizing hormone, which ripens the egg and allows it to be released, signal the ovaries to produce estrogen and progesterone so that you can have a normal menstrual cycle. It's a very complicated and complex system and must be in a very particular balance to function properly; for the egg to ripen and mature; for the egg to be released and travel through the fallopian tubes; and for progesterone to be there to build up the endometrial lining to nourish an egg, so that if it's fertilized it can be implanted and nourished and grow so that it doesn't miscarry. When you have too much estrogen that suppresses pituitary gland function, you disrupt the normal hormone balance."

CHLAMYDIA "Another reason the pill is bad for female infertility," notes Barbara Seaman, "is that it promotes the growth of chlamydia. This condition has reached epidemic proportions in the United States, with over half a million new cases yearly. Chlamydia causes pelvic inflammatory disease, which can then cause sterility. Usually, the first time it strikes, chlamydia does not render a woman sterile. Women who get the condition once should give up the pill right away."

NUTRITIONAL DEFICIENCY Seaman says there are a lot of nutritional issues involved with taking the pill. "If a woman has been on the pill for a long time, she may be very low in folic acid; vitamins B_1, B_2, B_6, B_{12}, C, and E; and trace minerals zinc and magnesium, all essential to normal fertility. Sometimes just getting on a really good diet with really good supplements can get her back into a fertile cycle without needing heavy-duty drugs. It should be noted, however, that any dietary supplements used should be low in vitamin A, niacin, copper, and iron, the levels of which tend to be elevated in pill users."

Assisted Reproductive Technology

"The laboratory options have just exploded in the past decade for infertile couples," Carla Harkness reports. "In 1978, the first 'test-tube' baby was born in England through a process called in vitro fertilization. Since then, the process has been instituted worldwide. There are now over 260 clinics practicing some form of that kind of laboratory fertilization, which is now called Assisted Reproductive Technology or ART.

"Now the boundaries have even exceeded menopause. Before, you had the practice of donor sperm for artificial insemination. Now there is the ability to fertilize donor eggs from younger women with the husband's sperm and to implant those eggs in an infertile woman who is over 45 or 50. She is able to carry a child to term that is not genetically related to her. These kinds of options have all become available, and they offer a great deal of hope to many couples."

ETHICAL ISSUES While modern advances in fertility treatments offer a wealth of new possibilities, they also raise new ethical concerns. "A number of religious groups have raised questions about the intervention of technology in the natural process of reproduction," Harkness explains. "There is also a theme of pronatalism at any cost here, emphasizing that to be complete as couples or as women, people absolutely must birth a biological child.

Another big issue revolves around extending maternal age past nature's deadline of menopause. Before, women in their mid-40s probably weren't able to get pregnant because their bodies would stop that function. Now, it is possible for women in their 50s and 60s to become pregnant. This raises a number of questions: Is that putting too much demand on their bodies? What about the age difference between them and their children? What about obligations to aging parents while having little ones in your midlife? Additionally, there is a legal and moral question revolving around the status of unused, frozen embryos in the event of death and divorce.

"There are further questions surrounding the availability of this expensive technology to those without the means or the medical insurance. Unfortunately, these treatments are quite expensive. From the moment you walk into a specialist's office asking for an evaluation, you start incurring costs in the hundreds of dollars for examinations and tests, all the way to thousands of dollars for the in vitro techniques. It's about $10,000 per cycle for a straight in vitro lab procedure, all the way up to $15,000 if egg donor in vitro fertilization is utilized."

Many women distrust scientific intervention in general. Problems with intrauterine devices (IUDs) have caused pelvic inflammatory disease resulting in infertility. Diethystilbestrol (DES), an estrogen replacement often used as a "morning-after" pill in the United States even after it was linked to cancer and anomalies of the vagina and cervix, has been another big problem, as has thalidomide. Now there is a concern about using female hormones to stimulate ovulation. With most infertility treatments, whether the problem is due to the man or woman, it is mainly the women who undergo the drug treatments, the surgeries, and so forth. What are the long-term effects of exposing women to these drugs?

Natural Options

Dr. Marjorie Ordene, a gynecologist from Brooklyn, New York, believes that while there is a place for technology in fertility, women are too quick to seek out these methods, and she suggests trying various natural options first.

PINPOINTING TIME OF OVULATION Women should learn to recognize their time of ovulation by taking their temperature first thing in the morning, before getting out of bed. Says Dr. Ordene, "Usually, temperature rises in the second half of the cycle, 2 weeks before menstruation. The mucus that is produced around the time of ovulation has a clear and slippery quality. This is the kind of mucus that is needed for the sperm to penetrate the cervix."

WHAT TO AVOID Robin Wald cautions that women trying to conceive should avoid exposure to toxic substances that not only may interfere with conception but have also been linked to miscarriage and birth defects.

"The first thing I tell people to avoid is tobacco smoke. If you're a cigarette smoker and you plan on getting pregnant, quit smoking. Tobacco is very high in chemicals, including cadmium, which is a toxic heavy metal that accumulates in the reproductive organs of both men and women. It interferes with sperm production in men and hormone production in women. Secondhand smoke can cause similar problems.

"I also encourage people to stop drinking, even if they only drink moderately. Alcohol interferes with fertility by causing liver toxicity. The liver is the primary organ for building up cholesterol to form the steroid hormones which are important to reproductive health. Marijuana and other drugs can also cause liver toxicity and should be avoided.

"In addition, I suggest that people eliminate caffeine, both in coffee and sodas; switch to decaf coffee or herbal teas, and increase your water intake.

Although the subject of caffeine and fertility is controversial, studies have shown that as few as two cups of coffee a day or two cans of caffeinated soda can increase your chance of a miscarriage by four times and your infertility by 50 percent.

Wald further cautions women to avoid taking some over-the-counter medications. "A lot of women who experience menstrual discomfort think nothing of taking an aspirin or ibuprofen. But nonsteroidal anti-inflammatory drugs are also harmful to the reproductive system.

"One thing to avoid that cannot be overemphasized is pesticides—both pesticides that have been sprayed in your garden and pesticide residue from food that you buy. Pesticides are very toxic to the reproductive system. This is because pesticides are in a class of chemicals called xenoestrogens, synthetic chemicals that act like estrogen on the body. Overexposure to xenoestrogens can result in a condition called estrogen dominance. In estrogen dominance there is too much estrogen circulating in the body, which throws off the balance and production of other hormones that are essential for fertility."

Other sources of xenoestrogens are food additives, preservatives, and meat from animals that have been fed hormones. Dairy products also contain xenoestrogens, both from the cows' own hormones and from hormones given to them to promote milk production.

DIET AND LIFESTYLE Women should maintain a healthy diet and follow a basic exercise program. Fertility specialists Dr. Talha Sawaf, Dr. Yehudi Gordon, and Marilyn Glenville, writing in *Positive Health* magazine, recommend eating organic foods as much as possible and avoiding food additives, coffee, and tea. They advise eliminating nonessential medications and avoiding exposure to radiation, hazardous substances in the workplace, pesticides, and pollutants such as toxic metals. They point out that becoming as healthy as possible before conception improves the quality of the egg and sperm, thereby maximizing fertility and reducing the risk of miscarriage. Conversely, fertility is decreased by poor nutrition, vitamin or mineral deficiencies, and too much alcohol, cigarettes, and stimulants.

Robin Wald, who suggests that the very first step in optimizing fertility is to examine your diet, says that the standard American diet does not promote either health or fertility. She recommends an organic, whole, live foods diet. "The advantage of eating live food is that the nutritional value and the quality are that much higher. Good nutrition is vital when you're trying to get pregnant. Vitamins, minerals, fats, amino acids, and other nutritional components from our foods are essential for keeping the reproductive system healthy. Eat fresh fruit and vegetables, especially leafy green vegetables like collard greens, kale, Swiss chard, red chard, and beet greens, which are very high in folic acids and loaded with calcium. Folic acid is essential for preventing birth defects like spina bifida, and calcium will aid in building your baby's skeleton as well as keeping your own bones healthy."

She suggests minimizing your intake of processed flour, bread, baked goods, and pasta, and incorporating more whole grains into your diet. She recommends brown rice, millet, quinoa, oats, and buckwheat. "Whole grains are loaded with fiber and have very high nutritional quality. Raw nuts and seeds are also good, as are chickpeas, lentils, black beans, and pinto beans, which are both high in fiber and a good source of nonanimal protein.

"Fiber is important in promoting the excretion of toxins and bound-up estrogens from the gut. If you have insufficient fiber to move things through your intestines in a timely way, these estrogens sit in the gut and get reabsorbed into the body. So instead of having environmental estrogens or estrogens your body has created circulating through your body once, they're now going through a second, third, or fourth time, which contributes to estrogen dominance."Wald advises eating soy products, like tempeh and miso. "Soy is a good source of phytoestrogens, which have a chemical structure similar to estrogen. Phytoestrogen tricks your body into thinking that it's getting estrogen, but the advantage of phytoestrogens is that they tell your body to lower its own estrogen production, which helps balance your estrogen levels. As well, phytoestrogens block the absorption of xenoestrogens."

EMOTIONAL AND SPIRITUAL ISSUES Often, a woman has apprehensions about becoming pregnant that need to be addressed. It may be reassuring to talk to the inner child and let her know that even though there will be another child, the little girl in her will still get the attention she needs. This kind of spiritual work is often important in achieving pregnancy.

Feelings of blame, guilt, anger, and frustration that infertile couples often experience will have a negative effect on their fertility. Discussing such issues, perhaps with a counselor, can resolve these negative feelings and improve the chances of conception.

Infertility is a very stressful, major life event, and stress can itself adversely affect fertility. Robin Wald describes how stress affects reproductive function. "Every time there is a stress response in your body, the adrenal glands secrete a group of hormones that have an inhibitory affect on the hypothalamus, which is the master gland that signals the production of the hormones needed for reproduction. When you have excessive stress, the hypothalamus does not function properly.

"Stress can also cause a condition called hypoprolactin anemia. Prolactin is another hormone that prepares the breasts for milk production. If a nonpregnant woman has high levels of prolactin, it will make conception difficult because it can shut down ovulation.

"If you're under a lot of stress, do whatever you can to reduce it," Wald suggests. She recommends yoga, meditation, breathing exercises, spiritual work and prayer, visualization and imagery, bodywork, and massage as ways to lower stress levels.

Nutritional supplements can also help. Wald recommends vitamins C and E, beta carotene, alpha carotene, coenzyme Q10, and antioxidants to protect against stress-induced free radical damage.

ASIAN NATUROPATHIC APPROACH The traditional Eastern approach to fertility depends less on modern technology and more on time-tested knowledge. Dr. Roger Hirsch, a naturopathic physician from California, explains Chinese philosophy and infertility treatments based on this point of view: "We look at making the abdomen happy. This is an aphorism for correcting the digestion, menstruation, and hormones, so that women can conceive. Of course, raising the man's sperm count and sperm motility is important as well, because it is not just the woman who is infertile in an infertility situation. A key to this is the way the blood flows in the pelvic cavity." Chinese medicine uses acupuncture, massage, heat, or crystals applied at points along the energy pathways, or meridians, to balance the flow of energy in the body. Changing the diet, decreasing emotional tension, and balancing heat and cold will increase the effectiveness of the basic treatment. Thus acupuncture is more effective when used together with herbs to regulate the menstrual cycle, promote ovulation, and increase general vitality, all of which enhance fertility. Chinese medicine can be combined with assisted reproductive technology to minimize stress and help women tolerate drugs and surgery.

HERBS "In Chinese medicine," says Dr. Hirsch, "herbs are used to tone renal/adrenal function because reproductive function is related to the kidney and to functions related to the kidney. The actual viability of the eggs for a woman over 40 is related to kidney yang function."

HERBA EPIMETI. One herb that is very good for kidney yang is an aphrodisiac called herba epimeti, which translates in English to "horny goat weed." The Chinese noticed that goats become sexually active after eating this particular plant. They put the plant into the herbal formula for women who are kidney yang–deficient, and they noted that it increased sexual desire.

LUTAIGOU. Lutaigou, the gelatin that comes from boiling the antlers of deer, is used by the Chinese to help women over 40 who are trying to extend their egg-producing years. It helps slow down the biological clock.

WORMWOOD. In the European system, we have wormwood, which creates more circulation in the pelvic cavity. The Chinese use this along with daughter seed and fructose litchi, a little red berry.

DONG-QUAI AND CORTEX CINNAMOMI. Both of these help the circulation in the pelvic cavity. Cortex cinnamomi is not the cinnamon you put in your mulled cider, but a cinnamon with a very thick bark.

ACUPUNCTURE In China, acupuncture has been used in the treatment of infertility for centuries. The Chinese look at five principal organs—the liver, spleen, heart, lung, and kidney—and use acupuncture to release blockages from these systems so that energy, or *chi*, can move freely. This helps the body return to good health. Promoting fertility is one benefit that can be obtained.

Acupuncture to kidney points releases psychological blocks that interfere with reproduction. Dr. Hirsch uses the treatment to help patients overcome deep-rooted fears connected to sexual abuse and low self-esteem. "In treating self-esteem issues, I work on the heart and kidney points. The acupuncture points that seem extremely valuable for this are pericardium 5 and 6. If a practitioner is having a problem with understanding whether or not a psychological issue is involved in the infertility, and the patient does not know what the issue is, pericardium 5 can be needled. If something is holding the person back, that will bring an event or dream to memory, and the patient will understand why she is stuck. In treating self-esteem issues, we may also release stress by needling the heart 7 point, heart 9, and sometimes heart 7 to heart 5.

"We also address conception vessel 17, which is between the breasts. This is a very important place for women because it opens their energy. It also helps relieve liver chi congestion or stuckness. Remember, the liver and the liver hormones, both in Chinese and Western medicine, govern the flow of blood in the pelvic cavity."

WESTERN NATUROPATHIC APPROACH Dr. Joseph Pizzorno says that as a naturopath and midwife he saw numerous infertile couples and discovered two causes of the condition that were not generally recognized by the orthodox medical profession: "The first was pituitary insufficiency. The pituitary gland was not secreting enough of the hormones needed to stimulate the ovaries to mature, ripen, and produce a viable ovum. Most of these women had been on birth control pills for long periods of time. Even though they had been off the pills for several years, their pituitary never functioned fully again.

"With these women I did two things. I gave them an herbal concoction using herbs that are commonly used for women's health problems, which are supposed to stimulate proper pituitary functioning. I also gave them raw pituitary gland from an animal. There were surprisingly good results with this treatment. A urine test beforehand measured the level of hormones from the pituitary. If a patient had low hormone levels, I would then use this protocol with them. A surprising number became pregnant once their urinary hormone levels returned to normal.

"The second major cause was pelvic inflammatory disease, where there were infections in the fallopian tubes, the little tubes that go from the uterus to the ovaries. Infections leave scars. Then the ovum cannot penetrate the tube and get into the uterus for fertilization.

"An age-old hydrotherapy procedure, called sitz bath, helps end this problem. A woman gets two big pots of water. (We use washtubs that are about 3 feet in diameter.) One tub gets filled with hot water (as hot as she can stand it). When a woman sits in it with her arms and legs out of the tub, the water level reaches her umbilicus. The other tub gets filled with ice cold water. That tub is filled to the point just below the umbilicus. In other words, there is more hot water than cold water. The woman sits in the hot water for 5 minutes, and then in the cold water for 1 minute. She alternates back and forth three times.

"The first time a woman does this, she will find it startling. But after a while she will actually start to like it. She does this every day. After a few treatments, she starts getting a discharge. As near as we can make out, this discharge is the body throwing off scar tissue and toxic material in the ovaries. This is a particularly dangerous time for a woman to have intercourse. The ovaries are starting to open up, and there is a high probability of an ectopic pregnancy. The egg will only be able to go partway down the tube since the tube is not yet open enough for it to get all the way into the uterus. We therefore tell women no unprotected intercourse for at least 3 months while doing these treatments every day. Again, a surprising number of them become pregnant."

RESTORING THYROID BALANCE Even as far back as the 1930s, alleviating low thyroid conditions was found effective against infertility. Dr. Ray Peat says, To keep thyroid levels up, women should snack frequently and eliminate unsaturated fats. Although unsaturated fats are often touted as beneficial, recent studies show them to inhibit thyroid secretion. More high-quality protein may be needed, especially by women following a weight-loss program or a vegetarian diet. A daily minimum of 40 grams is recommended. Taking a thyroid supplement for a short period of time can greatly help. "People whose thyroid function is suppressed can benefit from a week or two of thyroid supplementation," Dr. Peat advises. "They don't need to take this indefinitely."

NATURAL HYGIENE Dr. Anthony John Penepent, follows the principles of natural hygiene when treating any medical condition: "Over the years, I have seen many wonderful things happen with natural hygiene which would not have been possible with allopathic medicine." Explaining infertility, Dr. Penepent says there are many causes, but that all of them can be treated similarly: "There are many mechanisms that can come into play. You can have basic amenorrhea or failure to ovulate. You can have any variety of hormonal imbalances or fallopian tube obstruction. In 40 percent of the cases it is not the woman's fault, although she may take the blame to save her husband's ego. The man may have a low sperm count, depressed sperm motility, or abnormal sperm morphology. These are all possibilities. Then again, conception may occur but the egg or ovum may not have sufficient nutrients for the embryo to develop. What happens then is you have unrecognized spontaneous abortions that make it appear as if the woman is infertile, when in actuality she just has a nutritional deficiency.

"In many cases, an infertile woman can conceive and go on to have a successful pregnancy with a minor amount of dietary change. In the case of the fallopian tube obstruction, it may be necessary for her to fast for several days. I remember one patient, a rabbi's wife, who was childless. Because of their religious beliefs, it was absolutely essential for her to bear children. In her particular case, I put her on a fast for several days and followed that up with a nutritional regimen. She was able to conceive within 6 months."

CONSUMER ADVOCACY GROUPS Carla Harkness recommends becoming a part of a consumer advocacy group that can provide individuals and couples with support and information. One group, called Resolve, has its national office in Somerville, Massachusetts, and a string of chapters across the country: "Resolve is a great ally that provides literature, referrals, and legal advocacy to the infertile. Chances are, wherever you live, there's a chapter by you."

54

Endometriosis

Endometriosis is a condition in which the glands and tissues that line the inside of the uterus (the endometrium) grow outside the uterine wall. Normally, cells build up in the uterus each month in preparation for pregnancy, serving as a nest for an incoming embryo. When pregnancy does not occur, the lining is shed and appears as menstrual flow. In endometriosis, endometrial-type cells may attach themselves to the fallopian tubes, ovaries, urinary bladder, intestinal surfaces, rectum, part of the colon, and other structures in the area.

Between 7 and 15 percent of American women have endometriosis. One of the goals of the medical treatment of endometriosis is to reduce the stimulating effect of estrogen on these cell "implants." Since there is no cure for this illness, the most that natural care can do at present is to work on relieving the pain.

Dian Shepperson Mills, a nutritionist and tutor at the Institute for Optimal Nutrition in London, is the author of *Endometriosis: A Key to Healing through Nutrition*. She explains that the implants cause a problem "because the endometrium is designed to shed blood at the end of every month if a pregnancy has not been achieved. So these endometric implants which are scattered around on the bowel and the bladder and so on do likewise; they shed blood. When you are having a normal period, the blood comes out of the body down the vagina. However, with endometriosis, the implants bleed into the abdominal cavity, and the blood is trapped in there because it has no exit. Thus, people with endometriosis get considerable amounts of pain."

However, Mills explains, women with the tiniest spots of endometriosis often have far more pain than women who have large lumps of endometriosis.

There seems to be no rhyme or reason as to why all this pain occurs mainly in women who have small amounts of endometric implants.

She adds that there is a problem with this illness beyond the pain: "We also think that the reaction going on in the body, which is trying to remove the implants, which the body's immune system knows should not be there, may affect people's fertility in some way, although we don't know how. It's believed that it is mainly the chemical secretions by the immune cells which are trying to remove the endometrium that are affecting the sperm or the ova."

Women may experience menstrual pain, pain on ovulation, pain on intercourse, and problems with fertility. As Mills says, "It affects 1 in 10 women, so it's almost like looking at asthma or diabetes in that it is experienced by a lot of people. Yet it's not very well known, for it's very difficult for some women to talk about this, as it's such a personal thing."

Causes

The exact cause of the condition remains a mystery, though several theories exist as to why it happens. These are some possible explanations.

RETROGRADE MENSTRUATION. Blood flows backward instead of downward through the cervix and out of the body. It is thought to go out the fallopian tubes and into the pelvic and abdominal cavity. Once it is there, cells from the exiting blood implant themselves outside the uterus onto other tissues.

LYMPHATIC CHANNELS. Cells of the endometrium lining pass through lymphatic channels or migrate via blood and then implant themselves outside the uterine cavity.

GENETIC PREDISPOSITION. Certain families are predisposed to the condition.

IMMUNOLOGIC DISORDER. The immune system is deficient in some way, causing tissue to proliferate in abnormal areas. The idea is that through some type of immune deficiency, hormonal and chemical influences cause endometrial tissue to become activated at different times in the cycle.

CHILDBEARING. Childbearing in combination with methods of contraception may be responsible.

Symptoms

About 70 percent of women with endometriosis have severe, chronic symptoms. Endometriosis can produce slight or severe pain, ranging from mild cramps to agony and dysfunction. Endometrial implants produce chemicals, including prostaglandins, which cause the uterus to contract, resulting in cramping. Pain also results from swelling, inflammation, and scarring of affected tissues. It is usually cyclical and most commonly occurs just before menstruation. Some women have pain during sexual intercourse any time in the month.

Where and to what degree pain is felt depend on the location of the endometrial tissue and the degree to which it has spread outside the uterus. Some women have pain during urination as a result of implants on the bladder. Some have pain during bowel movements because of colon and rectal implants. There can be ovarian pain or pain radiating to the back or buttocks or down the legs. Upon a manual gynecological examination, there may be pelvic pain.

Internal bleeding may occur as well as nose bleeding or bleeding from another orifice at certain times of the month. Any cyclic bleeding is suspect for endometriosis. Other symptoms that sometimes appear include aggravated premenstrual syndrome (PMS), bladder infections, fatigue, and lower back pain. Endometriosis may result in infertility when it interferes with ovarian function.

Diagnosis

Endometriosis can be suspected in the presence of one or more of the symptoms listed above, but the only real way to confirm a diagnosis is with a surgical procedure known as a laparoscopy, which allows the doctor to actually see and biopsy tissue. Sonograms and magnetic resonance imaging (MRI) scans may be helpful, but they are not definitive in making the diagnosis.

The proper diagnosis is important, notes Dr. Anthony Aurigemma, because while endometriosis is considered benign, it can become malignant.

Conventional Therapy

Treatment usually consists of medical prescriptions for pain control and reduction of endometrial growth. Antiprostaglandin medicines such as indomethacin, ibuprofen, and naproxen are often given to reduce pain.

Another popular pharmaceutical, danazol, is also used for this purpose, but in some women it does not provide total or lasting relief. Studies show that danazol has a good effect after surgery to remove adhesions. After some of the adhesions have been removed, it may help an infertile woman become pregnant. A side effect of the drug is that it may increase cholesterol, especially the low-density lipoprotein (LDL) variety, which is implicated in accelerated arteriosclerosis. The adverse effects of all these drugs can include weight gain, edema, decreased or increased breast size, acne, excess hair growth on the face and perhaps even in a developing fetus, and deepening of the voice.

Hormones are sometimes given to fool the body into believing it is pregnant, since pregnancy seems to retard or prevent the development of endometriosis. This method appears to have some benefit, but the side effects include depression, painful breasts, nausea, weight gain, bloating, swelling, and migraine headaches. Since the side effects can be fairly severe, this is not a popular method.

Newer drugs, called gonadotropin-releasing hormone compounds, are sometimes given by injection. These agents suppress pituitary gland release of the female hormones follicle-stimulating hormone (FSH) and luteinizing hormone (LH), causing what is called a clinical pseudomenopause. They help reduce pain in many women and decrease the size and volume of endometrial tissue after surgery.

Through the advanced surgical technique of female reconstructive surgery (FRS) developed by Dr. Vicki Hufnagel, the uterus and ovaries can be repositioned, thus reducing the deep pelvic pain that is associated with endometriosis.

Alternative Therapies

PAIN RELIEF "When I started looking at nutrition for the endocrine system," Mills says, "I came across lot of research which suggests that if you are deficient in various nutrients, it may affect the way your body deals with pain. These nutrients would be the essential fatty acids, such as evening primrose oil, fish oil, linseed oil, safflower oil, and vitamins C, E, and K. All these are important in the body's control of pain. The B vitamins, particularly B_1, seem to be important in building up the endorphins, which are the body's natural painkillers. Also, there is an amino acid called DLPA, which is DL-phenylalanine, which seems to help in dulling pain. Also, there are zinc, selenium, and magnesium."

If you are deficient in many of these nutrients, your body may not be able to cope well with pain. Mills says, "If we look at, say, magnesium, we see that it is very important in allowing muscles to relax. Calcium and magnesium balance one another. Calcium causes muscles to contract, and magnesium allows them to relax. Seeing that the uterus is one of the largest muscles in the body, it would be quite important to make sure you are getting enough magnesium-rich foods, such as green leafy vegetables, nuts, and seeds. The same is true of B vitamins. There are lots of those in vegetables and fruits. That's also where you'll get vitamin C. Zinc will be found in nuts and seeds. Selenium would be in seafood."

DIGESTION AND THE REPRODUCTIVE SYSTEM "Once I have a patient who has a major endometriosis problem," Mills says, "the first thing I look at is her digestion. If she doesn't get the nutrients from food or any supplements she takes, nothing will work. So, you have to heal the digestion first. If she has constipation or diarrhea or heartburn indigestion, I will give her digestive enzymes, acidophilus, and possibly slippery elm. Then, once we've got that healed, you can try a digestive supplement, such as a multivitamin, and some magnesium, zinc, and vitamin C.

"You have to analyze what is wrong with each individual person and tailor the treatment specifically to her needs. Generally, for endometriosis, I try to ensure that the woman is taking evening primrose and fish oil. The supplements also must be wheat-, yeast-, sugar-, and dairy-free. By taking magnesium, zinc, the probiotics, and the digestive enzymes, you are working through the body system from different angles to try to relieve the pain while supporting the endocrine and immune systems."

NATUROPATHY Dr. Tori Hudson, a naturopath from Portland, Oregon, believes there is most support for the immunological weakness theory of endometriosis because women with this condition have altered immune cells and fewer T lymphocytes. By improving immune function with supplements, diet, and botanicals, she claims to help many patients: "I've seen women with severe pelvic pain who were scheduled for surgery one month from the date I saw them. My treatment helped them recover completely without the surgery." She adds that most, but not all, women respond to her protocol, which is designed to stimulate a maximal immune response. The basic program consists of the following.

Antioxidants
Vitamin C: to bowel tolerance, up to 10,000 mg
Beta carotene: 150,000 to 200,000 IU
Selenium: 400 mcg
Vitamin E: 800 to 1200 IU

Changes in the diet are made to further stimulate the immune system. This is accomplished by lowering fat; adding whole grains, vegetables, and fruits; and eliminating immune system inhibitors such as coffee, sugar, alcohol, and high-fat foods. Foods such as cheese and meat have high amounts of estrogen and are omitted, because estrogen aggravates the disease. A mostly vegetarian diet is best for lowering estrogen and stimulating the immune system.

Two botanical formulas are included. One contains chaste tree berry, dandelion root, motherwort, and prickly ash in equal amounts. A half teaspoon is taken three times daily. The other formula contains small doses of toxic herbs that must be carefully prescribed by a naturopathic physician.

In addition, Dr. Hudson sometimes prescribes natural progesterone made from wild yam. The wild yam extract is converted in the laboratory to natural progesterone.

OTHER NUTRITIONAL RECOMMENDATIONS Dr. Susan M. Lark, a physician who is the author of *The Women's Health Companion: Self-Help Nutrition Guide & Cookbook*, recommends vitamins, herbs, and minerals that will decrease estrogen stimulation of the endometrial cells.

VITAMIN A. In the form of beta carotene, a maximum daily dose of 5,000 units to help decrease the excess menstrual bleeding that may occur with endometriosis.

VITAMIN B COMPLEX. 50 to100 milligrams with an additional dose of up to 300 milligrams daily of vitamin B_6. These vitamins help the liver convert excess estrogen into less stimulating forms.

VITAMIN C. 1000 to 4000 milligrams of bioflavonoids daily. Vitamin C not only regulates estrogen levels but reduces cramps and bleeding by strengthening capillaries. You can get bioflavonoids by eating citrus fruits (including the inner peel), berries, the skins of grapes, alfalfa, buckwheat, and soybeans and taking 800 milligrams a day of vitamin C as a supplement.

VITAMIN E. 400 to 2,000 units a day. If you have high blood pressure, begin with 100 units and work up to the higher levels gradually. Vitamin E helps even out the effects of high levels of estrogen.

ESSENTIAL FATTY ACIDS. Essential fatty acids (EFAs), including linoleic and linolenic acids, are the source for the manufacture of prostaglandins, which prevent cramping of muscles and blood vessels. Good sources of EFAs are raw seeds, especially flax seed, nuts, salmon, mackerel, and trout. They can also be taken as dietary supplements.

HERBS. 100 milligrams per day maximum dose of fennel, anise, blessed thistle, black cohosh, and false unicorn root works to restore hormonal balance. You can also use white willow bark and meadowsweet to reduce pain, fever, cramps, and inflammation of the endometrial implants. Be sure to follow the directions on the label, since these herbs can cause an upset stomach and diarrhea.

ASIAN MEDICINE Dr. Roger Hirsch, a naturopathic doctor in California who specializes in Asian medicine, says that the Chinese diagnose endometriosis by looking at the way the blood flows in the body, specifically in the pelvic cavity. This is determined by the appearance of the root of the tongue, which represents the pelvic cavity. "If a woman has endometriosis, there will be raised bumps and papillae in the back of the tongue and perhaps a greasy yellow coating," Dr. Hirsch says. "If you look at the back of your tongue in the mirror and see raised bumps that are red and fiery, especially during the time of menstruation, you may well have endometriosis."

HELLERWORK Hellerwork is a bodywork technique derived from Rolfing. Both modalities use deep tissue work to improve body structure, but Hellerwork is different in that it is not painful. Certified Hellerwork practitioner Sarah Suatoni gives an overview of the process: "There are three components to

Hellerwork. There is a hands-on part, which feels much like a massage; a movement educational aspect; and a mind-body dialogue aspect.

"In the hands-on process, we analyze the body much as a chiropractor would, looking at the posture, or the structure, as we call it, to determine which parts of the body are out of balance. We look to see which myofascial tissue connections are creating this misalignment. Then we work with our hands to release it.

"The second part of the work is movement education, in which we do very simple everyday movements. We look at how a person sits or stands. In the case of computer programmers, we look at how they sit at the computer and use their arms. We look at whatever it is that may be contributing to the dysfunction in the body, and then we begin to look at how we can have the person move in a way that will not create the same problem.

"Last but certainly not least is mind-body dialogue. We work under the belief that our emotional patterns, memories, and attitudes are reflected in our bodies. In the same way one needs to look at a movement pattern in order to shift some sort of physical dysfunction, one needs to look at emotional patterns or beliefs in order to shift those as well.

"This work is a process where people come in for 11 sessions. Once a week for an hour and a half is ideal, although other time frames are possible. Each session touches upon a different part of the body and different aspects of the being."

Suatoni tells how she began using Hellerwork to treat endometriosis and similar chronic conditions: "I met Dr. David Kauffman, a urologist, who determined that women with interstitial cystitis had severe spasm of the pelvic muscles. He has since started working with patients with endometriosis, vulvodynia, vestibulitis, and a number of other conditions that show the same symptoms of severe spasm or contraction. Dr. Kauffman was using biofeedback and felt that he needed someone who did hands-on work to accompany the biofeedback treatments. That's how I began.

"Although this process deals with mind-body relationships, this does not imply that these diseases are imaginary. Some women have been told for years that their disease is all in their head, when there are all kinds of physical evidence for the disease. Rather, the disease is the result of a set of relationships between the mind and body. Hellerwork and other forms of bodywork help because they are process-oriented and look at relationships. Once women start understanding these relationships, they find that they have a whole lot of power to overcome disease and regain health."

HOMEOPATHY Homeopathy is another holistic therapy that addresses underlying emotional causes. Dr. Aurigemma has been treating his patients homeopathically for 10 years and claims that the therapy is completely safe and highly effective. "There is no doubt in my mind that something actually happens and that it helps people," he says. "I utilize the remedies because I see them work. What spurs me on is the continuous improvement of most of the patients I see."

Patient Story

One woman came to see me who was on prescription narcotic medication for the pain. The medicine gave her no relief, and she was at the point of wanting a hysterectomy to get relief from the pain. I put this woman on a natural hygienic regimen for a couple of weeks. First she fasted for 5 days. Then she followed up with a nutritional plan.

Let me briefly describe a typical hygienic regimen. The patient has a breakfast consisting of a vegetable juice or a vegetable and fruit juice combination, a blended salad, a piece of fruit, perhaps some hot cereal, and a couple of soft-boiled egg yolks. Lunch is a vegetable juice or vegetable and fruit juice combination, a blended salad, a cup or a little more than that, a piece of fruit, and then some raw nuts or unsalted raw-milk cheese. For the evening meal the patient starts with juice again, blended salad, tossed salad, and steamed vegetables such as string beans, broccoli, or escarole. Then she goes on with the main course, which includes a steamed potato or yam, natural brown rice or another whole grain, and a legume. I also might supplement the meal with egg or cheese, depending on the protein needs of the woman. Of course, there are variations for individual patients.

After following this general plan, this patient was pain-free at the end of a month. That was 10 years ago. Right now she is pregnant with her second child, whereas before she was infertile. Natural hygiene has tremendous implications for endometriosis. There is absolutely no reason why a woman should have pain or be infertile because of such a simple condition.

From my perusal of the literature I can see that endometriosis is plainly a condition of liver toxicity, where the liver is failing to completely break down the estrogen hormones that the body is manufacturing. These breakdown products wreak havoc in the form of endometrial tissue in the pelvic cavity. — Dr. Anthony Penepent

55

Infections and Diseases

Herpes

Some viral infections, such as a cold or the flu, are like bad party guests you can't persuade to go home. They seem to hang around forever, although you know they will eventually leave. After a few weeks of misery, the cold and flu depart. But there are other viruses, notably herpes, which come to the party with a bedroll and tablecloth, planning to take up permanent residence.

There are a number of types of herpes. One is the common cold sore, which usually occurs before another, more aggressive virus, such as a cold, is going to take hold in the body. That's why it is called a cold sore. Cold sores on the lips are usually referred to as fever blisters. A cold sore is classified as herpes simplex virus 1 (HSV-1). A more serious kind of herpes is genital, sexually transmitted herpes, called herpes simplex virus 2 (HSV-2). There is also herpes zoster, which used to be called shingles. Finally, Epstein-Barr virus is the form of herpes that causes mononucleosis.

Michele Picozzi, a health writer who specializes in natural medicine and the author of *Controlling Herpes Naturally*, points out that there is some controversy about the relationship between the two HSVs. There is no agreement on the status of "herpes simplex 1, which occurs, technically, above the waist, most often on the face or the lips, and simplex 2, which occurs below the waist. There is a body of evidence that they are actually different viruses, and they are classified as such. However, some researchers think they are both the same virus, which acts differently in different parts of the body. This would indicate that there is merely a herpes simplex 1 that is appearing at different sites."

Herpes can be pervasive, persistent, painful, and embarrassing. It also represents a fairly serious health risk both to the individual and to the community because many people who have herpes, particularly genital herpes—that is, anywhere from 20 to 25 percent—don't know they have the disease, since they don't experience symptoms. Even without symptoms, they can transmit the disease. Herpes is very contagious, and it has no cure.

As Picozzi notes, "Herpes has remarkable staying power. Once you contract herpes, you have it for life. It never leaves the body. It lies dormant in the nerve endings at the base of the spine. Thus the possibility of infecting people over a lifetime is considerable if there are recurrent outbreaks.

Aside from the facial and genital areas, herpes can affect the eyes and the brain, with more serious health consequences. Herpes sores can also increase a person's risk of contracting AIDS. In addition, for the numerous people who already have a diminished or compromised immune system, recurrent outbreaks of herpes can put a further strain on their immune reserves.

There is, however, some evidence that contracting facial herpes as a child lowers the risk of contracting genital herpes or even AIDS as an adult.

CAUSES Some factors involving both food and emotional and physical states can cause herpes to recur, although the exact mechanism by which this happens remains a medical mystery.

According to Picozzi, "Stress is considered to be the number one precursor to a herpes outbreak, and this applies to all types of stress: emotional, mental, or physical. Physical stress would include such things as overexertion, exercising too long, exercising in the sun, and doing a type of exercise which your body is not ready for. For example, you may be lifting weights and trying to increase your weight load. That may put a strain on the body. Stress inhibits the production of interferon, the body's antiviral agent. That's important, because herpes is a virus. Stress also inhibits the body from creating antibodies to fight off infection."

Certain foods have been found to cause herpes recurrences. These are primarily foods high in the amino acid arginine, including chocolate, peanuts, sunflower seeds, soy, and coconut. There are also some foods that raise the acidity of the blood. A high blood acidity level can irritate soft tissues, which is usually where herpes appears. These foods are sugar—that is, processed sugar—white flour, and red meats.

Exposure to strong sunlight—ultraviolet B (UVB)—has been shown to be a major factor in causing facial herpes, that which occurs on the lips, around the nose, or on other parts of the face.

Some people have a recurrence of facial herpes because there has been a trauma to the skin, for example, when they have dental work. Some people have a sensitive mouth, and so just the friction of the dentist working in that area can cause the virus to recur.

Also implicated are seasonal changes, particularly the transitions from winter to spring and summer to fall, when the body goes through certain adjustments and detoxifying periods. This can also cause herpes to recur, depending on how well you are taking care of yourself at that particular time.

Genital herpes can be sexually transmitted, and pregnant women can transmit the virus to their unborn children. Moreover, prescription drugs that lower immunity, such as antibiotics, steroids, and antidepressants, can set off an attack.

WARNING SIGNS About 50 percent of people who have recurrent infections of herpes virus experience warning signs. Medically, these signs are known as a prodrome. These sensations are usually experienced in the area where a previous infection has occurred.

Picozzi explains, "The most common of these is a tingling or an itching, twitching sensation. Some people feel heat or a crawling beneath the skin, or "pins and needles." Some feel as if they are coming down with the flu. They feel fatigued. Their lymph glands are swollen, and they have other muscular aches and pains throughout the body. These signals from the brain can last anywhere from a few seconds to a few days."

She describes some recent work on the emotional triggers of an outbreak: "The most interesting thing I have found in researching herpes is the mind-body connection. Most people with genital herpes will tell you that for them, stress is the biggest precursor for an outbreak. I have found that this connection goes even deeper. I call it the overlooked psychological connection.

SYMPTOMS Genital herpes causes surface sores on the skin and the lining of the genital area. In women, sores can appear on the cervix, vagina, or perineum and may be accompanied by a discharge or vaginal blisters. There is often a burning sensation, especially at the onset of an outbreak. Other symptoms may include urinary problems, fever, and lymphatic swelling. Intercourse is painful and should be avoided during an outbreak to prevent transmission. HSV-2 occurs intermittently and usually lasts 5 to 7 days.

As the name implies, facial or oral herpes tends to attack the skin and mucous membranes on the face, particularly around the mouth and nose. These cold sores tend to appear as pearl-like blisters. Although they don't last very long, they can be irritating and painful. Herpes zoster, the result of the varicella zoster virus, causes agonizing blisters on one side of the body, usually on the chest or abdomen. Pain is usually felt before effects are seen, the result of overly sensitive skin covering the affected nerve. The symptoms may last from a few days to several weeks.

CONVENTIONAL TREATMENT There is no conventional medical cure for herpes, although drugs are commonly given to lessen symptoms. The most often prescribed of these is drugs acyclovir (Zovirax), which supposedly reduces the rate of growth of the herpes virus. Herpes medications have many potential side effects, including dizziness, headaches, diarrhea, nausea, vomiting, general weakness, fatigue, ill health, sore throat, fever, insomnia, swelling, tenderness, and bleeding of the gums. In addition, acyclovir ointment can cause allergic skin reactions.

NATURAL REMEDIES Herpes sufferers will be glad to learn that natural remedies are often highly effective in shortening the length of outbreaks and diminishing their frequency. Here are some of the important ones to know about.

NUTRITION AND LIFESTYLE CHANGES

When herpes strikes, it is always a good idea to rest and eat lightly. Short fruit fasts, with plenty of pure water and cleansing herbal teas, can be very helpful. Good herbs to include are sage, rosemary, cayenne, echinacea, goldenseal, red clover, astragalus, and burdock root. Beneficial bacteria, such as those found in nondairy yogurt and in supplements containing lactobacillus and acidophilus, support the digestive processes necessary for the maintenance of the immune system. Other nutrients that directly enhance the immune system include garlic, quercetin, zinc gluconate, buffered vitamin C, and beta carotene (vitamin A). Bee propolis is anti-inflammatory, while B vitamins combat stress. Also good are bee pollen, blue-green algae, and pycnogenol.

Dr. Steven Whiting, author of *The Complete Guide to Optimal Wellness*, has spent a great deal of time looking at the value of lysine.

"Lysine is an isolated form of an amino acid. Herpes, like so many viruses, requires complete protein in which to replicate. The lysine molecule mimics the virus's favorite protein structure, yet it is missing several bonds that are vitally important to the virus's lifestyle. When you increase lysine in the blood, the herpes virus attaches itself quite quickly to the molecule, and then it is too late. It is unable to replicate. You can shorten the outbreak of herpes down to a matter of a few hours with this treatment. In fact, if you catch it soon enough, you can keep the outbreak from occurring."

He recommends a full-spectrum program for the management of herpes.

"First take vitamin C, which is a powerful antioxidant and should be used in the presence of all viral infections. Take 2,000 milligrams as a minimum per day. Vitamin E used topically, for example, on the lips, will relieve pressure and irritation quite rapidly. It also is a powerful antioxidant and helps prevent cross-linkage at the outbreak. Take zinc, 100 milligrams per day, and copper, 2 milligrams per day. Acidophilus is certainly very important in any viral condition because of the die-off of the viral material, which eventually has to be processed in the colon. Take four to six capsules once or twice a day. Finally, and most important, is L-lysine, which can be purchased at your health food store in isolated form. In order to achieve saturation at the cellular level, you'll need 1 to 3 grams a day, but take that only for an actual outbreak." ..However, as Picozzi notes, lysine is not useful for everyone. "Some people don't do as well as others using lysine alone to control herpes. Some dietary supplement manufacturers have come out with formulas containing lysine with some supporting herbs and vitamins that some people may find more effective."

Nervous system stressors, such as caffeine, alcohol, and hard-to-digest foods such as meat, should be avoided, especially at the onset of an attack. Foods high in the amino acid arginine, such as chocolate, peanut butter, nuts, and onions, are also associated with higher incidences of outbreaks.

Since stress promotes outbreaks, it is important to make time for activities that alleviate tension. Among the many possibilities are biofeedback, yoga, meditation, deep breathing, and exercise.

Toothbrushes should be changed frequently and completely dried before reuse to prevent reinfection. Soaking them in baking soda also fights germs.

HERBS

Picozzi also see herbs as an important part of the treatment." Some herbs are very good for building and maintaining immunity. They include echinacea and licorice root, both of which have been shown to have interferon-like properties. Echinacea also has some antiseptic qualities. It helps the body regulate the glandular system."

Also recommended is goldenseal, which is very important because it regulates liver function and in addition is reported to cleanse and dry the mucous membranes, the site where herpes often appears.

Siberian and American ginseng are invaluable in helping the body boost its resistance to stress and infection because they support the adrenal glands and the nervous system.

Tarragon is good because it contains caffeic acid, which has been found to prevent herpes. Tarragon has been shown to be beneficial for fatigue, particularly when taken in combination with lemon balm. Lemon balm has become very popular for both internal and topical use. It's best taken as a tea, two to four cups a day.

Herbs should only be taken for short periods, say 1 or 2 weeks, and under the supervision of a health care practitioner.

HOMEOPATHY

According to Dr. Erika Price, a practitioner of classical homeopathy and holistic healing, the following remedies may prove extremely helpful for cold sores:

Natrum muriaticum. When sores are on the lips, especially in the middle of the lips, the 30c potency of this remedy should be taken twice a day.

Phosphorus. Cold sores that manifest above the lips, accompanied by itching, cutting, and sharp pain, should be treated with the 30c potency of phosphorus twice a day.

Petroleum. For cold sores that erupt in patches and become crusty and loose around the lips and mouth, petroleum is indicated. A 9c potency is needed three times a day.

Apis. Apis helps cold sores around the mouth and lips that are accompanied by stinging; it also helps painful blisters that itch and burn. A 6c potency is needed three to four times daily.

The following remedies may be helpful for female genital herpes:

Natrum muriaticum. This remedy is indicated when the herpetic lesions are pearl-like blisters and the genital area feels puffy, hot, and very dry. A 6c potency, four times a day, may be beneficial.

Dulcamara (bittersweet). Women who tend to get a herpes outbreak in clusters on the vulva or the hair follicles around the labia and vulva every time they catch a cold or get their period probably need dulcamara in a 12c potency two to three times a day.

Petroleum. Petroleum may be beneficial if herpes eruptions form in patches and the sores become deep red and feel tender and moist. Outbreaks usually occur during menstrual periods, and most often affect the perineum, anus, labia, or vulva. A 9c potency should be taken three times a day.

The following remedies may be helpful for shingles:

Arsenicum album. This remedy benefits most cases of shingles, especially when the individual feels worse in the cold, worse after midnight, and better with warmth. If taken at the onset of an attack, it is best in a 30c potency twice a day for 2 to 3 days. After the first 3 days, it is indicated if there is a burning sensation in the areas that were affected by the zoster eruptions (typically the chest and abdomen). At this point 12c, taken two to three times a day, is best. This remedy is excellent for the getting rid of the burning sensation that is often present.

Hypericum perforatum (St. John's wort). This is a wonderful remedy for any kind of nerve pain. It is indicated whenever there is intense neuritis and neuralgia with burning, tingling, and numbness along the course of the affected nerves. Take this remedy in a 30c potency, two to three times a day, as needed.

AROMATHERAPY

The use of essential oils has recently gained popularity in the United States, where they are used widely in skin and body care products. However, the medicinal value of certain oils has long been accepted in other countries, particularly France, where in many instances, their antimicrobial properties make them an acceptable replacement for drug therapy.

Aromatherapist Valerie Cooksley, author of *Aromatherapy: A Lifetime Guide to Healing with Essential Oils,* says that pure essential oils, properly used, can heal cold and canker sores. One mouthwash she recommends combines 5 drops each of peppermint, bergamot, and tea tree oil with raw honey, which is used as a carrier. This is important, as oils do not mix with water. The mixture is then added to a strong sage or rosemary tea. Rinsing with the formula several times a day balances the pH of the mouth and helps heal infections. Using this daily may even prevent outbreaks.

Additional spot treatments alleviate pain and restore health. One that Cooksley recommends involves dabbing a cotton swab with myrrh oil and applying it directly onto cold and canker sores. Another aromatherapist, Sharon Olson, dabs a cotton swab with diluted tea tree oil and places it on the cold sore to kill the virus. She follows this up later with lavender, which soothes the sore and stimulates the growth of new skin. The addition of fresh aloe vera gel further promotes healing. A side benefit of the therapy is its ability to lift the spirits. "When I get a cold sore, I get depressed," reveals Olson, "so I usually inhale some rosemary or basil to lift my spirits and clear my mind."

Sexually Transmitted Diseases (STDs)

Sexually transmitted diseases (STDs) were once a scourge that could bring death or madness. As recently as the 1940s, they were deeply feared.

These diseases now are much better understood and more treatable. However, although many people realize that there has been progress in the conventional medical treatment of STDs, what they may not know is that there has also been progress in using alternative, particularly herbal, treatments for STDs.

GONORRHEA Gonorrhea is caused by the bacterium *Neisseria gonorrhoeae*; women are far more likely to become infected than men.

Carol Dalton, a nurse practitioner, says that because gonorrhea can cause pelvic inflammatory disease (PID) and other illnesses, as well as infertility, she believes in treating it by conventional means. "We don't want women who have the infection to pass it on. Gonorrhea can occur without any symptoms for a long time, so that you might be passing it on without being aware of it. We treat this very aggressively."

The first recourse is antibiotics. However, Dr. Allan Warshowsky cautions that antibiotics must be carefully monitored. Dr. Warshowsky is a board-certified obstetrician-gynecologist whose specialty is holistic gynecology.

He says, "Most of my treatment of this disease is fairly conventional. I use antibiotics unless patients specifically ask me not to use them. But it is also important to maintain and restore gut bacteria while treating a patient with antibiotics. I use bifidum, acidophilus, and some of the *Saccharomyces* strains of beneficial yeast to maintain normal gut biosis. I think this is paramount."

He combines this with herbal treatment and psychological counseling. "It is also important, especially if a patient is having recurrent problems with STDs, to look at her relationships, because whatever is going on physically is a manifestation of a deeper energy problem in the individual. If the patient is amenable to examining these deeper problems, it can really help lead to a much more lasting cure than just taking antibiotics.

"There are certainly people I see who prefer not to have antibiotics and, then, as long as the patient is a willing partner in her own therapy and not just looking to me to cure the disease, I use some herbal products, such as echinacea and goldenseal, and other herbs and supplements that can be helpful in enhancing immunity and fighting off infection."

Dr. Linda Page, a doctor of naturopathy who is the author of *Healthy Healing*, has found a variety of herbs useful in treating STD's, including gonorrhea. She uses a combination that includes goldenseal, myrrh, pau d'arco, vegetable acidophilus, ginkgo, and dandelion. Another combination she uses is burdock, juniper, squawvine, bayberry, dandelion, gentian, and black walnut.

She adds, "You can see where we are going with these herbs. This is obviously a broad-spectrum approach—antifungal, antiviral, and antibacterial. This is because these categories of STDs seem to exhibit symptoms of all these types of infections: fungal symptoms, such as discharge; bacterial symptoms, such as inflammation; and viral symptoms, in that these infections can migrate to other parts of the body."

CHLAMYDIA Amanda McQuade Crawford, an author and health expert whose new book is called *Herbal Remedies for Women*, describes chlamydia as one of the most widespread STDs in North America. The infecting organism, *Chlamydia trachomatis*, is a one-celled parasite with a rigid cell wall. Crawford notes that Chlamydia is harder to clear up with herbal agents than some other one-celled organisms, such as bacteria and yeast, which respond very well to herbal treatment. "It often goes undiagnosed and can cause an inflammation of the cervix in women. This is why it is one of the leading causes of more serious pelvic diseases, particularly PID [pelvic inflammatory disease]."

SYMPTOMS

"Usually the first symptom is a painless bump that goes unnoticed, followed by swollen lymph glands and headaches," Crawford says. "Some women get strange fleeting pains in their joints and muscles, as well as chills, and even weight loss, 1 to 4 weeks later.

"There will be a vaginal discharge that feels like mucus but has a bad odor. There may also be pain with sexual intercourse and some spotting after intercourse. If there is spotting between menstrual periods, a woman should see a licensed practitioner to look for signs of redness on the cervix.

"Other signs that women might experience are urinary frequency and painful urination, as well as some lower abdominal pain, although these symptoms may be caused by some other conditions as well."

Dalton emphasizes that chlamydia often leads to PID. "It can go up into the uterus, the fallopian tubes, and the ovarian area and cause very serious infections and scarring and, therefore, infertility." As with so many diseases, early detection is essential. It can also cause problems in pregnancy, including premature or difficult delivery.

TREATMENT

In conventional drug treatment, antibiotics are used. Crawford explains, "Which antibiotic is chosen, if any, will depend on whether a woman is pregnant or not. There are often secondary infections with bacteria or viruses and that can complicate the picture. That's another reason why chlamydia is difficult to treat with simple remedies."

In Dalton's practice, she uses antibiotics. "We use antibiotics because of the risk factor. I think in health care you always weigh the risks versus the benefits of treatment. In this case, you see that the risk is great. Even if someone isn't concerned about fertility, you still weigh the risk of damaging the woman's immune system because you have an active infection that could become very serious. So chlamydia is one of the things that we don't really fool around with. We treat it with antibiotics; and we recheck it to make sure it's gone."

Crawford has looked into herbal treatments for chlamydia. One is the anti-inflammatory herb calendula, or marigold—not the garden variety, but the medicinal single-flower kind. Demulcents such as plantain are also useful and often combined with herbs that help normalize the hormones. As she puts it, "Sometimes a hormonal imbalance will have led to a change in the reproductive tissues, so these rectifying herbs are needed to make it possible to clear up this infection."

Herbal douches can also be of some help with reproductive infections, though, according to Crawford, they really can't get to the source of the problem. While the douche is rinsing out the infectious agent, it is also rinsing away the helpful bacteria, which is why you should be cautious about using herbal douches with any kind of infection. Still, the antimicrobial herbs used in the douches can help reduce the infectious organisms. "What we normally do," Crawford explains, "is follow each douche with a rest period, because these douches can dry out the tissue, making the irritated vaginal walls more susceptible to other infections. Even plain water douches will have that effect."

Crawford describes a douche formula that uses 2 ounces of organic grape root (also know as barberry bark root) and 1 ounce of calendula flower. Steep 1 ounce of this mixture in a pint of boiling water for about 45 minutes. Strain it and let the tea cool to a comfortable temperature for vaginal use. To this mixture, add about 7 drops of essential oil of tea tree. You can use a wire whisk to help mix them together. Make sure all the containers used are sterilized. Use this as a douche twice a week for up to 3 weeks. It's not necessary to rinse the herbs out of the vaginal canal afterward, but Crawford says that it feels very comforting to get rid of some of the bad-smelling discharge from chlamydia.

Dr. Page uses vaginal ointments to treat chlamydia. She suggests a combination of berberine-compound herbs: goldenseal, barberry, and Oregon grape. Mix this with vitamin A oil and apply directly to the cervix on a tampon.

PELVIC INFLAMMATORY DISEASE (PID) Pelvic inflammatory disease generally originates from an infection, like chlamydia, that spreads out of control. Dalton says that chlamydia is the primary cause of PID. Because PID can be a "silent" infection, someone can have it for years, without knowing she is infected. "So, it's easily transmitted. It can fester in the cervical canal, and then, when the immune system is low, can creep up into the other pelvic organs and cause a major infection."

She adds that it was a shift in birth control methods that played a big part in the rise of PID. "We really saw a lot of this disease when IUDs became popular, particularly when the Dalkon Shield was still being used. The Dalkon Shield had a multifilament string; there were multiple threads within this string, and bacteria could climb up the threads more easily, and into the uterus. The problems with the Dalkon Shield brought about a greater understanding of PID: how to develop cultures for it, how to study it, and what treatment to use knowledge of the damage that PID could do."

SYMPTOMS

PID symptoms vary; some women have very severe symptoms, other women have symptoms so mild that they are unaware they are infected. The most common symptom is pain, which ranges from a dull ache to pain so debilitating that walking is impossible. Other symptoms are bleeding, a foul discharge, cramps, swelling in the abdominal area, fever, and chills.

In addition to damaging the internal organs, PID can also result in scarring, particularly of the fallopian tubes. As Dalton explains, "This is how PID causes infertility. Even after you have cleared the infection, even if it hasn't blocked the tubes completely with scarring, the wavelike, hairlike projections that sweep the sperm through the fallopian tube to the egg and which sweep the egg up into the fallopian tube to meet with the sperm are often damaged and flattened. So that even though you may have a good, clear tube, the system isn't working properly. When this happens, it's a very serious problem, particularly for young, fertile women. It's probably one of the major causes of infertility. That's why we have to be really aggressive in testing for chlamydia and in treating it. We can clear the infection. We can give women antibiotics, but if we don't catch it soon enough, it can do all of this damage may and result in infertility."

TREATMENT

Dalton explains that once a woman is at the point where PID has really taken hold, there is severe swelling and inflammation in the entire pelvic area. To heal properly, the woman has to rest her body completely, which means bed rest. "Because whenever we are standing or walking, just because of gravity and the weight of the body, the pelvic area is impinged upon and there is a lot of pressure. So we encourage a woman to go to bed and rest while she is being treated. We get a much better response, much better healing, quicker healing, and less reoccurrence when this is followed.

"The other thing we advise patients to do is use diet and supplements to encourage healing. We use zinc and vitamins C and E to encourage good oxygenation and tissue repair. We have to remember that the antibiotic just kills the bacteria, it does not cause healing to take place. Those tissues have to heal on their own, and if you give them a little extra encouragement with extra nutrients they are going to do that in a quicker and better fashion."

HUMAN PAPILLOMA VIRUS (HPV) Different strains of HPV (human papilloma virus) cause either genital warts, warts on other parts of the body, or cervical cancer. HPV is particularly hazardous, says Carol Dalton, because it often goes undetected. "People often have no idea that they have it because it's microscopic, so it's easily transmitted during sexual intercourse. One study showed that 75 percent of a group of women and men who were tested were positive for HPV, and most of them did not realize they were infected." HPV is diagnosed in women most frequently by a Pap smear. The pap smear results come back as "atypical, suspicious of HPV" or "dysplasia, suspicious of HPV," Dalton explains. She also underlines the possible consequences of getting HPV. "It's the primary cause of dysplasia. Probably over 90 percent of the time, dysplasia of the cervix or, eventually, cervical cancer, is caused by HPV. That's why it's so important to get a proper diagnosis."

The condition of the immune system is related to the health of a woman's vaginal and cervical cells. "Clearly, a woman can be infected with this, and we know it is in her system, but she is not having any problems. It's not invading the cells and growing and changing them into abnormal ones. Whether or not a woman will develop HPV depends on the response of the immune system.

"Once a woman develops abnormal cells, we diagnose it by doing a colposcopy and biopsy of any abnormal cells. A colposcope is an instrument we use to look at the cervix, vagina, and labia. It magnifies these areas so we can actually see the cells to identify the areas where abnormal cells are present. After we have identified the abnormal cells, we do small biopsies—pinhead size or smaller. The biopsies are sent to a pathology lab where they section them and examine them under a microscope to identify the cells and see what is going on there."

TREATMENT

There are several treatments for HPV. "The typical treatment can be to do nothing and watch for a while to see if the body can heal itself and reverse the process. Cryotherapy, freezing of the cells, may be used, as well as laser therapy or a procedure called LEEP (loop excisional electrosurgical procedure), which uses an electrical wire to cut out abnormal tissue. All of these destroy the abnormal cells."

The fortunate thing," Dalton continues, "is that the vagina and cervix produce a new surface of cells about every 6 to 8 weeks. So if we can remove the cells that are abnormal, new, healthy cells will hopefully grow in. One reason it is important to remove the abnormal cells is that new cells tend to be like the cells next to them, so if abnormal cells remain in the body the new cells will grow into abnormal cells too."

The unfortunate thing is that just removing these abnormal cells often does not end the problem. As Dalton notes, "You can't kill off the virus completely, since it is in the surrounding tissue. You can't cauterize or remove the whole lining of the vagina. We only remove the cells that have become abnormal. There is a very high recurrence rate, with HPV causing the same abnormal cell growth all over again, unless you improve the woman's immune system and strengthen those normal cells."

Oral supplements of zinc, vitamin C, beta carotene, folic acid, and general B complex, along with a multivitamin-mineral, may aid in this process. Dalton says, "We recommend larger than usual doses of these because we found that the new cell growth responds well to these nutrients. Moreover, many of these are antiviral nutrients. They help the woman's body fight the virus more readily and more systematically.

"We also use vitamin A suppositories. There's been a fair amount of work done on how cervical dysplasia can be treated with topical vitamin A. There are also suppositories we use called papillo suppositories that are made to fight the HPV virus topically. With these, we are treating the whole vaginal area and not just the cells that have become abnormal. We also use something called formula W, for wart virus, that contains herbs that help fight the HPV virus."

Her clinic uses both oral and topical treatments. They also examine patients' stress levels, their diet, and their lifestyle issues. This seems to be a successful approach, since, she maintains, "We have about a 1 to 2 percent recurrence rate with HPV, while the national average, when conventional methods are used exclusively, is 10 to 15 percent recurrence. So we feel that treating the whole person has made a huge difference in our ability to prevent recurrence, which is really the issue. HPV is not so hard to treat initially, but it's keeping it from coming back that is really the problem. I would encourage women who have this problem to look at the whole person."

HIV and AIDS have created a further difficulty in treatment." We've had to be very careful about screening for HIV and AIDS and treating those patients," Dalton points out, "because the immune system with HIV is so compromised that if a woman with HIV does contract HPV, it seems to grow at a very rapid rate. The cells can turn into cancerous cells much more easily on the vulva, labia, cervix and vagina. Practitioners treating patients who have HIV and AIDS need to be extremely cautious in doing colposcopies and biopsies. Even more than with the average patient, be aggressive with treatment and in building the immune system. Because having these other problems will greatly increase the risk factor of the abnormal cells turning into cancerous cells."

GENITAL WARTS Genital warts are caused by HPV. Symptoms of genital warts can take as little as 3 weeks and as long as 8 months to develop after exposure to the virus. Genital warts are contagious, even before they become symptomatic.

Dr. Page treats genital warts successfully with vitamin C therapy. "Up to 10,000 mg daily is used to enhance white blood cell activity and boost immune interferon. We use a mix of carotenes up to 200,000 IU daily." She also uses aloe vera gel as a topical application for genital warts. She particularly recommends an aloe vera/garlic mixture. "You steep garlic cloves in the aloe vera gel, so you have a very high sulfur mix. We ask patients to drink two glasses of aloe vera juice daily. We also use a 'vag-pack' for genital warts, which includes goldenseal, burdock, chaparral, and sarsaparilla. Blend the herbs and put them on a tampon and insert into the vagina. This is an internal poultice to draw out the infection. It is very effective, especially when you add B complex with extra folic acid. Both these supplements help normalize those abnormal cells." She adds, "This is a virus, so you would want to take antiviral herbs. The ones I use regularly are lomatium, St. John's wort, and bupleurum. Occasionally, I also use myrrh. Any combination of these works. It's best to use them in an extract if you want antiviral activity."

Dr. Warshowsky notes that genital warts should be treated creatively and holistically. "When a woman is willing to do an entire body-balancing protocol, where she is looking at what is going on in her life that is making her susceptible to infection, balancing out her gut bacteria, eating a nutrient-rich diet, and employing some of these beneficial herbs and supplements, I think there is good success in restoring order, restoring balance, and getting rid of infection."

Lupus

Lupus, or systemic lupus erythematosis, is an autoimmune disorder of the connective tissues that affects eight times more women than men. Lupus is the Latin word for "wolf," and erythema means "redness"; the typical red skin sores caused by the disorder are said to resemble a wolf's bite. Lupus can be mild or life-threatening; it affects 1 out of 130 women between the ages of 20 and 40.

Females of African, Native American, and Asian descent develop the condition more frequently than those of European ancestry.

Lupus occurs when antigen-antibody cell complexes circulating through the body are deposited in various body tissues such as the kidney and skin, causing inflammation. Symptoms may be exacerbated by infections, extreme stress, antibiotics, and certain other drugs. Although the exact cause of this disease is unknown, hormones are believed to aggravate it, particularly estrogen, which is why so many women are affected. According to an article by Anthony di Fabio, of the Arthritis Trust of America, which is posted on my website (www.garynull.com), lupus seems to be related to the use of estrogen therapy, indicating that it may be to some extent hormone-dependent.

SYMPTOMS Initial signs include arthritis, a red "butterfly" rash across the bridge of the nose and on the cheeks, weakness, prolonged and extreme fatigue, and weight loss. There may also be fever over 100 degrees, light sensitivity, skin sores on the neck, hair loss, chest pain, Raynaud's disease (a constriction of circulation in the extremities that causes fingers to turn white or blue in the cold), joint pain, muscle inflammation, anger, depression, and anemia. If the central nervous system is involved, seizures may occur.

Additional symptoms include mouth or nose ulcers and a nail fungus, which is an outgrowth of infection by *Candida albicans*. Often lupus sufferers have headaches. The characteristic skin sores are raised reddish patches that become scaly and crusted. When they fall off, they leave white scars. If these sores spread to other tissues in the body, tissue wasting may occur.

Lupus may begin abruptly with a fever, or slowly, with infrequent flare-ups. Those whose symptoms appear only in the skin have a better prognosis, while those whose kidneys and brains are affected have a poorer prognosis. In some patients, many different organs—lungs, heart, kidneys—are affected.

TRADITIONAL TREATMENT Mild cases of lupus are treated with nonsteroidal anti-inflammatory and analgesic drugs such as aspirin, ibuprofen, indomethacin, and sometimes phenylbutazone. Prednisone, a form of cortisone, may be given for arthritis and muscle aches. In severe cases of lupus, steroidal drugs are prescribed for internal and external use. However, long-term use of these medications can damage the liver and weaken the bones. Steroids depress the immune system, leaving the body vulnerable to infection.

For both mild and severe forms of lupus, says Anthony di Fabio, traditional treatments only relieve symptoms; they do not get at its causes.

NATURAL THERAPIES Alternative practitioners have successfully treated lupus with a variety of therapies, generally based on changes in diet and appropriate supplementation.

HERBS AND SUPPLEMENTS

To lessen inflammation, use pycnogenol, cat's claw, black walnut, omega-3 fatty acids, and flaxseed oil. Pau d'arco and aloe vera juice act as blood cleansers. A good nervous system tonic is gotu kola. Colloidal silver is antibacterial, antifungal, and antiarthritic.

According to Dr. Jonathan Wright, a physician and nutritionist from Washington, writing in the December 1995 issue of *Nutrition and Healing*, vitamin B_6, up to 500 milligrams three times a day, will help relieve symptoms. People with lupus also need supplementation with hydrochloric acid. He adds, "All lupus patients have food allergies, and will improve when this condition is handled." In addition, over half of women have low levels of DHEA and testosterone and need to take these hormones as supplements.

INTRAVENOUS THERAPIES

According to di Fabio, Dr. Ronald M. Davis of Texas reports success treating lupus patients using EDTA (edetate calcium disodium) chelation therapy with DMSO (dimethyl sulfoxide, an antioxidant), and intravenous hydrogen peroxide. Dr. Davis initiates treatment of lupus and other autoimmune diseases by giving antifungal drugs such as metronidazole, since it appears that some antibodies related to autoimmune disease are produced in response to fungal microorganisms found to be present in such diseases.

ACUPUNCTURE

Acupuncturist and massage therapist Gina Michaels, of New York City, explains that she individualizes her acupuncture treatments according to each patient's unique profile: "The Chinese recognize that there are different kinds of arthritis. One type is from heat and wind, another from cold and damp. Western pharmacopeia treat them all the same, but we make a differentiation according to the symptoms that the client is displaying. Then a strategy is formed.

"Each decision an acupuncturist makes looks at the large picture. For example, if the person has a headache, along which meridian is that headache located? Is it the gallbladder channel? The stomach channel? Are they having other symptoms, such as fever or sweat? Is the central nervous system affected? All of this is very, very important in deciding what treatment protocol to choose.

"There are eight meridians formed during conception that go to a very deep constitutional level. Treating these is very useful for illnesses that are systemic or of a much deeper nature."

DIET

The Arthritis Trust of America recommends that people with lupus avoid overeating; minimize intake of cow's milk and beef; eat more green, yellow, and orange vegetables; eat nonfarmed cold-water fish several times a week; avoid alfalfa sprouts and tablets containing L-canavanine sulfate, a substance that can worsen lupus; and avoid taking L-tryptophan, which can exacerbate the autoimmune reaction.

The diet should be high in vegetables and low in grains. Wheat grass is excellent for reducing inflammation. Foods detrimental to healing include peanuts, bread, corn, soybeans, and other foods that can produce fungi and molds. In addition, alcohol, spinach, and carrots may aggravate the condition. Acid-producing foods, such as orange juice, meat, and dairy products, can also be harmful.

FASTING

Di Fabio quotes Dr. Joel Fuhrman, who says, "Having fasted over a thousand patients with various diseases I can say without hesitation that fasting is very often the only avenue that a patient can use to establish a complete remission.

"This is especially true with autoimmune illnesses like lupus, where it is almost impossible to shut off the hyperactive immune system with nutritional modifications alone, without total fasting." Fasting, he explains, is not merely a method of detoxifying. "The body clearly has the mechanism to adequately handle the removal of endogenous wastes generated in the fasting state. In fact, fasting has been shown to improve or normalize abnormal liver function." No drugs of any sort should be taken while fasting.

EXERCISE

Regular exercise is important, because it helps to keep the joints moving.

STRESS MANAGEMENT

Lupus can flare up during times of extreme stress. Working at a job one dislikes can be a contributing factor, for example. It is important for people to examine their lives and to create circumstances that promote health and happiness.

AROMATHERAPY

Essential oils can help calm the emotions and eliminate flare-ups. Rubbing tree oils such as pine and cedar directly onto the joints can diminish swelling. A drop of chamomile, lavender, lilac, or neroli can be placed on the palms and breathed in for relaxation. When there is chest congestion, eucalyptus is excellent for clearing the nasal passages and lungs.

Thyroid Disease

Thyroid disease is about 15 or 20 times more prevalent in women than in men. About 1.5 million women are being treated for it in the United States, compared to only about 100,000 men. Thyroid disease is at once a hot-button issue and one of the most misunderstood illnesses facing us today. To cite just one example of the importance of thyroid disease: 70 percent of women with infertility and miscarriage have hypothyroidism.

IMPORTANCE OF THE THYROID The thyroid gland is an important component of the immune system. Dr. Stephen Langer, who practices preventive medicine in Berkeley, California, explains that the thyroid gland is a small, butterfly-shaped organ at the base of the neck that releases about a teaspoon of hormone a year which affects the metabolism and acts as a cellular carburetor for every cell in the body—from our hair follicles down to our toenails. The thyroid can be implicated in just about any condition.

Dr. Langer says, "If a person's metabolism is hypo-functioning, everything is going to be slow. In a book I wrote called *Solve the Riddle of Illness*, I explain why upward of 40 percent of the population may have subclinical hypothyroidism and not detect it by the traditional blood chemistry work that is done at their general practitioner's office. The symptoms of low thyroid include weakness, dry, coarse skin, slow speech, coarse hair, hair loss, weight gain, difficulty breathing, problems with menstruation, nervousness, heart palpitations, brittle nails, and severe chronic fatigue and depression. "If you have a patient with a constellation of symptoms like that, they're going to be sick and tired of feeling sick and tired. Plus they're going to feel depressed all the time because they're going from one doctor to another, sometimes with two or three or four pages worth of complaints, and the doctors tell them it's all in their head, or that they should go home and learn to live with it."

Dr. Hyla Cass, a holistic psychiatrist, emphasizes the importance of thyroid inflammation, or thyroiditis, as a root cause of a variety of emotional and physical problems. She also describes the difficulty today of establishing the diagnosis of thyroid disorder in the face of continuing skepticism from conventional physicians. According to Dr. Cass, "When the thyroid isn't working properly, the immune system is impaired, and this sets up a vicious cycle. You have a person whose immune system is depleted and who is anxious; they're told by regular doctors that the problem is all in their head, that there's nothing physically wrong with them. So then they feel worse."

HYPOTHYROIDISM

SYMPTOMS

Dr. Mark Lader is the supervisor of nutritional services at the Natural Wellness Center in New York. He's been in practice for over 10 years and is coauthor of *The Encyclopedia of Women's Health: Herbal and Nutritional Health*. He describes some of the history of hypothyroidism, a disease whose prevalence and dangers were already noted in the 1970s, although, since that time, it has remained a puzzle to scientists.

Dr. Lader says, "A milestone in the study of the disease was the publication of Broda Barnes's *Hypothyroidism: The Unsuspected Illness*. Back in 1976 when she wrote the book, so many of the symptoms that so many people were experiencing—ones which appeared to have no obvious cause—were called hypothyroidism. Some of those symptoms were tiredness, sluggishness, lethargy, weakness, slow speech, dry, coarse skin, bumpy skin on the back of the arm, intolerance of cold, puffy face or hands, loss of the outer third of the eyebrow, cramping, infertility, absence of period, excessive menstrual bleeding, loss of appetite, thinning of hair on the scalp, face, or genitals, swelling of the neck, gaining weight easily, and abdominal swelling. There are so many symptoms of hypothyroidism that are related to dysfunctions in so many organ systems of the body."

Broda Barnes was convinced that as many as 40 percent of Americans were affected by some form of hypothyroidism. But the effects of hypothyroidism go even beyond the multiple symptoms recognized by Broda Barnes. According to an article in the online magazine *Alternative Medicine* (www.alternativemedicine.com), hypothyroidism can also aggravate many female problems, including miscarriage, fibrocystic breast disease, ovarian fibroids, cystic ovaries, endometriosis, PMS, and menopausal symptoms. All of these, the article asserts, can be caused or aggravated by hypothyroidism.

Although the exact cause-and-effect connection is not worked out, it is known that hypothyroidism is linked to hormonal imbalances, particularly an excess of estrogen over the other female hormone, progesterone. Normally, a woman's ratio of progesterone to estrogen is 10 to 1. If she has too much estrogen, this is bad for the thyroid, since estrogen inhibits thyroid production while progesterone promotes it. The connection between thyroid production and female hormones indicates that a disruption in one sphere will affect the other.

TESTING

In conventional medicine, hypothyroidism is diagnosed by serum testing of the hormones thyroxine (T4), triiodothyronine (T3), and thyrotropin or thyroid-stimulating hormone (TSH). The textbook explanation is that low T4 and T3 levels along with high TSH indicate hypothyroidism. Dr. Lader comments, "On the face of it, hypothyroidism seems to be a real simple illness. The symptoms and blood values seem to correlate very well to a hypothyroid case, and then when we give levothyroxin, the symptoms seem to go away."

However, these tests are not as accurate as they might seem. An *Alternative Medicine* article points out that "most of the standard thyroid tests (for T3, T4, and TSH levels) often fail to pinpoint an underfunctioning thyroid, leading physicians to make erroneous diagnoses." The article goes on to say that doctors diagnose by symptoms, even while they remain unaware of the medical cause. So a patient with depression gets Prozac; one with weight gain is prescribed a weight loss drug; and one who is continually tired is said to suffer from chronic fatigue syndrome and gets no treatment.

In Dr. Lader's opinion, the standard blood tests do little to pinpoint the actual cause of the thyroid problem. Instead, he looks at the patient's overall environment to locate key problem sectors. The first step is ascertaining the patient's body temperature.

"For my own diagnosis, I ask the women about their symptoms and also use something called a basal temperature test, which is a very simple way to learn if the body is running cold. [Basal body temperature is a person's resting temperature upon waking up in the morning.] We ask the woman to use an oral thermometer. She shakes it down before she goes to sleep at night. The first thing upon arising in the morning, she puts it under her armpit for about 7 minutes.

"The temperature should be above 97.8. If it's below that level, many doctors will say that is diagnostic for hypothyroidism. However, we must remember that some people have a lower body temperature than others. They tend to run a little cool but don't have the hypothyroid symptoms. Some people's underarm temperature doesn't even rise after they have a significant improvement in their symptoms."......Dr. Lader looks at the whole body and a person's whole environment. In his experience, most of the symptoms that people with hypothyroidism come in with are lethargy, weakness, dryness, and cold intolerance. By studying both the temperature and the patient's whole history, he is able to assess the patient's condition.

CONVENTIONAL TREATMENT

Conventional treatment relies on prescription drugs. According to Dr. Lader, on the surface, it would seem reasonable to treat the symptoms of hypothyroidism with synthroid or armorthyroid, (the natural form of thyroid), or levothyroxin. These drugs make the symptoms disappear in a high percentage of cases. "But," he asks, "are we really getting to the true causes of the problem?" He cautions that there are certain drawbacks to these medicines.

Dr. Lader explains: "We know that in conventional treatment the patient will be on the medication for her whole life. Natural doctors believe we don't need to medicate people that long. Moreover, the increasingly larger doses these people are getting over the course of a lifetime cause more and more adverse symptoms."If we look at the big picture, according to Dr. Lader, we see it's important to treat the whole body. "One of the true hallmarks of an alternative, natural practitioner is that she or he believes that eliminating symptoms is not really enough to determine if a successful therapy has been carried out." He adds, "Probably most readers realize that we have a medical tradition in this country of relegating hypothyroidism to the idiopathic trash heap. 'Idiopathic' is a term used when traditional medicine does not know what the cause is. In my opinion, though, it means we are not asking the right questions. Saying that this problem has unknown causes or ones that cannot be addressed nutritionally is really a copout. At the same time, many doctors just whip out the hormone replacement therapy prescription pad in order to treat the symptoms while ignoring the cause. To me this is sad, a sad commentary on our whole health care system in this country."

Dr. Lader notes that there are many different agents in our environment that decrease thyroid function, ranging from stress to food. And, says Dr. Lader, treating environmentally induced hypothyroidism by using hormones or drugs is an excuse for those who are not willing to do the right work to get people well. He argues that to treat hypothyroidism, "We have to use a natural approach to make the body stronger and healthier. To really give optimal treatment for hypothyroidism, we have to treat the ultimate cause of the illness. So we will have to deal with diet, nutrition, and all the environmental factors that can affect our thyroid gland."

CAUSES

Dr. Lader believes that nutritional deficiencies and stress are the two major keys to hypothyroidism. He says that although iodine deficiency or excess has been fully documented as a causal factor, in the United States, unlike other countries, iodine deficiency is not significant because most of the salt consumed in the United States is iodized.

Micronutrient deficiencies are important. Some of the major nutrients involved in thyroid metabolism are selenium, glutathione, and zinc, which are known to be required for proper conversion of T4 into T3, the form of thyroid hormone that is active in the tissues. Dr. Lader says that we also should examine protein, fat, and carbohydrate consumption to really get an idea of what's happening with the thyroid gland. With hypothyroidism, as with so many other chronic illnesses, excess carbohydrate intake can be a major contributing factor. Too much carbohydrate can push blood sugar high and stimulate cortisol production, leading to hypoglycemia, and this increases thyroid production.

Dr. Lader also notes that suboptimal intake of calories, especially in women, may contribute to hypothyroidism. Diets high in caffeine may also adversely affect thyroid function. In addition, Dr. Lader notes, "Food allergies affect our thyroid glands, and that is why we see so many people with allergies who commonly have other systemic endocrine problems in their bodies. You also have to stop and look at chemical and medical toxicity. People whose cholesterol rises year after year may have hypothyroidism."

The gut is another place where problems can start. Our bodies detoxify and eliminate thyroid hormones through the gut, where certain enzymes in a healthy intestine help to break apart the soluble thyroid hormones so that we can reabsorb them through our intestines. Many people have had a lot of antibiotic therapy, and poor diet or intestinal problems have led to imbalances in microflora. This imbalance decreases the body's ability to reuptake active thyroid hormone. It's very important to establish a healthy environment in the intestines in order to maintain normal levels of thyroid hormones.

"We also have to look at the liver," Dr. Lader continues, "which is probably the most abused, overworked, and stressed organ in the body. Our liver is exposed to a number of toxins, which we have to make soluble so that we can excrete them out of our bodies. The same enzymes that break down many environmental toxins also break down thyroid chemicals. If our livers are overworked due to exposure to toxins, and those enzymes speed up, we are also going to be moving lots of thyroid hormone out of the body. This is really the X factor in thyroid illness."

Dr. Lader says that many drugs that people take also interfere with thyroid function. These include antidepressants and interferon, which is taken to treat hepatitis C but can affect thyroid function.

ALTERNATIVE TREATMENT

"The first thing I like to have my patients do is take the underarm temperature test," continues Dr. Lader. "Women who are menstruating need to do it on day two, day three, and day four of their blood flow. Remember if the temperature's 97.8 or below, they might have hypothyroidism.

"The next step is to keep a seven-day diary, which records foods eaten, stress, symptoms, and physical conditions. This diary can sometimes convert what appears to be a very difficult case into one that's obvious by giving you an idea of what is really happening in the body."

Next he concentrates on developing a healthier lifestyle. This includes eating right. "One thing I urge my patients to try to avoid is the brassica family foods—cabbage, broccoli, cauliflower." He acknowledges that these foods have many health benefits, but says that some people are eating way too many of them, especially if they are exhibiting thyroid symptoms. Stress management is also important. One of the major problems of hypothyroidism, as noted, is inadequate conversion of inactive thyroid (thyroxine) into active thyroid (triiodothyronine). Stress elevates cortisol, which inhibits this conversion process. Heavy activity, exercise, and different stress-reduction methods are needed. One also has to take a good, high-quality multiple vitamin and eat a healthy, balanced diet.

Another aspect of treatment is nutritional supplementation. The creation of a supplement program has to be handled carefully, Lader explains. "It comes down to the fact that every hypothyroid patient is different and requires a different approach. Supplemental programs need to be customized so that they address all the factors that have been ascertained during the diagnosis and the workup. In general, we have to make sure people are taking in adequate amounts of selenium, glutathione, and zinc."

Dr. Lader concludes, "People who are suffering from hypothyroidism should view the disease as a chance to make some positive changes in their lifestyle. especially in terms of stress and toxicity."

THYROIDITIS Over the past 15 years or so, it has become apparent that some people with thyroid conditions have normal thyroid hormone levels and are suffering from another condition, known as Hashimoto's disease, or autoimmune thyroiditis.

What triggers an autoimmune response? Dr. Langer explains, "Imagine autoimmune thyroiditis to be like rheumatoid arthritis of the thyroid gland. A person can have rheumatoid arthritis, which is an autoimmune condition where the body puts out antibodies to the joints. Frequently people with rheumatoid arthritis can experience long periods of remission. When they are under a great deal of stress, the body puts out antibodies to the joints and all their joints swell up. A similar things happens with thyroiditis; if a person gets stressed out for any reason whatsoever, the body can start pumping out antibodies to the thyroid gland. The thyroid becomes acutely inflamed, and thyroid hormone which under normal circumstances would not be released starts escaping. It's almost like pumping speed into your system.

Dr. Langer notes, "There is a very precise blood test that any doctor can order called the autoimmune thyroid antibody test, and most of the people who I suspect have thyroid conditions and have normal thyroid hormone levels will have an elevation in their antithyroid antibodies. If they have an elevated antithyroid antibody level, they have the symptoms that go along with low thyroid, which can be any one of 125 symptoms that we enumerate in *Solve the Riddle of Illness*."

Like hypothyroidism, thyroiditis can cause a number of psychological symptoms. Dr. Langer explains: "With thyroiditis people get anxiety attacks and panic attacks for no apparent reason. They could be sitting and reading a book. All of a sudden they will develop a cascade of heart palpitations and fearfulness.

I've had a number of patients who have been rushed, almost on a monthly basis, to the emergency room to be worked up by cardiologists because their heart was pounding over 200 beats a minute. Cardiologists would do EKGs and echocardiograms and then tell them to go see a psychiatrist. The psychiatrist would work them up, not find anything, and then put them on an antidepressant or a tranquilizer, and actually make the condition worse. When you have an undiscovered organic basis for a psychological problem, being put on psychotropic medication is like sitting on a thumbtack and being put on pain pills for the rest of your life. It has about the same effect. It wears the system down, and as a result the patient's condition not only does not improve but will in fact deteriorate, because the underlying cause is not being treated.

"To treat patients with thyroiditis, I put them on a trial dose of thyroid and continue to monitor their thyroid hormone levels. Most of these people wind up taking between one and two grains of thyroid a day and their thyroid hormone levels still stay normal despite the fact that their levels were supposedly normal to begin with. More importantly, they get a complete remission of symptoms, many of which manifest themselves as psychological symptoms.".A large number of Dr. Cass's patients also have thyroiditis. I really can't emphasize the importance of this problem enough," she says, "because thyroiditis often accompanies the mixed infection syndrome, which can consist of any combination of the following: parasites, candidiasis, and the viral syndromes, including Epstein-Barr virus and cytomegalovirus. Psychological components include depression, anxiety, and even panic attacks.

"To treat thyroiditis, I've done nutritional consults on people that were under the care of other physicians. When I suggested that they had thyroiditis and that it was to be treated with low doses of thyroid hormones, I was met with skepticism from the other doctors.

"When people have these long-standing chronic conditions, they can become extremely depressed. They feel like they can't go on anymore, particularly when their body has been so racked by the continuing illness. Also, some of the mixed infection of thyroiditis and the parasites or other viruses can actually affect the brain directly. Thyroiditis and its accompanying infections affect the central nervous system along with every other organ of the body. So people come in extremely depressed, both as a reaction to their prolonged illness and as a primary symptom of the illness, and this is usually totally overlooked. That's why it's crucial to do a good medical workup on a patient whose disorder may at first appear purely psychological in origin."

"There is one more connection to be drawn between depression and thyroid dysfunction," Dr. Langer adds, "poor libido. One of the classic symptoms of depression is a loss of interest in sex. Those people who in the past were sexually active, but who all of a sudden or gradually started to lose interest in sex, will be diagnosed as being depressed right away. Men come into my office by the score—many of them young—who have potency problems, and they can't figure it out because they have no apparent organic illness. As a result, they get performance anxiety, and if that continues long enough, they wind up getting severely depressed. But I have found that if you go to the root cause of their depression, very often it's the thyroid that's malfunctioning.

"If a person develops an acute depression that leads to a sexual dysfunction —which it frequently does—a doctor would be remiss if he or she didn't look for an imbalance in the thyroid. Patients have got to start taking their health destinies into their own hands and demanding that doctors do thyroid testing and look for autoimmune thyroid disorders and nutritional imbalances, which are frequently the underlying causes of sexual dysfunction and depression."

WHO IS AFFECTED?

"The constellation of problems associated with thyroid disorders occurs not only in middle-aged people but also in young people, and not only in women, but also in men," Dr. Langer says. "While thyroid disease, particularly autoimmune thyroiditis, is classically considered to be primarily a disease of women, this is just not true. I have seen as many men as women who are suffering from autoimmune thyroiditis and, I might add, from hypothyroidism. Men are really given short shrift and aren't even given the requisite diagnostic tests in many instances to rule out thyroid disease because the medical profession thinks that this is strictly a woman's disorder.

"Moreover, I have seen teenagers and children who are acting out, who are written off as hyperactive, when they may be suffering from a thyroid disorder. Very young children or teenagers express their emotions differently from adults. Sometimes they get written off as being mentally retarded or having minimal brain dysfunction. Then they're given any one of a number of different drugs and placed in special classes. Many times, these young people have thyroid disorders that can be easily treated. But because thyroid dysfunction often leads to frequent infections, these kids are placed on antibiotics. Then they wind up with an overgrowth of yeast in their gut that in turn causes a low-grade inflammation in their gastrointestinal system. As a result, they don't adequately digest their food, so the body starts regarding the food as a foreign invader and puts out antibodies to the food. The child starts exhibiting the classic symptoms of food allergies, which are psychiatric complaints: anxiety attacks, depression, forgetfulness, inability to concentrate, even full-blown panic attacks.

"In a lot of these cases, you can actually isolate and eliminate the foods that cause an anxiety attack, but merely removing the food is not enough to get to the underlying cause of the disorder. Frequently patients have food allergies because of a preexisting condition in their digestive systems which has to be addressed. The presence of such a preexisting condition can cause immune system alterations which result in autoimmune dysfunction. So this is a vicious circle. One of the chief target organs of autoimmune dysfunction is the thyroid gland. You get autoimmune thyroiditis."

ALTERNATIVE THERAPIES

"The question for holistic clinicians to ask themselves, regarding each individual patient, is where they're going to intervene," Dr. Langer says. "Different physicians will intervene at different places, depending upon their background and interests. I try, to the best of my ability, to get to the root cause of what's going on. If I am having difficulty figuring out the cause, then I try to intervene at a point in a person's imbalance that will cause the least disruption to their lifestyle and give them the best results for the least amount of money in the quickest period of time. Frequently, that turns out to be treating with small doses of thyroid and altering eating habits. In my clinical experience, I have found that with the thyroid and nutritional support, very often a person will get better. The thyroid is not a lifetime treatment and can be removed after the person's condition has been stabilized. Thyroid treatment is inexpensive, works rapidly, and when done properly it is absolutely nontoxic.".Dr. Allan Spreen, a general practitioner who specializes in nutrition-based medicine, reminds us that while thyroid supplementation is an important modality, it is not fail-safe. "I'd love to say that correcting thyroid function is a panacea. While it doesn't work 100 percent of the time, if a patient comes in complaining of fatigue and depression that is linked with the physical findings of foods not digesting well, and cold extremities, then an underactive thyroid may be the root cause. People come and say, 'Oh, my husband says, "Don't touch me with your feet at night because they're just ice cold."' These are the same people who are comfortable in a room when everybody else is boiling and who are freezing in a room when everybody else is comfortable. Their thinking seems to have slowed down. They just don't seem to be able to concentrate like they used to, and they don't remember lists the way they used to.

"In this kind of a situation, once I find that their blood levels of thyroid are normal, I go back to the old school of Broda Barnes, who, 40 or 50 years ago, did axillary temperature testing. I ask my patients to keep a record of their early morning basal body temperature. If their basal metabolic rate based on early-morning body temperatures is really low, then I consider them to be candidates for thyroid supplementation. In axillary testing, Broda Barnes talked about temperature ranges between 97.8 and 98.2 degrees Fahrenheit, which is lower than the 98.6 people think of as normal. But the axillary temperature is taken in the armpit first thing in the morning, using a mercury thermometer that stays there for 10 minutes before they get up. If their temperature is, much of the time, down in the 96.8, 96.7, 96.5 range, I at least consider the possibility that the person needs low doses of natural thyroid, which is still available.

"Thyroid is a prescription drug. Some doctors who use this type of testing use synthetic thyroid. I prefer to prescribe natural thyroid in very low doses. If a person responds—either their temperature rises or their symptoms lift—then I retest them to see if their blood levels of thyroid have changed. Many times a person with this profile of symptoms who takes thyroid begins to feel better, but their blood tests remain unchanged, including levels of thyroid stimulating hormone (TSH) and actual thyroid hormone. This means that the blood testing has missed the diagnosis, and yet the person feels well with the increased, but undetectable, dose of thyroid hormone."

Patient Stories

I came to be treated by Dr. Spreen only after first following the conventional route in medical treatment. In 1988, I was in my fifth year of infertility treatments, had taken multiple infertility drugs, and wound up severely depressed, which caused me to lose 35 pounds in 2 months. I couldn't sleep, I had panic attacks, the whole horrible group of symptoms associated with depression. The doctors put me on the conventional Xanax treatment for 3 years before I met Dr. Spreen, who was helping me with some other related medical problems. I had hair loss, skin problems, nail-biting problems. I had aches all over my body, especially in my legs. Dr. Spreen got me on a vitamin regimen, which made me feel somewhat better.

Then Dr. Spreen put me on very low doses of thyroid and immediately— within 2 to 3 weeks—all the problems I just mentioned were gone. Now I had had thyroid checks three times during the whole time when I was being treated for infertility, and the blood tests had always come up negative. But I knew that in my family there were thyroid problems. There are at least six members of my family that I can think of who have thyroid disorders, but mine just never showed up on my tests. After taking these very low doses of thyroid, my skin problem cleared up, I stopped biting my nails, and my legs stopped aching. The mild depression I was still suffering from all of a sudden in August vanished. I felt great. I slept like a normal person again. I had energy. People started commenting on how I seemed to be like my old self again. It was like getting a new lease on life!

I feel rather fed up with the original doctors I went to see. They treated me like I was a hysterical woman who needed to get a grip on things. I have never told them about my recovery using alternative methods because I don't think they'd be receptive to it.—Jenny

I had hives, some kind of an allergic response, about 5 years ago and it progressed to the point where I had hives on my vocal cords. It was a pretty serious allergic reaction, for which I was first treated with antihistamines. Later, I was treated with prednisone. When small doses of prednisone given every other day didn't help, my doctor began increasing the dosage until I was taking 70 milligrams every day. After about 6 weeks I started declining physically from taking this tremendous dose. I gained about 50 pounds. I had conjunctivitis in both of my eyes. I had open sores.

I was so weak I was almost bedridden. I did find another doctor who slowly weaned me off of the prednisone. But when it was all over, my immune system had been damaged. I had a lot of viral illnesses that are usually associated with chronic fatigue syndrome. I could scarcely get out of bed, and I couldn't lose all the weight I had gained. So I went from doctor to doctor. I was living in the Midwest at the time and many of these doctors said, "Your metabolic system has been altered by prednisone. Too bad, but you will never lose that weight. And prednisone can damage the immune system. Too bad, but your immune system has been damaged." No one could offer me any help at all.

I first went to Dr. Atkins in New York and he was a lot of help to me. It was through Dr. Atkins and his association with Dr. Huggins that I learned about dental amalgams, because when your immune system is depleted you are much more susceptible to any kind of toxins, including mercury leaching from mercury amalgam fillings. It was causing me a great deal of trouble and I did have those removed.

Then I moved to California and I had heard, previous to my moving, about Dr. Slagle and her work with depression. In fact, I referred friends to her, friends I had made in California, and they had these miraculous cures from depression after 2 weeks of taking B-complex vitamins and amino acids. But I didn't think of going to her myself for quite a while because I thought of her as someone who only treated depression. In fact, like many alternative physicians, she treats the whole person. She had worked with fatigue a lot, and she first tested me thoroughly and found that my thyroid and, in fact, my whole endocrine system, was not functioning properly, most likely as a result of prednisone. She picked up subtleties in the test that other doctors ignored. She has the philosophy that a body should be healthy and whole. She doesn't need gross parameters of unusual test results to say something is wrong here. So she was able to discover that I had a rather unusual problem in my thyroid and she was able to treat it.

When I began seeing her I still had very limited energy. Even though Dr. Atkins had helped me lose weight so I looked normal, I still didn't feel normal. In one day, I could either go to the grocery store or go to a doctor's appointment. That was all I could do. The remainder of the day I had to rest. I went to Dr. Slagle and after she began treating my thyroid I had a leap of improvement. I regained my energy. She also gave me amino acids, which heightened my mood. Even though I hadn't thought I was depressed—and I still don't think I was—generally the amino acids made me feel healthier. And while I don't have the energy of a lot of people around me, I can pretty much function normally, which is a miracle. It has been a five-year struggle and I'm finally living practically a normal life.

Here's what I have learned from my experience. You simply cannot go to a traditional physician and carelessly allow that doctor to treat your symptoms with drugs. Traditional physicians tend not to look at the whole person, but to give drugs to ameliorate the symptoms, or to treat individual problems without regard to what that treatment does to the rest of the body. I learned to use tremendous caution when entrusting my body to someone. If you're going to trust your body to someone, you should know a lot about the physician. You should know whether the physician treats the whole person and sees you as more than an allergy or a gallbladder.—Helen

I recently saw a young woman who came in depressed, tired, unable to get up in the morning, and feeling overwhelmed by her work responsibilities. Her history revealed that she was often cold, especially in her hands and feet (she even wore socks to bed), had thinning hair, dry skin, constipation, and was losing the outer part of her eyebrows. I suspected an imbalance in her thyroid. When I asked about thyroid disease, she said that it had been suspected before, but her tests had been normal. I checked her thyroid hormones, including thy-roid antibody levels.

Often despite "normal" blood tests, there is an underactive thyroid. Dr. Broda Barnes's technique of monitoring thyroid function through body tem-perature is used by many alternative practitioners. Although this patient's thyroid hormone blood levels were normal, she did, in fact, have antithyroid antibodies, confirming a diagnosis of Hashimoto's thyroiditis. This is an autoimmune disease, treatable with thyroid hormone, antioxidants, and adrenal support. Her signs were those of hypothyroidism, indicating that the circulating hormone was being rendered ineffective. With Hashimoto's thy-roiditis, there are often also intermittent signs of hyperthyroidism, or overac-tive thyroid, such as irritability or heart palpitations.

I prescribed thyroid hormone from natural (animal) sources, and asked her to monitor her body temperature, so I could adjust the dosage. She asked whether this supplementation would suppress her own thyroid function, and whether she would be taking it for the rest of her life. The answer was no on both counts. The treatment actually supported her own gland, allowing it to heal. Within 10 days of starting the program she was feeling alive again.
—Dr. Hyla Cass

56

Breast Cancer and
Other Breast Diseases

Breast cancer is the most frequently occurring cancer in women. We see 182,000 new cases a year, along with 46,000 fatalities. In 1950, 1 in 20 women was diagnosed with the disease; today, the number has risen to 1 in 8. Yet even the new conventional medical treatment for preventing breast cancer —the drug tamoxifen—is basically flawed.

Causes

Dr. Michael Schachter, a complementary physician from New York, describes some of the key factors in the development of the disease.

ESTROGEN "Women whose menstrual periods start when they are relatively young have an increased risk for developing breast cancer, as do women who have a late menopause," explains Dr. Schachter. "This suggests that a woman who has a longer exposure to female sex hormones during her lifetime is at greater risk for developing breast cancer and that estrogen, the female sex hormone that stimulates cell growth, may play a role in its formation. Women who have no children and women who have children but do not breast-feed also have an increased risk. This suggests that the other female sex hormone, progesterone, may have a protective effect.

"Other known and accepted risk factors include an increased alcohol intake, a diet high in fat, being overweight, and a family history of breast cancer. This is because fat tissue can make estrogen and alcohol tends to stimulate its production. In summary, most risk factors seem to be associated with increased lifetime exposure to estrogen, decreased lifetime exposure to progesterone, or a combination of the two.

"Estrogen and progesterone tend to balance each other in the body. Excessive estrogen or reduced progesterone may lead to a condition known as estrogen dominance. The symptoms of estrogen dominance include water retention, breast swelling, fibrocystic breasts, premenstrual mood swings and depression, loss of sex drive, heavy or irregular periods, uterine fibroids, craving for sweets, and fat deposition in the hips and thighs.

"Estrogen tends to be transformed into two major metabolites in the body. They can be called the good and the bad estrogen, just as there are the so-called good and bad cholesterol. The bad estrogen, known as 16-alphahydroxyestrone, favors the development of breast cancer, whereas 2-hydroxyestrone seems to protect against it. Certain chemicals stimulate the formation of one or the other."

XENOESTROGENS "Now that we've seen that the role of estrogen is very important," Dr. Schachter continues, "this leads to a discussion of something called xenoestrogens. *Xeno* means 'foreign,' and xenoestrogens are chemical substances that are foreign to the body but behave like estrogens. These substances mimic estrogen's actions. Some xenoestrogens can reduce estrogen's effects. These varieties, which are rapidly degraded in the body, usually occur in plant foods such as soy, cauliflower, and broccoli. They protect against the development of breast cancer. Other xenoestrogens, typically synthetic ones, appear to stimulate cancer growth.

"We are living in the petrochemical era. This period began in the 1940s as a result of technological advances in the procurement of oil and the manufacture of its products. In 1940 1 billion pounds of synthetic chemicals were manufactured; by 1950 the amount had increased to 50 billion pounds; and by the late 1980s 500 billion pounds of synthetic chemicals were being produced annually. Many of these compounds are toxic, mutagenic, and carcinogenic. The majority have not been adequately tested for toxicity, let alone for their environmental and ecological effects.

"Approximately 600 chemicals have been shown to be carcinogenic in well-designed, controlled, and validated animal experiments. And within the scientific community the overwhelming consensus is that chemicals carcinogenic to animals are also carcinogenic to humans. In large-scale epidemiological human studies, approximately 25 chemicals have been proved to be carcinogenic. For each of these 25 chemicals, animal research established carcinogenicity one to three decades earlier, making the animal studies all the more significant.

"Many synthetic chemicals behave as bad xenoestrogens, particularly pesticides, fuels, and plastics. They do so in various ways. Some enhance the production of the so-called bad estrogens that I mentioned earlier, and others bind to estrogen receptors, inducing them to issue unneeded signals to increase cellular growth. Xenoestrogens may enter the body through animal fat, since they tend to accumulate in fatty tissue and tend to concentrate as you go up in the food chain.

"Xenoestrogens tend to be synergistic so that a mixture of tiny amounts of many chemicals may have dire effects."

POOR LYMPHATIC DRAINAGE Another possible cause of breast cancer is poor lymphatic drainage, which may be caused by constrictions such as those caused by wearing a bra. Dr. Sidney Ross Singer, a medical anthropologist who did graduate work at Duke University, specializing in biochemistry, has championed this point in his book *Dressed to Kill: The Link between Bras and Breast Cancer.*

Dr. Singer explains: "The lymphatic system is so underemphasized by modern medicine. When I was in medical school, there was not even 10 minutes discussion of it. Yet it is a critical part of the body."

It's the circulatory part of the immune system. It consists of tiny vessels, like capillaries, microscopic in size and originating in all the tissues of the body. They drain the tissue of fluid, toxins, debris, cancer cells, bacteria, and so forth. The blood flowing through the blood vessels delivers oxygen and nutrition through capillaries under pressure. The fluid in the blood oozes out to bathe the tissues. This fluid is called lymph fluid. It is the medium of exchange through which nutrients are delivered to the cells.

As the cells take in oxygen and food and give off their waste, some of the cell debris is flushed out through this other channel, the lymphatic system. For the breast, most of the lymph nodes are located in the armpits. These nodes are tiny factories for white blood cell production in response to infection. They filter out the lymph fluid, which then goes back to the bloodstream and through the heart.

This pattern of flow is how the body works normally, Dr. Singer says. However, "when you wear a constrictive garment, the pressure of the garment, like the elastic of a bra, presses on these tiny vessels, shutting them off and preventing them from draining. They have no internal pressure; they are passive drains. They are not like the blood capillaries, which are under pressure from the heart. As soon as they are constricted because the bra lifts the breasts and gives them a different shape—which requires pressure—there is a backup of fluid in the breast, which is a condition called lymphedema, or edema for short." This pressure and backup can cause pain and tenderness in the breasts.

Before a woman has her period, her estrogen level is very high, and this causes generalized body fluid retention. This is what premenstrual syndrome is all about, a generalized, all-over-the-body edema. That goes away after the hormones drop and the woman starts having her period. But during that time of elevated fluids she has typically been wearing the same size bra she wore all month, yet her breasts have been a little bigger. As a result of the constriction from the bra, which has become like a tourniquet, the breast cannot drain the fluid, and it backs up, causing congestion in the breast tissue.

The end result, Singer explains, is that "the cells are sitting in their own waste and debris. The pressure builds, there's tenderness, and cysts form. That's why women get cysts in their breasts. These cysts, which are filled with lymph fluid, eventually become hard. This condition is called fibrocystic breast disease. Eighty percent of American women have it, and it's because of the bra."

X-RAYS Dr. John Gofman, professor emeritus of molecular and cell biology at the University of California, Berkeley, sounds the alarm on the harmful effects of x-rays in his book *Preventing Breast Cancer.*

The effects of x-rays take years, even decades, to manifest, which is why orthodox medicine does not pay attention to this danger. Indeed, x-rays are standard practice for medical diagnosis and treatment. "The incubation time is what has led organized medicine exactly in the wrong direction," says Dr. Gofman.

"In the first half of the twentieth century medicine looked at treatments in this way: If you gave someone poison, the effects would be seen in weeks or months. They did not think in terms of years or decades. What we have learned about x-ray-induced cancer is that a very small proportion occurs in the first few years after the x-rays are administered. But most of them take 10, 20, even 50 years. Women with breast cancer who are 45, 50, or 60 are thinking, Why me? I haven't done anything wrong. What these women are not thinking about is what they were exposed to early in life."

It is not the radiation itself that persists but chromosomal damage, Dr. Gofman says. "Inside the nucleus of every one of our cells is a string of DNA organized into 46 chromosomes. That's a treasure. Damage to your chromosomes is going to be there for the rest of your life.

"A couple of years ago, I tried to answer this question—not whether x-rays cause breast cancer but what part of all breast cancers are being caused by x-rays? My estimate was about 75 percent. Everybody said, 'Oh, that's too high. It must be much lower.' Since that time I've done much more extensive work, and I have changed my numbers from 75 percent to more than 90 percent. Moreover, I now have enough data on a variety of other cancers to say that most cancers, not just breast cancer, are caused by medical x-rays."

Whether Dr. Gofman is 100 percent right or just partly right, whether medical x-rays are a primary cause of breast cancer and other types of cancer or merely an important secondary factor that until now has been ignored by our government and the medical establishment—in either case women need to recognize the seriousness of the problem and insist that radiation exposures be as minimal as possible.

DIET Earlier, Dr. Schachter gave one explanation of how fat can cause breast cancer. Here Dr. Charles Simone, director of the Protective Cancer Institute in Lawrenceville, New Jersey, gives another reason why fats generate disease: "We know that fatty foods actually convert normal cells into problematic cells. Consuming high-fat foods, particularly unsaturated fats, increases free radical production, damaging the cell membrane. At this point the damaged cell has two choices. It can die. That's fine, because if it dies, you make another one. Or it can repair itself. In the repair process, a cell can go awry and metamorphose into a cancer cell. So fats cause free radicals, which damage cells, which in turn try to repair themselves and transform themselves into cancer cells."

Robin Keuneke, a natural food counselor and the author of *Total Breast Health*, points to another factor: essential fatty acid deficiencies. These fatty acids are found, for example, in extra-virgin olive oil. Many studies have linked Italian diets, which contain lots of extra-virgin olive oil, to lower rates of breast cancer. Italian women do not have a low-fat diet, but neither do they have trans-fats in their diets. (Trans-fats are unstable, highly reactive molecules that promote free radical oxidation and therefore can have mutagenic effects. They are found in margarines and other processed oils, shortenings, and confections such as cookies and candy.) A study of the relation of trans-fats and breast cancer in 1997 found that women with breast cancer have higher amounts of trans-fats in their body fats compared with women without the disease.

Other diet choices that seem connected to higher rates of cancer are cooked meat and fried foods. Keuneke notes: "One of the theses of my book is that burned meat and fried foods are linked to breast cancer. I found four studies linking burned meat, such as bacon, to cancer. Yet although the most recent study was published in November 1998, the so-called experts said there was not enough information to recommend changes in cooking. They went on to claim there was only one study out making the connection between fried foods and cancer."

This is not true. The first study was published in 1972. It was a population study looking at Seventh-Day Adventist women, who have a relatively clean diet. It found that women who ate the greatest amount of fried potatoes had the highest rate of breast cancer.

Hot, spicy foods, oily foods, and stimulants such as coffee, black tea, drugs, and alcohol also should be avoided. Water should be pure, free from fluoride, chlorine, pesticides, and other synthetic chemicals.

TOBACCO AND ALCOHOL Dr. Simone cites two other factors as leading contributors: "We know that tobacco is the number two cause of cancer in our country and the number two cause of breast cancer as well. Regarding alcohol, we know that two to three drinks per week is enough to confer a two- to threefold risk of getting cancer of the breast independently of everything else. So the number one, two, and three causes of breast cancer—a high-fat diet, smoking, and alcohol consumption—are totally within our control."

Symptoms

The initial symptoms of breast cancer include thickening, a lump in the breast, and dimpled skin. Later on there may be nipple discharge, pain, ulcers, and swollen lymph glands under the arms.

Once breast cancer is diagnosed, the prognosis depends on the course of the disease. Dr. Schachter explains, "The staging of breast cancer involves the size of the cancer in the breast, whether it has spread or metastasized to regional lymph nodes, and whether it has metastasized to distant organs. The more lymph nodes involved and the greater the size of the tumor, the worse the prognosis. Stage zero is limited to the topmost layer, and the five-year survival rate is about 90 percent. In stage 4, in which cancer has metastasized to lymph nodes above the collarbone or has distant metastases to organs such as the liver, lungs, and brain, the five-year survival rate drops to 10 percent."

Prevention

While the possibility of a positive diagnosis for breast cancer is terrifying, it is empowering to know that there are steps that can be taken to prevent the condition, that minimally invasive treatments are often beneficial, and that it is possible to avoid a recurrence.

Before we outline the steps you can take to prevent breast cancer, let's look at one step that is highly touted by conventional medicine, but which I would not recommend. This is the use of tamoxifen. We saw earlier that excessive estrogen production is held responsible by some for breast cancer. This is the rationale for prescribing tamoxifen. However, asserts Sherrill Sellman, psychotherapist and author of the best-selling book *Hormone Heresy*, this treatment is far from the panacea it is claimed to be.

THE TAMOXIFEN DEBATE Tamoxifen has been used for over 20 years as a treatment to prevent a recurrence of breast cancer. It has been only moderately successful in preventing new tumors, but even this moderate success has come at a cost. While tamoxifen may benefit some women with breast cancer, it is also a highly toxic drug with serious side effects.

Tamoxifen, Sellman explains, "is the leading drug being given to women with breast cancer. Millions of women are on it." Tamoxifen is in a class of drugs collectively known as SERMs, serum estrogen receptor modulators. Although the way these drugs work is not totally understood, it is believed that SERMs block the action of estrogen on the breast tissue, which in turn inhibits the growth of tumors.

So how does tamoxifen prevent breast cancer? Sellman says, "The theory is that it works like a weaker estrogen." Estrogen is a major factor in the growth of breast tumors. Many but not all breast cancers require estrogen to grow.

These types of tumors have a site on the cell called an estrogen receptor. Tamoxifen competes with estrogen to reach these receptors, where it creates a barrier that prevents estrogen from binding to the cell.

In theory, then, tamoxifen acts like a phytoestrogen, although it has contradictory effects. In the breast it seems to reduce the effects of estrogen on tumor growth, yet in other parts of the body it acts like one of these estrogens, stimulating growth, for example in the uterus, where it can cause endometrial cancer. "It's unpredictable," Sellman stresses, "in the sense that we don't really know what are going to be the consequences in a woman's body."

HISTORY OF TAMOXIFEN

In the early 1980s American researchers began to speculate about whether tamoxifen might actually prevent breast cancer in women who had never had the disease. So in 1992 the National Cancer Institute initiated a $60 million clinical trial to test tamoxifen as a cancer preventative. Thirteen thousand healthy women who were at higher than average risk for breast cancer were enrolled in the trial. Half the women took tamoxifen (20 milligrams a day); the other half received a placebo.

From the beginning, the Breast Cancer Prevention Trial was controversial. Critics of the trial were outraged that healthy women would be exposed to the health risks associated with tamoxifen.

Results of the trial were made public in April 1998. At first glance, the trial results seem impressive. Women in the trial who took tamoxifen had a 44 percent reduction in breast cancers compared with the placebo group. But these results are misleading; tamoxifen also caused uterine cancer, blood clots, and cataracts. In fact, women who got tamoxifen had almost 3 times the rate of endometrial cancers and blood clots. Two prominent health groups, the National Women's Health Network and Public Citizen, have calculated that for every 1,000 women who take tamoxifen, there will be 2.9 fewer cases of breast cancer, but 2.8 more cases of extremely serious health problems. Even more important, results of the trial show there is no difference in overall survival rates or in the number of women who died of breast cancer.

In addition to cancers, blood clots, and cataracts, tamoxifen also caused strokes, hot flashes, vaginal discharge, mood changes, menstrual irregularities, and skin rashes.

In October 1998, the Food and Drug Administration (FDA) approved the use of tamoxifen to reduce the risk of breast cancer in healthy women. But even members of the FDA's own advisory committee voiced concerns about giving tamoxifen to healthy women. One committee member noted that every woman who took tamoxifen was exposed to the health risks, but only a few women would benefit from the drug.

Critics of the FDA say that approval of tamoxifen as an anticancer drug is premature. Two European studies found tamoxifen provided no benefit as a preventive measure. Still other criticism focuses on the statistical model (known as the Gail model) used to assess breast cancer risk for women considering taking tamoxifen as a cancer preventative. Opponents say this model greatly overstates risk, putting large numbers of women into a high-risk category and therefore eligible to take the drug.

HEALTH RISKS

The health risks associated with tamoxifen, some of which are mentioned above, are the same for women who have breast cancer as for those who take it as a treatment to prevent a recurrence. Tamoxifen may also cause liver damage and liver cancer. Animal studies found a link between tamoxifen and liver cancer in rats, but the results of human studies have been less conclusive.

A Swedish study looked at 1,327 breast cancer patients who took 40 milligrams of tamoxifen each day for 2 to 5 years. Comparing this group to one of the same size that didn't take the drug, it was found the tamoxifen users upped their chances for getting uterine cancer sixfold.

Strangely enough, many women's groups are supporting and advocating this treatment. Most of the time, however, these are groups that take money from the pharmaceutical industry. But other women's groups have been the primary activists opposing tamoxifen, the lead group being the National Women's Health Network. And there have been so many false reports and so much misinformation that unless you really investigate the issue thoroughly, you will very seldom get access to truthful data. As Sellman says, "It's very easy to play with results, stats, and studies to make it look like something wonderful is occurring when in fact it is a scam. This drug has the potential to be such a big money spinner. It is already the number one drug given to women with breast cancer. The industry will stop at nothing to get its drug out there. Health is not their primary concern."

DIET AND LIFESTYLE Dr. Tori Hudson, a naturopathic physician in Portland, Oregon, says, "I believe that breast cancer is a preventable disease. Just look around the world. Women in our culture have one of the highest—if not the highest—incidences of breast cancer, while women in Asia have the lowest.

"The reason is diet. To make a big story simple to understand, cultures that have a vegetarian diet or are closest to a vegetarian diet have the least breast cancer. That's how it all pans out no matter how you look at it. This implies that cultures that eat less fat, especially less animal fat, have the least breast cancer. So the big picture is really clear. Eat a lot of vegetables, fruits, and whole grains and beans. Those foods provide protection."

Letha Hadady, an herbalist and educator in New York City, visited China to learn why Chinese women have such a low incidence of breast cancer compared with American women and those in other Western nations. While diet was a big part of the picture, she learned that other factors came into play as well. To prevent breast cancer, Asians build immunity through diet, cleansing herbs, and the avoidance of pollution, stress, negative emotions, smoking, alcohol, and radiation: "They have much cleaner habits than we do." In addition, Hadady made this important discovery: "I found it quite interesting that breast cancer is considered a disease of melancholy in China. That feeling of heaviness in the chest leads to poor circulation and excess phlegm. This leads to two conclusions: Increase circulation and you have a better chance of prevention, and reduce phlegm. The easiest way to reduce phlegm is to stay away from foods such as cheese, chocolate, fried foods, and milk. You will not find dairy in the diet in China. Their diet tends to consist of grains and greens."

Certain foods are medicinal in their ability to protect against breast cancer. They include soybeans, soy products, and lima beans. Isoflavones and phytoestrogens found in soybeans, soy products, and lima beans protect against cancer. The low incidence of breast cancer among Japanese women is largely attributed to the widespread eating of soybeans. Other cancer-fighting foods include flax, fish that is high in omega-3 fatty acids (salmon, tuna, sardines, mackerel, and herring), cruciferous vegetables (broccoli, cauliflower, and brussels sprouts), mushrooms (Reiki, shiitake, and maitake), and onions.

Many herbs have been shown to help in both preventing and treating the disease. Some of these are listed in the next section.

In his book *Breast Health: A Ten Point Prevention Program*, Dr. Simone outlines the following plan for optimal breast health:

Optimize nutrition.

Take antioxidant supplements.

Avoid tobacco.

Avoid alcohol.

Avoid estrogens.

Exercise.

Minimize stress.

Become spiritually involved.

Increase your awareness of sexuality.

Get a good regular physical examination starting at age 35.

Dr. Schachter states that trace minerals play a vital role in the prevention of free radical damage: "The body contains certain antioxidant proteins, such as SOD (superoxide dismutase), which help neutralize oxidatively induced free radicals. SOD requires three minerals—zinc, copper, and manganese—to function properly. Deficiencies of any one of these minerals may predispose to oxidation damage, with a resulting increase of susceptibility to breast cancer.

"Adequate amounts of calcium and magnesium are also important. Considerable evidence exists supporting the role of selenium in preventing and treating cancer. A dose of 200 micrograms daily is safe, and large amounts may be given with monitoring. Chromium and molybdenum may be supplemented as well, and these are also important.

"Recently I have begun to use the whole range of trace minerals in colloidal form as a supplement. That's a liquid form where the minerals are bound to organic chemicals. We use about 70 different minerals. Many of these minerals are in trace amounts, have already been shown to be essential, and are probably lacking in our synthetically fertilized soil. I believe these colloidal trace minerals will play an important role in bolstering the immune system."

Alternative Treatment Approaches

REEXAMINING CONVENTIONAL ASSUMPTIONS When a diagnosis of breast cancer is made, minimally invasive therapy may be just as effective as more intrusive standard medical approaches, according to Dr. Robert Atkins, a well-known advocate of holistic medicine: "Women develop a lump in their breast and appropriately have a mammogram or biopsy which leads to the diagnosis. At this point the trouble begins. The doctor gives the patient two choices: a mastectomy or a lumpectomy with radiation. A paper just published on this reported a third option that was every bit as good regarding survival rate and life expectancy. That was simply to do a lumpectomy without the radiation."

DIET AND NUTRITION Dr. Atkins goes on to say that women don't realize that after the diagnosis and treatment there is much they can do to regain total health: "The biggest fallacy of all is when doctors tell patients after therapy that they've done all they can do and there is nothing left to do. This ignores the whole concept that people can get healthier by enhancing all their internal systems to make sure that the neoplasia, the process of forming cancer, no longer takes place. In other words, cancer is not the tumor itself; cancer is a process.

"Once you know that, you can ask, 'What can nutrition do?' You will learn that it can help in multiple ways. First and foremost, free radicals trigger the formation of cancer and the recurrence of cancer. Nutritional antioxidants can help slow down the formation of free radicals. Additionally, plant foods have antioxidant and immune-enhancing properties."

To prevent and reverse free radical damage to breast tissue, Dr. Steven Rachlin, an internist in Syosset, Long Island, New York, has his cancer patients follow this daily protocol:

Emulsified vitamin A (up to 50,000 IU)
Beta carotene (up to 100 mg)
Vitamin B_1(400 mg)
Vitamin B_6 (500 mg)
Folic acid (3,200 mcg)
Vitamin C (up to 5 g)

Coenzyme Q10 (270 mg)
Flaxseed oil (1 tbsp)
Cat's claw (1,800 mg)
Melatonin (up to 10 mg)
Shark cartilage (1 mg/kg of patient's weight)
Pycnogenol (150 mg)
Essiac tea (several ounces)
Pancreatic digestive enzymes (up to 40 g)
Aloe vera juice (9–12 oz)
Minerals

HERBS

Natural herbal substances are a veritable gold mine for treating as well as preventing breast cancer. Some herbs to know about are listed below:

CARNIVORA (VENUS FLYTRAP). This powerful herb is popular in Europe but less known in the United States. In Germany it is even used to wipe out cancer that already exists.

ESSIAC. Essiac is a Native American herbal combination that has a synergistic effect in putting an end to cancer and aiding in its prevention.

CAT'S CLAW. A cat's claw formula is used by the Peruvian Indians for the prevention and treatment of cancer.

EVENING PRIMROSE, BORAGE, AND BLACK CURRANT SEED OILS. All these herbs supply gamma-linolenic acid, which is known for its strong anticancer activity.

XIAO YAO WAN. This combination of digestive herbs increases circulation, builds blood, and breaks apart fibroids. The Chinese say it prevents breast cancer caused by phlegm and feelings of melancholy, which impede circulation to the chest. *Xiao yao wan* is available in Chinatowns throughout America.

DANDELION. Dandelion helps prevents cancer by breaking up phlegm and eliminating it from the system. Excess phlegm can turn into tumors.

ASTRAGALUS. Astragalus is a wonderful immune-system-strengthening herb that can be used in cancer prevention or as an adjunct to cancer treatments. Add a teaspoon of astragalus powder to some pure water and drink once or twice a day. Or try Astra-8, a combination of astragalus and other immune-system-strengthening remedies in capsule form that is found in health food stores.

ROSEMARY. Rosemary has been highly researched and is recommended even more than soy for its breast-protecting qualities. According to Keuneke, "Use rosemary in a vinaigrette or to marinate fish. Try to buy rosemary on a regular basis. Perhaps make a salad dressing with rosemary and garlic, fresh lemon, and extravirgin olive oil. All those ingredients are wonderful foods that are eaten throughout the Mediterranean."

MINT. Include mint in your diet on a regular basis. Mint has a phytochemical in it called limonene, which is effective in fighting breast cancer. In one study, it was found to reduce mammary tumors in animals up to 80 percent. The foods containing limonene are mint, dill, sage, celery seed, caraway, and organic citrus peel. The last item is also found in the Thai diet, which uses a lot of lime peels.

TURMERIC. Turmeric also contains a vital phytochemical that has been found to prevent mammary tumors in animals.

ENZYMES Enzymes are organic substances that help create reactions in the body, such as breaking down fats. They are linked to breathing and all the bodily functions we need to live and stay well. There are 3,000 enzymes in the body. A healthy person can produce enough enzymes to fight off cancer cells, but things such as free radicals from smoke, pollutants, junk foods, and medications interfere with enzyme production.

"So, as you can imagine," Robin Keuneke says, "there are many people who are low on enzymes. To combat this people can increase the amount of raw foods in their diet and increase fresh juice—juice all kinds of fruits and vegetables."

Numerous studies, she recounts, link enzymes and breast health. Over 90 were conducted by universities throughout the world regarding the beneficial effects of enzymes. Much of this work has been done in Germany.

EXERCISE Dr. Schachter notes, "Any activity that removes accumulated toxins in the breast reduces the chance of women developing breast cancer. Studies show that aerobic exercise is associated with decreased cancer risk, as exercise promotes lymphatic drainage and sweating helps remove toxins from the tissues.

"Although I am not aware of any direct studies showing reduction of breast cancer with a detoxification program using saunas and certain nutrients as is done with the Hubbard method of detoxification," says Dr. Schachter, "I do know that this procedure has been clearly shown to reduce pesticides and other toxic chemicals in the bloodstream and in fat tissues. Since high levels of these substances increase the risk of breast cancer in women, reducing them with this detoxification method should help reduce the risk of breast cancer to women."

MASSAGE Lymphatic detoxification is aided by manual lymphatic drainage (MLD), a simple method of massage that uses light, slow rhythmic movements to stimulate the flow of lymph in the body. Massage therapist James Kresse notes that this is especially important for women suffering from lymphedema, a condition that often occurs after a mastectomy: "When our lymph nodes are not functioning properly or have been irradiated or removed, an excessive accumulation of stagnant waste occurs. The lymph system becomes overloaded, thus forming lymphedema.

"MLD should be applied directly after surgery rather than when a massive edema has formed. This will guard against any possibility of a blockage in the system or alleviate any that exists. Studies in Europe show that severed lymph vessels regenerate with constant MLD therapy. The therapy makes the scars from the mastectomy more subtle, which increases the mobility of the arm. It also lessens pain from surgery and the uncomfortable sensitivity that occurs."

IMMUNO-AUGMENTATIVE THERAPY In the 1950s Dr. Lawrence Burton and a team of researchers discovered Immuno-Augmentative Therapy (IAT), a nontoxic, noninvasive method of controlling cancer by restoring the patient's own immune system. Although the therapy was successful, Dr. Burton left the United States after medical politics prohibited him from practicing here. In 1977 he opened the Immunology Research Center in Freeport in the Grand Bahama Islands, where thousands receive treatment for the disease.

Since Dr. Burton's death, Dr. John Clement, an internationally respected cancer specialist who studied with Dr. Burton, heads the center. Dr. Clement gives an overview of the treatment: "The intellectual basis of the treatment is that many cancers can be controlled by restoring the competence of the patient's immune system, as the body's complex immune-fighting system may well be the first, best, and last line of defense against many cancers.

"The method we use is similar in any type of cancer we treat, although each patient has her treatment tailored to the results of her own blood test. We do not deal with toxic chemicals in any way. We assay the blood for the factors we believe are aiding the patient's cancer. By identifying these factors, we are able to control them, put them back into balance, and hopefully destroy the patient's cancer."

Regarding breast cancer, Dr. Clement says: "We have had patients with breast cancer who have had no other treatment but IAT for upward of 20 years who have no recurrence of disease. While we are still claiming only to control their cancer, you will see that to all intents and purposes, by any kind of medical description, they have been cured."

Dr. Clement reports less success with patients who come to him after extremely arduous chemotherapy and those with advanced cancer where there is a loss of bone marrow and fluid collection in the abdomen or pleural effusions in the lungs.

See chapter 39 for more information on IAT.

THE MIND-BODY CONNECTION Dr. Carl Simonton, medical director of the Simonton Cancer Center in California and coauthor of *Getting Well Again* and *The Healing Journey*, firmly believes that emotions drive healing systems and that the imagination and standard counseling can be used to increase a patient's will to live. "I would like to give an example of a patient I have worked with for over 20 years," he says. "This 36-year-old woman came to me in 1976 with metastatic breast cancer that had spread to her ribs and spine. Her father was a physician, and her husband's family had run a retail store for three generations. She was involved in helping her husband run the family business.

"Her religious and spiritual life was important to her. It was a great source of strength. She wanted more time to be involved in religious administration and spiritual counseling. As she began to pursue these areas, her beliefs about how she should be the good daughter, the good wife, and the good mother came into play. These beliefs were all quite rigid, allowing virtually no freedom for her own creativity. Over time we helped her make a shift in these beliefs and behaviors that was central to her recovery.

"She has been free of disease for 15 years. Currently, she is weller than well and runs marathons. The family store burned down about 10 years ago. Now she works primarily in church administration, doing religious and spiritual counseling, which is what she always wanted to do."

Patient Stories

I have always been interested in holistic medicine, and I was a great fan of Carlton Fredericks. In 1989, when I discovered a lump in my breast, I sought help directly from a holistic doctor, Dr. Robert Atkins. I went to him before any diagnosis because I knew that if I had to have surgery, I wanted to see someone who was open-minded about alternative therapies.

The lump was malignant, and I had a modified radical mastectomy. Fortunately, my lymph nodes were clean, but the tumor was not a hormonal tumor and it was a very aggressive one.

I started therapy with Dr. Atkins that consisted of a low-carbohydrate diet. That meant absolutely no caffeine and no sugar of any kind. I was also on a program of vitamins and nutrients targeted to my specific problem. Once a week I was given an intravenous drip of an anticancer formula developed by Dr. Atkins that was largely vitamin C.

Soon after surgery I had a problem. The tumor grew back into the incision. Both the surgeon and Dr. Atkins advised radiation, which I was given for 5 weeks. While I was undergoing radiation, I did the IV weekly, and it alleviated any side effects of the radiation. I wasn't tired, and I was able to work half days.

A month or so after the radiation, the tumor came back again in the area of the incision, and again it was removed. I continued Dr. Atkins's therapy. That was almost 7 years ago, and I haven't had a problem since. I am still on the diet and the vitamin program. The intervals between the IVs have been extended to two months.

There is no question in my mind that Dr. Atkins saved my life.—Marylou

I got breast cancer 10 years ago, when I was 39. I had conventional surgery but would not undergo chemotherapy or radiation. Since I had no positive node involvement and no metastases after surgery, I was told that I was fine and that there was nothing else to do. But because it was a very large tumor and an aggressive one, I was concerned about it. Since I had been involved with natural medicine for a long time and was pretty well educated in it, I started to search for ways to prevent the return of the cancer.

I discovered a lot of things. I went on a 1-year program of injections of a formula that was mostly mistletoe. I had to get the prescription for the vials and send away to Switzerland for the formula. I injected myself with the herbal formula.

I did a lot of reading, and I took courses in Chinese herbology. I learned about several herbalists and studied with Letha Hadady over the years. I took several workshops with her where I learned about Chinese herbs and the whole philosophy of Asian medicine as well as the Ayurvedic and Tibetan systems. Over the years, I have taken formulas of Chinese and Western herbs.

The results are difficult to show concretely. All I can tell you is that I don't have cancer and that 10 years later, after having had a very aggressive kind of tumor, I am still fine.

I believe in natural medicine. I also believe very firmly that it is important to have a practitioner, to not use the local health food store as your medical adviser. Everybody has to be examined individually.—Rita

Fibrocystic Breast Disease

Fibrocystic breast disease is caused by overcongestion from foods that clog the system, such as wheat, dairy products, refined foods, and fats. Caffeinated products such as coffee, tea, chocolate, and soft drinks are hard on the body and add to the problem, as does a sluggish thyroid gland, which makes metabolism more difficult and leads to constipation, causing a buildup of toxins. Toxic accumulations worsen congestion and can manifest as breast lumps (cysts). Stress worsens the condition.

SYMPTOMS Fibrocystic breast disease shows up as single or multiple breast lumps. Cysts are usually harmless but are related to a higher than normal chance of contracting breast cancer later. Mammograms determine whether breast lumps are benign.

Drs. Ruth Bar-Shalom and John Soileau, naturopaths from Fairbanks, Alaska, add that the symptoms may also include tenderness and pain in the breast. In an article on the American Association of Naturopathic Physicians website (www.naturopathic.org) they stress the importance of learning breast self-examination and performing it every month, a week to 10 days after the menstrual period starts. This enables you to recognize the cystic areas. If you are not sure whether a lump is a cyst or something else or if there is a discharge from the nipples, consult a physician.

DIET AND NUTRITION A diet high in complex carbohydrates can make a difference; fruits, vegetables, grains, beans, and some fish are recommended. Red-hot peppers, cayenne pepper, and regular or daikon radishes cut through mucus and help eliminate breast lumps.

According to Drs. Bar-Shalom and Soileau, the most important dietary measure for reducing cysts is to eliminate from the diet all forms of caffeine, including coffee, tea, chocolate, and soda. Meat, especially the hormone-containing commercial type, should be avoided as much as possible. Finally, since constipation can aggravate fibrocystic breast disease, it is important to eat more vegetables, fruits, and whole grains and drink 8 to 10 glasses of water a day.

SUPPLEMENTS The following nutrients offer extra help when combined with a cleansing diet: selenium, vitamins A, C, and E, magnesium, and iodine drops. Iodine speeds the metabolism of the thyroid gland. As the metabolism perks up, breast lumps tend to disappear. Iodine drops from seaweed can be obtained in the drugstore in a saturated solution of potassium iodide or Lugol's solution. There is also an Edgar Cayce remedy called Atomodine. In addition, health food stores sell iodine drops in the form of liquid kelp. Before you use iodine, a thyroid blood test should be done to check for thyroid antibodies. This ensures that there is no thyroiditis, an inflammation of the thyroid gland. Drs. Bar-Shalom and Soileau suggest the following supplements:

Multivitamin.

Vitamin B complex. 50 milligrams twice a day.

Vitamin B_6.100 milligrams twice a day.

Vitamin E. 600 units per day.

Flaxseed oil. 2 capsules or 1 tablespoon a day.

Beta carotene. 150,000 units per day. If you are pregnant or of childbearing age, take no more than 15,000 units a day.

Amino acids. Take 1,000 milligrams each of choline and methionine a day to remedy the hormonal imbalance which is said to result in formation of cysts.

HERBS Herbalist Letha Hadady recommends the following plant remedies to break up congestion in the chest and release phlegm and mucus from the system before they lead to more serious problems:

XIAO YAO WAN. This formula is a combination of digestive herbs that increase circulation, build blood, and break apart fibroids. *Xiao yao wan* is available in Chinatowns throughout America.

DANDELION. Dandelion tea or capsules can be taken every day to break apart fibroids.

Dr. Bar-Shalom and Soileau recommend in addition poke root and iris versicolor taken as tinctures. Take 5 drops of each three times daily for up to 3 months. Do not take these herbs if you are pregnant.

EXTERNAL TREATMENTS

CASTOR OIL PACKS. According to the medical psychic Edgar Cayce, stimulating liver circulation ends constipation. Substances that clog the body and form breast lumps are then eliminated. To do this, rub castor oil on the skin over the liver. Cover this area with a towel and place a heating pad over it. Do this for 20 minutes each day.

PEPPERMINT OIL. Rubbing peppermint oil on breast lumps diminishes them by stimulating the circulation.

PHYTOLACCA OIL AND HYDROTHERAPY. Joseph Pizzorno has found success with this combination treatment: "We have a woman put a hot compress on her breast so that it gets real warm. She then covers the area with phytolacca oil. After the application, she covers it with a cold pack. We combine herbal medicine with hydrotherapy to help the cysts drain out of the breasts. I use that treatment with a lot of women and have had quite a good response."

HOMEOPATHY Drs. Bar-Shalom and Soileau suggest the following homeopathic remedies. Choose one based on how well it matches your symptoms and then take it under the tongue three times a day, stopping when the symptoms are relieved.

PHYTOLACCA. Use phytolacca, 6c potency, for hard, sensitive breasts or when you have multiple nodules.

CONIUM MACULATUM. For sharp pain in the nipples and for breast swelling, take conium, 12c potency.

SEPIA. When irritability accompanies breast swelling, take 6c potency.

YOGA Dr. Gary Ross, a family physician and certified yoga instructor from San Francisco, recommends yoga poses, meditation, and breathing exercises to alleviate fibrocystic breast disease brought on by stress and a sluggish thyroid. In addition, he advocates deep-breathing exercises to bring more energy into the chest area. Visualization creates a mind-set that helps make lumps disappear. Further, meditation creates spiritual and mental tranquillity that is conducive to healing.

Lymphedema

Lymphedema, a swelling of the limbs caused by an accumulation of lymph fluid, affects 1 percent of the U.S. population. Health practitioner James Kresse explains, "There are two types of lymphedema. The first is *primary lymphostatic lymphedema*, an inherent condition that predominantly affects women in their mid-30s but can manifest at birth or during adolescence. The second is more common and frequently occurs in patients who have had mastectomies or the removal of malignant tumors. The large increase in the incidence of breast cancer and subsequent mastectomy operations is one of the major reasons for the rise in lymphedema today. Secondary lymphostatic lymphedema can occur from 6 months to 3 years after the initial surgery."

SYMPTOMS Lymphedema appears as a swelling or skin thickening in a limb. It is important to detect the condition early, and this can be done in several ways. Kresse advises, "Notice any jewelry becoming tighter on the affected limb over a short period of time. Or squeeze the affected limb for 10 seconds. If an indentation is noticed, notify your surgeon immediately or measure your arm with a cloth tape measure around your wrist and forearm. If you notice an increase in the circumference of your arm, call your surgeon right away."

MANUAL LYMPHATIC DRAINAGE Lymphatic detoxification is aided by manual lymphatic drainage (MLD), a simple method of massage that uses light, slow rhythmic movements to stimulate the flow of lymph in the body. "This type of therapy is very, very light," says Kresse. "It's almost featherlike. We're working on the parasympathetic nervous system. A regular massage stimulates the sympathetic nervous system. That is our fight-or-flight nerve. The parasympathetic nervous system is our night nerve, our rest and relax nerve. This is the nerve that lymph drainage affects in order to calm the patient down."

COMPRESSION BANDAGING In addition to MLD, compression bandaging is used to apply pressure around the affected limb. Exercises performed with the bandage enhance muscular contractions that help with lymph flow.

LIFESTYLE CHANGES Kresse states, "There are dos and don'ts that a person should be aware of. Just to mention a couple, as far as the dos are concerned, the person needs to practice meticulous skin care with the use of pH-balanced lotions and creams to protect the skin. Following a good nutritional program consisting of lots of fruits and vegetables is helpful. Salt and fatty foods should be eliminated, and protein intake should be limited. It is important to maintain an optimum weight, as obesity contributes to lymphedema. Exercise such as swimming, walking, and stretching is excellent. Incorporating deep diaphragmatic breathing techniques, along with specific exercises taught by an MLD therapist, is good. While sleeping, the patient can elevate the limb by tilting the mattress or by placing pillows under the arm. Antibiotic solutions should be carried at all times for incidental cuts, scratches, or bites. Infection should be treated at the first sign.

"Precautions to take include not subjecting oneself to extreme temperature changes such as hot tubs, saunas, steam baths, and other thermal treatments. Care must be taken when using instruments on the affected limb, such as the instruments used in manicures and pedicures. Pets must be watched to see that they don't scratch or bite. Blood pressure readings, injections, vaccinations, and acupuncture should be avoided on the infected arm. Constrictive clothing and jewelry should not be worn. Heavy prostheses can cause excess pressure on the affected limb. Care must be taken when cooking, gardening, and doing daily chores. Finally, heavy objects must not be lifted. This can cause a lymphedema right away or somewhere down the line."

Other therapies that help lymphatic conditions include rebound exercise, ozone therapy, enzyme therapy, colon hydrotherapy, deep breathing exercises, and a good vitamin and herbal program.

57

Cervical Dysplasia, Fibroids, and Reproductive System Cancers

Cervical Dysplasia

Cervical dysplasia is an abnormal growth of cervical tissue caused by the sexually transmitted human papillomavirus (HPV), the same virus that is responsible for cervicitis, genital warts, and cervical cancer. These conditions can be detected with a Pap smear.

The likelihood of a woman contracting cervical dysplasia increases with intercourse at an early age, unprotected sex with several male partners, smoking, birth control pills, and weak immunity. Dr. Tori Hudson explains, "Women who have intercourse at an early age are more vulnerable to getting genital warts and cervical dysplasia because the cells of the cervix at that age are more susceptible to being infected by the virus.

"Smoking is the biggest factor in acquiring cervical dysplasia and cervical cancer. If you smoke, and you are exposed to the virus, you are much more likely to develop dysplasia, and you are much more likely to develop cervical cancer from your dysplasia. We know that nicotine actually lodges in the glands of the cells of the cervix. When exposed to the virus, the DNA can change to take on more abnormal features. If you have genital warts and you smoke, it is much more likely that they will turn cancerous as well.

"Oral contraceptives are known for creating a folic acid deficiency, and folic acid deficiency is associated with acquiring cervical dysplasia and having the disease progress to cancer."

SYMPTOMS Dr. Hudson describes cervical dysplasia as a progressive syndrome that develops over time: "After initial exposure to the virus, there is no indication that anything has changed. Later, immune changes may occur. Warty tissue may develop, then mild dysplasia, moderate dysplasia, severe dysplasia, carcinoma in situ, and then invasive cancer." Since these symptoms are not evident upon physical examination, Pap smears are necessary.

PREVENTION Since HPV is sexually transmitted, the conditions associated with it are preventable. Notes Dr. Hudson, "Cervical dysplasia, genital warts, and cervical cancer are all sexually transmitted diseases. That should make an impression on all of us, because it really dictates how we should protect ourselves.

"Obviously, we shouldn't smoke. We should protect ourselves by having safe sex and a healthy immune system. If you take birth control pills, it is advisable to take folic acid. A good maintenance dose would be 800 mcg daily. Those are the main ways to protect against cervical dysplasia and genital warts." Additional preventive daily supplementation may include 1,000 milligrams of vitamin C and 25,000 units of beta carotene.

To catch the condition early, Dr. Hudson stresses yearly Pap smear exams. Statistics show that the longer women wait between Pap smears, the higher the incidence of cervical dysplasia and cervical cancer.

DIAGNOSIS Before treatment, it is essential to get fully diagnosed to determine the stage of the illness. If a woman has an abnormal Pap smear, her partner needs to be examined by a urologist for warty tissue. Otherwise, they will pass the virus back and forth, reinfecting each other. Diagnosis by a licensed, well-trained alternative practitioner will determine whether a woman is a candidate for natural treatments only or needs to integrate these approaches with conventional methods.

CONVENTIONAL TREATMENTS Conventional medicine usually does nothing to treat mild dysplasias and genital warts. "Basically, they wait to see if it gets worse," says Dr. Hudson. "Often the body can reverse mildly abnormal states to normal on its own, as the body has an extraordinary ability to heal itself. But when it can't, then the disease progresses, and the downside of waiting becomes apparent."

In the later stages, aggressive measures may be taken. The preferred conventional treatment is known as LEEP (loop excisional electrosurgical procedure), which uses an electrical wire to cut out abnormal tissue. This is less expensive and less traumatic than the method of treatment previously used, called cone biopsy or conization. In advanced disease states, a hysterectomy may be needed to save a woman's life.

ALTERNATIVE TREATMENTS

NATUROPATHIC APPROACH

Women with cervical dysplasia often have excellent results using naturopathic approaches. Dr. Hudson notes, "In the results of a research study that I conducted at the College of Naturopathic Medicine in Portland, we treated 43 women with varying degrees of cervical dysplasia. Through my treatment protocol, 38 of the 43 reverted to normal, three partially improved, and two had no change, meaning that they didn't get better and they didn't get worse."

Dr. Hudson's protocol consists of three parts: systemic, local, and constitutional treatment. She stresses that after a woman follows the protocol for 3 months, it is important for her to once again be examined by a health practitioner and to obtain another Pap smear. Sometimes a biopsy is also needed.

SYSTEMIC TREATMENT
Beta carotene, 150,000 IU daily

Vitamin C, 3,000–6,000 mg daily

Folic acid, 2.5–10 mg daily. (Note: High doses of folic acid must be prescribed by a naturopathic physician. After 3 months, the amount of folic acid is decreased.)

Immune herbal formulation

LOCAL TREATMENT
Vitamin A suppositories

Herbal suppositories

CONSTITUTIONAL TREATMENT
Diet: An optimal immunity diet is low in fat and high in whole grains, vegetables, and fruits. Immune system inhibitors such as coffee, sugar, alcohol, and fat are omitted.

Use of condoms

Avoidance of smoking

HERBAL TREATMENT

Amanda McQuade Crawford, a medical herbalist, uses herbal infusions to treat cervical dysplasia. In her book *Herbal Remedies for Women*, Crawford also recommends herbal douches. Her favorite douche uses 1 ounce of wheatgrass juice for every 6 ounces of sterile water. If wheatgrass is not available, she recommends the following douche solution:

1 ounce marshmallow root

4 ounces periwinkle leaf

1 ounce goldenseal root

1 ounce *gotu kola* herb

Grind the herbs and mix with 4 ounces of boiling water. Strain, and allow the mixture to cool to room temperature before using.

Here's another one:
1 cup warm, but not hot, sterilized water
15 drops of thuja essential oil
1 ounce calendula oil
15 drops vitamin E oil
You can also add:
4–6 drops of blue chamomile essential oil
4–6 drops of geranium essential oil
Dilute the oils in water and mix together well.

IMMUNO-AUGMENTATIVE THERAPY (IAT)

Treating cervical cancer by restoring the patient's own immune system has also proved successful at Dr. John Clement's Immunology Research Center in Freeport in the Bahamas. Dr. Clement specifies that success can occur if the treatment is begun early, even after surgery. (See chapter 56 for more information.)

Fibroids and Uterine Bleeding

Fibroids are growths composed of muscle tissue that are usually benign. They attach themselves to the inner or outer wall of the uterus. One in five women over 35 has them; the majority of these women are African-American. These tumors grow in response to estrogen levels. Medically, they are also referred to as fibromyoma uteri and leiomyoma uteri.

Complementary physician Dr. Robert Sorge says that fibroids are nature's way of encapsulating toxins that result from an unhealthy diet and lifestyle: "Most of our patients with this condition consume tremendous amounts of coffee. As far as I'm concerned, this is something that every person concerned about their health must stop drinking. Diet sodas, greasy fries, pizza, potato chips, doughnuts and Danishes, and other devitalized foods add to the problem."

Registered nurse and licensed acupuncturist Abigail Rist-Podrecca, of New York City and Kingston, New York, adds that Asian medicine sees fibroids as the result of blockage to the uterine area: "This can be caused by anger, emotional upset, or a history of problems with menstruation, where it is either late or prolonged. Sometimes, after an abortion, the endometrial wall will still have some cells from that particular pregnancy. Further down the line, that can develop into fibroids."

SYMPTOMS Small fibroids are symptomless, but when they grow, they may result in painful periods, bladder infections, and infertility. Uterine bleeding is another common symptom, explains Rist-Podrecca: "If the fibroid is located on the inside of the uterus lining, then you will have this uterine bleeding, which usually sends women to the gynecologist, where she opts for hysterectomy. If the fibroid is located on the muscle wall, there is not so much bleeding but the fibroid will continue to grow."

Dr. Sorge adds that bleeding is the body's attempt to restore balance, according to naturopathic medicine: "Circulation and oxygenation of the uterine muscles and blood vessels are diminished, and metabolic waste products begin to build up. Bleeding is the sign of a highly toxic condition attempting to correct itself."

CONVENTIONAL APPROACH Small fibroids that do not cause problems are sometimes removed by a procedure known as a myomectomy. This procedure removes the fibroid only and does not interfere with a woman's ability to have children.

For larger tumors or fibroids that cause heavy bleeding, hysterectomies are the standard treatment. Dr. Herbert Goldfarb, a gynecologist and assistant clinical professor at New York University's School of Medicine, reports that the majority of these operations are unnecessary, as well as dangerous. In addition, hysterectomy can be psychologically destructive.

"A new laser procedure, called myoma coagulation, has the potential to end the use of hysterectomy for fibroids once and for all, but most people don't know about it," Dr. Goldfarb says. "My book *The No Hysterectomy Option* was written in response to my frustration at having a technology to help women avoid hysterectomies, but women not knowing about it. Sometimes women need hysterectomies, but often they are told they need them for frivolous reasons. My book is designed to help women understand when a hysterectomy is needed and when other options are available. I always like to say that a hysterectomy may be indicated, but may not be *necessary*. Our best customer is an informed consumer."

According to Dr. Tori Hudson, one alternative to hysterectomy is hysteroscopic surgery, which is used when a fibroid is protruding into the uterus. The surgeon inserts a hysteroscope (a tubular instrument that allows the surgeon to visualize the interior of the uterus) through the cervix and shaves away the fibroid with instruments passed through the hysteroscope. The hysteroscope is also used to shrink larger fibroids with lasers or electric currents.

An alternative for relatively small fibroids on the outside of the uterus is laparoscopic surgery. The laparoscope, an instrument used to visualize the interior of the abdomen, is inserted through an incision in the abdomen, and the fibroid is vaporized by an electric current or removed surgically, using instruments passed through the tube.

Dr. Vicki Hufnagel, using the new technique of female reconstructive surgery (FRS), has been successful in removing uterine fibroids regardless of the size or number of tumors, limiting both blood loss and surgical complications.

ALTERNATIVE THERAPIES

MYOMA COAGULATION

Dr. Goldfarb lectures extensively to doctors on this new technology, which has enabled him to successfully prevent hysterectomies in hundreds of women with fibroids and uterine bleeding. The typical candidate for this procedure is a woman uninterested in reproduction, since the uterine wall may become too weak to support a pregnancy. Also, the size of the tumor must be 10 centimeters or less (approximately 6 inches). If the fibroid exceeds this size, it can be reduced with the medication Lupron: "Lupron reduces estrogen levels in the body, and temporarily reduces the size of fibroids," Dr. Goldfarb says. "With Lupron, we get a 30 to 50 percent reduction in size."

Once the tumor has become smaller, coagulation can be performed, which shrinks it another 50 to 75 percent and puts an end to the problem: "When we do this procedure, we literally undermine the tumor by destroying its blood supply. As we put needles around the fibroid, it turns blue, showing that the blood supply has been interrupted. Fluid and blood go out, and the tumor shrinks. It becomes stringy tissue and just sits there, becoming very small, eliminating the need for removal. The patient has no symptoms and can go about her life without the need for further surgery."

DIET AND EXERCISE

Fibroids grow in response to estrogen, and so nutritionist Gracia Perlstein advocates the natural lowering of estrogen through diet and exercise as a first-line defense against fibroid growth.

As Perlstein explains, "Research shows that an over-fatty diet increases estrogen in the diet, and we know overweight women produce more estrogen. So the first approach would be dietary.

"The best diet for a woman attempting to decrease the size of her fibroids, or at the very least keep them from getting any larger, consists of whole foods and is semivegetarian or vegetarian. The best protein sources are from vegetables and include whole grains, especially millet, amaranth, quinoa, buckwheat, whole-grain oats, and brown rice.

"Eat small quantities of legumes daily. Soybeans and foods made from soy, in particular, contain isoflavones that discourage tumor growth. Foods made from soy include tofu, fortified soy milk, miso, and tempeh. A variety of other beans can be used to make wonderful ethnic dishes: black beans, adzukis, pinto beans, chickpeas, mung beans, lentils, and lima beans. Grains and beans are your best source of proteins.

"The liver detoxifies excess estrogen, so you want to support liver function by avoiding all recreational drugs, alcohol, fried foods, coffee, and any processed or refined foods. Be sure to drink at least two quarts of pure water a day to help your bowels and kidneys. You are trying to remove excess estrogen from the system, and this is supported when your organs of elimination work properly."

Exercise is also very important, says Perlstein. "Regular exercise will reduce excessive estrogen levels. Most people are familiar with the fact that hard-training women athletes sometimes reduce their estrogen levels to the point where they stop menstruating. We are not after that kind of effect, but regular exercise is very beneficial and helps the body remove excess estrogen."

For further uterine support, Perlstein recommends the following supplements and herbs:

➤Balanced oil supplement (a mixture of flax, borage, and other unrefined, natural, organic oils), 1 tablespoon daily

➤Multiple vitamin/mineral supplement

➤Iron and herb supplement. This should be taken if there is anemia from heavy bleeding. Avoid high doses of iron as they are implicated in cancer and heart disease

➤Vitamin E, 400 units, twice daily

➤Silica supplement

➤Vitamin C with bioflavonoids, 1,000 milligrams five times daily, divided over the course of the day

➤Evening primrose oil, 100 milligrams three times daily

➤False unicorn root tincture, 15 drops in a small amount of water, taken every hour, for acute uterine problems

➤Shepherd's purse tincture, 15 drops in a small amount of water three times a day, may stop excessive bleeding

➤White ash may reduce size of fibroids

Perlstein asserts that such a comprehensive program of diet and lifestyle changes, geared toward reducing excess estrogen, gives the body the tools it needs to shrink fibroids or keep them from growing any larger.

NATUROPATHIC TREATMENTS

Complementary physician Dr. Anthony Penepent recommends fasting for excessive uterine bleeding, excluding life-threatening situations where a woman needs hospitalization: "This condition signals liver poisoning. During the course of the month, a little fasting might be in order, in addition to a very strict hygienic regimen, to straighten out the condition. I have had patients with all forms of dysfunctional uterine bleeding, and I cannot remember any woman who followed my instructions who did not have a good result."

Dr. Joseph Pizzorno, president of John Bastyr College of Naturopathic Medicine, recommends oil-soluble liquid chlorophyll. He says this old natural therapy can quite effectively put an end to abnormal uterine bleeding. Oil-soluble liquid chlorophyll is available in capsules. Two to three are usually taken two to three times a day. Dr. Pizzorno says that for some reason, the chlorophyll seems to relieve this condition: "Many people think this works because it improves clotting, but it turns out that women with abnormal uterine bleeding do not have clotting abnormalities. So why it works is not clear, but the bottom line is, it works quite well."

HERBS

According to Judy Griffin, an herbalist from Texas and author of *The Woman's Herbal*, as quoted in *Positive Health* magazine, treating fibroids involves decongesting the liver by using safe herbs that can be taken over an extended period of time, including dandelion and vitex berries. Vitex is particularly beneficial for fibrocystic disease because it lowers estrogen levels.

Abigail Rist-Podrecca says the following herbs are good for stopping dysfunctional uterine bleeding when taken under the supervision of a Chinese herbal practitioner:

Poo wha. Made from bee pollen.

Er jow. From the hide of an animal.

Chuan xiong (Ligusticum wallichi). Regulates bleeding by the amount taken. Too much causes uterine bleeding, and too little stops it.

Han lian cao (Warrior's grass). Helps tone the spleen and uterus and stops intense uterine bleeding.

ACUPUNCTURE

Acupuncture points that relate to the uterus are found on the ankle. Rist-Podrecca explains how electrical acupuncture to this area helps reduce fibroids: "We use a small electrical current. This makes the uterus contract and expand. It palpates the area slightly to get the body to recognize that the fibroids are there, increase circulation, and start vibrating the fibroids so that they are released."

HOMEOPATHY

Beth MacEoin, a homeopath and the author of *Homeopathy for Women*, as quoted in *Positive Health* magazine, says that since fibroids are a chronic condition, they are best treated by a practitioner. For acute symptoms, however, a number of remedies may be effective; these must be chosen based on the specific symptoms a woman is experiencing at a given moment. "The idea is that for a remedy to be active, the remedy chosen must match the symptoms as closely as possible. So it would be very important to select that remedy with the help of either a practitioner's support or a very good, solid self-help manual."

With that in mind, consider the following remedies for uterine bleeding and fibroids:

Ipecac. Dr. Marjorie Ordene, recommends this remedy to stop acute hemor-rhaging with bright red blood. "When given in the 200 potency, every 15 min-utes, ipecac slows down the bleeding. That's two pellets under the tongue, until the bleeding actually stops. I have had success with a number of patients, and other physicians have reported this as well."

Shina and sabina. Dr. Ken Korins says the two remedies to think of first for heavy bleeding are shina and sabina. Shina is for heavy, dark blood that forms clots and leads to debility and exhaustion. Sabina is also for clots, but here the blood is bright red. When large clots are being expelled, there is a laborlike pain that radiates from the sacrum to the pubis.

Secale. Women who need secale have dark blood that is almost black. Periods are profuse and prolonged.

Phosphorus. Phosphorus is indicated when there is bright red blood with no clots.

Trillium. Trillium is indicated when bleeding is very heavy and bright red. The person characteristically feels faint and dizzy after bleeding. Periods occur biweekly, and the woman feels worse with even slight movement.

Aurum muriaticum. This remedy may reduce the size of fibroids. It should be used when there are no other symptoms, such as heavy bleeding, and there is no particular discomfort.

Hydrastinum muriaticum. This remedy has been known to cure large fibroids, especially when they seem to be on the anterior wall of the uterus, pushing on the bladder and causing symptoms of urinary frequency and pain.

Reproductive System Cancers

Women are susceptible to ovarian cancer, uterine or endometrial cancer, and carcinomas of the uterine cervix. Of the three, ovarian cancer occurs most often and is increasing in frequency. Uterine cancers are easier to detect in the begin-ning stages and tend to be more treatable, whereas ovarian cancers are rarely discovered early on, and are terribly damaging to the woman's quality of life.

OVARIAN CANCER Women who are sedentary and don't exercise have an increased risk of ovarian cancer, explains Dr. Susanna Reid, a naturopathic physician at the Center for Women's Health in Connecticut. Dr. Reid also believes that being overweight, smoking—especially if you are postmenopausal —consuming alcohol and milk, eating meat (especially fried meat), and eating a diet lacking in fruits, vegetables, and fiber also increase the risk of ovarian cancer. The drug tamoxifen is associated with ovarian cancer, and hormone replacement therapy may also increase the risk of this cancer.

Ovarian cancer usually manifests after menopause, especially in women who have few or no children, were unable to conceive, or gave birth later than the average age. Other factors that place women at risk include a past history of spontaneous abortions, endometriosis, type A blood, radiation to the pelvic region, and exposure to cancer-causing chemicals, such as asbestos.

Women should look for the following early indications of ovarian carcinomas: abnormal vaginal bleeding, weight loss, and changes in patterns of urination and bowel movements. While a Pap smear will not detect ovarian cancer in the beginning stages, ovarian cancer can be diagnosed through annual pelvic exams.

Dr. Reid emphasizes therapies to help prevent reproductive cancers. Once reproductive cancer has appeared, she believes the role of natural medicine is to help heal the body after any surgery, for, she says, most reproductive cancers are not curable with natural remedies.

"I focus a lot on lifestyle. Fruits and vegetables have been shown in epidemiologic studies to protect against ovarian cancer, so I suggest that people put a lot of fruit and vegetables in their diet. Carotenoid-containing foods appear to specifically protect against ovarian cancer, carrot consumption in particular. Vegetable fiber is also important. Green vegetables and carrots seems to have a particular affinity for the ovaries and help protect them from reproductive cancers. Cruciferous vegetables in particular are very important in increasing natural killer cell toxicity. Whole grains also provide protection."

One of Dr. Reid's guiding principles is to have people return to natural or raw foods as much as possible. She says that animal products have a strong association with ovarian cancer and recommends eliminating animal products from the diet. "That even includes yogurt, which many people think is one of the best dairy products to eat. I don't think a person can be too careful. Ovarian cancer doesn't have a very positive prognosis, so if anything, a person should do too many things rather than not enough.

"Legumes seem to help as well and also help eliminate alcohol; wine consumption is associated with an increased risk of ovarian cancer. Although green tea isn't specific for ovarian cancer, it does act specifically on breast cancer, so that might be something a woman would want to add to her diet. Also, moderate exercise increases immune function and is an important aspect of treatment."

Dr. Reid says that women with ovarian cancer seem to have a problem with the antioxidative mechanism in their bodies, and suggests using antioxidants like vitamin E and selenium to help deal with oxidative conditions in the body. Indole-3-carbonyl may also be useful. "There is a new herb called *Camptotheca acuminata* that the National Cancer Institute is studying that seems to show some promise in the treatment of ovarian cancer."

CERVICAL CANCER Cervical cancer is associated with cervical dysplasia. Although not all cervical dysplasia results in cancer, it can be the first stage of a malignancy.

Oral contraceptives and DES (diethylstilbestrol), reduced physical activity, multiple sexual partners or having the first intercourse at a young age, smoking, frequent douching, genital herpes, and multiple pregnancies are all associated with cervical cancer.

In the early stages of cervical cancer symptoms are usually absent, although there may be a watery vaginal discharge or spotty bleeding. Signs of advanced cervical cancer include dark, odorous vaginal discharges, fistulas, weight loss, and back and leg pain. One's chance of survival increases with early discovery through yearly Pap tests.

Dr. Reid warns that cervical cancer can begin as a chronic inflammation that, if not treated, becomes cervical dysplasia and eventually becomes cervical cancer. She says that cervical conditions may be related to a virus. "Natural medicine has a really good track record in treating cervical dysplasia before it gets to cancer. I would not treat cervical cancer with natural remedies. A woman would normally have the cervix removed surgically.

"To treat cervical dysplasia, we use a diet high in fiber as well as flax seeds, olives, and avocados. There is some recent research that shows that olives contain immune-enhancing substances. And of course, I recommend a lot of fruits and vegetables."

Dr. Reid also recommends using supplements and botanicals. These include folic acid, beta carotene, and vitamins E and C with bioflavonoids. She also has a six-week set protocol that utilizes suppositories. It begins with mild herbal suppositories, which she alternates with more intense herbal suppositories followed by a healing herbal suppository. In one study, 38 of 43 patients with cervical dysplasia using this treatment had their Pap smears revert to normal.

ENDOMETRIAL CANCER Endometrial cancer is associated with hormones, including hormone replacement therapy with or without progesterone, a history of infertility, failure to ovulate, the use of drugs containing estrogen, and uterine growths. Tamoxifen is one drug that significantly increases the risk for endometrial cancer.

According to Dr. Reid, other risks include not having given birth to any children, beginning menopause after age 55, being overweight, using alcohol, and eating a diet high in calories, especially when you are postmenopausal. Eating meat and saturated fats—even fat from fish, especially processed fish—and low consumption of vegetables, fruit, fiber, and legumes, are also risk factors. Other poor dietary habits that increase risk are drinking soft drinks and consuming sugar. Oral contraceptives seem to decrease the risk of endometrial cancer.

The symptoms of endometrial cancer are abnormal bleeding in the vaginal area, especially after menopause, and pain in the lower abdomen or back. A Pap smear does not always catch endometrial cancer early, but the cancer can be detected with a surgical examination of the uterus.

As with other reproductive cancers, Dr. Reid believes that endometrial cancer has to be surgically treated. "It's not something that we would ever treat in natural medicine."

Dr. Reid says that natural treatment is focused on helping the patient heal from surgery. She uses therapies that facilitate healing, such as zinc and antioxidants and anti-inflammatories such as bioflavonoids and quercetin and bromelain. The specific therapy depends on how the surgery was done. "If it was done vaginally you can use hydrotherapy treatments on the abdomen. There is a time in during which you have to be quiescent because clots are setting, so you don't want to encourage bleeding. Patients should drink lots of fluids and eat very light foods, so their bowels are minimally taxed and their digestive systems can rest as the abdomen is healing."

COMBINATION TREATMENTS Gar Hildebrand, of the Gerson Research Organization in San Diego, California, says that more patients would triumph over reproductive system cancers if a combination of approaches were employed. This is the case because contemporary treatments for ovarian cancer are disappointing. While they can make cancers disappear for weeks or months at a time, they fail in the end as the cancer returns with a vengeance to finish the job. In fact, orthodox survival rates for ovarian cancer patients are only between 5 and 10 percent.

Cancers of the uterine cervix initially exhibit higher success rates with surgery, which may involve the removal of the uterus (hysterectomy), as well as both ovaries and the fallopian tubes (salpingo-oophorectomy), in addition to x-ray and hormone therapies. But there is no guarantee that the cancer will not return. He states, "No one should be treated by a single specialty, and then watched in hopes that the cancer will not come back. It's not scientifically justifiable, nor is it acceptable to the patient. Sitting and waiting just causes horrible, immune-suppressing anxiety." Among the multiple modalities that work best for patients with ovarian and uterine cancer are nutrition, coffee enemas, hyperbaric oxygen, and Coley's toxins (see chapter 41 for more information).

Patient Stories

I still have cervical cancer, but I am working on overcoming it through a number of approaches. I watch my diet very carefully. I feel that my condition is in an early enough stage where I can handle it nutritionally. But it's not just nutrition that I have to deal with. I have to deal with all the emotions that help to create disease in the body. It's also a matter of detoxing. I do colonics and a lot of juicing. I take supplements. And I do meditation, and exercise.

The major reason I started to see a nutritionist was, of course, the wake-up call, the cervical cancer, which was just diagnosed 3 months ago. But I had also had ulcerative colitis for almost 20 years.

I feel like I now have energy again. I exercise at least several times a week, which was literally impossible before. I even had trouble getting up a flight of subway steps without feeling exhausted at the top. So I have several different things that I am working with: nutrition, meditation, and detoxification. I'm working on it.

Now I have to find a gynecologist who is holistically oriented because my primary care physician dropped me after I refused to have a hysterectomy. I feel very lucky. I feel that someone else trying to deal with this would have followed the recommended course of action and would have given up her reproductive rights, allowing herself to be mutilated, and always being fearful of having the cancer reappear.

Also, I feel that the cancer is nothing more than a wake-up call. Your body is saying, "Hey, something is wrong here. You're out of balance. You need to address this, this and this." If you don't, disease is the end result. Now I am vegetarian and doing a lot of things differently. If I didn't, I might not be alive now.

I might be at a higher risk for the cancer to spread throughout more of the body. This doesn't mean that I am 100 percent there. I still have a lot of work to do. But I feel very hopeful.—Morgan

58

Menopause

Menopause marks the end of the female reproductive cycle, which typically occurs between the ages of 45 and 50 but can happen anywhere from 40 to 60, or even earlier as a result of surgery or illness. Menopause is said to begin when a woman goes through one complete year without a period. The stage before menopause, called perimenopause, may last as long as 10 years. Many women harbor misconceptions about the nature and effects of menopause. Yet in cultures where menopause is less feared, symptoms are virtually nonexistent, and in fact menopause is anticipated as a rite of passage into a stronger, wiser time of life.

Causes

"It is a myth to imagine that the ovaries fail at menopause," says Sherrill Sellman, international seminar leader, psychotherapist, and author of numerous articles on women's health and of the best-selling book *Hormone Heresy*. "During perimenopause, the ovaries go through a last hurrah. The body is making very high levels of estrogen, trying to kick-start the ovaries so they can keep going. There is no winding down, but rather very high levels at this time, though they tend to fluctuate quite erratically, causing hot flashes.

"Nature produced the ovaries, which are endocrine glands, to keep working throughout a woman's life. There will be a reduction in hormone levels because during this period she is shifting out of her reproductive nature into a new stage of life. She does not need to be producing the hormones required for ovulation. At menopause her body shifts just enough so she is no longer able to produce eggs, but she is still producing adequate levels of estrogen to maintain the functions of her body. The two main estrogens are estradiol and estrone. The estradiol drops only about 15 percent from what it would be during perimenopause, and the estrone drops about 40 to 50 percent. But the body does continue to produce hormones.

"At menopause the outer part of the ovaries, which has been more responsible for producing eggs, begins to shrink because eggs are no longer being created, but the inner part, called the inner stroma, actually gets switched on for the first time. It produces hormones that look after the heart, blood vessels, skin, and libido, protecting the woman's body and her well being.

"Furthermore, when estrogen production by the ovaries declines, other parts of the body are switched on, such as the adrenals, which help turn body fat into estrogen. So even women who have hysterectomies, if they are healthy, are able to create enough estrogen to keep themselves vital without needing supplementation." Sellman adds that progesterone levels do seem to be low at perimenopause and low progesterone affects a woman more at this stage than does low estrogen. These levels can be assessed through saliva assay tests—which, she asserts, should be the gold standard for assessing hormone levels, not blood assay tests, which are now widely used. "Saliva tests are widely available in the United States and give accurate readings. Blood tests generally show only 1 percent to 9 percent of the hormones circulating in a woman's body, which will lead doctors to think women are deficient. It's this type of misdiagnosis that leads to mistreatment."

Symptoms

One of the first changes perimenopausal women experience is in the frequency of their menstrual cycle. The time between cycles may increase or decrease, or they may skip a month. Usually blood flow is reduced, but women may also experience heavy, irregular bleeding. Other common symptoms associated with menopause are hot flashes, dry skin, mood swings, depression, irritability, vaginal dryness, night sweats, bladder infection, fatigue, and sleep disturbances.

"Many changes appear in perimenopausal women, but the negative ones usually arise from stress, bad diet, pharmaceutical drugs, exhausted adrenal glands, and other things—not from lowered estrogen levels," says Sellman. "I believe, based on my own experience, that the symptoms of menopause—and also those of PMS, which are produced by the same imbalances—are really the result of poor health. When we can correct these imbalances, our hormones automatically go back into balance and we receive all the benefits. Women need to understand that a healthy liver, a healthy digestive system, a healthy adrenal system, and getting the colon working are the factors that contribute to healthy hormone production."

Dangers of Hormone Replacement Therapy

"Hormone replacement therapy is based on deceit," asserts Sherrill Sellman. In the 1970s, women turned their backs on supplementation with estrogen alone because it had been found to cause endometrial cancer. So the drug companies came up with hormone replacement therapy (HRT), which used a combination of estrogen and a synthetic progestin like Provera. They used a synthetic because natural progesterone, which has no toxic side effects, cannot be patented. To sell HRT to women, who were scared of hormones after the revelations of the 1970s, the companies claimed that HRT reduced the risk of a condition most women were unaware of: osteoporosis.

In the early 1990s, a new reason for healthy women to take this powerful carcinogenic steroid was introduced. HRT was said to be a way to protect the heart. A Harvard study of about 46,000 female nurses found that those who had taken HRT had a lower incidence of heart disease by up to 50 percent. However, when that study was more fully investigated, it turned out that the women with lower rates of heart disease were actually women who were healthier in general. Compared to the group who were supposed to have a greater incidence of heart disease, they were wealthier, more likely to exercise, and had better diets; fewer of them had diabetes; and they smoked less. The women who didn't take HRT were more likely to have diabetes, smoked, were poorer, and didn't visit their doctors. Also not reported in the study was the fact that the women who took HRT had a 50 percent increase in strokes. This, then, was a flawed, biased study.

By now HRT, originally supposed to be only a short-term treatment for relief of menopausal symptoms, had become a long-term treatment given to prevent other conditions, conditions which only might occur. But giving it to healthy women with no history of heart disease, to perhaps prevent them from one day getting it, is dangerous. In truth, according to Sellman, the use of hormone replacement therapy is actually killing women because it is increasing their risk of cardiovascular disease.

"Recent studies have challenged the theory that hormone replacement therapy is beneficial to the heart. A study that came out in August 1998—sponsored by Ayerst, the company that manufactures the number-one replacement estrogen, Premarin—used estrogen and progesterone in an attempt to show the benefits of HRT as a secondary treatment for the women in the study who already had some sort of heart disease. They gave half the women hormone replacement therapy and the other half a placebo. After 5 years, they discovered that in the first year of treatment, the women taking the HRT had a 50 percent increase in heart attacks. Over the 5 years, the risk decreased. The conclusion was that women who already had heart conditions got no overall benefit from HRT. But this glossed over the horrible fact that HRT increased heart problems the first year. What was more, women taking it had three times as many blood clots in the legs than women taking the placebo. There was also an increase in gallbladder disease.

"The estrogen and synthetic progestin used in HRT are not natural substances, but powerful steroid drugs. About 120 risks and side effects are associated with this combination, some of which are life-threatening, including not just heart problems but cancers of the reproductive organs, breast cancer, increased risk of diabetes, asthma, thyroid imbalance, and immune dysfunction.

The manufacturers' own package inserts warn that these drugs should not be taken by women who have current problems with or a past history of clotting, thrombosis, stroke, cardiovascular disorders, high lipoproteins (a specific type of blood fats), severe hypertension, or lipid metabolism disorders. Estrogen and progestin will increase the possibility of strokes and clotting, since they thicken the blood and raise blood pressure. And these factors all contribute to the possibility of heart disease."

Progestin also contributes to birth deformities. That is why women on the pill are told not to get pregnant. It also impairs the liver and the gallbladder, and may contribute to depression and headaches. It promotes increased facial hair, fluid retention, infertility, and miscarriage. A large number of women now have endometriosis, which is at least exacerbated, if not caused, by synthetic estrogens and progestins. Progestin interferes with blood sugar, increasing the risk of diabetes. Progestins are just as dangerous as estrogens in causing a range of serious health problems.

Another important point is that estrogen and progesterone are not just sex hormones. They regulate and influence all the systems of a woman's body, including the digestive, immune, circulatory, and nervous systems. Because tampering with these hormones has grave consequences for a woman's physiological and psychological health, it must be done with great awareness and concern. Instead, what happens is that HRT plays havoc with her physiology.

One of the more serious consequences of a prolonged excess of estrogen, as mentioned, is an increase in breast cancer. The latest finding from the Boston nurses study, which has been going on for 18 years, is that women on HRT who have been taking synthetic estrogens and progestins for 10 years or more have a 100 percent increased risk of breast cancer. The combination of progestin with estrogen was even more deadly than taking estrogen alone, for progestin, as mentioned, is also carcinogenic, associated with a higher incidence of reproductive cancers: breast, endometrial, and ovarian.

With respect to osteoporosis, Dr. Bruce Hedendal of Boca Raton, Florida, comments, "Most people are told that estrogen prevents osteoporosis. This is true to some degree. Around menopause, synthetic estrogen replacement therapy is effective for 5 to 7 years only. It slows down the bone loss, but it does not reverse it in any way, shape, or form. The studies have shown that 8 to 10 years after menopause is finished, there are no benefits to estrogen replacement therapy on bone loss."

Dr. Robert Atkins, director of the Atkins Centers for Complementary Medicine, confirms that one side effect of estrogen therapy is insulin resistance. "This syndrome is characterized by low blood sugar, high blood pressure, or high insulin levels. But the most frightening one of all to most women has to do with upper body obesity."

Natural Therapies

Natural therapies can make HRT unnecessary. I completed a year and a half study of people who went on a strict program of cleansing and detoxifying, eating no animal proteins, no meat, no sugar, no caffeine, no processed food. They exercised 6 days a week for an hour. They drank lots of fresh organic juices, sometimes as much as a gallon a day, and certain herbs.

Three women in that group who had been postmenopausal—one who had been so for 18 years and had had a hysterectomy—returned to a premenopausal state of health. Skin wrinkles were gone, energy restored, human growth hormone was back, and hormones were balanced. The gray, thinning hair of one 71-year-old woman grew back brown and thick. Another woman had a low libido, and her mucus membranes were dry, as was her skin. Her skin and mucus membranes regained moisture, and she enjoyed a level of health and energy that she hadn't experienced for years. Her toenails and fingernails, which had been brittle, yellow, and cracked, became pink and fresh. This was all without medication or any hormone replacement therapy. We just gave her body a chance to rebalance itself; we honored it by not giving it anything that would have led to an imbalance.

DIET Dr. Jane Guiltinan, a naturopathic physician from Washington, says, "A lot of women don't know that there may be alternatives to estrogen replacement therapy. There are some very good plant sources of estrogens in some of our foods. In fact, you can get significant amounts of plant estrogens. They have been shown in several research studies to improve menopausal symptoms. "The food that has the highest content of estrogen is soy. Soybeans, tofu, tempeh—anything made with soy—will contain plant estrogens. Oats, cashews, almonds, alfalfa, apples, and flaxseeds contain smaller amounts of estrogen. A woman emphasizing those foods in the diet can experience significant decreases in her hot flashes." Studies suggest that too little magnesium in the diet is one cause of hot flashes. Magnesium can be found in whole grains, beans, and soy products.

Sugar, which can cause hot flashes and other menopausal symptoms, should be avoided. Sugar, coffee, and alcohol adversely affect the blood sugar and can disturb the emotions.

Ann Louise Gittelman, author of *Before the Change: Take Charge of Your Perimenopause*, notes that weight gain, a common problem in perimenopausal and menopausal women, can be minimized by eating the right kinds of foods.

These foods are incorporated in Gittelman's Changing diet plan. "Low-glycemic, or slow-acting, carbohydrates will supply lots of energy for their calories. My favorites are those that are lower on the glycemic index, which is a list of carbohydrates ranked as to how they develop into blood sugar in your system. I like yams rather than white potatoes, and I like whole rye meal rather than wheat. I choose unprocessed carbohydrates that are moderate to low on the index, which also provide high-quality fiber to help eliminate excess estrogen from the system by lowering blood levels of this hormone.

"In addition, a number of fruits and vegetables are particularly high in phytochemicals and phytohormones. These include apples, grapefruits, lemons, pears, peaches, and a wide variety of vegetables that are high in fiber and loaded with phytochemicals.

"Fats are important on the Changing diet plan. We need to add essential and beneficial fats, not take them away. These come in the form of the high-lignan flaxseed oil, olive oil, toasted nut seeds, and avocado. These fats stabilize blood sugar levels.

VITAMINS AND MINERALS The following nutrients provide an additional boost to good health in the menopausal years:

MULTIVITAMINS. Women need a natural multivitamin/mineral supplement containing higher amounts of magnesium than calcium and high amounts of B and C vitamins. A good multiple vitamin helps build the adrenal glands, which lessens emotional symptoms.

VITAMIN E. This vitamin is known for its ability to rejuvenate the reproductive system and alleviate hot flashes. It also helps lessen vaginal thinning and dryness. Mixed (beta-, delta-, and gamma-) tocopherols are best as they are found together in nature. D-alphatocopherol is also preferred over synthetic vitamin E. Generally, 400 units per day should be taken in the beginning. The dosage can be gradually increased to 600 units, although some women may need up to 800 units.

ZINC. This mineral supports ovarian function. A good source is zinc picolinate. It can also be taken as an amino acid chelate or as zinc methionine. The recommended dosage is 25 to 30 milligrams per day.

B COMPLEX. B-complex vitamins are important throughout life, but there is an extra need for these during menopause. They can be obtained from whole grains and green vegetables. B_5 (300–400 mg/day) and B_6 (150 mg/day) are especially helpful during menopause. Folic acid, in prescription doses, is a valuable replacement for female hormones, according to Dr. Carlton Fredericks.

ESSENTIAL FATTY ACIDS (EFAS). EFAs, which are precursors to the natural hormones in the body, are very important for both men and women. People on low-fat diets should pay special attention to this. A diet too low in fats can lead to an increased risk of cancer and aging. Omega-6 fatty acids can be found in flaxseed, sesame, pumpkin, and safflower oils. Omega-3 fatty acids are found in fish oil capsules or fish. Both are needed. EFAs help prevent or treat vaginal dryness.

VITAMIN D. The best source of vitamin D is sunlight. It can also be taken in supplementation (400–600 IU/day), although caution should be taken not to get too much of this vitamin. Another source of vitamin D is salmon oil. People living in polluted environments need more vitamin D.

CALCIUM. Calcium is essential to prevent osteoporosis; supplementation should begin before the onset of menopause. There are many forms to choose from. Dairy is a poor source because many people have an intolerance to it. Calcium citrate is easy to digest, as it is already in an acidic medium. Calcium carbonates are alkaline and therefore more difficult to digest. Amino acid chelate is an excellent source of calcium. Calcium lactate is another good source. Calcium gluconate can be made into a powder and mixed into drinks; 1300 milligrams per day, from food and supplemental sources, is the recommended dosage.

GAMMALINOLENIC ACID (GLA). This is available as evening primrose oil, borage oil, or blackcurrant seed oil; 200 milligrams per day is recommended.

BORON. Research shows boron to be a precursor of both female and male hormones.

SUPPLEMENTS THAT HELP CREATE HORMONES Sherrill Sellman advocates natural progesterone, which is an identical match to what the body makes, as opposed to the synthetic progestins, like Provera, which are molecularly altered and thus don't fit exactly with the body's hormone receptors. Instead, these synthetics give instructions that are out of harmony with a woman's physiology. By increasing progesterone levels with natural progesterone, women can eliminate and reverse many of the conditions resulting from estrogen dominance, such as hot flashes, depression, low libido, breast tenderness, fluid retention, and digestive problems. Progesterone helps normalize thyroid function and blood clotting. Progesterone is the hormone that is predominant right after ovulation, and it increases women's libido. Finally, progesterone oxygenates the cells.

PREGNENOLONE. Taking 25 to 30 milligrams a day helps the body create female hormones.

DHEA. Natural DHEA, found in wild yam extract preparations, rejuvenates the body.

PROGESTERONE CREAM OR SERUM. Progesterone is a woman's rejuvenating hormone; it protects against cancer and fibrocystic cysts and increases the beneficial effects of thyroid hormone. In addition, it guards against osteoporosis by putting calcium back in the bones. After menopause, progesterone can be taken 3 or 4 weeks out of the month. Wild yam cream contains progesterone and can be purchased over the counter. Natural progesterone can also be taken orally.

ESTRIOL. This natural, friendly estrogen has been shown to inhibit breast tumors in animals. Some gynecologists are beginning to recommend estriol for menopausal women because it is safer and more effective than synthetics.

TRIPLE ESTROGEN. This formula is 80 percent estriol and 20 percent estrone plus estradiol. Estriol affords protection against breast tumors. Together, estrone and estradiol help reduce the risk of osteoporosis and cardiovascular problems. There are no negative side-effects.

HERBS A number of herbs on the market help relieve perimenopausal and menopausal symptoms by restoring the progesterone-estrogen balance. They include alfalfa, black cohosh, blue cohosh, damiana, fennel, licorice root, motherwort, red clover, red raspberry leaves, sarsparilla, and certain forms of wild yam. Flaxseed contains lignan, a phytohormone fiber that removes excess estrogen from the system. This is particularly important, since too much estrogen is believed to fuel breast cancer. Whole flaxseeds can be ground up or can be taken as flaxseed oil.

Vitex, or chaste berry, is commonly referred to as the menopausal herb because it alleviates many symptoms, including hot flashes, vaginal dryness, and mood swings. It works by raising the progesterone level. Ginkgo biloba has been shown to be effective in leveling mood swings.

The Chinese have been using herbs to treat women's problems for 5,000 years. Roberta Certner, President of the New York State Association of Professional Acupuncturists, says that Chinese medicine sees a woman as giving birth to herself at menopause, since she no longer has an obligation to her children. This philosophy thinks in terms of cycles of 7 years. When a woman is 49—often the age when menopause begins—it sees her lifespan as half-finished. "The next half of the lifespan is for self-growth." Certner explains that "Chinese medicine is adamant that women shouldn't be suffering from night sweats, insomnia, mood changes, and other symptoms, and herbal formulas are good for this purpose. They help to rebalance the energies of the body so that a woman doesn't feel at the mercy of these tremendous moods and powerless over bodily changes."

According to Certner, one virtue of Chinese medicine is gentleness: "People aren't forced to take medications which reduce libido function, which set up terrain for heart conditions. It really addresses the mechanism itself and not just the symptoms. The reason Chinese medicine works is that it goes to the root of the problem. If progesterone is low, you enhance the progesterone, using something like dioscorea or leonorus, whose name itself means 'mother root.'" Many different herbs are available to the practitioner, who chooses the ones to use in a given case according to the nature of the particular person involved. As Certner says, "Chinese medicine doesn't really treat conditions—it treats people."

Important tonic herbs in Chinese medicine include astragalus, *Dong quai*, ginseng, and licorice root.

HOMEOPATHY The homeopathic remedy chosen should correspond to the symptoms described. According to Ken Korins, a classically trained homeopathic physician in New York City, only one should be used for best results. Sometimes it's a matter of trial and error; if one does not work, another can be tried. These are some of the remedies Dr. Korins recommends for menopause.

The following remedies are recommended for hot flashes:

LACHESIS. Heat is felt all day long, while cold flashes may be experienced at night. Once the menstrual flow begins, all the symptoms disappear. Symptoms are worse with pressure and heat, and better with the onset of discharges or flows. Increased sexual desire is also associated with a need for lachesis.

BELLADONNA. There are many hot flashes. The face looks red and feels hot, and there is hot perspiration coming from the face and a pounding, throbbing, congested feeling in the head. Often there is dryness. Condition improves with resting quietly in the dark. Symptoms worsen with light, cold air, and sudden jolts. The emotional state can border on hysteria with rages.

GLONINE. Hot flashes are focused, with pressure in the head and feelings of congestion. There may be an associated rise in blood pressure at the time of the flashes. Symptoms are worse with heat and better with cold air. Emotionally, there is a fear of death; there is mental agitation.

AMYL NITRATE. Flashes of heat are accompanied by headaches. Often they are associated with anxiety and heart palpitations.

MANGANUM. Hot flashes are associated with nervous system depression. The body does not want to move. Symptoms improve when patient is lying down. Emotional state is peevish and fretful. There is a loss of pleasure in joyful music, but a profound reaction to sad music.

The term "flooding" refers to irregular periods which stop for a while but are very heavy when they return. The following remedies may also help younger women with extremely heavy periods:

CHINA. There is heavy bleeding, with dark, clotted blood, leading to debilitating fatigue. Symptoms get worse with drafts and light pressure, but better with strong pressure and heat. Emotional symptoms are apathy with a strong disposition toward hurting other people's feelings (not the normal state).

SABINA. The period is characterized by heavy, bright red, clotted blood. Expelling the clots is painful, and pain radiates from the sacrum to the pubis. Emotional symptoms are irritability and a dislike for music.

SECALE. Periods are profuse and prolonged. Blood is almost black. Symptoms worsen with heat and improve with cold.

PHOSPHORUS. There is easy, frequent bleeding of bright red blood, often with no clots. The patient is low-spirited, with multiple fears. Also, memory may decrease. Another symptom is constant chilliness.

Remedies for vaginal dryness and thinning include:

SEPIA. The vaginal area is itchy and dry. There is a sense that the uterus is falling out of the vagina. There is also a loss of libido. Symptoms tend to be worse with standing, cold and rest, anything that causes venous congestion. Symptoms are improved with anything that increases venous flow, such as motion. Emotionally, there is an indifference to loved ones, sadness, and a tendency to weep easily.

NATRUM MURIATICUM. Vaginal dryness makes sexual intercourse very painful. Discharges tend to be acrid and burning. There is often a loss of pubic hair. Emotional state is one of depression and irritability, which is worse with consolation. Symptoms also tend to worsen around 10 o'clock in the morning.

BRYONIA. Vaginal dryness is accompanied by severe headaches. Any motion is painful and distressing. Condition improves with rest.

NITRIC ACID. Vaginal dryness reaches the point where the mucosa fissures, causing splinterlike sensations in the vaginal area.

EXERCISE Regular exercise can reduce the frequency and severity of hot flashes. For best results, it is a good idea to begin exercising before menopause begins. Otherwise, exercise may trigger hot flashes. Exercise also alleviates mood swings and depression by naturally raising serotonin and endorphin levels in the brain. The best exercises to engage in are dancing, brisk walking, running, swimming, biking, and tai chi. Additional benefit is derived from cross-training, doing different exercises on different days. This prevents any one part of the body from becoming overdeveloped or overstressed.

AROMATHERAPY "Aromatherapy is truly holistic because it is a mind and body treatment," states Ann Berwick, author of *Holistic Aromatherapy and Women's*

Health. "I think this is part of the secret of its power." Berwick uses essential oils to help alleviate a number of conditions, including hormonal imbalance in women going through menopause. "Cyprus, fennel, and clary sage are believed to have estrogenlike effects. For overall balancing, I recommend to my clients that they use these oils in a lotion or body oil, and apply it to their body two or three times a day. When women are experiencing hot flashes, I also suggest that they breathe in peppermint or basil on a tissue throughout the day. I find that a great help for most of my clients."

AYURVEDIC MEDICINE Menopausal women report relief and rejuvenation from Ayurvedic formulas using herbal phytoestrogens and phytoprogesterones. Ayurveda believes that balance is the key to perfect health. It basically determines which body/mind type a person is and helps people choose the type of foods they should eat and the type of exercise that is best for them. Chapter 43, Chronic Fatigue Syndrome, discusses some Ayurvedic principles in detail. You can also read *Perfect Health* and *Ageless Body, Timeless Mind* by Deepak Chopra.

REFLEXOLOGY Laura Norman, a certified reflexologist from New York City, says, "For menopause, in addition to working the reproductive organs, I also would encourage you to work your thyroid gland, as this will help take over when the ovaries produce less estrogen. This is how to find this point: the base of the toes reflects the neck area where the thyroid is located. Press your thumbs into the base of your toes and thumb-walk across that ridge, particularly in the base of the big toe.

"Another area to massage is the adrenal gland reflex point. You are on the big toe side of the foot. Go about a third of the way down your foot. You are under the ball of the foot, in line with the big toe. If you press your thumb into that area, it will provide energy when you feel fatigued.

"Also, the pituitary gland, which helps all the other glands to work, is located in the center of the big toe. Pressure applied there helps stimulate that area. Both feet should be massaged equally."

PART ELEVEN

Of Special Concern to Men

When many people think of the Hong Kong cinema, what immediately comes to mind are gangsters or kung fu fighters. However, the Chinese, whose doctors have given great attention to sexual dysfunctions such as impotence and infertility, also have created many films that dwell, often in a comic manner, on these matters. I'm not talking about pornography but raunchy ribaldry as in the film *Sex and Zen*. At the beginning of the film, the hapless hero accidentally has his penis cut off. He wanders from magician to quack to alchemist, trying to find a replacement. One offers to take one from an animal, and another fashions a prosthesis out of tin.

The earthy comedy's underlying comment is on the importance of sexual expression to Chinese culture, something we will have reason to be thankful for in these next few chapters as we note, among other remedies, Chinese herbal formulas used for men's health problems.

59

Sexual Dysfunction in Men

Impotence is of concern to men everywhere as has recently been highlighted by the sensation caused by Viagra, the "wonder drug" that has restored potency to millions of men. Soon after its introduction in the late 1990s it turned out that Viagra was not as wonderful as it was cracked up to be. For one thing, Viagra has limited value, helping only certain forms of impotence and addressing the symptoms but not the underlying cause. Moreover, there are side effects, ranging from flushing and headaches, to hazy vision and even death. But this hasn't stopped the Viagra bandwagon. As of 2000, 4 million American men were taking the drug, and worldwide sales exceeded $1 billion annually. Given that some 30 million American men are believed to have some degree of erectile dysfunction, it's not surprising that other impotence pills will soon be added to this primed market.

We will begin this chapter with a few remarks about Viagra in a discussion that will also delve into the psychological causes often behind impotence. We will also make some mention of the natural slowing down in sexual activity that accompanies aging. At a certain stage, we will see, repeatedly using Viagra or other drugs to stimulate an erection may be an unwise act of forcing the body to go beyond its natural bounds. We will also bring up the subject of male menopause, which is not just a time for a man to look backward at what he has lost in aging, but to look ahead at what positive changes he can make and new plateaus he can reach. Then we will look at herbal and other natural remedies for impotence.

Impotence, Aging, and Viagra

Dr. Michael Tierra is a consultant who has 25 years of experience with Chinese medicine. His East West Clinic is located in Santa Cruz, California. He is the founder of the American Herbalists Guild and has written a number of books on herbal medicine, including *Chinese Traditional Herbal Medicine*.

He told me told me about a patient he was seeing. "I had a gentleman about 70 years old, who had tried Viagra with poor results. He would get an erection but he had no desire for his partner. I had him check on the drugs he was taking."

Dr. Tierra explains that the drugs an older man will take often have impotence as a side effect. A doctor imagines a man of 75 or so shouldn't even think about sex, so he won't mention the side effect. "This particular gentleman was taking Coumadin, a blood thinner to prevent heart attack. I think this particular drug may have been causing the impotency."

This doesn't mean, Dr. Tierra cautions, that once the patient had adjusted his medication, he should return to Viagra. "With Viagra, the body is being forced to do something it is not naturally inclined to do. This is asking for trouble. If you don't find the cause of your impotence, and you just force your organ to perform, you may be exhausting some latent resources in your body." Moreover, Viagra has side effects, such as heart attacks.

"The issue here," according to Dr. Tierra, "is a man needs to recognize that as he ages, he needs to slow down. But there is so much ego involved in sexual performance [that he refuses to acknowledge aging]."

I spoke further about this with Jed Diamond, a licensed psychotherapist and leader in the men's movement, who has published all over, in *The Wall Street Journal*, *The New York Times*, and other places. His latest book is *Male Menopause*.

He points out that to think of Viagra as the only treatment for impotence is stifling the possibilities. Impotence affects nearly 30 million American men. "Erectile dysfunction is very common," he says. "There are a number of viable treatments. Viagra is only one way." He mentions the many natural alternatives such as those discussed below. L-arginine and ginkgo, for example, release the nitrous oxide mechanism in the same way Viagra does, allowing for a relaxation of the blood vessels in the penis, which allows for erection to occur.

Diamond continues, "Right now the situation around Viagra is bad. It's being prescribed like candy, rather than, as it should be, recognized as a very potent drug."

Dr. Michael Tierra notes that the Viagra craze is partially ego-based. Men feel a psychological pressure to perform. "But few men are good lovers because they don't realize that women are slower to get aroused and so these men are not catering to the women's needs."

Such attitudes make them think they should have sex more often than they are really capable of having it. According to Dr. Tierra, a man at age 50 should be having sex once a week. By 60 or 70, he should cut back to once or twice a month. That's sex with ejaculation. He points out, in Chinese erotic thought there is a concept unknown in the West: sex without ejaculation is a gratifying possibility. Women can have sexual fulfillment without ejaculation, and men need to learn more about this path. Men need to become better lovers.

Moreover, there is a physical reason to occasionally practice this type of sex. Chinese doctors argue that ejaculation depletes energy and so should be done with moderation. As one ages, there is a natural drying process and the vital secretions will lessen. That's why people wrinkle as they get older. There are not enough vital secretions in the body. Women will have dryness of the vagina as they age.

You've heard of young people being referred to as "ripe" or "luscious." These folk idioms contain the observational truth that the body is touched by plentiful secretions when we are young. As we age, these secretions are at much more of a premium. You don't want to waste these secretions.

Male Menopause

The aging as it first becomes evident in the middle of middle age is now being called "male menopause." Think about this. Every 6 seconds another baby boomer turns 50. With these tens of millions of people aging, there is a wake-up call going out. Say you're an average guy, who's just hit 50. You worked on your career, your family. You got the best education that's available. But did you pay attention to your health? Maybe you misconstrued what it means not to be overweight. You think because you're not overweight, then you're not sick. But you must know that there are people who are processing cancer or diabetes or heart disease, and they are not overweight.

A man's midlife crisis is now called male menopause. The symptoms of the crisis, according to Diamond, are drops in testosterone, and DHEA, among other things. These are measurable changes, but their significance varies as does the rate of drop. As a man reaches this stage, there is also increased fatigue, and a loss of memory, especially short-term memory. There's going to be a weight gain, even for those who exercise and keep fit. There will be emotional changes, often increased indecisiveness, fearfulness, anxiety, and depression. There will be sexual changes, including a lowering of sexual desire, particularly toward a partner a man has been with for a long time. There are difficulties with erections and less of a general feeling of well being.

How Aging Affects Sexuality

Dr. Eric Braverman, author of *Male Sexual Fitness*, gives more details on how aging affects sexuality. "Men begin to experience a sexual decline after age 30.

The biological reasons for this decline are a falling testosterone level, falling amounts of growth hormones, and lower DHEA levels. These declines are programmed into the body in the same way a woman is programmed to experience menopause around age 50." At that age, women are no longer fertile and their bodily changes reflect this. Men can be fertile till age 80, but their sperm counts start declining by age 40 or even at 35."

Sexual frequency also begins to slow down, although men may not notice this change until age 50 or 60. But a majority will begin to experience a deficiency in the hormones mentioned from about age 40. There is a reduction in the ability of the gastrointestinal tract to absorb nutrients. The brain slows down, losing 10 milliseconds of speed per decade, and losing alpha waves.

Diamond says there are a number of courses a man can take as he experiences these changes "Some men will react by saying, 'This is old age. We have to accept it.' Other men react by trying to go backward to return to their youth. Maybe they try to find a younger woman or buy a sports car. Whatever the attitude, there's much more positive ability to move ahead if a man takes care of his health." As he sees it, this is the crucial period that determines if the second half of a man's life will be powerful, productive, and passionate or whether it will be a time of ill health, despair, and depression.

Male menopause comes along from about age 40 to 55, although, in unusual cases it could range from as early as 30 to as late as 65. With men there is more of a bell-shaped curve for its onset than there is for female menopause. For the female, it takes place in a much narrower time period, around age 45.

Now these are not just hormonal and physical changes, but they are accompanied by psychological changes. A man begins to question, asking, "What have I done with my life?" and "What have I done that was significant?" There are also spiritual changes as the man begins to ask bigger questions, such as, "Is there something to life beyond just acquiring things?" Suddenly, a man may feel the need to pursue a calling, not just a career. Often at this age, a man becomes a mentor, teaching some of the things he has learned to younger men. This is so essential because without that you have younger men growing up without role models, with a feeling that older men don't care about them. And you have older men who are saying, "I've had a career. I've raised a family. But there's something missing." That missing component is the feeling of giving something back.

Society needs this mentoring. This is an opportunity the male menopause can offer. The chance to take on something larger, which will not only be good for the man but for youth and society. Also at this stage, friendship and intimacy grow more important as well as having a partner one can get to know more deeply.

"Now I'm often asked," Diamond told me, 'what can women do to help men who are going through male menopause?' For one, they have to try to understand what is going on. Second, women have to take this seriously, because there can be erection problems, depression problems. This is not just a mild transition. "And third," Diamond added, "this time can be looked forward to. We don't have to look at this period as if doors were only being closed. They are also being opened. It can be a wonderful time if we will understand it."

Diet and Lifestyle

Let's look at some recommended guidelines and therapies for impotence. Eating a highly nutritious whole-foods diet, as described throughout this book, is the best way to build the foundation for good health. Eating properly means selecting unprocessed or minimally processed foods, and having the right balance of vitamins and minerals. Vitamins C and E, zinc, and essential fatty acids are especially important for a man's sexual health. Amanda Crawford, an herbalist from California, says, "I recommend eating six pieces of organic fruit every day. Any fruit a man likes: oranges, apples, papayas, blueberries, pears, all through the list. Go out and spend money on the most inviting fruits available in the market."

You might want to also work on preventing cardiovascular disease with the supplements that are good in that area. B vitamins can be obtained by eating whole grains. Garlic can be taken—two to four cloves a day or 1,000 milligrams as a supplement. Also take magnesium, from 50 to 100 milligrams a day. This is also rich in many foods.

Tobacco, alcohol, and high cholesterol levels have been linked to erectile dysfunction. Nicotine can constrict blood vessels in the penis and thus prevent it from becoming rigid. Dr. Neil Baum, associate clinical professor of urology, in an article posted on the Healthwell website (www.healthwell.com), says that penile blood supply can be increased by reducing total cholesterol levels and by increasing your HDL ("good') cholesterol.

Dr. Baum notes that exercise, while important, should be done in moderation. He provides a special warning, and some advice to bicyclists: Excessive biking can diminish blood supply to the penis by compressing the blood vessels between the rectum and scrotum, which is where you sit when riding a bike. Active bicyclists might want to consider investing in a seat designed to transfer the pressure from the scrotum to the buttocks.

Many over-the-counter and prescription medications can affect a man's sexual potency. Dr. Baum says that more than 500 drugs, including diuretics, sedatives, and antihistamines, are associated with sexual dysfunction. Men older than 50 are at greatest risk. You should talk with your doctor about adjusting your dosage or changing medications if you think a drug may be causing your impotence.

Holistic Approaches

Dr. Braverman recommends a holistic approach, saying, "My practice is holistic toward treating sexual dysfunction. The penis is an organ like any other organ in the body so we follow the key principles of healing we would with any other organ." When he finds a man is having a problem, he checks a number of physical functions. He checks blood flow. "If it is retarded, we will use niacin, chelation, even Viagra, to increase blood flow to the penis."

He also looks at whether the nerves to the penis are healthy. Here he looks for any influence of diabetes or neuropathy.

Careful measurement must precede treatment. "There is no substitute for measuring," Dr. Braverman says. "No one can manipulate a patient's testicles and say, 'Yep, there's enough testosterone there.' No doctor or healer can look at someone's belly and say, 'The liver is certainly making enough growth hormone.' It just can't be identified without tests. We have to measure it all."

There are markers whereby doctors can measure statistically the level of anxiety or the level of depression that may be associated with sexual dysfunction. They can accurately determine the levels of testosterone, DHEA, and so on. "This is no guessing game," Dr. Braverman says.

Dr. Braverman's practice differs from that of conventional physicians in that he looks at the whole picture. Sexuality is not just related to the penis. Where testosterone is low, of course, the penis is affected, but also the general health levels are going down. The DHEA, which is coming from the pancreas, liver, and brain, is dropping, and these organs are also touched. Also, when a person is anxious, depressed, has insomnia or emotional upsets, this will have an effect on the brain. Any failure in the bodily system will weaken sexual functioning.

After looking at the circulation and the nerves, Dr. Braverman's major concerns are the adrenal glands, the growth hormone axis (brain, pancreas, and liver), the gastrointestinal tract, and the brain. If there is weak absorption in the intestine, for instance, this will cause an overall bodily imbalance.

"What's exciting about all this," Dr. Braverman says, "is that if we look at the body as a whole and work with that, we can get better results than from just treating the genitals alone."

According to his experience, growth hormones can yield dramatic results in men in their 50s, 60s, and 70s. And DHEA can also be very impressive. To help sustain an erection, there are various agents that make the erection last longer, so men can have better sexual experiences. He sees these and other new treatments creating "a new age in the treatment of sexual dysfunctions."

Dr. Braverman recounts some of the more dramatic cures he has witnessed. There was a man who hadn't had sex in 9 years. He was the victim of a stroke. He went on DHEA growth hormone and testosterone. This restored him sexually.

"I had a 72-year-old man," Dr. Braverman says, "who told me he was interested in having sex once a week. After we got him started on growth hormones and other substances, he found himself having it six times a week."

The funny thing, he mentions, is that usually when you treat men and improve their libido and performance, you end up treating their partners too, because the partners are not ready for this.

In another case, a man in his 60s was having memory problems. Dr. Braverman began treating his hormonal imbalances, which also affected his sex drive. His wife had mentioned that, in 30 years of marriage, he had been a low sex person. The treatment had gone on a while and his wife came in. She couldn't believe the change. "'Wow,' she said, 'I wish we had come to you earlier.' This was a low sex man who seemed to have little need for human warmth. We changed around his whole attitude. Not just his desire for sex, but he was hugging, touching, feeling, experiencing a sensual relation to another person in a way he never had before."

Chinese Herbal Medicine

Herbalist Letha Hadady, author of *Asian Health Secrets* and *Personal Renewal*, in an article posted on the Healthwell website (www.healthwell.com) explains that the Chinese treat sexual dysfunction by increasing adrenal energy, muscle strength, and endurance with herbs that boost vitality and immunity. Dr. Michael Tierra adds that Chinese therapy begins by trying to uncover the root causes of the problem. *Yin* and *yang* are the two basic energy principles seen by Chinese medicine as guiding life. The terms describe the opposing physical conditions of the body. *Yin* is connected to the parasympathetic nervous system, which is responsible for maintaining and calming the body, serving to conserve and restore energy. *Yang* is connected to the sympathetic nervous system, which is the body's alerting system, sometimes referred to as the fight-or-flight system. This system is responsible for preparing the body to respond to stressful challenges.

Impotency is said to stem from one of three possible debilities intimately involved with the *yin-yang* duality:

BLOOD DEFICIENCY AND STAGNATION, ARISING FROM POOR CIRCULA-
TION. The indications of this state are weakness, anemia, and paleness. *Dong quai* is recommended here. Although it is commonly given to women after menstruation to restore the blood, it can also be useful in this instance.

YANG DEFICIENCY is due to an androgenic hormone deficiency. Here the male hormones need to be strengthened. This type of impotency can be recognized by coldness, weakness, and spontaneous perspiration. What would be useful here might be rehmannia and eucommia. They should be taken in combination at 15 grams per day, broken into two doses. Dr. Tierra adds, "They are regularly taken together because the Chinese don't see one herb as totally answering a medical problem. Chinese herbs act to augment systems in the body. Often a preparation will avail itself of a primary herb and a helping herb that reduces possible side effects of the primary herb." Such formulas are especially indicated for complex conditions, which involve more than one system in the body, or when a strong effect is needed, since a combination of herbs will generally be stronger than a single herb. Deer antler and Chinese ginseng are also helpful in this situation. Take 3 or 4 grams of both twice a day.

YIN DEFICIENCY. This is the evident cause of impotency when the person is run-down, weakened, often thirsty and suffers from night sweats, dryness, and insomnia. Rehmannia Six is indicated in this case. Ashwagandha can also come in handy. This is an herb that builds potency. It is not a stimulant but a gradual enhancer. It needs to be taken over a few months. After 1 or 2 weeks, there will be increased vitality accompanied by less tension, a good combination. Take 3 drops in a teaspoon twice a day.

Chinese ginseng (Panax) has long been used in Chinese medicine to restore sexual health to both men and women. Modern-day studies have confirmed its benefits. Hadady cites a1997 report from Yale University stating that Chinese ginseng stimulates the production of nitric oxide. Nitric oxide helps to relax smooth muscles and allows blood to flow to all parts of the body, including the penis. It functions like Viagra but without the side effects. And, Hadady says, "While Viagra emphasizes sexual performance, ginseng is said to tone the entire endocrine system for a more holistic beneficial effect."

Panax must be used with caution in people with high blood pressure, chronic headaches, or insomnia, Hadady warns. Side effects may include fever, facial flushing, or dizziness. Panax may be combined with other herbs such as Solomon's seal (Polygonum multiflorum) or *he shou wu.*

A couple of Chinese herbal formulas have proven generally useful. One is schisandra chinensis, which helps with excessive sweating, excessive urination, and discharges of all kinds. It is like a mortar that holds the *chi* energy of the body.

A second useful one is epimedium grandiflorum. The epimedium is a flower that is grown in shady areas and used as an ornamental. Its Chinese name, *yin yang huo,* translates as the "horny goat herb." It was used to increase the sexual activity of animals. Use 6 to 12 dried leaves, boiled in 2 or 3 cups of water for one half hour. Drink 1 or 2 cups twice a day.

This problem of premature ejaculation often has a psychological basis, but it may have physiological causes also. The Chinese would say it is due to a *yang* deficiency and its associated coldness. It can be treated with a rehmannia/eucommia combination called *you qui wan* or with Rehmannia six. Astragalus would also be effective. *You qui wan* can be brewed as a tea, with 4 or 5 cups decocted down to 2 cups. It can also be taken as a dried extract, where a person swallows a teaspoon with water.

Other Herbal Remedies

C.J. Puotinen, a noted herbalist, explains that the best herb to choose depends on the cause of the problem. If the problem is an arterial blockage, ginkgo biloba, widely regarded as a memory tonic, can help increase circulation, as has been documented in European studies. If you take 240 milligrams of ginkgo daily, it should relieve impotence due to arterial blockage. Puotinen says that ginkgo biloba is best taken as a standardized extract because the constituents are not readily assimilated by the body. It does not break down well with alcohol either so it's not effective as a tincture or crude extract.

More generally, Puotinen's two most common recommendations are yohimbe bark, which is a strong aphrodisiac, and damiana, "which is a gentler, more romantic, milder herb. The latter is suggested as a first choice when dealing with problems of impotence, since it has fewer adverse side effects."

Yohimbe bark, because of its strength and side effects, is often taken in combination with other herbs. It should not be taken by people with high blood pressure, heart or liver disease, diabetes, kidney problems, or by anyone who uses alcohol, tranquilizers, or antihistamines. When you are taking it, you should not be consuming such things as liver, cheese, or red wine. In fact, with all these restrictions, the bark sounds more like a pharmaceutical than some of the other herbal preparations. It is best taken in one of the combinations available in health food or herbalist stores. These combinations should be used according to the directions on the label.

Incidentally, a few years ago, a Chinese corporation accidentally fed carp it was raising these last two herbs, and the fish's reproduction increased.

Puotinen says that in *The Male Herbal*, author James Green recommends the following: "Take 2 tablespoons of yohimbe bark and add them to 2 cups of water. Make a tea by simmering for 10 minutes. Add 1 gram of vitamin C to stop nausea and aid in assimilation. Drink one or two cups. If you feel any side effects, such as gastrointestinal problems, then try smaller dosages or take the bark in blends. This bark should only be used for a short period of time. It's not something you want to repeat more than once in a day. This is not a tonic."

Rosemary Gladstar, former director of the California School of Herbal Studies and author of *Herbal Remedies for Men's Health*, relates her concerns about yohimbe. "I know yohimbe is getting quite well known in this country and men are using it, but very improperly. As an herbalist I am seeing men who are developing quite a bit of problems. It can make them feel nauseated and very headachy. I am really trying to stir men away from using yohimbe unless they are using it under the guidance of a practitioner and for more serious health problems. Muira puama [an herb from Brazil] does not have those harmful side effects and has a great reputation as a sexual stimulant for men. I would [even] recommend more common herbs like sarsaparilla and sassafras which don't have quite the marked effects but will have a longer safer use if men are feeling like their hormonal levels or low or their vitality is low."

Here is my protocol for an alternative to Viagra:

yohimbe bark extract	100 mg
anise	20 mg
velvet bean	20 mg
cardamom	20 mg
cinnamon	20 mg
ginkgo	30 mg
ginseng	30 mg
muira puama	400 mg
oat	30 mg
wolf berry	30 mg
ashwagnanda	30 mg
country mallow	30 mg
saw palmetto	30 mg
nettle root	100 mg
ginger root extract	50 mg
zinc L-monomethionine	10 mg
L-arginine	1,000 mg
phoshatidyl choline	500 mg

60

Male Infertility and Related Problems

In chapter 53, we discussed infertility from the female perspective. In this chapter, we look at some of the alternatives now available to address male infertility. This chapter will also include some recommendations for the treatment of infections and other problems of the male genitalia.

Causes

Male infertility is caused most often by a deficiency of sperm creation or by the sperm's lack of motility. Sperm motility does make a difference. Without that capacity to move in the seminal fluid, there will not be a high probability of conception since the sperm is not getting where it has to go. The form and structure of the sperm itself, known as its morphology, also may play a role. Among other things, saunas and excessive vigorous exercise can diminish sperm production.

The Chinese Perspective

Dr. Michael Tierra, a consultant with years of experience with Chinese medicine, says that because the balancing of *yin* and *yang* is so important, an herb should be taken that addresses both sides of the energy equation. "Infertility," he explains, "will be caused either by a *yin* or *yang* deficiency. In this case, though, there is a planetary, that is, broadly effective, Chinese formula that addresses both sides of the deficiency at once. Called, *wu zi wan* (The Five Herbs of Creation), it will tonify both kidney yin and kidney yang equally."

Also useful for this problem is ashwagandha. Avoid the imports of this herb from India, though, because they may have a high bacteria count.

Dr. Tierra notes that ginseng is also valuable for those with an energy deficiency. If you have little energy or a weak digestion, 6 to 9 grams taken in two doses should prove valuable. It can be taken as tea. Try the Chinese or Korean red varieties, not American. "The little bottles you can buy in stores are not serious helps to our health because the amount of ginseng in them is too minute," he warns. "You'd have to drink a case of them to feel any effect."

If you get the ginseng root, you can break off a chunk with a hammer and suck on it all day. You can also brew it up as the Chinese do in a ginseng cooker. A cooker, which can be purchased in Chinatown, is a ceramic cylinder with little feet on the bottom so it will stand up in boiling water. You fill it with water and the root, then place it inside a second pot that is filled with water itself. Place it on the stove and bring the water in the outer pot to a boil. It functions like a double boiler. You leave the little jar inside the pan and leave it to simmer for hours. You don't actually have to buy the Chinese pot. You could put a Mason jar in a pot of water and achieve the same effect. This is also a fine way to make herbal teas since it seems to combine decoction and infusion all in one.

Herbalist Letha Hadady, in an article posted on the Healthwell website (www.healthwell.com), recommends epimedium to boost sperm production. This herb has also been found to stimulate the sensory nerves. You can make a tea by simmering about a handful of the dried leaves in a quart of water for 15 minutes. Hadady warns that epimedium should not be used for long periods or by people with high sex drives. Side effects associated with overuse include dizziness, dry mouth, and nosebleed. Epimedium may be combined with Schisandra chinensis, or *wu wei zi*, and lycium fruit (Lycii chinensis), *gou qi zi*, or Solomon's seal.

Dr. David Molony, author of *The Complete Guide to Chinese Herbal Medicine*, makes the following recommendations:

TZE PAO SAN PIEN. Dr. Molony says that this Chinese formula, which increases potency, is one of the best methods to treat infertility.

DEER ANTLER. A useful herb but, Dr. Molony cautions, not if you have a lot of heat, are irritable, and have high blood pressure. It is a stimulating preparation. It has to be counterbalanced with a *yin* element that will cool you down.

REHMANNIA. If you are *yin* deficient, on the other hand, you will need a tonic such as Rehmannia Eight or Rehmannia Six. "In general," Dr. Molony says, "the problem of Americans is that they are too hot. They overdo stimulants, even overdo vitamins. People will take so many vitamins that the *yin*, the cooling element in the physiology, is sucked up. With extreme *yin* deficiency, you will not be able to ejaculate or even relax enough to get an erection."

The tonic and adaptogen herbs are also quite helpful. Tonics are herbs that act to restore and strengthen the whole system. They produce normal tone, gradually improving overall function. The adaptogens are a type of the tonics. They gradually correct imbalances. The most widely known adaptogen is ginseng. These tonics lower or raise blood pressure that is out of whack, and bring blood sugar into the normal range. They will slow a too-rapid pulse or, alternately, speed up and strengthen a sluggish one. In the same manner, they will recalibrate a reproductive system imbalance.

Other helpful adaptogens recommended for men with fertility problems are astragalus, Siberian ginseng, and the Chinese herb *fo-ti*. All of these have followings among herbalists, who believe that over long periods, they correct imbalances that lead to infertility and other health problems.

Other Herbal and Nutritional Remedies

Herbalist Amanda Crawford has some additional advice. For one, she thinks we should all be eating a more Mediterranean diet. "This would be one rich in garlic, rosemary leaves, and olives, taking them not as supplements but as part of eating a wide variety of natural foods." She says we should add to that the herbs that help the liver, such as dandelion root and leaf. Taken as a tea, dandelion will make you feel more grounded and will have untold benefits. Take 1 cup a day for 3 weeks. Its effects will start subtly but become clearer after drinking the tea every day for a week. In the second week, the man will feel an increase in power. In the third week, he will feel as invincible as the dandelions that keep coming up on the lawn.

Blue vervain is another herb for the liver. It has a bitter taste. Take one half of a teaspoon, diluted in water before meals, morning and night for 6 weeks to get the best benefits. It acts to balance hormones, liver, and blood. "In the pre-Christian herbal traditions," Crawford says, "it was said to make you true to your self. When we talk about infertility, it's never far from questions that pertain to both the emotional and spiritual sphere."

Tribulus is an herb used in the body-building and sports community. It increases testosterone and growth hormone in the body as well as sperm count. It was traditionally used in India as a counter to infertility and as an aphrodisiac. It can be taken in a 250 milligram capsule twice a day. However, Crawford says, "This is a fairly strong herb. It may not be your best option to increase testosterone without knowing why you have low testosterone in the first place. Doing that may be asking for trouble. I urge men, especially those who may not be as fit as body builders, not to begin with this herb without first consulting your physician."

A safer way to improve infertility is with zinc. Its helps with spermatogenesis and prostate problems.

Arginine is an amino acid. Again, don't take this by the bucketful. Too large a dose can exacerbate dormant infections. Since there are small but appropriate amounts of arginine in organic whole foods, such as oatmeal, sunflower seeds, and even cocoa, avail yourself of those ways of ingesting it.

Crawford makes this suggestion for a good cold-morning breakfast containing the amino acid arginine as well as other nutrients: old-fashioned oatmeal, not the instant type which is of no value to your body but that made from rolled oats, organic when possible. On top you can put some flax seeds and some dried fruits, such as blueberries for the bioflavonoids. Eating that morning medicine will help nourish your reproductive health and anchor your sense of health from the inside out.

There are a number of other herbal remedies that are useful in relation to infertility, according to herbalist C.J. Puotinen. If the problem seems to stem from the circulatory system use gotu kola and ginkgo. Also said to enhance fertility are stinging nettles and green oats. Although there have been no clinical studies on these substances, anecdotal evidence certainly supports their value.

Rosemary Gladstar, former director of the California School of Herbal Studies and author of *Herbal Remedies for Men's Health*, adds one more herb to the list: pumpkin seed. "I always recommend it to men to use as a supplement because it helps to completely restore the male reproductive system," she says.

Infections

The herbal approach can also be used for other common problems of the bladder and urethra. "For urinary tract infection," herbalist C.J. Puotinen says, "cranberry juice is recommended." It is often thought of as a source for women with these infections, but it can also be used with men. It helps maintain a healthy pH balance within the urinary tract, preventing bacteria from adhering to the lining or walls of the tract. So infections can't get a foothold.

One can also used buchu to treat infection as well as small stones and fluid retention. Buchu is both a diuretic and urinary tonic. It can be taken for long periods of time. Puotinen also talks about corn silk, "which is simply that found on the ears of corn," as another tonic. "One can't overdose on corn silk," she says. European goldenrod also can be taken.

Other useful herbs are juniper berries, which can be taken in small quantities, and barberry. Any infection in the bladder area can be cleared up very easily by using barberry, especially when it is taken in combination with cranberry juice, which will cover its offensive taste, or in capsule form. Few would take it as a tea, although that is a possibility. It should be made as a decoction, not brewed, tea.

Other Problems of the Male Genitalia

Dr. Michael Tierra gives the following recommendations for handling inflammation of the testicles and discharge from the penis. "These conditions require herbs that are anti-inflammatory and diuretic at the same time. These would include yellow dock root, chaparral, and goldenseal. Use 30 drops of each. Ideally, they should be taken in combination to get a broader, synergistic effect."

One good combination is:
   30 drops of verbaris
   30 drops of goldenrod
   30 drops of yellow dock root
   30 drops of gentiana
   Garlic should be taken separately, one or two cloves a day to combat infection.

61

Prostate Conditons

In 2000, prostate cancer killed an estimated 37,000 American men. Some180,000 new cases were diagnosed. The risk of developing prostate cancer—as well as other prostate problems—rises greatly with age. As our country matures demographically, with older people making up an increasingly larger segment of the population, the number of people affected will continue to climb. Fortunately, there are many proven alternative therapies to prevent and treat prostate problems. In fact, the results from alternative medicine have been so conclusive that even the orthodox medical community is taking notice.

In 1998, a study of 29,000 male smokers revealed that those who took 50 milligrams of vitamin E per day for 5 to 8 years had 32 percent fewer diagnoses of prostate cancer as compared with men who did not take the vitamin. In addition, there were 41 percent fewer deaths from prostate cancer in the vitamin E group. Another large, 10-year study, this one of the effects of selenium on skin cancer, found serendipitously that people who took 200 micrograms of the antioxidant daily had 63 percent fewer cases of prostate cancer. Of course—as usual—these impressive results are still not convincing enough for mainstream medicine. It needs more data. So a 12-year, government-sponsored trial of more than 32,000 men will begin soon to, in the words of one of the organizers, "establish how safe and effective vitamin E and selenium really are for prostate cancer prevention."

What is the Prostate?

The prostate is a small, walnut-shaped gland between the bladder and the penis. It surrounds the urethra, the passageway from the bladder through which urine is excreted. It provides the seminal fluid that nourishes and transports sperm.

The prostate gland has to be considered in relation to the whole body. A healthy body has a healthy prostate. Among the conditions that can affect the prostate are prostatitis, prostate enlargement (prostatic hypertrophy, benign prostatic hyperplasia), and prostate cancer.

Warning Signs of Prostate Problems

According to Dr. Lawrence Clapp, the author of *Prostate Health in 90 Days* who has a background in homeopathy and body work, typical warning signs of prostate problems include hesitation in urination, undue urgency in urination, and the feeling that you have to get up at night to urinate. Evidence of an inflamed prostate can also be back pain. A lot of men don't realize that back pain can be produced by prostate difficulties.

If you have pain with fever, pain with stools or with cloudy urine, then that's prostatitis. Benign prostatic hyperplasia (BPH) refers to the noncancerous enlargement of the gland. This gland encircles the urethra, and as it enlarges it can put pressure on it, pushing it shut; this is what causes urination problems. Prostate cancer, one of America's leading malignancies, may or may not be associated with symptoms. This generally slow-growing cancer often goes unrecognized in many older men, who ultimately die of other causes. Some men experience urinary or other problems. A PSA (prostate specific antigen) test—although not always reliable—is often used to diagnose the disease.

Who is Affected and Why?

At about age 40, 10 percent of men have a slight enlargement of the gland. By age 50, 50 percent have some enlargement. By age 80, 90 percent show symptoms. "Surprisingly," Dr. Clapp says, "prostate problems are occurring in younger and younger men. Many traditional doctors are even saying, prostate problems are inevitable," Dr. Clapp says, adding, "I don't agree."

What causes a prostate difficulty? "One way this problem begins," Dr. Clapp explains, "is that in our sex lives we pick up bacteria from our partners. These bacteria remain in the prostate." The prostate can't handle them all or handle the variety of them so this causes infection. And this infection languishes until the prostate becomes inflamed or enlarged.

A second reason for prostate problems is diet. In most countries in the world, men do not have these problems. But in the United States, their occurrence is partly conditioned by the use of tobacco, alcohol, rich and spicy foods, fats in red meat, and by overeating. All these things weaken the prostate, so it can't fight back against bacteria so well.

Prostate problems have also been tied to the pesticides we use. These pesticides are loaded with estrogens and chemicals designed to work on the reproductive systems of insects. Unfortunately, they build up in our systems. "I remember," Dr. Clapp recalls, "as a boy growing up, we kids used to run behind the DDT truck that sprayed the neighborhood [to kill mosquitoes]. They still do that spraying in Florida." These pesticides get into all our foods. It's on the grass the animals eat. Even if you wash your vegetables very carefully, which is helpful, you'll still be getting the pesticides that have worked their way into the inner membranes of the plants.

Israel outlawed the use of pesticides more than 10 years ago. Now cancer is down 60 percent. That's highly suggestive.

A swollen prostate also can be caused when pituitary production, stimulated by stress or alcohol consumption, converts testosterone into dehydrotestosterone, which is harmful.

One final reason for some prostate problems, which is almost comic, is tight underwear. Frequently this underwear will cut off circulation.

Conventional Treatments

Dr. Harry Preuss, professor of medicine and pathology at Georgetown University Medical Center, and author of *The Prostate Cure*, tells us about the conventional treatment for prostate problems. "The standard approaches are through surgery or drugs. There is an operation in which the prostate is reamed down to a good size. There are also laser and microwave approaches in use. There are also drugs that can be taken to relax the prostate and allow the urine to flow out. These will be administered over a matter of months and may have quite adverse side effects."

In the case of prostate cancer, the conventional options include radical prostatectomy (surgical removal of the prostate gland), external-beam radiation (conventional radiation), radioactive seed implantation (insertion of radioactive seeds that kill the cancer), cryosurgery (freezing of tissue), hormone therapy (to stop the production of testosterone) and bilateral orchietomy (removal of the testes to eliminate the body's testosterone). For elderly or very sick men, the doctor may recommend a wait-and-see approach.

Alternative and Complementary Approaches

DIETARY REMEDIES According to herbalist Amanda Crawford, good prostate health requires avoidance of alcohol, tobacco, sugar, red meat, and dairy products. It is also imperative to avoid processed foods. At the same time, increase the amount of fiber you eat. Look for organic fruits, vegetables, and whole grains. You'll also want to cut out the coffee. Try green tea instead. Crawford explains: "It has a little bit of caffeine. Caffeine in small doses helps our body. This green tea gives us a gentle lift and it has fewer negative side effects than coffee." A Harvard study of 48,000 men found that those consuming the most tomatoes, tomato sauce, and pizza were up to 45 percent less likely than other men to develop prostate cancer. Lycopene, the pigment in the tomatoes, has been found to help prevent prostate cancer. Lycopene is also found in watermelon and pink grapefruit. Vitamin E and selenium, as noted at the beginning of this chapter, also are beneficial against prostate cancer.

Anne Louise Gittleman, author of *Super Nutrition for Men*, who has a private practice and consults around the country, believes that a lack of trace minerals is connected to prostate problems. First, let us recall the importance of these minerals. They allow us to use ingested proteins by helping produce the enzymes that break down these proteins into amino acids. If they are not broken down, these incoming proteins are toxic to the body. These elements are precursors to all hormonal functions and so are especially important to men.

Most people in our society assimilate only 20 percent of the protein they take in because they are deficient in trace minerals. They may lack them because the purifying and processing of food in our current agricultural methods, along with acid rain and other environmental factors, mean that these minerals are being lost from our plants and diet. We are a mineral-deficient society, which compromises our overall health.

Gittleman highly recommends that men include supplemental trace minerals in their health plan. These minerals will help balance pH, detoxify lymph, and build and re-establish enzyme and hydrochloric acid production. They will also aid in carrying oxygen to the cells.For many men, they may be the missing link to a healthy prostate.

One important trace mineral is zinc. It is vital in the production of testosterone and for muscle strength, which declines with age. Zinc can be depleted from the body by the use of sugar, coffee, and alcohol.

Herbalist Amanda Crawford also recommends increasing zinc. She says you can get this by eating pumpkin seeds. If you're taking the zinc in tablet form, you might need to take 30 to 50 milligrams a day, which is a high dose. So she says it's better to get the mineral through the seeds. Pumpkin seeds, aside from being high in fiber, have the essential fatty acid cucurbitacin. We know this has a beneficial effect on men's health generally and on the prostate in particular. The pumpkin seeds can be taken with almonds, sesame seeds, flax seeds, or milk thistle seeds. The latter are good for the liver and protect the body against some of the compounds that have been associated with prostate cancer. Six hundred to 1,200 milligrams a day of milk thistle seeds are indicated.

You could take a handful a day of each of these seeds: pumpkin, flax, and milk thistle. Crawford says not to tie yourself to one or the other. "Perhaps you could have them in a protein shake each morning or sprinkled on a salad. So you are eating these foods as your medicine and it becomes interesting. You don't have to swallow yet another pill."

Manganese is another valuable mineral. It acts to stabilize blood sugar. It can be obtained from nuts and seeds. Selenium and chromium are two other necessary minerals. Chromium contributes to keeping muscle mass lean, balancing blood sugar, and helping individuals lose weight. Vanadium is a favorite of weight lifters and also helps with blood sugar metabolism.

HERBAL SOLUTIONS Herbalist C.J. Puotinen states that the standard herbal remedy for prostate problems is saw palmetto. It is the easiest herb to find, the easiest to use, and the most likely to bring fast results. It may have gastrointestinal side effects, however. The majority of users experiencing serious prostate symptoms will experience benefits 5 to 10 days after beginning its use.

Amanda Crawford adds that saw palmetto will actually decrease the size of a gland that is already swollen. The way it works is this: As a man ages, his testosterone drops and his estrogen levels begin to rise. The prostate absorbs some of this estrogen but saw palmetto will inhibit the absorption so the gland either reduces in size or ceases to swell.

The saw palmetto is a berry native to Florida and South Carolina. It smells funny and doesn't taste very good but it's rich in oils and beneficial plant compounds. It used to be given to livestock or people after a period of high stress, such as a drought. It has a nourishing effect on men, aiding the essential fatty acids, although its effects are not yet fully understood.

Crawford advises taking 2 grams of the dried berry per day. "You need to get the extract in a kind of solvent that is natural but good at extracting oils. There are some very good extracts on the market today. If you're using the extract, take 320 milligrams a day. Take this for a minimum of a month to see if it's working well. It works best at a minimum of 3 months of consistent use. For many men, they may be taking it a year to see the best benefits. In capsule form, take 160 milligrams, two or three times a day. It is useful to combine it with pygeum Africanum, which is excellent at 40 milligrams three times a day. This can be mixed with pumpkin seed oil as the three work together."

Pygeum, though, may have side effects, including vomiting, nausea, indigestion, and other gastrointestinal difficulties. There are further costs. Pygeum is taken from areas in Africa where the environment has been weakened by industrial farming. People who are politically conscious about how they spend their consumer dollars may not want to support some of the things going on where these plants are harvested. It might be better to use plants that are indigenous to North America, ones that are abundant and not endangered.

Saw palmetto also works very well with nettle root. One teaspoon of the root extract two times a day, morning and night, will reduce the nocturnal need to rise and urinate.

Prostatitis, with painful urination, discharge, and other problems, requires an appropriate diagnosis from a doctor. In addition to what the doctor prescribes, one might want to take a tea of mixed herbs. The recipe is as follows:

damiana leaf	*2 ounces*
echinacea root	*4 ounces*
ginger root	*1/3 ounce*

HOW TO MAKE HERBAL EXTRACTS

In these chapters on men's health, and other chapters throughout the book, we have repeatedly talked about the vital use of herbs in the healing process. It might be worthwhile to pause briefly and talk a little more about herbs. Since we have dwelt on the value of herbal extracts, we'd like to mention how you would go about making your own extract if you so desired. Herbalist C.J. Puotinen tells us, "One way these herbs are available is in raw or crude tinctures." A tincture of this sort is an alcohol extract made by putting one of these herbs in combination with vodka or another grain spirit. These extracts are called crude because they are not chemically manufactured in the laboratory.

You can make these crude extracts on your own in forms that often are more effective than products you can buy over the counter. Let's explain how you would go about doing that, using as an example the preparation of saw palmetto berry, which, as we have seen, is a useful substance to use to work on prostate problems.

You can find the saw palmetto berry in any herbal store. It has a distinctive aroma. Select high quality berries, ones that look like real berries, not shredded wheat. They have a discernible taste and color. These will be dried herbs unless you live in the Southeast or Florida, where they grow.

Take a small amount, say 1 cup of the dried herb for a 4 quart jar. Fill the jar one quarter full with the berry, then half or three quarters full with the vodka, rum, brandy or a neutral grain spirit. Many U.S. herbalists prefer 80 proof vodka.

Cover the herbs with the alcohol for a period of several hours to a few days. They will expand as they absorb the alcohol. Keep an eye on the alcohol level so that you always have a margin of a couple of inches above the dried plant material. Then leave the jar sealed in a warm place, but out of direct sunlight for 4 to 6 weeks. Some herbalists will even prefer 8 weeks. Some will go by the lunar cycle, bottling it at the new moon and keeping it in the container for two full moons, which is about 6 weeks. Shake it every couple of days. By this time the alcohol has absorbed as much of the plant's constituents as it is likely to. Now strain the liquid into a measuring cup and then pour it into amber glass bottles for long-term storage.

You might also choose to pour the liquid into another jar with dried palmetto berries in order to create a double or, eventually, triple strength extract. That would be very effective and can be taken in a smaller dosage. With the double strength extract, you can read the recommended dosage and cut it in half.

It is a time-consuming process, but the extract prepared in this manner will be of better quality than what is bought in stores.

Some people are afraid of using extracts that have been prepared in this way because they anticipate negative effects from the alcohol on their biochemistry. Don't forget, though, that the more concentrated the extract, the less alcohol it has in it. Also remember the dosages are measured in droppers or teaspoons. You will not be taking a large amount. However, if you want to avoid alcohol, you can use other liquids such as vegetable glycerin or cider vinegar, using the same count you would use for spirits. These substances are not as effective because they don't dissolve all the constituents of the herb as alcohol would, nor do they have the preservative qualities. Alcohol tinctures will last for years.

hydrangea root	1 ounce
licorice root	1/3 ounce
stinging nettles	1/3 ounce

Take one ounce of this mixture and steep it—don't boil it—for 15 minutes. Then strain that out. It should be taken for 8 days. The tea nourishes the immune cells and decreases inflammation. And it won't get in the body's way of healing itself.

Dr. Preuss calls our attention to another herb-based remedy, sernatin. Sernatin is a water-soluble extract from flower pollen, mainly derived from rye, dried, mixed, and given in a capsule. This extract has been proven, in double-blind studies, to be as good as or better than pharmacological agents. There are 10 good clinical studies done in Europe and Japan that show the benefits of sernatin. It has been shown that 60 to 80 percent of sufferers get some relief from symptoms without side effects. The only downside is a mild upset stomach, which is reversible by stopping the sernatin or reducing the dosage. This adverse reaction affects 3 percent of takers, which is not that high, since it is a reaction that would affect 1 or 2 percent of those taking a placebo. The dosage is two pills two or three times a day, amounting to about 63 milligrams in total. This extract is commonly used in Europe and Japan, but not so much in the United States.

For the inflamed prostate, hydrangea extract in doses of 20 drops or 30 milligrams is recommended. Herbalist Letha Hadady, in an article posted on the Healthwell website (www.healthwell.com), recommends a Chinese formula called *Kai Kit Wan* for prostate discomfort. She explains that this formula increases circulation, reduces water retention, and relaxes smooth muscles.

THE CHINESE PERSPECTIVE Dr. Michael Tierra, author of *Chinese Traditional Herbal Medicine*, also recommends saw palmetto as herbal treatment for the prostate. However, drawing on the wisdom of Chinese medicine, he points out that there are different causes for prostate dysfunction. Thus, to treat the problem correctly, one must begin with the cause.

If kidney deficiency is to blame, indicating a problem in the endocrine system, it is necessary to strengthen this system. Rehmannia Six or Eight, both Chinese herbal preparations, are called for. Six if for a *yin* deficiency; eight for a *yang* deficiency. The basis of Chinese medicine is not, as in Western medicine, to see the prostate problem as a single disease, but to break the disease down into components and see how it is individually manifesting. Each symptom is addressed by an herb, and the symptom picture in general is handled by an herbal combination.

Kidney deficiency that creates a prostate problem can be further divided into three basic types. First, there are problems due to poor circulation in the pelvic region. These can be treated with lovage, Chinese salvia, red sage, or red peony. Second are problems in the urine flow, so that it is slow or incomplete. These problems should be treated with diuretic herbs, such as water plantain, which is grown in the United States, or *fu ling*. Third, there may be problems with swelling. These should be treated with utilizing herbs, such as seaweed, particularly kelp. Another incredibly effective herbal remedy from China is Kit Kat pills, which will treat swelling as well as frequent urination.

In all cases, about 9 grams a day of the herbs should be taken. Dr. Tierra suggests that his patients take the herbs in a tea. He gives them a combination that will include several herbs. A patient takes 4 or 5 cups of water, cooks them down to 2, and then drinks 1 cup in the morning and one in the evening.

David Molony—herbalist, acupuncturist, and author of *The Complete Guide to Chinese Herbal Medicine*— adds that for an inflamed prostate, gentiana formula is helpful because it includes herbs that cool the inflammation, as would antibiotics, and has a diuretic effect, increasing urination. This formula can be purchased in a Chinese herb store. The usual dose is eight pills, three times a day.

MASSAGE Prostate problems can also be treated with massage. For the massage oil, you'll need a carrier oil to which small amounts of the essential oils will be added. For the carrier oil, use olive oil, almond oil, or any cold-pressed oil. Don't use a vegetable oil. Add to this oil the essential oils; these are aromatherapy oils, derived by steam distillation from herbs. Take a few drops of these herbal oils. One recipe calls for 5 drops of either lavender or thyme oil. Then add 10 drops of cypress or fir to add an evergreen fragrance. To that add 10 drops of eucalyptus and rosemary, for a cleansing fragrance. Put this in 1 fluid ounce (2 tablespoons) of the carrier oil.

Massage this into the prostate area and into the whole lower abdomen and even into the back. Massage the gland, which is four or five inches into the rectum, for 15 or 20 minutes. The swelling frequently goes down immediately as fluids are cleared by finger pressure. You may see a shiny black waste that is liberated.

Massage the deep muscles around the prostate gland between the testes and the rectum. This will have an uplifting and antidepressant effect.

An even simpler way to pamper the prostate requires little effort. Invert your posture. Get a slant board and lie on it for 20 to 30 minutes a day or use yoga to take some of the pressure off the area. Let gravity give you a massage.

You may also try an enema, using first hot water and then cold water to expel stagnant fluids.

ACUPUNCTURE Dr. Michael Tierra also has found acupuncture to be helpful in relation to prostate problems. "It should be done on a weekly basis," he states. "There are points to be touched on the inner legs and abdomen. This will not be as effectively reached by acupressure. Acupuncture must be done."

PART TWELVE
Aging Well

In the largely unread, fourth book of *Gulliver's Travels*, the hero comes to an island, near Japan, where a race has realized mankind's dream of living forever. The irony is that these immortals all wish they were dead because, though they have lived hundreds of years, these have been miserable years, since they have all the infirmities of the aged, such as blindness, deafness, arthritis, and senility. Jonathan Swift's satirical thrust can be applied today, when we consider the following facts. Americans are living longer than ever before, but many are unable to enjoy longevity because its potential pleasures are canceled out by the prematurely early encroachments of aging.

In the following chapters, we look at how aging affects many of the body's systems, including the brain, and the natural techniques now being used to reverse it. In addition, we look specifically at two "health and beauty" areas that are not only affected by the aging process but also are cause for concern at other times of life: teeth and hair.

62

Reversing the Aging Process Naturally

The idea that aging inevitably means gaining weight and having high blood pressure, high triglycerides, high cholesterol levels, and arthritis is widely accepted. Since so many people have these problems, we think of them as normal. Even doctors are likely to say that when you get to be a certain age, these conditions are to be expected and, since they are irreversible, accepted.

Fortunately, research over the last decade has given us a better understanding of the causes of aging; in particular, several theories have led to new therapies offering older people opportunities not only to improve their health but to actually slow down the aging processes. We now know that it's possible to live to 100 and beyond and to stay healthy throughout our life spans, thus "rectangularizing" the aging curve. Dr. Martin Feldman, a traditionally trained physician who practices complementary medicine, supports this stand.

"We need to have optimum energy as we grow old, not accept the diminishment many find encroaching as they grow older." Dr. Feldman cites joint disease as an example of a condition that medicine has accepted as inevitable, a condition that is reversible. There is now an epidemic of joint disease in the United States. The majority of people over 60 have early, moderate, or late osteoarthritis. Conventional doctors call osteoarthritis a wear-and-tear disease, as if the joints wore out like the parts of a car. That sounds plausible, but it is nonsense. The disease is a product of deficiencies and occurs when the joint is not being nourished. A nourished joint will remain healthy. Dr. Feldman has seen marathon runners in their 70s and 80s who use their joints 10-fold or even 50-fold more than a normal person does, yet their joints remain robust.

Causes of Aging

FREE RADICAL DAMAGE It is widely accepted that aging and degenerative diseases are the result of cellular damage brought on by free radicals, molecules that have become unstable after losing one of their orbiting electrons. The unpaired electrons of these molecules make the molecules highly reactive, and in an attempt to restore balance, a free radical will steal electrons from other molecules, causing cellular damage and destruction.

Free radicals are produced through normal metabolism in the body, but increase with exposure to animal fat, alcohol, cigarettes, and other toxic chemicals. Dr. Christopher Calapai, a proponent of complementary medicine who has a medical practice in New York City, gives an example of how this damage can occur: "Free radicals generated by cigarette smoke are huge in number. They steal healthy electrons from the lining of the lungs, thereby oxidizing lung tissue. When lung tissue is oxidized, cells break down and die. As hundreds of thousands of cells become oxidized and damaged, tissues and organs throughout the body are affected. Aging and disease are magnified."

LOW THYROID FUNCTION Low thyroid functioning can prompt diseases associated with aging. Dr. Ray Peat, a distinguished research scientist from Eugene, Oregon, says that doctors in the first part of the 20th century were better informed than today's doctors about the importance of correcting this condition: "Most of the basic research on the thyroid was done before World War II. Pharmaceutical companies came in after the war with what they thought was the latest word in understanding the thyroid. It turns out they were wrong. Until 1940, it was accepted that 40 percent of Americans benefited from taking thyroid supplements. After faulty tests were established, it was believed that only 5 percent of Americans needed or benefited from thyroid supplements. In the 1930s indications of hypothyroidism included such things as too much cholesterol in the blood, insomnia, emphysema, arthritis, and failure of the immune system. Many conditions now considered mysterious diseases were recognized as traits of low thyroid. Very often these conditions would simply disappear when thyroid supplements were given.

"When the thyroid is low we have to rely on emergency systems—such as the production of adrenaline and cortisone—to adapt to stress. Cortisone and adrenaline are now recognized as factors that cause damage, setting degenerative diseases in motion and causing damage to the lining of blood vessels and brain cells, but very often people don't realize that it is the thyroid that keeps us from relying excessively on these stress hormones."

BIOLOGICAL CLOCK Another theory holds that the body has a built-in cellular "biological clock" that is set so that cells self-destruct after a certain amount of time. Dr. Lance Morris, a naturopathic physician from Tucson, Arizona, notes that since the theory was first propounded, the proposed upper limits for the clock's running time have increased. "At this time," he says, "there is a feeling that the top limit is pushing 140 years. Individuals have actually lived to that age, and even longer."

SHRINKING THYMUS GLAND Another theory relates aging to atrophy of the thymus gland, which plays a role in maintaining a healthy immune system and fighting infection. As Dr. Morris explains, "When we are born, this gland covers our entire chest. It's huge. As we grow older, it diminishes in size, a process known as thymic involution. One of the theories of aging is that if we could stop thymic shrinking we could stop the aging process altogether."

MERCURY Dr. Hal A. Huggins of Colorado Springs, Colorado, highlights another cause of premature aging, the mercury in silver amalgam fillings. According to Dr. Huggins, the mercury in your fillings does not just sit there—you inhale it and it goes into your lungs. Every time you eat and chew, minute amounts of mercury get into your stomach and digestive system and from there to cells in all parts of your body, where it can undergo oxidation, forming methyl mercury, a highly toxic substance.

OTHER THEORIES Dr. Elton Haas, an integrated medicine physician, is director of the Preventive Medical Center in San Rafael, California, and author of *The Staying Healthy Shopper's Guide*, among other best-selling books. In an article on the HealthWorld Online website (www.healthy.net), he summarizes a few other theories of aging: errors in DNA, possibly caused by free radicals; alterations in brain function; imbalance in the hormonal and nervous systems; a breakdown in immune system function; and stress. His own theory, he explains, is that all these processes combine in various ways in each person to result in aging, with the key factor being "stagnation of bioenergy circulation and stagnation of the digestive tract and bowels."

Symptoms

A wide variety of gradual bodily changes are associated with aging, such as an increased susceptibility to weight gain and fatigue. But there is no physiological reason why most people should become obese or get tired more easily as they grow older: these are society's, not nature's, norms. It can be just as natural, for example, for people to eat and sleep a little less as they grow older, compensating for any slowing down of metabolic processes and thus maintaining stable weight and energy levels.

Typical signs of aging also include changes in skin, hair, nails, and connective tissue. Decreases in memory, concentration, and sharpness may also accompany aging. Again, it is not inevitable that these changes take place.

As people age, they may suffer from elevated blood sugar, an increase in cholesterol and triglycerides, and other chemical imbalances. The risk of contracting degenerative diseases such as cancer and heart disease, and suffering from thyroid dysfunction, musculoskeletal problems, and gastrointestinal disorders, also typically increases with age.

Diagnosing Problems

Aging well means being healthy and balanced from within. To check that all systems are running optimally, Dr. Calapai recommends a full spectrum of diagnostic tests, with special attention to adrenal function, vitamin and mineral levels, blood chemistry, pancreatic enzymes, and stool. "The adrenal glands produce our antiaging hormones. With age, some people start producing less. This can be from free radical damage, excessive stress, injuries, and all sorts of reasons. As a result we see changes in memory, concentration, skin, hair, hormonal fluctuations, and energy levels. We start to see problems with immune response and increases in blood sugar, cholesterol, and abdominal deposition of body fat. So we need to look at adrenal function.

"Certainly, tests should look at vitamin and mineral levels to check our digestive and absorptive abilities. Looking at the basic blood chemistry tells us how well we are absorbing protein. We need to look at the fat-soluble vitamins and cholesterol, triglycerides, and the ratio of good HDL cholesterol to bad LDL cholesterol, which can provide information about our fat absorption. I also recommend looking at enzymes of the pancreas to assess function and having a comprehensive stool analysis done to see whether or not there are too many undigested particles in the stool. If parasites are present, this can decrease our absorptive ability. These are some of the main tests we need to perform to get a thorough picture of the individual."

Natural Approach to Aging

ANTIAGING DIET A basic healthy diet will vastly improve the quality of life and reduce the aging process in people of all ages. This diet should consist of high-quality organic foods, emphasizing complex carbohydrates such as beans and whole grains, fruits, and vegetables. Adolescents, who are still growing, may need more of certain nutrients, and people in specific age groups may have specific nutrient requirements that can be addressed through supplements.

Antiaging diets contain few, if any, animal-based proteins; fats are minimized and high-fiber foods are emphasized. High-fiber diets help prevent common afflictions associated with aging, such as constipation, hemorrhoids, pressure in the intestines, ulcers, high blood pressure, colorectal cancer, and overall body toxemia. One of the principles of longevity is eating to the point of being not quite full. As we get older, it is advisable to eat small servings more frequently. Uneaten portions can be frozen for later use.

At least eight 8-ounce glasses of water should be drunk daily. Many senior citizens suffer from dehydration because their intake of fluid is inadequate. Dehydration adversely affects the body's electrolytes, which carry electricity and are important for normal functioning of the nervous system. Additionally, fresh juices, which are high in enzymes, should be a regular part of the diet. Recommended intake is two to three 6-ounce glasses of fresh, organic mixed vegetable juice per day, with 1 to 2 milligrams of buffered vitamin C added to each glass, or up to bowel tolerance.

VEGETARIAN DIETS A number of doctors stress the benefits of a healthy vegetarian diet. For example, participants in Dr. Martin Feldman's nutritional program, who are on a vegetarian diet, are doing better lowering their cholesterol than any comparable group. He states, "We did not select people to come in to work on cholesterol problems. We are using a total assault on the lifestyle without focusing on cholesterol. The level of reduction is superior to that found in any prior drug study [studies in which drugs were used to cut down on cholesterol]. It is extremely important that we can achieve this reduction without drugs. Drugs are expensive and have side effects. Also, we do not know what long-term problems may arise with them."

Dr. Dean Ornish has shown that a vegetarian diet can help clear the arteries.

SUPPLEMENTS The first thing to look at as a means of reversing the symptoms of aging is supplements. Most people do not understand the effective use of vitamins and minerals as dietary supplements. Basically, you must follow the law of compensation. If you smoked, used sugar, caffeine, or alcohol, if you were an angry person who held in your anger, if you have not honored the life force, if you have not exercised, if you have felt unfulfilled, you must work to compensate for these deficiencies.

One-a-day supplements are the easy way out. I have met people who say, "I eat meat. I eat sugar. But it's all right because I take my one-a-day vitamin." My friend, that does not work. The body cannot be lied to. After 30 or 40 years of the body's being debilitated by an unhealthy lifestyle and environment, a little pill will not do the trick. You need to detoxify and cleanse the body.

You have to know what your bodily state is and plan accordingly. I would suggest one level of usage for healthy people who know they are healthy, and a very different level for those processing diseases. A person becoming conscious of his or her health will need to consult a nutritionist who can design a personalized supplement program to meet his or her individual needs.

The reason that supplements are even more crucial as we get older is that as we age, certain fatty acids, amino acids, and members of the main groups of nutrients are lost. Scientists looking into this issue already know that choline, tyrosine, glutathione, cysteine, vitamin E, zinc, and chromium are poorly absorbed and deficient in older people. Meanwhile, as these substances grow scarce, there is a buildup of heavy metals, such as aluminum and lead. These metals can be removed from the body through a process known as chelation. Vitamin C and zinc are also useful in flushing them out. Most importantly, all the nutrients that are lost, for whatever reason, must be restored for optimum physical and mental functioning.

At the same time, the free radicals in our bodies, which grow in number as we age, have to be fought. Remember, when you eat meat, drink alcohol, and are exposed to pollutants, the body creates free radicals. They cause the skin to wrinkle in the sun, and they foster cancer, arthritis, and heart disease. However, antioxidants, such as beta carotene and vitamin A, are able to neutralize the effect of the free radicals, slowing down the aging process.

ANTIOXIDANTS

Dr. Morris calls aging a catch-22: "Oxygen is the great substance that sustains and gives life, but unfortunately it is also the substance that destroys us through oxidation." For this reason, antioxidants are essential. Here are the most important ones.

VITAMIN E. 400–1,600 international units (IU), taken at the largest meal. People with herpes, chronic fatigue syndrome, hepatitis, and even AIDS have dramatically improved after taking large doses of this vitamin on a regular basis. Dr. Wilfred Shute, who works with his brother Evan in Canada, has treated over 30,000 patients in his decades of medical practice. He has helped patients with intermittent claudication, diabetes, gangrene, and many other conditions. Vitamin E is best in its natural form (as a mixed tocopherol or d-alphatocopherol). Synthetic vitamin E (dl-alpha) should be avoided.

BETA CAROTENE. 25,000 IU per meal. Beta carotenes can be obtained in all the green, red, and orange fruits and vegetables. They help slow down aging and lessen cancer risk. They are nontoxic, since the body converts beta carotenes into vitamin A and will not convert more than it can use.

VITAMIN A. 1,000–3,000 IU per meal. Blood tests will determine whether or not a person is getting too much vitamin A, which can be toxic.

SELENIUM. 100 micrograms per meal. One cause of premature aging and even death, particularly in professional athletes, is cardiomyopathy, an enlargement of the heart. This is usually associated with selenium deficiency. Adequate amounts of this critical nutrient are needed to help the body produce the antioxidant enzyme glutathione peroxidase, which is on the front line of aging defense.

ZINC. 30 to 90 milligrams daily. Zinc feeds over 100 enzyme systems in the brain, as well as various systems throughout the body. It is essential in the formation of stomach acid; without sufficient zinc, malabsorption syndrome occurs. Most older people are zinc-deficient.

VITAMIN C. 2,000 to 5,000 milligrams daily, higher doses for antiaging protocols and fighting disease (under medical supervision, up to 150,000 milligrams via intravenous drips). The single most important dietary supplement is vitamin C. Its benefits are multiple. This vitamin is important for the skin, giving it youthful elasticity. This is because it produces collagen, a type of connective tissue that holds the muscles and skin together. It helps the body produce interferon (an antiviral glycoprotein) and increases leukocyte activity. It aids the thymus gland, the liver, and the brain, while acting to prevent arthritis, cataracts, and heart disease.

At the Healing Center of New York City, drips of vitamin C and other nutrients are used to counteract the aging process. Dr. Howard Robins points out that toxins and free radicals are stressful to both the body and mind. A body in pain, fatigued, and under attack from heavy metal and other pollutants is weakened, and the mind is adversely affected. Dr. Robins asserts that intravenously administered vitamin C cleanses the body. The Healing Center also uses drips with other nutrients, such as EDTA (ethylenediaminetetra-acetic acid) to cleanse the heavy metals from the body, and destroy viruses and keep them from replicating. These drips will also help boost energy levels.

GRAPESEED EXTRACT. 50 milligrams per day, up to 200 milligrams per day for people in a disease state. This bioflavonoid has the highest known antioxidant properties of any nutrient.

SUPEROXIDE DISMUTASE. This important antienzyme nutrient is produced by the body. It is not effective when taken orally unless it is enteric-coated. According to Dr. Haas, manganese and copper, together with zinc, support the action of superoxide dismutase.

HORMONES Dr. Richard Ash has talked to his large New York City radio audience about the revivifying power of DHEA (dihydroepiandrosterone), which is a key ingredient underlying the normal functioning of the adrenal gland. He tells us that when the body is under stress, the adrenal gland requires higher amounts of cortisone and adrenaline. If these hormones are overused, they will become depleted as will DHEA, their precursor.

An 80-year-old woman may have only one-twentieth of the DHEA she had at age 20. According to Dr. Ash, this can result in all sorts of negative consequences for the immune system, leading to a weakened capacity to fight diseases. One of the earliest signs of DHEA depletion is an inability to get REM sleep, which can lead to insomnia and chronic fatigue. An uninformed doctor may prescribe sleeping pills for a patient with insomnia, which will not get at the root of the problem. Other symptoms of low DHEA levels are hyperglycemia (an excess of glucose in the blood), palpitations, sweating, confusion, poor concentration, and the inability to cope with everyday stress.

Another effect of low DHEA is a reduction in salivary IgA, an antibody that fights infection in the gastrointestinal (GI) tract. When IgA is depleted or absent, there will be more antigen penetration in this area as well as increased sensitivity reactions to foods and chemicals There may be inflammation of the GI tract, a condition called "leaky gut," in which certain foods and chemicals are not absorbed but pass out into the bloodstream. When the body tries to defend itself against these unexpected intruders, autoimmune disease may arise. Dr. Ash notes that by administering DHEA and building back up salivary IgA, we can diminish food sensitivity, lower toxic load, and repair the GI tract, restoring normal immune system functioning by treating the cause not the symptoms.

Dr. Eric Braverman, founder and director of Princeton Associates for Total Health in Princeton, New Jersey, has found that counteracting the aging process has to be undertaken on an individual basis. His treatments are personalized on the basis of each patient's specific hormone balance, brain function, attention span, memory capacity, and cardiac and exercise capacities. Once these have been evaluated, the patient's nutritional needs are assessed. He recommends natural yam extract, which contains progesterone, estrogen, and testosterone (PET), the three hormones he considers essential. Progesterone has anticancer properties and helps calm the brain. Estrogen strengthens the bones, has anticancer effects, especially in the colon, aids memory, and gives cardiovascular protection.

Testosterone reduces the side effects of other hormones, and helps keep the sex drive vigorous through a person's fifties, sixties, and beyond. For a woman, the ovary produces all three of these substances, but, as Dr. Braverman puts it, "If the ovary dies, you must resurrect it. If you permit an organ to die, you allow yourself to die. We must stop this if we want abundant life. We replace depleted hormones with PET, and missing adrenal with DHEA."

BIOFLAVONOID COMPLEX Another invaluable supplement group is the citrus bioflavonoid complex, which can be obtained from lemons, plums, and oranges, among other fruits. With an orange, one can cut open the skin and right below is the nutrient, the bioflavonoid. Another good bioflavonoid is rutin, which comes from buckwheat. To take the bioflavonoid in pill form, I recommend 300 milligrams per day for a healthy person, while someone in poor health should take 500 milligrams. As for the rutin, the proper dosage for a healthy person is 25 milligrams per day, while the ill person may take up to 50 milligrams.

BLUEBERRY AND RED CABBAGE EXTRACTS. Blueberry extract is good for the eyes. During World War II, the Royal Air Force gave this to its pilots to improve night vision and strengthen the immune system. Red cabbage extract is also important. There are cultures that lack a variety of foodstuffs, but those peoples eat cabbage and obtain its antibacterial, antiulcer properties. Cabbage, eaten juiced or steamed, is very healthful.

GREEN TEA. If you lived in China, you would probably be drinking green tea and taking green tea extract. We know it has anticancer properties. It is an immune system stimulator. Decaffeinated green tea is very beneficial.

GLUTATHIONE. Glutathione is good for the immune system, but it is not easily assimilated by the body, so it should be taken with something that produces it in the body, such as N-acetylcysteine. The recommended dose is 200 milligrams a day for the healthy and up to 400 milligrams for those not in the best of health.

OTHER SUPPLEMENTS

CALCIUM. Calcium protects against osteoporosis and colon cancer, is important for strong teeth, and helps energy (production as well as heart and nerve function.

CHROMIUM. Chromium supports glucose tolerance, decreasing the craving for sugar, and plays a role in preventing atherosclerosis by helping to lower blood cholesterol.

COENZYME Q10. Every cell in the body needs this coenzyme to create energy and build stamina.

L-CARNITINE. L-carnitine, a nonessential amino acid involved in fat metabolism, may help reduce fat and weight.

L-CYSTEINE. This amino acid, which scavenges free radicals, protects the tissues from chemicals and aids detoxification, partly by helping the liver produce and store glutathione. Most often it is taken with vitamin C to prevent the formation of kidney stones of cysteine, which is produced when cysteine is metabolized. Take 250 milligrams with a gram of vitamin C twice a day. When you take L-cysteine on a regular basis, you should also take a formula that contains the other amino acids the body needs.

DIGESTIVE AIDS. *Lactobacillus acidophilus*, along with other intestinal bacteria, may be needed occasionally to support the balance of bacteria in the colon. Similarly, supplements of hydrochloric acid and digestive enzymes aid digestion and metabolism of food, and thus prevent both nutritional deficiencies and free-radical formation due to food reactions.

ESSENTIAL FATTY ACIDS. Essential fatty acids, such as EPA (eicosapentaenoic acid) and DHA (docosahexaenoic acid), diminish the risk of cardiovascular disease. Flaxseed oil is a good source of both omega-3 and omega-6 essential fatty acids.

FOLIC ACID. Folic acid also helps in RNA, DNA, and red blood cell synthesis.

MAGNESIUM. Magnesium supports the cardiovascular system and decreases nervous tension.

MOLYBDENUM. Molybdenum is a trace mineral that may help prevent cancer.

NIACIN. Niacin, a form of vitamin B_3, decreases cholesterol and helps improve circulation.

NADH (NICOTINAMIDE ADENINE DINUCLEATIDE). Also known as coenzyme 1, NADH is a naturally occurring substance in the body that supplies energy to the cells, allowing them to live longer.

RNA. RNA, taken in blue-green algae, spirulina, chlorella, and wheatgrass (all of which also are rich in chlorophyll), can decelerate the aging process.

SEA ALGAE. High in trace elements, antioxidant cofactors, flavonoids, and carotenoid.

THYMUS EXTRACT. Pure oral thymus extract enhances immune function and helps reverse the aging process.

TYROSINE. Strengthens the thyroid and adrenal glands, protecting against stress.

VITAMIN B_{12}. Vitamin B_{12} boosts energy and protects the fatty sheaths that cover the nerves. It is involved in synthesis of red blood cells and DNA and RNA, which are needed for important rebuilding processes.

HERBS Herbs are an important part of any antiaging nutritional protocol, and can be taken as capsules, powders, teas, or tinctures.

FO-TI. *Fo-ti* rejuvenates the endocrine system and is an excellent digestive tonic.

GINKGO BILOBA. The ginkgo tree has survived for hundreds of thousands of years due to its powerful immune system. An extract of the leaf of the tree improves circulation to the microcapillaries of the brain and heart so that needed nutrients and oxygen can get to all the tissues.

GINSENG. Ginseng is the best-known longevity herb. For centuries, the Chinese have revered ginseng for its rejuvenating effects. Research has shown that ginseng can stop the free radical damage associated with aging. It helps people focus better when under stress and increases overall energy levels.

GOTU KOLA. Elephants, which graze on gotu kola, are known to have excellent memories and to be long-lived. Gotu kola is useful for increasing vitality and endurance, and may lower blood pressure.

HAWTHORN BERRIES. Hawthorn berries support circulation and cardiac function.

MILK THISTLE. Milk thistle protects liver function. The liver releases toxins from the body, promoting health and youthfulness.

YAM. Wild yam supports adrenal gland production of DHEA, a building block for the development of estrogen, progesterone, testosterone, and cortisols, which decrease with age. As an adaptogen, wild yam balances the body's hormonal functions. It has been shown to ameliorate numerous chronic conditions, including heart disease, cancer, arthritis, and autoimmune diseases. DHEA is extremely safe, with no known side effects.

Dr. Haas mentions two other beneficial herbs: *Capsicum* stimulates elimination and circulation, and its mild diuretic properties help cleanse the kidneys. *Garlic* is antiviral, antibacterial, and antifungal. It boosts energy but—unlike coffee—helps lower cholesterol and blood pressure. Garlic also stimulates liver and colon detoxification and may have anticancer properties.

DETOXIFICATION THERAPIES The more toxic we are, the faster we age. Cosmetic changes such as face-lifts and hair dye may temporarily make people appear younger, but they do not make a real difference. To keep youthful and healthy, we must address what is happening inside. "Everyone needs detoxification," says Susan Lombardi, founder and president of the We Care Health Center in Palm Springs, California, and author of *Ten Easy Steps for Complete Wellness.* "I am vegetarian, and I take care of myself. Do I still need detoxification? Yes, because the air that we breathe is polluted, the water that we drink is full of chlorine, the clothing we wear is made of artificial fabrics and chemicals, the lotions and shampoos that we use all contain chemicals. Once these chemicals are inside us, we never fully eliminate them unless we go through a detoxification procedure." Lombardi recommends rejuvenating the system from the inside out by limiting food intake to fresh raw vegetable juices once a week, along with the following simple, yet effective, detoxification therapies.

JUICE FASTING
Juice fasting is detailed in chapter 9, Detoxification.

CHELATION THERAPY

Dr. Martin Dayton, who is board-certified in family medicine, chelation therapy, and clinical nutrition, says that chelation therapy has multiple benefits, and long life is one of them:

"Dramatic increases in life span are found with chelation. While there are no longevity studies per se, this conclusion is implied indirectly by studies which show a lessening of killer degenerative diseases. In fact, chelation favorably impacts all four major causes of death in the United States [heart disease, cancer, cerebrovascular disease, and lung disease]." In chelation therapy, a synthetic amino acid, EDTA, is administered to the patient through an intravenous drip. The EDTA moves through the blood vessels and attaches itself to heavy metals in the blood such as mercury and lead, holding onto these substances until they are washed out of the body in the urine.

Aside from its overall benefits, chelation therapy specifically helps aging individuals by improving brain function. Dr. Dayton cites the following evidence: "Research shows that circulation improves greatly in the brain and to the brain. One study of 15 patients who had 20 infusions of chelation therapy found that 14 out of 15 demonstrated significant cerebral blood flow. Some showed dramatic improvement in cognitive abilities.

"In another study, 30 patients with carotid blockages were given 30 chelation treatments over a 10-month period. The carotid artery extends from the chest through the neck to the brain. It is the brain's main source of blood flow. Blockage decreased between 20 and 40 percent.

"Unclogging carotid blockage is vitally important because the American College of Physicians states that patients with an obstruction of 70 percent or greater are at a high risk for stroke. They even recommend chelation therapy as a preferred treatment. I take that to heart and use chelation therapy on these individuals. People who have carotid artery disease improve as their arteries open up. I see this happen over and over again." (See chapter 32 for more on chelation.)

COLON CLEANSING

Colon cleansing refers to washing out of the colon in order to remove toxic buildups. The procedure is described in detail in chapter 9.

ENZYME THERAPY

Nina Anderson, author of *Over Fifty, Looking Thirty: The Secrets of Staying Young*, attributes slow aging to sufficient enzyme levels: "Many scientists say that people get old before their time due to enzyme exhaustion. Some people are old at 40 because of the lack of enzymes, while others are young at 80 because of an abundance. Above all else, I would advise anybody who is trying to avoid looking and feeling older as they get older to take supplemental enzymes."

She goes on to explain that enzymes allow nutrients to be used. For example, you have enzymes in the heart that allow magnesium to be used. Without those enzymes, magnesium cannot get to the heart: "Enzymes are molecule catalysts found everywhere in your body. In fact, there are over 1,300 different ones. They make everything happen. In my book I use this analogy: minerals are building blocks of your body. They are the nose, eyes, ears, bones, all the things that hold you together. Something has to build this. Enzymes are the construction workers that facilitate everything in the body going together."

Anderson recommends eating more raw foods, mineral supplements, and digestive plant enzymes to increase enzyme levels. Raw foods are loaded with enzymes. Fruit and vegetable juices are filled with enzymes. When food is processed, the first things taken out are enzymes. Why? Because the enzymes are what allow the food to ripen. However, if the food becomes too ripe, it rots. To stop it from ripening and rotting so that it can be sold longer, these enzymes must be destroyed. But if you destroy the enzymes, you destroy the food's life force. It will have carbohydrates, vitamins, fats, and minerals, but not its life force.

"The mineral supplements to take," Anderson adds, "should be in crystalloid form, with electrolytes. The crystalloid form goes right into the cell walls. This fortifies your body.

"Plant enzymes assist in the digestion of food right on through the intestinal tract. You want to help the digestive process for the whole length of the digestive tract. With supplemental enzymes, you won't have an upset stomach anymore or feel bloated and exhausted after a big meal. The skin will start to improve too. The skin manifests everything that happens inside. If your inner organs start to degenerate, if they are not functioning properly, this kind of stress shows up on your face. The first thing people do when they start getting older is look in the mirror and go, 'Oh my God, I've got wrinkles.' They spend millions trying to get rid of them. But what they have to realize is that wrinkles start from inside. You have to work on the inside to get the outside to reflect that good health.

"Without the proper enzymes, none of the other good things you do matter. For example, the fat-soluble vitamins A, D, E, and K require fat for absorption. That fat has to be broken down by an enzyme, lipase. If lipase is not present in sufficient quantities, that fat will not be broken down. If the fat isn't broken down, the vitamins will not be released. Therefore, you can spend a fortune on vitamin pills, and if you don't have the proper enzymes to release those vitamins into your system, they are just going to be flushed out."

Enzymes can be used externally as well as internally for youthful effects: "There are amazing enzyme treatments for the skin. Papaya enzymes are wonderful. Or you can mix a plant enzyme powder and put it on as a mask. Not only does it take the lines out of your face, but it fills them in and builds up collagen. It can also get rid of age spots and shrink moles. When you use enzymes as a mud pack when you come in from the sun, it fights free radicals that otherwise might foster melanoma."

EXERCISE AND OTHER PHYSICAL TECHNIQUES When we exercise, we detoxify as we sweat through our skin and exhale from our lungs. Some good exercises include jogging or daily brisk walks, yoga stretches, and jumping on a minitrampoline, which exercises every cell in the body. Exercise slows down the aging process because it stimulates detoxification.

Chiropractor Mitch Proffman says that traditional cultures have appreciated the connection between physical fitness and longevity, making athletic activities a part of women's ritual ceremonies: "In traditional Navajo society women would run three times daily as a formal part of the 4-day rites of passage after the onset of menstruation. The first run was at dawn, and each subsequent run would be for a longer distance. It was believed that the total distance a woman could run would determine her longevity."

He goes on to state that recent research supports the connection between exercise and a longer life: "The *Journal of the American Medical Association* has reported that exercise increases people's life spans. Women walking 40 to 50 minutes, three to four times per week, live longer. The same article claims that exercise decreases the chance of dying from all known diseases. This can be attributed to the fact that most major diseases, such as cancer, diabetes, and heart disease, are stress-related, and exercise reduces stress.

"Another important function of exercising is that people's mental abilities improve. In a recent study at the University of Illinois, Dr. William Greenboro, studied four different groups of rats. One group led a sedentary life. Another group played aimlessly on wood and plastic in their cages. A third group was on a special motorized wheel, and a fourth group walked through intricate mazes and ropes. The finding was that all rats that exercised in any manner had more capillaries in their brains and better brain function. This suggests that exercise fuels the brain with more oxygen and increases natural growth factors, in humans as well as in rats."

Dr. Joseph Pizzorno, president of John Bastyr College of Naturopathic Medicine in Seattle, Washington, says that strengthening exercises are the best defense against the increased frailty people face as they age: "It turns out that the majority of the debility of old age is simply due to people not using their muscles. The full strength of what one had at twenty and thirty is almost completely returned with weight strengthening exercises. There are a lot of different weight training programs out there. I have been doing some research. The one I find most effective, and am now using personally, is something called Super Slow. Weights are used in a very, very controlled, very, very intense way to get maximum effects from the exercise. I am quite impressed with what I have seen."

STRESS RELEASE "In my personal opinion, the single most important factor influencing aging and disease is stress," says Dr. Morris. "We need to control emotional anxieties and tensions, and learn how to not let life get to us. It is important to learn to let go and enjoy life." Methods Dr. Morris suggests to overcome stress include deep breathing exercises, tai chi, yoga, meditation, qi gong, mantras, massage, Reiki, and biofeedback. "These are things I recommend that all of us do in the pursuit of health, longevity and wellness." Although exercise strengthens muscle and increases suppleness, sometimes bad patterns of movement or chronic tensions create problems in the joints or muscles. One practice that helps eliminate the problem of poor movement habits is the Feldenkrais method.

Since exercise increases oxygenation, it also has the potential to foster free radical damage. To prevent undesirable effects, women may want to combine exercise with sufficient amounts of antioxidants in the diet and/or as dietary supplements. (See "Antioxidants," above.)

BREATHING EXERCISES Breathing exercises combined with physical activity increase the action of lymphatic cleansing. Detoxification expert Susan Lombardi explains: "For lymphatic cleansing, you want to synchronize your breathing with the movement of your legs and arms. When you are walking or jumping on the trampoline, inhale four times and exhale four times. Move your arms and legs each time you take a little breath. Inhale through your nose and exhale through your nose or mouth.

"This breathing technique was learned from the Taromaro Indians, who live in the northern part of Mexico. They are famous for their fantastic health. They have no need of hospitals or homes for the elderly. They have no disease, no police force, no jails, and no mental institutions."

SKIN BRUSHING Using a natural brush on dry skin removes dead cells and leaves pores open, so that more toxins can be expelled. Lombardi explains why this is so important: "We are supposed to eliminate two pounds of toxins through the pores of the skin. Due to pollution, smog, the creams we use, the clothes we wear, and so forth, our pores are more closed than open. Always brush toward the heart."

SAUNAS The sauna is a good follow-up to dry skin brushing because it pushes toxins out through the skin. The main thing to remember with saunas is to be prudent. You want to perspire but not remain there for too long. Nor do you want too much heat. "Follow the directions," says Lombardi. "And wear a cooling drape on your head. You don't want to heat up the brain area."

There are multiple benefits from sauna detoxification, explains Lombardi: "You will look and feel better. Your skin will be clear and you will not have constipation. Your nails will improve as well as your heart and digestive system. It will clear your mind and improve concentration. Nothing will de-stress your body like a sauna."

MAGNETIC HEALING Susan Bucci is a holistically trained nurse who has spearheaded the development of magnetic healing products. "Magnets oxygenate tissues and allow cell walls to absorb more oxygen," she explains. "They promote mental acuity and normalize pH balance by increasing alkalinity. Restorative sleep is enhanced. Therapeutically, they stop pain, fight infection, and reduce inflammation and fluid retention. Over time, fatty and calcium deposits dissolve and the circulatory system opens up. Put that all together and you've got healing from A to Z. Take that a step further: If you achieve optimal well-being, you can actually live a long, productive life."

In addition to promoting overall well-being, magnets can eliminate many specific signs and symptoms of old age. Bucci reports these antiaging benefits from her own use of magnetic healing techniques: "My energy level has increased. I used to have chronic fatigue in the worst way, but now that's gone. My immune system is functioning much better, so my susceptibility to viruses and colds has decreased dramatically. Allergies are basically gone, and there are no more killer sinus headaches. My circulation has improved so that I withstand weather a whole lot easier. Wounds heal quickly, and my spider veins have disappeared. Also, I was headed for an early menopause, but now my menstrual cycle is very much on track, very regular.

"Hair, skin, and nails have definitely improved. My hair grows faster and has a much better quality to it. Within 2 weeks of using magnets on a daily basis, I was able to see new, thick, dark hair growing. My grays started falling out and disappearing. I was going to color my hair about 4 years ago, and I still haven't touched it with an ounce of anything. My skin definitely looks and feels younger. And my nails grow so well that if I break one, it doesn't upset me. I know that it will grow right back."

How can magnets do so much? Simply stated, magnets confer a wide range of benefits because we are magnetic beings who derive energy from the earth's magnetic field. Bucci explains: "One reason we get sick is that the earth has lost a good deal of its magnetism, which leaves the body in an unbalanced state. Additionally, we are bombarded by unhealthy energies." Magnets create overall benefit by restoring internal harmony.

It is important to realize that not just any old magnet will do. The negative pole restores health and good energy to the system, while exposure to the positive pole is detrimental. This has been proved repeatedly in studies where a variety of creatures, from earthworms, mice, and chickens to larger animals, live twice as long as untested control groups when exposed to negative field magnets, and half as long when exposed to positive fields. Bucci recommends unipolar magnets, marked by the Davis and Rawls system with an "N" or the word "negative" and a green label. "That's the healthy side, and that's the one we face toward the body." Negative field ions support biological systems, which help the body to heal itself. "The body is an amazing machine with a remarkable capacity to cure itself," Bucci says. "Give it a boost in the right direction and it does the rest on its own. The negative field is completely safe and risk-free."

Bucci finds that magnets work best when worn on a daily basis. During the day she wears a magnet over her heart to improve circulation and oxygenation. "It keeps the heart open and flowing and sends all that wonderful oxygen throughout my body," she says. At night, she takes the magnet off and sleeps with her head on a magnetic mattress pad. She does this because the most important benefit while sleeping is increased melatonin production from the brain's pineal gland: "People are running out to buy melatonin, but guess what? We can encourage our own melatonin production.

"People ask me how long magnets should be worn. Generally speaking, the longer you wear them, the more healing takes place. You can wear them all night and during the day. Generally, the body will tell you when it has had enough. It also will tell you when a condition has healed, although you should check with a physician just to make sure."

63

Brain Aging

One of the most disturbing symptoms of aging is diminished brain function, which can cause everything from forgetfulness and loss of concentration to Alzheimer's and other serious diseases. (Alzheimer's disease is discussed in chapter 49.) Fortunately, modern research reveals that much can be done to keep the brain in top form your entire life. Below, several experts in antiaging discuss new advances in the field.

Dr. Eric Braverman says that brain aging affects people differently and that brain health is a preventative process. "Even when you feel halfway decent in your 50s, 60s, and 70s, parts of your body may be breaking down," he cautions.

The part of the brain affected determines which symptoms manifest themselves. "Individuals age in all different shapes and forms, just as a face can have wrinkles on the brow or wrinkles under the eye," Dr. Braverman says. "The area of the brain that slows down can affect such things as general memory, concentration, and logic."

Another leading researcher in the field of antiaging, Dr. Ross Pelton of San Diego, author of *Mind, Food, and Smart Pills*, agrees that our brains do not have to deteriorate as we age: "It is simply poor nutrition and abuse that allows this condition to develop. Virtually everyone can enhance their memory, learning capabilities, and intelligence." Dr. Pelton helps his patients optimize brain functioning with two goals in mind: to slow down or stop the brain aging process and to optimize the function that they do have.

Dr. Dharma Singh Khalsa is a physician trained at Creighton University School of Medicine and Harvard Medical School, and the author of *Brain*

Longevity. "There are many simple things that we can do right now to improve our memories, to forestall any degeneration, to be at our highest mental potential no matter what age or what stage of life we are in," Dr. Khalsa says. "We just have to look at the brain as a physical organ. We have to give it the oxygen it needs, the blood flow it needs, the nutrients it needs. We have to eat right, lower our fat intake, take supplements, meditate or do something to lower the stress in our lives, get physical exercise, think positively, and use our brain. If we do all of these things we can improve our brains. Combine this with a knowledgeable doctor in the field of antiaging medicine and look at hormone replacement therapy. I think hormone replacement therapy is coming into its own now and there is no question that it is definitely beneficial. It is a matter of picking the right person and the right dose. I think that we are going to go a long way toward beating this disease."

How the Brain Works

Dr. Khalsa explains how the brain works. "We have energy in the brain in the form of a power plant called the mitochondria. We have the synapse, a very important juncture where electrical-chemical energy is transferred from one cell to another to create memory or help us produce other memories, draw up old memories or restore new memories."

The endocrine system affects our emotions and we see a decline in mood and sex drive that normally occur as people age. Dr. Khalsa highlights some of the changes in the endocrine system.

"The endocrine system is primarily the hypothalamus, which is the brain's brain that controls just about everything including aging. It sends hormones called releasing hormones or factors down to the pituitary gland, which is the master gland of the brain. It orchestrates the secretions of all the glands in your body: the thyroid gland, the adrenal gland, the gonads (in men the testicles, in women the ovaries) and this causes the release of various hormones. When you are young it is responsible for growth and development and as we get older it is responsible for reproductive functions. Then after we reach a certain age when these hormones decline and that is when we start to devitalize. They peak at age 30 and start to decline at around 40 and at about 50 they really start to plateau. Don't forget the pineal gland, which is so important in creating a healing environment in the body so we can regenerate ourselves daily and have more energy and vitality as we get older. And you have DHEA released by the adrenal gland. There is an exquisite intimate relationship between all these hormones. These hormones affect our emotions, our mood, the sex drive, our overall feeling of well-being and our feeling of vitality as we get older. That is why it is so important to follow a brain longevity program."

Diet and Nutrition

Dr. Pelton recommends building total body health with a healthy diet. An organic vegetarian diet supplies the body with more protective nutrients and healthful fiber, and at the same time decreases toxins. Additionally, he believes that people should take a high-potency multivitamin and/or mineral supplement and extra antioxidants with each meal: "We are no longer looking at the Recommended Daily Allowance (RDA) as the level of nutrients appropriate for people. I say RDA stands for Really Dumb Allowance. It's more like the minimum wage, the minimal amount you can get by on. If we want to get into lifestyles of antiaging and life extension, we need to consider not only healthy diets but a program of optimal nutritional supplementation. Antioxidants are among the most important protectors against the aging process in general and against brain aging in particular. They will stop the onset of senility, Alzheimer's disease, and other brain injuries."

Dr. Khalsa elaborates, "What works for the heart works for the head. We know that high fat in the diet will contribute to hardening of the arteries in the heart, the large arteries in the neck, and the small arteries in the brain. Therefore it is critical to move away from these high fat diets and follow a more holistic type of diet. We construct a diet according to the patient's preferences that has about 15 to 20 percent fat so it is tasty. But it is not the 30 to 40 percent fat that you see in the standard American diet. Some of the high protein diets may be effective short-term for weight loss and I think in the long term they are not going to prove to be healthy."

SUPPLEMENTS Dr. Khalsa goes on to talk about vitamin and mineral supplements that affect the brain. "An all-purpose insurance policy multiple vitamin/mineral pill has vitamin E, vitamin C, vitamin A in all its forms, the B vitamins, and the minerals is very useful day to day. Then we use brain-specific nutrients backed by strong scientific research. Vitamin E slows the progression of memory loss. Ginkgo is a good brain specific nutrient. Coenzyme Q10, which is still not that well known to the general public, is a very energetic cofactor that works in the brain's power plant, the mitochondria. Phosphotidyl serine, or PS, from bovine brains has some excellent results even with patients with dementia. Newer types of phosphotidyl serine synthesized from soybeans is excellent in reversing memory loss and rejuvenating the brain. It is great for depression and mood and has even been shown to improve seasonal affective disorder. There are some other nutrients as well that I like, like fish oil or DHA. It is an algae or you can get it from salmon."

Flaxseed oil, an important brain nutrient, is the greatest source of the essential fatty acid omega-3 (EPA). Omega-3 is converted into another fatty acid, which nourishes the fat cells in the brain. Dr. Pelton says that 1 tablespoon of flaxseed oil is needed daily. It should be refrigerated, not cooked, and taken with the largest meal of the day.

DMAE (dimethylaminoethynol) is a naturally occurring but little-known B vitamin that enhances memory, boosts natural energy, and improves sleep. Additionally, it helps learning problems in children who have short attention spans. DMAE is safe, but if too much is taken, it can produce mild headaches, insomnia, and muscle tension.

Melatonin is a substance from the armamentarium of alternative medicine that has attracted attention in the mainstream media recently. This is a brain hormone produced by the pineal gland, and it diminishes with age. A dose of 3 milligrams once daily taken at bedtime can help normalize sleep cycles and support the pineal gland

Dr. Khalsa describes two new compounds. "There are two compounds I use for 60 year olds who have early memory loss. I don't use them for everybody. The compounds I spoke of before are regenerating or protective, not stimulating like these two. Hypericin A in combination with vitamin E can be as effective as some of the drugs that are mildly effective or moderately effective. Hypericin has the same effect. It blocks the enzyme that destroys the memory compound. Hypericin A, from Chinese cub moss, can be taken in capsule form, 50 micrograms to 100 micrograms twice a day. Combine it with vitamin E and you have a very good reversal compound. I don't think hypericin should be taken by everybody because most normal people have enough of this memory compound. We must be much more scientific and much more specific about how we use these supplements.

"There is another one and that is vincristine. This is from the periwinkle plant. It increases metabolism in the brain and oxygenation. It can be overstimulating so you have to be careful. Select a program, hopefully in concert with a holistic practitioner. See how to create your own brain longevity program because not each one of these supplements is right for everybody."

There are two minerals that also affect memory: zinc and boron. "Studies showed that those who had the right amounts of these minerals did better on short-term memory tests than those who had low amounts," Dr. Khalsa says. "However taking megadoses didn't have any further improvement. A good source of zinc: oysters. Good sources of boron: apples, prunes, dates, raisin and peanuts."

OTHER NUTRIENTS Dr. Pelton utilizes some additional nutrients to enhance brain function. Hydergine (co-dergocrine mesylate) increases oxygen to brain cells and makes a person less susceptible to free radical damage and aging. Dr. Pelton says this is one of the most important substances for preventing brain aging because of its oxygenating capabilities. Hydergine is available in the United States, although as a prescription drug.

Lucidril (meclofenoxate hydrochloride), as its name suggests, makes you more lucid. This exciting drug can actually reverse brain aging. Dr. Pelton explains: "The primary yardstick in brain aging is the buildup of lipofuscin, the result of free radical damage over the years. This buildup is really cellular garbage that collects and coalesces inside the cells into a black, tarlike mass. In elderly people you can see this in the skin as liver spots or age pigment. It is theorized that when 60 to 70 percent of the brain cell is clogged, it breaks down and stops working. That's when the symptoms of senility kick in very quickly. Lucidril actually dissolves and flushes out these garbage deposits from brain cells and restores the brain cell to a much younger state." Lucidril has been shown to extend the life of laboratory animals and to enhance intelligence, learning, and recall.

Piracetam is not available in the United States; however, it is available in over 85 other countries worldwide, where it is appreciated for its remarkable qualities and its complete lack of toxicity. Like Hydergine, piracetam prevents brain cell destruction caused by a lack of oxygen. Piracetam also can increase the flow of electrical information between the left and right hemispheres of the brain, a process known as superconnecting. It has proven effective in treating the learning disorder dyslexia. When used in conjunction with high-potency lecithin, piracetam is highly effective in helping some Alzheimer's patients improve cognition, memory, and recall.

Lucidril and piracetam must be ordered from overseas. Although classified as drugs by the FDA, Hydergine, Lucidril, and piracetam have few, if any, negative side effects, according to Dr. Pelton—only positive effects on memory and the prevention of brain aging. Overseas mail order sources sell Hydergine in 4.5 milligram tablets, while in the United States it is available only in 1 milligram tablets. The higher dose, taken twice a day, is highly effective in helping people with early signs of memory loss.

Deprenyl (selegiline hydrochloride) has been shown in animal studies to prevent the destruction of a specific group of neurons in the substantia nigra, the area of the brain that goes bad when people develop Parkinson's disease. Moreover, it helps enhance intelligence and cognition when 5 milligrams is taken once daily.

Brain Electronic Activity Map (BEAM)

Dr. Eric Braverman has mapped brain aging and studied how nutrients influence this process. Using a test called the Brain Electronic Activity Map (or BEAM), a technique developed at Harvard Medical School and refined, strengthened, and expanded by Dr. Braverman, the brain's level of electric activity is studied. This is a crucial area of concern because such things as substance abuse, hormonal imbalance, chronic fatigue, anxiety, hypertension, and even Lyme disease may affect the brain and cause premature aging. Often electroencephalography (EEG) or magnetic resonance imaging (MRI) will show nothing wrong, while the BEAM test reveals that the brain has been suffering from stress. It gives a window on the brain and how it is aging. So, as Dr. Braverman says, he is using "the BEAM that lights the path to wellness."

He says that one thing this test registers is the speed of brain cycles, since slowing is a key marker of aging. The normal, healthy rhythm of the brain is 10 cycles per second of alpha waves, considerably faster than the heart's normal rate of one cycle per second. As people age, their brain rhythm decreases to nine, eight, or seven beats per second. There is a decrease in alpha rhythms and an increase in theta waves.

This can occur prematurely for many reasons, including head trauma, Alzheimer's disease, and abuse of such substances as cocaine, marijuana, and alcohol. Any one of these conditions can cause the frontal and temporal lobes to age in an accelerated manner. Aging is also accelerated by whiplash, metabolic disorders, loss of circulation, and "toxic home syndrome," which refers to the damage that can be done to the body by substances, such as cleansers, that vaporize; pesticides; and herbicides found around the house or garden. Add to that possible harm from fluorescent lights and electromagnetic pollution. The latter is that which may be caused by the electromagnetic grid that characterizes our environment, surrounded as we all are by digital clocks, VCRs, CD players, computers, electric blankets, cellular phones and beepers, and microwave ovens.

Dr. Braverman notes that a computerized spectral analysis will pick up how these factors have affected the brain. A PET (positron emission tomography) scan, which provides data about the metabolism of the brain, can be correlated with a BEAM test, which may record not only weaker brain electrical activity but a loss of metabolism of the neurotransmitters.

Exercise

Research shows that the whole neurotransmitter system of the brain can be improved through exercise. Exercise boosts your ability to think because it increases the blood circulation to the brain. This brings more oxygen to the brain. It also increases the production of brain chemicals that are needed for information processing. It may also promote nerve synapses—the bridges between the brain cells—and make information coding faster and more efficient.

Mental Stimulation and Stress Management

"Combine physical exercise with some type of mental stimulation," Dr. Khalsa says. "Mental stimulation like reading a book, listening to a book on tape, or listening to an informational show and then discussing it with someone else.

Reading a newspaper and doing headline discussion or what I call column discussion where your first read the headline and then read the column to the right of it and then talk about it to somebody. Combine this with some physical exercise, sometimes at the same time, for example riding on a stationary bike and reading the newspapers or listening to a book on tape and you can actually make new connections. Our brains are hungry for connections, hungry to communicate, hungry to reach out and make new neuronal connections so that we can maintain our intelligence. The greatest way to do that is to keep using your brain, mental exercise, and to combine that with physical exercise"

Depression slows the brain processing. Relaxation and de-stressing helps memory. There are lots of ways to reduce stress. Something as easy as taking a deep, long breath and holding it for a moment will not only relax you but bring some oxygen to the brain and make it easier to think and concentrate. Yoga and meditation do the same thing. Listening to music can also be very relaxing.

A good night's sleep allows the entire body to recharge. If you get some quality sleep you are better able to concentrate. Research shows that people who are awakened during dream sleep fail to process memories from the day before and thus forget more. Dr. Khalsa points out that "recent studies have shown that you don't need to sleep as much as you think because in the last 2 hours you have very weird dreams and the rapid eye movement sleep is very intense. This raises cortisol levels and can actually cause some problems. In fact, people who have heart attacks have them most often in the morning. High amounts of REM sleep produce high levels of cortisol, which is why many people awaken with morning stress and anxiety. This particular feeling has been found to lead to memory loss specifically and other illnesses perhaps as well."

Dr. Khalsa emphasizes the need for a stress management program. "Anyone who does not have regular stress management program that is proactive, like a daily or almost daily practice of meditation, won't enjoy good health. Stress management tools that reduce the stress in your life and reduce the nasty chemicals such as cortisol. Cortisol attacks the memory center of the brain. It is like battery acid there.

"Start your day in a positive way, what I call 'Wake Up to Wellness.' There have been so many studies lately talking about prayer or meditation. Just take 10, 15, 20 minutes in the morning before you rush headlong into your day."

Other Alternative Therapies

Dr. Braverman believes that each person must be individually tested to determine weak areas of brain function and to devise a program that addresses specific needs. For overall general improvement, he endorses exercise and the following important therapies.

CHELATION THERAPY As described in the previous chapter, chelation therapy pulls out aluminum and other heavy metals from the bloodstream, resulting in improved memory. It can also reverse or prevent other destructive conditions associated with the aging process, such as arthritis, hardening of the arteries, cataracts, and strokes.

ELECTROSTIMULATION Amino acids and neurotransmitter precursors are more effective when accompanied by electrostimulation of the brain. A transcutaneous electrical nerve stimulation (TENS) unit, worn on the forehead and left wrist, helps drive these substances along a good pathway. A cranioelectrical stimulation (CES) device also helps electrical fields and enhances the entire neurotransmitter system.

REIKI Reiki is a type of massage therapy or bodywork in which pressure point techniques are used to move energy through the body, achieving balance and harmony. Reiki therapist Nilsa Vergara reports below on her clients' experiences with Reiki therapy.

"My first example is a 59-year-old woman who came to our healing circle feeling old and tired. She suffered from aches and severe pain in her neck and knee from car accidents. She was also going through job changes, and was estranged from her adult son.

"Each week she received a 15-minute session, and she quickly began feeling better. She released a lot of emotional toxins via crying and verbal expression of what she was feeling. She decided to take a Reiki class so that she could give herself daily treatments.

"Within a month, her changes were quite dramatic. She had a tremendous increase in energy and vigor. She told me she now feels like she is 28. With the Reiki, she now has very little pain. She feels emotional and vital. Her attitude has changed. She feels self-fulfilled and in control of her life. Her relationship with her son has greatly improved. To quote her, 'I feel like my whole life is as it should be.'

"My next client is a 65-year-old woman. When she first came to see us, she was depressed. She had been in therapy for years, but nothing seemed to lift the depression. She felt tired all the time and would catch colds easily. Emotionally, she felt like a victim, and others treated her like one.

"After her first 15-minute session she felt immediately better. She knew that something powerful was happening. She returned and eventually studied Reiki. Today, she reports feeling much healthier. She has more energy and an optimistic outlook. She no longer feels like a victim, and if anyone tries to put her in that role, she is no longer afraid to set limits. In addition, she is much more able to tolerate cold weather, which indicates that her body has improved its oxygen intake.

"One of my students has an 83-year-old mother who fell and broke her hip bone as well as bones in her wrist and arm. She decided to give her mother

Reiki regularly, and her mother responded quite well. She began feeling stronger and stronger. Within 4 weeks she was out of her cast, walking with just the aid of a cane, not a walker. This is pretty remarkable for an 83-year-old, because a broken hip does not always lead to a good outcome. So, as you can see, Reiki really enhances the body's ability to recuperate.

"Another client is a 53-year-old woman who had some serious memory problems. Her thinking was scattered; emotionally, she was fearful and guilt-ridden; and she was estranged from her adult children.

"I recommended Reiki to her to see if we could work through some of these emotional blockages and change these negative patterns. She took a Reiki class, and within 6 months, her memory improved tremendously. She was much more focused in her thinking, and her job performance improved greatly. She became more insightful and much less fearful. Now she can speak with her adult children and set limits, and she no longer feels anxious and guilt-ridden. In addition to using Reiki, she uses herbal teas for detoxification, drinks vegetable juices, fasts, and gets colonics."

64

Vision Concerns

Contrary to popular belief, eye problems are not an inevitable result of aging. Many eye diseases, including macular degeneration, cataracts, and glaucoma, can be prevented. Dr. Marc Grossman, an optometrist and licensed acupuncturist who lectures internationally on natural eye care, nutrition, and Chinese medicine, explains that it is not only the general public that has been misled.

"Eye care in this country is very symptom-oriented. In our training as eye doctors, we are taught that once something goes wrong with your eyes there is not much that we can do to try to improve it. We are not really taught much in school about prevention of eye problems. We are taught that eye problems are just a natural consequence of aging."

Dr. Grossman, the co-author of *Natural Eye Care—An Encyclopedia*, is among a small but growing group of eye care specialists who hold a different view. "We tend to treat eye diseases in a more holistic way," incorporating lifestyle, exercise, emotional well-being, nutrition, and herbs.

Diet and Lifestyle

There are a lot of things we can do to prevent or slow down some of the most common diseases that affect our eyes. Start with sunglasses that block both ultraviolet A and B and visible blue light because they may help decrease the risk of cataracts.

Routine eye exams are important if you are older than 50. Go to the ophthalmologist when you turn 50 to check for glaucoma or diabetic eye disease.

Don't wait until you are 50 if you are African American because you are much more likely to have these diseases, which can lead to blindness.

There is a strong relationship between nutrition and vision. It's not just carrots that are good for the eyes. A diet that emphasizes unrefined, natural foods is essential. Dr. Grossman says that more than 25 percent of the nutrients we absorb from our food nourish our visual system. He especially recommends whole grains, brown rice, spelt, buckwheat, and sea vegetables.

There are vitamins that are known specifically to help with vision. The best known vitamin for the eyes is beta carotene, a form of vitamin A, which has been found to protect against both cataracts and macular degeneration. A daily intake of 500 milligrams of vitamin C may help prevent cataracts. Take a supplement or eat a diet rich in vitamin C, with foods such as citrus fruits, sweet potatoes, and corn. Beta carotene foods are carrots, peaches, apricots, cantaloupes, beets, yams, and dark green, leafy vegetable such as spinach, collard greens, and Romaine lettuce.

Among the other important nutrients are vitamin E, zinc, selenium, taurine, riboflavin, and glutathione. The pigments lutein, zeaxanthin, anthocyanin, and the carotenes also are beneficial for preserving eyesight and protecting vision.

Sugar, alcohol, caffeine, and smoking all deplete the body of many essential nutrients. "Probably the number one problem for people with eye problems is smoking," Dr. Grossman says. "You increase your risk for eye disease by over 100 percent if you are a smoker."

Macular Degeneration

Macular degeneration, also known as age-related macular degeneration (AMD), is a condition marked by deterioration of the macula, the central area of the retina responsible for keen vision. It destroys a person's central vision and affects the ability to read, drive, and recognize colors and faces. It is the leading cause of irreversible blindness in the people older than 50, and currently affects some 13 million Americans.

Early signs of AMD are yellowish deposits beneath the retina called drusen. Few, if any, symptoms are present at this stage. Over time, there may be loss of parts of the retina and underlying structures. New blood vessels may develop around the retina, which may leak and scar.

"Macular degeneration is probably the most important eye disease that we can help prevent naturally because it is very slow in progressing and we really don't have good treatments for it in the medical world," Dr. Grossman says. "The most important nutrients for preventing macular degeneration are lutein and zeaxanthin." Lutein is a carotene found in kale, spinach, and collard greens, and zeaxanthin is contained in corn, egg yolks, and spinach. Studies have shown that 6 milligrams of lutein a day can reduce the risk of macular degeneration by as much as 50 percent, Dr. Grossman says. "Beta carotene is important to take with it, possibly about 15,000 to 25,000 IUs. When you are taking beta carotene and lutein, you need to take them at different times since they compete for the same receptors."

Other important nutrients are taurine, at least 500 milligrams, and zinc, about 30 milligrams. Dr. Grossman adds that "in all eye conditions it is important to have your thyroid levels checked because if you have low thyroid it is hard to convert beta carotene to vitamin A."

There has been some evidence that glutathione may help control the spread of macular degeneration. It can be found in fresh green, red and yellow vegetables. Canned or frozen vegetables lose all their glutathione in processing.

In an article posted on the HealthWorld Online website (www.healthy.net),

Donald J. Brown, author of *Herbal Prescriptions for Better Health*, offers some additional recommendations. He suggests taking ginkgo biloba extract, 120 to 240 milligrams per day in two or three divided doses, for early-stage macular degeneration. Bilberry extract is recommended for prevention of macular degeneration, as well as cataracts and other vision disorders. Bilberry contains potent antioxidants known as anthocyanins. Anthocyanins are the blue-red pigments or natural dyes that give bilberries, blueberries, cranberries, and cherries their color. The anthocyanins in bilberries help protect the lens and retinal cells of the eye.

Cataracts

A cataract is a clouding of the crystalline lens that prevents light rays from entering the eye. The clouding can be partial or complete, and usually progresses over a period of years. A person with a cataract gradually becomes less able to see objects clearly and may lose his or her peripheral vision. Cataract is a primary cause of blindness in the United States. Each year, about 1.35 million surgeries are performed to remove cataracts in the hopes of restoring vision.

The standard conventional medical procedure is to wait and watch a developing cataract until it becomes "mature" or "ripe." At this point, an operation is performed to remove the affected lens and replace it with an implant. Phacoemulsification is a newer procedure that uses high-frequency ultrasound to break up, liquefy, and suck out the cataract.

Dr. Grossman and his colleagues take a more proactive approach to cataracts by looking at the reasons why they develop in the first place. "Almost all [people with] cataracts have been shown to be low in glutathione," he says. "We recommend different nutrients to help build the glutathione levels, such as n-acetyl cysteine, alpha lypoic acid, vitamin C, vitamin B$_2$, vitamin B$_6$, selenium, and zinc." Lutein, zeaxanthin, beta carotene and vitamin E also are important in preventing cataracts.

Like other parts of the body, the eyes need to be exercised to maintain good health. "As we get older we get reading glasses that actually do the work for us so that we don't have to exercise the lens of the eye," Dr. Grossman explains. "I give all my cataract patients certain exercises as simple as focusing back and forth, like looking at their thumb 6 inches away and then looking across the room."

Emotional issues are addressed as well. "We find that fear is most associated with cataracts," Dr. Grossman says. "In Chinese medicine that relates to the kidney meridian. We will talk to people about their natural fear of death, getting older, and what they don't want to look at in the world or look at in their future."

Glaucoma

In glaucoma, there is a rise in the pressure of the fluid within the eye (intraocular pressure). Peripheral vision is lost, and increased pressure on the optic nerve causes eventual wasting and blindness. Glaucoma affects nearly 2 million older adults in the United States.

"A high pressure in Chinese medicine means a stagnation of energy in the liver," Dr. Grossman says. "We treat the liver with herbs such as milk thistle, dandelion, bilberry, and gingko to get the circulation moving." To help with heart and blood circulation, he uses coenzyme Q10, 50 to 100 milligrams. Exercise is also important. This includes aerobic exercise as well as eye exercises. "Just 20 minutes of aerobic exercise every day or at least 4 or 5 times a week has been shown to increase circulation and therefore help with lowering the pressure."

Dr. Grossman also recommends vitamin C and magnesium. "Magnesium is very important in glaucoma because magnesium will relax the smooth muscle, and it's the smooth muscles in the inner eye that help regulate the outflow of the aqueous humor."

Emotional stress has been linked to glaucoma in research going back many years, Dr. Grossman says. "Above average stress has been shown to increase the risk for high eye pressure by almost three times....[W]e would say that reducing the stress in your life and living more harmoniously will reduce the internal pressure that produces anger and frustration. Those are the emotions most associated with glaucoma. Instead of trying to suppress that anger we recommend that you feel it. Don't indulge in it, but learn when to express it and when to say nothing." Meditation and tai chi also may be helpful.

"Sometimes glaucoma might be an indication that the neck area is really tight and chiropractic care or acupuncture might help to relieve that," Dr. Grossman says.

PART THIRTEEN

Everyday Health for the Whole Family

65

The Well Baby and Child

Many childhood conditions can be treated naturally to build up the immune system and avoid the negative side effects of over-the-counter or prescription medicines. Dr. Mary Bove is a naturopathic physician, licensed midwife, and former chair of Botanical Medicine at Pasteur University. She is also the author of *Encyclopedia of Natural Healing for Children and Infants*.

Dr. Bove says, "Children are born with an immature immune system that matures during the neonatal period. One of the reasons I choose natural remedies is because many of the natural remedies support immune system development rather than inhibiting it or stimulating it in a way that might not be appropriate. The other reason is because they give the parents a sense of empowerment to be able to work with things that are healthy and effective and that have little side effects."

Herbal Remedies

Dr. Bove shares some of her herbal remedies. First, she says, "we have to remember that children are not adults so they have to be dosed properly for their weight, their metabolism, and their age. Also the herbs and remedies used are often not the stronger ones or the ones that might have an adverse effect or influence on the body that is too strong for the child. The whole key is to make a form that the child will take because if the child will not take the medicine it is not going to work. If they have a fever with sore throat making an herbal remedy in the form of a frozen Popsicle is a nice way for the child to take the remedy. The cold soothes the throat and they will comply with taking the medicine. Making herbal teas with fruit juices is a great way to address flu and fever.

"Usually for a child I use 1 teaspoon of the bulk herb to 1 cup of water. Pour the boiling water over and steep for 5 to 10 minutes."

FEVER "Fever, a symptom that accompanies acute sickness, is a vital response of the immune system and something we want to work with," Dr. Bove says. "If the child is sick and feeling a chill, it means the body is trying to warm itself up. Herbal remedies like ginger or peppermint warm the body up, and help the fever do its job. You use an herbal remedy that helps the body continue its sweating and that work with the process that is already going on. The popular echinacea is appropriate to use at the beginning of an illness as an immune boosting remedy."

UPSET STOMACH Dr. Bove recommends a few herbs for an upset stomach. Chamomile "has a relaxing effect on the stomach and helps the stomach get rid of gas or bloating, and diminishes the nausea. Sometimes I use anise seed or fennel seed because they warm up the stomach particularly if the stomach has been cold or sluggish."

For stomach upset caused by emotional factors, Dr. Bove uses chamomile or lemon balm. For stomach upset caused by motion sickness, she recommends ginger. "Ginger is probably the most common thing I use with children. I use it in the form of ginger honey syrup that can be bought over the counter and mixed with seltzer water to make a natural ginger ale. They can sip it slowly during the time in the car or before getting in the car."

SKIN CONDITIONS "For diaper rash, a skin rash like atopic dermatitis, or eczema I use shaya butter," Dr. Bove says. "Shaya butter comes from an African tree and is used to hydrate the skin and diminish flaking. It is oily and protects the skin with a coating. Mixed with this are things like cholangiole flower or yeara flowers to diminish infection and improve healing. Cholangiole flowers have a strong effect on normal cell proliferation. Make sure the area is kept dry using different herbal powders such as combinations of lavender flowers, cholangiole flowers, or slippery elm. Another great suggestion is powdered bentonite clay. Put it lightly in the diaper area to diminish the risk of yeast infection or candida. The clay keeps the yeast from being able to grow."

Impetigo is due to infectious agents. Dr. Bove remarks, "Make sure the skin is kept very clean by washing with cholangiole soap or tea tree soap frequently. Then I usually use a combination of myrrh and goldenseal, a half a teaspoon of the extract diluted in 8 ounces of water. Use it as a wash and wash frequently over the infected area soaked in the wash substance itself."

What about burns? Dr. Bove says, "If it is a burn, I like St. John's wort. Traditionally this herb has been used for the skin to revitalize normal nerve tissue and vascular tissue, although we hear about its use as an antidepressant or as an antiviral. After the burn has cooled for 10 to 15 minutes under cold water I suggest saturating a gauze pad with St. John's wort and apply for an hour. It helps diminish blistering."

CHRONIC CONDITIONS When a child is exposed to an allergen over a period of time, the immune system becomes weakened and this is when you see chronic types of problems, such as a chronic runny nose, earaches, rash, and asthma. In these cases, it is particularly important to determine the underlying cause of the recurring symptoms.

"Chronic things recur over several months and this means the immune system is being compromised and something is triggering that," Dr. Bove says. "I look at environmental allergens, stress factors, food allergens, or nutritional deficiencies. Could it be secondary smoke, too much cow's milk, or things that drain the immune system, called antinutrients, such as sugars, preservatives, hydrogenated fats? Do they have nutritional substances in their diet or do they need to be supplemented? I look at possible allergens, like dairy products, peanuts, oranges, bananas, chocolate, soy and wheat."

After eliminating or reducing exposure to allergens, Dr. Bove boosts the immune system with immune nutrients such as bioflavonoids. She explains, "Bioflavonoids are substances found in nature that give color to plants, the yellow in squash, the purple in plums, the blue in blueberries. These substances are extremely useful to the immune system and to the collagen, vascular tissues of the body, skin, lungs, mucous membranes, and are diminished by processing or preserving foods.

"I'll supplement these with essential fatty acids. I'm talking about good fats, the fish oil fats or raw vegetable oil fats. We tend to eat hydrogenated fats, which are in solid forms like margarine, that I classify as antinutrients because they cause the body to rid itself of important nutrients such as magnesium or zinc. Do not expose the child to these types of fats. Give them good essential fatty acids, such as cod liver oil. Cod liver oil is one of my favorite things to boost the immune system of a child.

"So we give essential fatty acids and the bioflavonoids in combination with vitamin C. I give 500 milligrams of bioflavonoids for a child 5 years or older. If the child is younger I will dose it depending on the age and weight of the child. I also consider zinc deficiency, common in children with chronic respiratory problems, chronic earaches, chronic runny noses, or sore throats. These children do well with zinc supplementation of 7 to 15 milligrams a day over a period of several months."

URINARY TRACT INFECTIONS Urinary tract infections can be acute or chronic. "Acute urinary tract infection can be caused by yeast or bacteria and sometimes because of infiltration of bacteria from the rectal area from improper wiping. If the infection is chronic it might be a sign that the child is intolerant to a food so I consider allergies, looking for the culprit, looking at the immune system as well as treating the urinary tract itself.

"With children urinary tract infections can get serious fast. This is a time [for the medical professional] to assess whether this child should be on antibiotics or can this child respond to natural medicines. For nonserious acute urinary tract infections I use unsweetened cranberry juice because the sugar in the cranberry juice perpetuates the yeast or bacteria. Children don't like this because it is bitter. I suggest freezing it in the form of a Popsicle or mixing it with some other herbal teas that taste nice like anise seed or peppermint or spearmint or licorice. Most children will not necessarily take 3 or 4 cups of tea if they are under age 3 or 4 so you may need to make a syrup or elixir for the child in which they would be taking an extract of the herb. Typically used are corn silk or marshmallow root. They are very soothing to the irritation and the symptoms of burning or itchiness. Antibacterial herbs to flush out the urinary tract are thyme and oregano, which are culinary herbs that have medicinal properties."

Dr. Bove cautions that "certainly natural medicines have their limitations with acute illness."

Homeopathy

Dr. Paul Herscu is a graduate of the National College of Naturopathic Medicine and founder and director of New England School of Homeopathy. He has authored three books on homeopathy and children. He shares his views on the basic principals of how homeopathy helps in the healing process for children.

"When we treat a child for an earache we are not really treating the earache we are treating the whole child," says Dr. Herscu. "When we treat a child for a Strep throat we are not treating the Strep infection, we are treating the child so that child can get rid of the Strep infection. Treat the whole individual and treat their susceptibilities so they can deal with the complaint by themselves is a central tenant of homeopathy. Homeopathy looks at each child as having their own susceptibilities and predisposition toward illness. There is no such thing as an average kid. The whole idea of average doesn't exist for us. In homeopathy you try to treat the whole individual as opposed to any one part of them or any disease going on. This is opposed to the medical view of the body as a battlefield between the drug and the microbe.

"Constitutional homeopathy should not be practiced on one's own child. Have somebody else treat your child and you treat somebody else's child. What you are looking for is to change the whole nature of the child, the whole culture of the child, their whole predisposition—mental, emotional and physical. It's hard to get that kind of perspective if you are treating your own child."

Dr. Herscu continues, "Some children go to their physician with an ear infection and get an antibiotic and the ear infection goes away. Another child has an ear infection and gets the same antibiotic and it doesn't work so he is given a stronger antibiotic and it doesn't work and so on. Homeopathy looks at the predisposition toward illness that needs to be addressed. The antibiotics kill off certain cells that come back because the underlying cause of the infection is not addressed. By treating children homeopathically you can change the predisposition so they don't get the ear infection.

"Yes, you can use homeopathy acutely. Go to the health food store and find a homeopathic remedy for earaches or colds or bronchitis. The best of all circumstances would be that the cold would go away. But what I am talking about is constitutional homeopathy in which you take away the predisposition so they stop getting ear infections."

Dr. Herscu shares his homeopathic recommendations for children, reminding us that these remedies are aimed at multiple symptoms, not specific illnesses.

CALCAREA CARBONIC

"The most common homeopathic remedy is calcarea carbonic. This particular remedy has been used for at least 12,000 or 13,000 different symptoms, anything from recurrent ear infections to epilepsy. This type of child tends to be placid, obstinate, diligent. This type of temperament has recurrent infection, recurrent bronchitis, and difficulty learning to walk or talk. I have treated children with epilepsy with this type of temperament where the epilepsy has been much diminished or has gone. It is not specific for ear infections as much as specific for children with that temperament."

LYCOPODIUM

"Lycopodium is for the children that tend to be a combination of irritable and insecure, who lose their insecurities by being bossy. They tend to be anxious with new situations and worried about being picked on at school. The typical example is the child that is picked on at school and is shy around older children and then comes home and mercilessly picks on younger children. The children that need this remedy have a weakness in the digestive tract, anything from irritable bowel to constipation to infant intolerance of breast milk and repeated colic."

MEDORRHINUM

"Medorrhinum is for the child with temper tantrums, one after another. Bossy and feisty with repeated infections, they have everything from eczema at birth to autoimmune diseases near birth. For example, asthma at 2 months and arthritis at 6 months."

NATRIUM MURIATICUM

"Natrium muriaticum is a remedy for kids who tend toward depression. They don't like to be consoled, want to be by themselves, and have either one grief or repeated griefs and have pretty much shut down. I treated a 6 year old in New York who had anorexia and had not eaten in a couple of months. Her uncle or grandfather had passed away and that led to depression. Two days after the remedy she started eating."

PHOSPHORUS

"This is for children with a general temperament like Goldie Hawn—upbeat, friendly, bubbly, easy to make contact, fun-loving. They have tendencies to bleed, have nose bleeds, have diarrhea, and tend to be thin."

PULSATILLA

"Pulsatilla is one of the most common remedies for children who get repeated ear infections. This is the very clingy child who doesn't want to be put down, wants to be carried constantly. A warm blooded, thirstless child who cries a lot but the kind of crying that makes you want to pick them up and take care of them."

Jaundice

Kathi Kemper is director of the Center for Holistic Pediatric Education and Research at Children's Hospital in Boston. She is the author of *The Holistic Pediatrician*, and was a former instructor at the Yale University School of Nursing. She gives us her thoughts on a few common childhood concerns.

Jaundice is a common condition in newborn babies. Kemper explains, "The yellow skin color is simply from the breakdown products of the red blood cells. Babies are born with a lot of red blood cells which they need to get all the oxygen that mom has in her blood. So they have a much higher number of red blood cells before they are born than they actually need. They gradually turn over these excess red blood cells and the liver breaks them down into bilirubin, a yellow pigment. The bilirubin goes from the liver to the gallbladder into the intestines and then it is excreted in the stool. Babies who aren't taking in enough fluid or nutrition because they are having trouble nursing sometimes have a slow time getting the bilirubin out of their systems. So their skin can turn yellow.

"If you notice your child is yellow in the first day of life, take the child to the pediatrician. I know more and more people are birthing at home or leaving a hospital or birth center within 24 hours after the birth. But if you notice the baby looks yellow within that first 24 hours, that could be a sign of a more serious condition where the red blood cells are breaking down too fast and that has to be evaluated by a pediatrician. Most of the time jaundice appears when the baby is 3 or 4 days old and reaches its maximum when the baby is 4 or 5 days old. This is the kind of jaundice that comes while the intestines get working and everything is flowing through. The best treatment for that is nursing frequently and exposing the baby to sunlight. You don't need to take them outside. Just rest the baby in your arms near a sunny window for 15 minutes a day if it is cold outside and that will help the bilirubin break down in the skin so it can be eliminated through the intestines. If the baby is jaundiced for more than 10 to 14 days that is a red flag. Take him [back] to the doctor to make sure they don't have a serious problem with their thyroid or liver, things that are easily tested.

"Only very high bilirubin levels of 18 to 20 (the average in an adult is less than 2) are treated and most of that treatment involves making sure the baby is eating right and getting extra exposure to light. The light therapy might be sunlight or special phototherapy to get the baby's skin to break down the bilirubin faster. This is definitely not a time to use herbal remedies. In China and Hong Kong they used herbs that made the babies look less jaundiced but the researchers found out that the herbs made the bilirubin go directly to the brain. Even though the babies looked like they were getting better they were in fact getting the damaging effects of the bilirubin rather than being healed. Many herbs can affect the function of the liver and this is not the time you want to be experimenting, particularly with very new babies whose systems are still developing. This is a time to avoid herbs and strong nutritional supplements and just go with breast feeding very often."

Cradle Cap

What about cradle cap? "Cradle cap is a scaly rash on the scalp and is a very common condition," Kemper remarks. "Some people use nutritional supplements and B vitamins. There may be a little bit of fungal infection along with the cradle cap that can be treated with antifungal remedies. But most of the time it is just unsightly. The baby will not be bald. Treat it with plain old olive oil and rub it in gently, then get a soft toothbrush and brush the flakes out of the hair. If you do that two or three times a day before shampooing with a mild baby shampoo, that will be helpful.

"Some parents use a very mild hydrocortisone cream, 0.5 percent hydrocortisone cream, to help with the inflammation, the redness and swelling that sometimes goes along with this rash. This kind of steroid is very mild and not absorbed through the skin and into the body. It just works on the skin. But my favorite remedy is olive or any vegetable oil, as I described."

Bedwetting

Another common concern is bed wetting. "Bed wetting is a very common condition in childhood," Kemper says. "In fact we are all born as bed wetters. Most of us grow out of it by the time we are 3, 4 or 5 years old but a certain percentage of children do not. The first thing is to reassure the parents that it is a developmental process that they will eventually grow out of. The parents are not doing anything wrong and the child is not doing this on purpose. If the child is also wetting during the day take them to a physician to make sure they don't have diabetes or another serious condition. When there is extra sugar in your urine, as in diabetes, you urinate more often than usual and the child will be thirsty. For very young children, they need their urine tested for sugar and to make sure they don't have an infection in their bladder or kidney. Adults who have bladder infections go to the bathroom more often and that continues through the night and it can be painful. Children may not be able to tell you that they have to go more frequently or that it hurts when they urinate and just end up wetting the bed more often.

"Once you are sure it is not one of these serious conditions, the situation is simply getting some help to outgrow the problem. Common sense things are useful, like limiting the amount of fluids they take after dinner and waking the child during the night to use the toilet. The cheapest thing is to use an alarm clock to wake your children up 3 hours after they go to sleep. Wake them up at 11:00 before you go to bed and help them to the toilet. Then set the alarm for 2:00 in the morning and again at 5:00 in the morning. Older children can actually manage this on their own, having the alarm clock go off, getting up, emptying their bladder and then going back to bed. Eventually the intervals can be spaced out to every 3 to 4 hours and then 4 to 5 hours. I also use hypnosis and guided imagery. It is helpful to connect the child's mind to the full bladder and waking up so they can go to the bathroom to urinate and not go in their beds.

"Stretching the bladder may be helpful as many children who wet the bed also have a small bladder in addition to a delayed development in the hormones that regulate urine production. This means when your child says they have to go to the bathroom during the day, ask them if they can wait another minute or two so that their bladder gets gradually stretched just a little bit. They could also urinate into a measuring cup and see how much they get and how much is the most they can do. An average bladder size in a child is their age plus 2 ounces."

66

Natural Medicine Cabinet

M any times we want to be able to go to our home medicine cabinet and find what we need for our day-to-day ills and problems. In this chapter we describe some of the components of a well-stocked natural medicine cabinet.

Herbal Antibiotics

The widespread use of antibiotics in this country has created a serious problem. The danger now is that bacteria have become immune to some of our most common antibiotics. The way this happened is that bacteria communicate with each other and actually teach each other how to become immune to medications. They have become resistant to so many antibiotics. What does this tell us about further attempts to create stronger antibiotics? Steven Harrod Buhner, the author of *Herbal Antibiotics*, explains.

"Five million people a year are coming down with antibiotic resistant infections. The Centers for Disease Control and many epidemiologists are warning that in the next 10 to 15 years most of our antibiotic arsenal will fail. People will have to turn to more natural alternatives that are more ecologically sound, as herbs are. Things that naturally stimulate the immune system, that help us from getting ill in the first place.

"As our antibiotic arsenal fails, it becomes more and more important for everybody to stimulate their immune system and to keep it healthy and balanced. Whether it is bubonic plague or Ebola river virus some people never become ill because their immune system is potentiated and healthy."

Western medicine has been predicated on a certain type of thinking. This type of thinking is "that human beings can create whatever they want to, and kill anything that can harm us. If it is bears, we will kill bears. If it's bacteria, we kill bacteria. Antibiotics are exceptionally powerful. It is difficult for many physicians to change their thinking and realize they have to work with nature and not view diseases as the enemy.

"We only get sick when our bodies are out of balance. Our natural immune system should deal with almost all diseases we encounter. Plant medicines are not something bacteria can become resistant to. Herbal medicines are so much more effective than antibiotics and are a lot gentler on the body. Herbs are so complex. For instance yarrow, which has a lot of antibacterial qualities, has over 120 identified compounds, whereas penicillin has only one. The bacteria cannot respond to it, it's too complex. Antibiotics are very simple substances, which makes it easy for bacteria to learn how to shift, change and adapt, which they do with incredible frequency."

To identify the most useful herbal antibiotics, Buhner studied each individually. "When I assessed the most powerful herbs, I had three criteria. One was the length of time it had been used in different cultures. Second was the amount used by indigenous and folk practitioners around the world. Third was the effectiveness in clinical trials and laboratory studies. There are quite a few herbs that fell into all of those categories."

ALOE. "Aloe comes from a Southwestern American plant. Aloe is directly effective against Staphylococcus bacteria, even resistant Staph bacteria. Staph bacteria like to infect burns because the skin is not available to protect them. So aloe is used on burns and it softens the skin, keeps it moist and is soothing. Honey can be used almost identically. In China they have been using honey on second and third degree burns and seeing healing with no scarring or muscle loss."

ECHINACEA. "Echinacea is exceptionally effective against Streptococcal bacteria, those that cause Strep throat. It is well known and popular."

GOLDENSEAL. "Goldenseal is good in the mucous membrane system. Goldenseal is an amazing plant for E. coli infections that can cause severe, sometimes bloody diarrhea that can be fatal in children."

CRYPTOCOCCOIS. "This is a West African plant used traditionally for malaria for thousands of years. It is effective against all antibiotic resistant bacteria as well as malaria. It is equally good as the pharmaceuticals that are used for malaria but it doesn't have any of their side effects."

GARLIC. "Garlic is effective against every antibiotic resistant bacteria except for malaria. If you eat it regularly, it helps stimulate the immune system so that helps prevent infection. Use it raw as a juice or eat the raw cloves when you have a bacterial infection. If you have severe lung infections or tuberculosis, which centers in the lungs, garlic is excreted though the lungs. The body always takes it right to there, which is why so many people that eat garlic have garlic smelling breath. Many clinicians who are using herbs for difficult diseases like AIDS, use juiced garlic. They give people between 2 to 9 bulbs of garlic a day, not just the cloves. It is usually taken in a quarter to a half teaspoon in about 12 ounces of a binder like tomato or carrot juice. You drink it throughout the day."

LICORICE. "Licorice is one of the most potent herbs. It is an immune stimulant and immune modulator, which means it helps the immune system become more functional. It is very antibacterial against many bacteria. By the way, the rubbery candies we call licorice candies often contain no licorice and are mostly flavored with anise or fennel."

ESTONIA. "Estonia is a lichen that grows on trees throughout the world and has been found to be more powerful than penicillin. In dilute concentrations of 1 to 20,000 it completely inhibits both tuberculosis and resistant Staphylococcus bacteria. It is two plants in one, a symbiotic plant. The inner white thread is an immune enhancer and an immune stimulant, and the outside green part is strongly antibacterial. You not only fight bacterial disease directly but also enhance your immune functioning."

Homeopathic Remedies

A number of homeopathic remedies also belong in the natural medicine cabinet. According to Food and Drug Administration regulations, a natural remedy cannot be labeled safe and effective for treating a specific ailment even if study after study has proven that it is more effective than over-the-counter or doctor-prescribed medications. Therefore the average American will only see television commercials for products such as Anacin or Tylenol to treat a headache even though a simple homeopathic remedy may be safer and just as effective.

Millions of Americans suffer from a myriad of everyday health conditions and they do not know about natural remedies. Dr. Lynn Page Walker is a doctor of homeopathy and has a master's degree in Chinese herbology, and acupuncture. She has specific recommendations for what ought to be in everyone's medicine chest, especially if your access to a doctor or medical care is limited.

TEA TREE OIL. Dr. Walker's first recommendation is tea tree oil. "Tea tree oil is an oil from Australia, also called melaluka oil. It is a strong antiviral, antifungal and antibacterial. You could use it on any cut, for any kind of fungus in the mouth and for fungus under the nail. It works as a gargle for sore throat and for gum problems. There is a tea tree oil toothpaste for those with ongoing gum problems. It works on canker sores, cuts and abrasions, insect bites, and even as an astringent for the face. Tea tree oil is a good basic remedy to have around the house."

RESCUE REMEDY. "The next thing I recommend is rescue remedy, a boxflower essence that is a combination of five different flower essences. It is excellent for relieving stress so in emergency situations it calms children. It is safe for small children and animals. When there is a crisis I recommend that every member of the family, not just the sick one, take rescue to see things a little bit clearer."

BITING INSECT. "The next home useful remedy to have around the house actually prevents insect bites. It is Biting Insect by Molecular Biologicals. It is good for flea bites, mosquito bites, and any kind of bug bites. Although it helps with some spider bites, it is not as effective. If you know you will be exposed to bugs, take 10 drops three times a day."

PEPPERMINT OIL. "I recommend peppermint oil for a number of things. You can mix it in warm water and drink it for a stomachache or rub it directly on the forehead for a headache.

BLACK OINTMENT. "Black ointment is made by Nature's Way and some other companies. Anytime you have a splinter or any little sliver that won't come out, black ointment can draw it out. It is also a very healing salve for any kind of cut."

ARNICA. Dr. Walker also recommends "Arnica homeopathic in low potency, either a 6x or 30x, for any kind of trauma to the body. It stops the body from over-reacting to the trauma. It's good for muscle aches and pains such as on days when you have worked really hard physically. Some people take it before surgery but just take one dose to help your body not over-react."

TRAUMA OINTMENT OR TRAMMEL OINTMENT. These are "combinations of homeopathic remedies specifically for trauma. They are nice combinations to use on your muscles if you are sore."

CHOLANGIOLE TINCTURE. "Cholangiole tincture is a healing oil made from marigold flower. It is good for cleansing wounds and promotes healing. I've seen wounds heal in a day or two."

NUX VOMICA. "Nux vomica in a low potency, 6x or 30x is for hangover and also for upset stomach from overeating or overdrinking. When you feel bloated and your digestion feels off, nux vomica is a good remedy. It also works well for hemorrhoids."

CHOLANGIOLE HYPERICUM. "Cholangiole hypericum ointment, especially the brand made by Boron, promotes healing. The cholangiole promotes the healing and the hypericum helps with any kind of pain. Together they work for cold sores, any kind of sore on the face or mouth, cuts or abrasions to heal them fast and take away the pain."

GUNPOWDER 6X. "One of my favorites is not well known. It is called gunpowder 6x. This is for any minor infection like tooth abscesses or any infection on the skin. I find it useful for those who are getting their ears or bellybuttons pierced and they get infected. You can't get any sustainable antibiotic levels at those sites if you get an infection there. Take three gunpowder pills three times a day and the infection will resolve in 2 or 3 days."

VACTICIME DROPS. "Vacticime drops are a combination made by Complemed that stimulates your body to fight bacterial infection. If you had an abscess or sore throat or any kind of bacterial infection take 10 drops 3 to 5 times a day. This will clear the infection in a short period by boosting your own immune system."

ABC DROPS. "ABC drops is a combination of aconite, belladonna and chamomile homeopathic medications. Popular in Europe, it is good for colds, earaches and sometimes when your children are irritable such as when they are teething."

Headache

A pounding headache happens to most people at some time. It interferes with our lives and keeps us from functioning at our best. If you are a migraine headache sufferer, you know what I'm talking about. (See chapter 46 for a discussion of migraines.) Doctors offer powerful medications that may or may not help and have side effects of their own. And what causes our headaches? And how can we get rid of them without making ourselves sicker?

A new book called *No More Headaches, No More Migraines*, by Dr. Zuzana Bic has some of the answers. Dr. Bic is an assistant adjunct professor of medicine at UCLA at Irvine and is in private practice. In her research and work using integrative lifestyle medicine in the prevention of chronic diseases, she has been able to identify headache "triggers." There are many things that trigger headaches. If we know what the triggers are we can avoid them and cut down on headaches without pain medications. She describes changes we can make in our day-to-day lives to make headaches a thing of the past.

"Where my research is unique," says Dr. Bic, "is trying to identify the common denominator for all the lifestyle factors. I have a group I call diet-related triggers. In this group belong all food that is high in fat, high in refined sugar, most processed or refined food and food that is low in complex carbohydrates. A related group is obesity, which is connected to not eating properly, and also hypoinsulinemia or insulin resistance, one of the first signs of diabetes. Hypoglycemia, which means low levels of sugar, is another trigger for headaches. Prolonged hunger and dehydration can cause headache as can alcohol and caffeine intake.

"So what could be the common denominator of all these that lead to headaches? This is the question I have addressed in my studies. What I have found I try to explain to the patients. As you know the cells in the blood, platelets, red blood cells, and white blood cells, all coexist in the blood vessels. A high level of fat in the blood will crowd up the vessels, similar to a crowded freeway with one car bumping into another car. A process like platelet congregation occurs and there is a little bit of damage to the platelet, causing it to release serotonin. The body acts to excrete this excess serotonin and you have lower levels of serotonin. Serotonin is a very important neurotransmitter and important factor in triggering headache.

"There are other lifestyle triggers. These include smoking, a sedentary lifestyle, and physical exertion that is the exhausting type. Some patients who suffer from anorexia nervosa or bulimia exercise excessively and this is the type that can result in headache. Stress and oral contraceptives or hormone replacement also trigger headaches".

"There are 13 different types of headaches, the majority of which can be influenced by lifestyle modification."

But Dr. Bic points out that some types of headaches are caused by things other than triggers and these types of headaches are unaffected by lifestyle changes. Headaches caused by head trauma, infection or tumors in the brain, or problems with eyes or ears cannot be resolved with lifestyle modification.

She hits the nail on the head by identifying imbalanced diet as one of the main headache triggers. It makes sense that if you eat an unbalanced, unhealthy diet, your body will react by giving you a headache. In Dr. Bic's research she found that putting her patients on a low fat diet and combating their hunger with fruit, vegetables, grains, beans, and a higher amount of fiber helps. She also recommends increasing the daily intake of water. "They think they drink enough water but if they monitor it in their food diaries, there is not enough water. They are always surprised.

"I also recommend starting an exercise program or increasing the level of physical activity. Start walking 10 minutes in the morning and 10 minutes in the evening. Or park the car as far away as possible and walk to the office. To cut down on stress I recommend meditation or 1-minute relaxation techniques such as breathing exercises or changing how they perceive situations to a more objective point of view.

In her research she also elucidates the timing of the trigger and the headache. "Some of my patients are more sensitive and can have a headache immediately, 1 hour after the trigger. For others it can be 72 hours after the trigger. I think it is the accumulation of unbalanced lifestyle factors. It is possible for a person to be sedentary, eat a high fat diet, have a very stressful situation, and not be drinking enough water. All these things accumulate and they can have that headache from 3 hours to 72 hours."

So a good plan to avoid headache triggers is a low fat diet, lots of water, exercise, and stress-reduction.

Hangover

The alcohol hangover is an old problem. It's even referred to in the Bible: "Woe unto them that rise up early in the morning, that they may follow strong drink" (Isaiah 5:11). It may not happen too often but there are always those big celebrations—weddings, graduations, office parties, New Year's Eve—when we may drink too much alcohol. The doctors call it by a fancy name: veisalgia, meaning "uneasiness following debauchery" and "pain." The symptoms are headache, tremulousness, nausea, diarrhea, and fatigue combined with decreased cognitive and visual-spatial skills and work loss.

Alcohol in high doses can be toxic and also can dehydrate and have effects on the heart. Anyone who drives a car or has to operate machinery is going to have a problem when they have a hangover. Anyone who has to run a meeting or get the chores done is going to have a problem the next day. In a word they are going to feel lousy even after the alcohol is gone from their body. The alcohol leaves behind its toxic effects when you drink too much.

We know it has something to do with what's in the alcohol you overdose on. Dark-colored liquors, like brandy, wine, whiskey, give a much worse hangover. Drinking vodka or gin or other clear liquors does not cause the worst symptoms. Sulfites found especially in dark wines can make you sicker. Alcohol causes a diuresis, meaning dehydration, meaning you go to the bathroom and the fluids in your body are depleted.

Are there any ways to prevent hangover? In a non-blinded study an herbal preparation called Liv.52 from the Himalaya Drug Co. in Bombay decreased hangover symptoms. How did it work? The investigators thought it might be because the herb blocked the conversion of ethanol to acetaldehyde. Acetaldehyde is created from the byproducts of ethanol (which is alcohol) is our stomachs. It can act like a poison in some people. Women are more susceptible to this because they have lower levels of the enzyme needed to convert alcohol to something less toxic.

In another study, vitamin B_6 was given before, during, and after parties where the participants drank enough to get intoxicated. Those who took the vitamin reduced the number of hangover symptoms by 50 percent.

One thing everybody agrees on is to drink lots of fluids before, during, and after drinking alcohol. It helps to dilute the alcohol in the first place and replaces the fluids that are excreted by the kidneys. The diuresis or excessive fluid excretion caused by the alcohol causes the dehydration that leads to a lot of the symptoms of the hangover. And, of course, limit the number of times you get intoxicated with alcohol in the first place.

Aphrodisiacs

Aphrodisiacs enhance sexual desire, arousal, and performance. There are foods, herbs, vitamins and minerals, amino acids, hormones, and aromatic oils that can all directly affect our biochemistry and hence could affect our sexuality. There are over a dozen herbs that act as aphrodisiacs but they work in different ways and produce different results. For example, there are fast-acting herbs, which affect one or more of the stages of sexual response. Then there are herbs that, if taken over a long period of time, boost a person's overall physical and emotional readiness. Although herbal preparations do not carry the same risk as pharmaceuticals taken to enhance sexual performance, it is important to understand how to take them for maximum effectiveness. Overall, herbs can vary tremendously in their strength and effectiveness depending on where they are grown, when they are harvested, how they are processed, and so on. It can be challenging to sort it all out.

Nancy Nickel, the author of *Nature's Aphrodisiacs*, has studied food, nutrition, and alternative therapies for over 25 years. She is a member of the Holistic Health Association. Using her expertise as an educational writer, lecturer and researcher in nutrition, and molecular therapy, she offers a review of nature's aphrodisiacs.

She says, "Natural aphrodisiacs have been a source of legend for centuries. Oysters and shrimp actually contain nutrients that benefit the reproductive system. There have been some scientific studies of natural aphrodisiacs but not too many. Most research is done by pharmaceutical manufacturers and it doesn't pay them to research a product they cannot patent. But we have some scientific evidence on why several natural products and natural aphrodisiacs work. Three of these are damiana, yohimbe, and muira puama (also called potency wood)." These herbs are discussed in chapter 59.

As we all know sex is hardly ever just about sex. Emotions and psychological health have a direct impact on sexual health. Feelings like anger, worry, tension and depression all affect sexual encounters for both men and women. There are quite a few herbs that are useful for addressing this aspect of sex and pleasure.

Ms. Nickel helps us to identify what they are and how they work. "To reduce anxiety and elevate mood, there is kava kava, valerian, which is widely used in Europe, gotu kola, lemon balm, angelica, skull cap, and vervain. These work quickly. St. John's wort is also very good but take several weeks to have an effect. Kava kava tea has a physical effect on sexual performance; however it is also an unbeatable tension reducer. If makes you feel happy, relaxed and sociable. You can buy tea bags or make it from an extract. Put 10 to30 drops in juice or water. It is fairly safe although slightly narcotic. Because it affects the nervous system it should not be used by people who have Parkinson's disease or those taking an antidepressant.

"Gotu kola is an excellent nerve tonic. It stimulates the central nervous system, decreases depression and fatigue, and stimulates the sex drive. If you take it regularly, which you can do, gotu kola tea has a cumulative effect as a sex drive booster. Unlike herbs that contain caffeine it doesn't cause insomnia or nervousness. You can take up to one to three capsules a day. As an extract, you can mix 5 to 10 drops in a liquid and drink it. Take it about three times a day. Excessive doses can make you feel faint and sometimes it can cause a headache.

"Lemon balm can be grown in your own garden. It relaxes the nervous system and elevates your mood. It is one of the most gentle herbs and one of the most pleasant tasting. In Europe it is customary to drink lemon balm tea to calm stress and frayed nerves. It is available as a tea, a dried herb and as an extract. If you buy it as an extract, mix a half to one teaspoon in liquid. Use the dried herb to make tea. Avoid lemon balm if you have a thyroid condition because it could interfere with a hormone that stimulates the thyroid. They are not sure about this, but I say be on the safe side.

"Angelica is a versatile herb that increases blood circulation. It acts as an aphrodisiac and is especially good for tension headaches. The dose is between 10 or 30 drops in a liquid. It should not be used by pregnant women because in strong doses it can bring on a period. And, because it contains sugars, diabetics should not use it.

"Another excellent tranquilizing herb is skull cap. It is called skull cap because the flower looks like a little cap. Excellent for relieving stress or nervousness associated with sex, or any kind of performance anxiety. It is very safe and mild, relaxes the muscles, and produces inner calm.

"Just one more reminder: Because these herbs are potent and have chemical compounds that work, there are side effects so you have to be careful."

Viagra has been on the market for 2 years and has been astonishingly successful for erectile dysfunction. But it has side effects and contraindications. A full discussion of Viagra including my alternative protocol can be found in chapter 59.

67

The Common Cold

Colds are around us throughout the year. Sneezing, runny nose and congestion, fevers, fatigue, aches and pains. So far there has been no cure for the
common cold even though lots of money has been spent on medical
research. Keeping healthy in the first place is the best defense. Besides aspirin
and other decongestants, which have side effects of their own, there are other
things we can do to maintain and optimize our immune systems. A healthy
immune system can tackle the bacteria and viruses better than any antibiotic or
medication. Dr. Ray Sahelian is a board-certified family practice physician and
graduate of Thomas Jefferson School of Medicine. In his book, *Finally the
Common Cold Cure*, he recommends an approach for getting rid of the cold
before it takes too much out of us.

Immune System "Busters"

As Dr. Sahelian points out, the primary cause of the cold is a virus. There are
at least a couple of hundred types of viruses that cause colds. But, as we know,
not everybody comes down with the common cold when they are exposed to
the virus. The most likely reason why people don't get sick is that they are
maintaining healthy living habits.

Dr. Sahelian has identified four immune system "busters" that cause some
people to come down with a cold when they are exposed to the virus. The first
is sleep. "People come down with a cold when they are not getting 6 to 8 hours
of restful sleep. It is during the time of our deepest sleep that the immune cells
are regenerated. One particular type of immune cell, called the natural killer
cell, is very important. It is during deep sleep that the natural killer cell is acti-

vated. If it is not activated, then we are more vulnerable to getting a cold. Everyone is going to be exposed to the virus sooner or later, by shaking the hand of someone who has a cold or being exposed to children who are sneezing or coughing. If we have a good, activated immune system it is going to knock out that virus.

"Besides sleep, stress is another immune system buster, whether it be from relationship difficulties, financial worries, stress at work, physical stress, intense athletic competition—sometimes running a marathon can do it—or from illness. Stress can lower temporarily the immune system and that can cause the virus to take a foothold. Poor diet is going to lower the immune system, particularly a lot of sugars, potato chips, cookie, pies, and junk foods are going to interfere with the immune system."

The third immune system buster is smoking. "Smoking damages the lining of the respiratory tract," Dr. Sahelian says. "There are hairlike structures called cilia that are constantly sweeping out the germs that we inhale. If the cilia are damaged from smoking they are not going to be able to sweep out the bacteria or viruses and they settle in to start a cold or another type of infection."

The final immune system buster is taking antibiotics when you don't need them.

Dr. Sahelian explains, "Whenever someone comes down with a cold, as a rule they wait it out a day or two, take some over-the-counter pills if they are not into natural medicine, and then go to their doctor. The doctor examines them, says, 'You have a cold, take some more over-the-counter medicines, and you are going to be okay in a week.' Well, the patient is not satisfied if they made the effort to go all the way to the doctor, wait in the office waiting room, pay $60 to $200 to see a doctor, and then be told to use an over-the-counter medicine. So they are going to request an antibiotic prescription.

"So, even though 90 percent of all upper respiratory infections are caused by a virus, over 50 percent of the time the patient will come out with a prescription for an antibiotic. *Antibiotics do not kill viruses.* And antibiotics are going to be harmful because they can cause side effects. They can cause yeast infections, killing all the good bacteria in the gut. They can cause fatigue, allergic reactions, diarrhea and sometimes even more harmful things. So, that is not the answer."

Immune System Boosters

What is the answer then? "In addition to having a good healthy diet, taking some supplements on a regular basis, like vitamin C, vitamin E and juices and fish oils will help you stay healthy," says Dr. Sahelian.

Gail Ulrich, the founder and director of Blazing Star Herbal School in Shelbourn Falls, Massachusetts, and the author of *Herbs to Boost Immunity*, tells us more.

"Diet in our culture is high in fats and refined sugars and sodium as well as in processed foods. We now know that these foods produce free radicals in the body that create toxicity and weaken immunity. It is important to first of all eliminate refined sugar and refined flours, as well as caffeine, cigarettes, alcohol and processed or deep fried foods. It goes without saying to avoid tobacco, commercially raised red meats, especially because of the high pesticide and hormone content in these products, and to minimize alcohol consumption.

"An immune-enhancing diet would include a wide variety of organically grown fruits and vegetables or wild fruits and vegetables as well. You also need whole grains and legumes along with adequate amounts of protein from soy, grains or fish. The more you get back to a simple diet based on whole foods as they occur in nature, the better off you will be. It is important to include super-foods or nutrient-dense foods like miso soup, garlic, sea vegetables such as kelp. Wild foods are important in greens like dandelion greens, mustard greens, watercress, astragalus. and steamed nettle greens. There are some delicious medicinal immune-enhancing mushrooms like shitake and reishi. Yogurt that contains acidophilus is important for balancing the garden of the intestinal flora, if you don't have lactose intolerance. Other immune-enhancing foods include dates, almonds, buckwheat, chicken soup, chickpeas, burdock root, and parsley."

Other lifestyle changes can be in order. "They always say, eat like a king at breakfast, a prince at lunch and a pauper at dinner. Drink at least eight glasses of pure water daily and exercise adequately.

"There are many herbs we can use to enhance immunity. Echinacea is well known. I also recommend garlic, osha root, and milk thistle. These protect the mucus membranes and stimulate production of white blood cells. There are also deep immune tonic herbs that would be helpful to build the bone marrow and increase deep immunity. These are astragalus, Siberian ginseng, and shitake and reishi mushrooms. These herbs are especially helpful when we have immune deficiency and long term stress on the immune system.

"There are also herbs called adaptogens that help the body cope with stress on many levels, including not only physical stress, but environmental and emotional stressors. In this category is Siberian ginseng, panax ginseng, which is American and Korean ginseng, licorice, borage, and milk thistle, to name a few."

Fighting Colds the Natural Way

What should you do at the first signs of a cold? "Sometimes a cold can come on mildly—a scratchy throat, a runny nose or even just a tingling sensation in the nose or throat. But as soon as you notice the very first symptom, do not wait to act. Immediately take between 3 to 5 grams of vitamin C. You may wish to keep the 500 milligram capsules on your kitchen counter and take about 6 to 10 of these which would equal about 3 to 5 grams of vitamin C. Right after that immediately put a zinc lozenge in your mouth. The zinc lozenge should contain between 10 to 25 milligrams of zinc. Many people chew it and within a brief period swallow it but this is a mistake. The zinc is fighting the cold by acting locally in the throat and palate and the nasopharyngeal area. It has to stay in the mouth for as long as you can tolerate it, generally 5 to 10 minutes. You can bite it but keep the pieces in your mouth before you swallow it. Keep these at home because you never know, a cold can start at 2 in the morning and by the time you have gone to the health food store in the morning to buy these supplements, the cold might have taken a foothold.

"Another common mistake is stopping the medications too soon. The symptoms may have eased and then you forget to take the supplements. They have to be taken continuously. With the vitamin C you can lower the dose from 3 to 5 grams to one to 2 grams every few hours. I recommend the zinc at least every hour or two for the first half day and then every 2 to 3 hours after that. The problem with the zinc lozenge is that it can irritate the palate and cause soreness. But I would rather have that than allow the virus to settle in. These suggestions are crucial and timing is very important here.

"You may travel somewhere where zinc and vitamin C are not available so I recommend taking them with you when traveling. I also recommend using the zinc lozenge right before you go to bed. If you wake up take it again. Don't let 6 or 8 hours pass without doing it.

"People often ask how can I tell the difference between a virus, bacteria or allergy when I am having these symptoms? Even doctors have trouble differentiating them because the symptoms overlap. Viruses and bacteria will give fever but allergies do not. Runny nose is common with the common cold virus and allergies but bacteria will rarely if ever give you a runny nose. Nasal congestion is common with the virus and allergies, but bacteria rarely. Another way to differentiate viruses from allergies is muscle aches and pains. If you have bad muscle aches and pains it is more commonly a virus and hardly ever an allergy. Allergies will rarely give you yellow-green mucus but bacteria commonly will and all the viruses.

"I want to mention children and zinc. One study done recently did not show zinc to be effective in children. The kids probably swallowed the zinc tablets and didn't let the zinc stay in their mouth and throat long enough for it to kill the viruses. I still feel that in a clinical sense when used appropriately older children can use zinc effectively.

"It is not inevitable that we all come down with colds. By eating the right foods, getting a good night's rest, reducing stress, not smoking, taking some of the supplements on a regular basis, like vitamin C and fish oils, garlic, onions and then taking the immediate steps right away when coming down with a cold, you can, as a rule, either eliminate or decrease the frequency of viruses severely."

68

Holistic Dentistry

Turn-of-the-century author and editor Frank Harris wrote, "Doctors tell us that men commonly dig their graves with their teeth." Not only is this caused by improper diet, but by not taking care of one's teeth and even by putting poisons in one's mouth. In this chapter, we look at how dental health affects the health of the body and how the health of the body affects the teeth. We also evaluate the way people treat their teeth when they are diseased. You will find that typical treatments for repairing damage and maintaining healthy teeth, such as silver amalgam fillings and fluoridation of water, are much more hazardous than claimed. You will also learn that there is a group of dentists practicing what we've been preaching throughout this book, a nontoxic, whole body approach to health. It's called holistic dentistry.

What is Holistic Dentistry?

Dr. Joyal Taylor offers an overview of holistic dentistry in an article posted on the HealthWorld Online website (www.healthy.net). Holistic dentistry, also known as biological dentistry and environmental dentistry "involves far more than technique," Dr. Taylor says, adding "it encompasses a total awareness relating to the mind and body."

A holistic dentist starts with the assumption that patients must be educated and aware. Patients learn how their teeth and gums are affected by their body chemistry, eating habits, lifestyle, and genetic make-up. They learn how to prevent dental problems. They are told about possible side effects of dental materials. And they participate in the process of deciding on a treatment program.

Body chemistry analysis and nutritional guidance are important components of holistic dentistry. Holistic dentists avoid materials and procedures that they believe are toxic to the body. For example, they use porcelain, gold, or composite (plastic) restorations instead of mercury-based silver fillings. They use x-rays sparingly not routinely. They avoid the use of fluoride. Among the broad-based treatment methods they favor are nutrition, homeopathy, and acupuncture.

How Dental Problems Affect the Rest of the Body

Dental problems and procedures such as cavities, infections, fillings, and root canals can cause illness and injury throughout the body. Perhaps the most well-known danger is that dental fillings can release toxic metals into the body and disrupt normal functions. These metals can travel from teeth into bone, connective tissues, and nerves. Infections under and around the teeth can travel to other parts and affect the overall functioning of the body's immune system. Root canals can leave hidden bacterial pockets that prove a breeding ground for disease. A study some years ago took teeth that had root canals and ground them up. Some of the powder was placed under the skin of rabbits. The researchers found that if the patient from whom the tooth was taken had arthritis, the rabbit developed arthritis. If the patient had heart disease, the rabbit developed that. Clearly, toxins were still carried in the teeth after the root canal had been performed.

Healthy Diet, Healthy Teeth

The first thing to think about when it comes to healthy teeth is diet. A good diet will be reflected in the condition of the gums and teeth. Think of the general practitioner of yesteryear. One imagines this doctor making a house call on an ailing patient. His first request on seeing this patient was "Stick out your tongue." He wanted to see the tongue's color.

Dr. Victor Zeines, the author of *The Natural Dentist*, reminds us that this practice, far from being quaint and outdated, can still be used to make a good, first diagnosis of medical problems. In fact, Chinese doctors, who also ask to see the patient's tongue, have a book that discusses 280 diseases that can be detected from the state of the tongue. For example, a white tongue indicates that toxins are coming out of the body (this will be observed in people with a cold or the flu), cracks in the tongue indicate vitamin deficiency, a yellowish gray or yellowish green tongue indicates gallbladder or liver trouble, and a brownish or grayish green tongue indicates intestinal or stomach problems.

The mouth is indicative of the body's general state of health. If you have a cavity, it is the end result of general physical problems of the whole body, not just the isolated tooth.

Famed dental researcher Weston Price wrote a book, which he worked on in the 1920s and 1930s, based on studies of the teeth in people in native cultures. People who followed traditional ways, eating simply prepared food indigenous to the region where they lived had healthy teeth. As soon as they adopted a Western diet of canned processed food with white sugar and white flour, their dental health deteriorated. Children born to parents on a Western diet had occlusion and malformed teeth. Price even saw that children born before the introduction of Western foods had healthy teeth, while children in the same family born after the new diet was instituted had poor teeth.

When a person is not eating properly, the body becomes acidic. Minerals are pulled out of the mouth to travel into other parts of the body. The teeth weaken in an acid environment while acid-based bacteria increase. A cavity may arise from a mineral deficiency followed by an invasion of bacteria.

Sugar is a main culprit in this process, though not in the way popularly understood. Many people believe sugar gets in the mouth and sits on the tooth, wearing it down. The real problem with sugar is that it reverses the fluid flow. This flow normally goes from the tooth's pulp chamber into the mouth. Sugar alters this process, sending materials in the mouth into the tooth's internal environment, irritating the inside of the tooth.

Many Americans contend daily with high levels of stress, pollution, and a deficient diet. Food often comes to us shipped over long distances, losing many of its nutrients along the way. We need to make up for those lost qualities with vitamins and minerals.

Calcium and magnesium are especially important for healthy teeth. Folic acid can help the body utilize nutrients. Coenzyme Q10 and vitamin C also are recommended.

Green leafy vegetables and carrot juice are also high in calcium. Traditional culture held that chewing on kale was the fastest way to get white teeth. This idea probably is based on recognition of kale's high calcium content. Kale can be juiced and mixed with carrot or apple juice, perhaps with a drop of lemon.

The Truth About Mercury Fillings

Mercury is widely used in common dental fillings. The "silver" filling is actually a mixture of silver, tin, copper, and mercury. Mercury makes up about 50 percent of the filling. Eighty-five percent of the American population has these fillings.

For over 150 years we have been told these fillings are safe, the most durable available. This is not true. Until 1985, the American Dental Association (ADA) repeatedly declared that mercury never escapes from fillings. Then they had to acknowledge that it did leak. Still, even with the leakage, the ADA still declares the fillings safe.

SYSTEMIC EFFECTS OF MERCURY Dentist Flora Para Stay, in an article posted in the HealthWorld Online website (www.healthy.net), summarizes some of the research on the mercury in dental fillings going back at least 30 years. One of the first reports, published in 1970 in the *Journal of the American Dental Association*, concluded that mercury is not stable but rather "vaporizes at ordinary temperatures." In 1985, a report in the *Journal of Dental Research* stated that mercury vapor from fillings travels through the body and accumulates mostly in the brain, kidneys, and gastrointestinal tract.

According to Dr. Stay, researchers have also described a "battery effect" that occurs when mercury gets into the saliva. She explains that "currents are generated, causing mercury molecules from the surface of the fillings to be released into the tissues."

Mercury can also damage the immune system. Dr. Stay cites another report from the 1980s that concluded that amalgam and nickel-based fillings are associated with a reduction in the number of T-lymphocytes, a type of white blood cell.

The effects of mercury toxicity range from a metallic taste in the mouth, brittle nails, and dry skin, to fatigue, anxiety, depression, headaches, memory loss, gastrointestinal problems, kidney disease, heart problems, and more. Mercury can stop nutrients from entering the cells and prevent wastes from being eliminated. High mercury levels have been found in people with multiple sclerosis and other autoimmune diseases. Mercury also can produce spontaneous abortions. Because of these wide-ranging symptoms, mercury toxicity often goes undetected.

REMOVAL OF FILLINGS Many people aware of the dangers of amalgam fillings have had them removed and replaced with safer alternatives. Gold, porcelain, or composite restorations may be used. Upon removal of the silver filling, they often see improvement, although it may be constrained by the mercury already in the body. Dr. Michael Schachter has seen patients whose blood tests have gone from abnormal to normal once silver fillings were removed. He also seen people with multiple sclerosis and chronic fatigue syndrome markedly improved once fillings were taken out. Dr. Zeines has seen improved memory, better sleep, and less nervousness in patients following removal of mercury fillings.

Removing these fillings is not an easy task and the process is potentially dangerous since taking out the amalgam could accidentally release mercury.

Dr. Howard Hinton, a holistic dentist, stresses that the removal must be done under the care of both a physician and a dentist. The patient must be on a good diet and should undergo laboratory tests to determine how he or she is eliminating the mercury. Ideally, the removal should be carried out in a sterile, bubble chamber—a round room with a laminar air flow circulating through the space; negative ion generators, to charge particulates in the air; and processed water and air. A rubber dam is used in the mouth to reduce exposure and the filling is removed with extreme care. (The highest absorption in the body is in the mouth.) During the procedure, high suction and a lot of water are used to reduce the presence of mercury vapor.

Once the fillings are removed, the body should be detoxified. A lack of health improvement may be due to the fact that mercury is still in the body.

Dr. Elmira Gadol, another practitioner of holistic dentistry, says that garlic supplements will help the body eliminate the existing mercury toxins and selenium can be taken to neutralize the metal. Once the fillings are removed, hair analysis should be done to see what other heavy metals are in the body. These metals interfere with cell processes, such as the oxygen going in and the carbon dioxide going out. These metals also have to be drawn out or problems will remain.

Some patients can be helped by taking intravenous vitamin C. Also, various chelating agents can be prescribed. These agents will attach to the mercury and take it out of the body in urine or feces.

Hot baths with Epsom salts and baking soda are also recommended as a way to bring out the mercury. In working on detoxification, various methods should be tried alone and in combination.

The Fluoride Debate

We don't have to look too far to find fluoride these days—it's there in our toothpastes, our mouthwashes, and much of our drinking water. In fact, 50 percent of the people in the United States drink fluoridated water. Proponents of fluoride say we need it to prevent tooth decay. But many health experts say otherwise.

Dr. David Kennedy, from the International Academy of Oral Medicine and Toxicology, puts it quite well when he states that fluoride is a poison. It kills rats and insects so, certainly, it will kill bacteria if it is scrubbed on the teeth.

Dr. Taylor, in an article posted on the HealthWorld Online website (www.healthy.net), adds that fluoride is retained in the body, where it amasses over time. Small exposures now may not pose problems. But gradually, "you accumulate levels that may be dangerous to your health."

Many people are concerned about the lack of scientific research in this area. To date, there have been no long-term studies exploring how fluoride affects the body over time. Furthermore, Dr. Taylor says, the beneficial affects of fluoride have not been proven.

Dr. Mark Breiner, the author of *Whole Body Dentistry*, who has been practicing holistic dentistry for 20 years, says that putting fluoride into toothpaste or mouthwash will probably cut down on decay somewhat because it is such a potent toxin. However, he asks, while it may cause a decrease in tooth decay, what else is it causing? "I think there are better ways to prevent tooth decay, the main way being proper nutrition and if need be, some supplementation. But to go and use a potent toxin like that just doesn't make any sense."

HOW IT ALL BEGAN How did this potentially dangerous substance, with no real protective qualities, become so widely adopted? It all started back in 1939, when Trendley Dean, D.D.S., found that fluoride contributed to higher than normal levels of staining of the teeth. During the course of his research for the U.S. Public Health Service (PHS), Dr. Dean also found that the people with the most staining had the fewest cavities.

Following this discovery, in 1945 the PHS initiated what was to be a decade-long study of fluoridation and cavity rates in two U.S. cities. As Dr. Taylor explains, halfway through the study, public health officials began touting fluoridation, saying that the fluoridated city (Grand Rapids) was showing a drop in cavity rates. The cavity rate in the nonfluoridated city also dropped, by about the same amount. However, for unknown reasons, the latter city was taken out of the study. When the research was published at the end of the decade, Dr. Taylor says, it only included the findings from Grand Rapids.

Although it soon became clear that there were problems with the research—and despite the fact that there were no studies of possible side effects from long-term use—the fluoride bandwagon had taken off. No matter that two decades later it was found that the tooth decay rate in Grand Rapids was no different from the national average, or that dental costs in fluoridated states were no different from those in nonfluoridated states. These findings were ignored. As Dr. Taylor says, "The machinery was already in place and there was no turning back."

Around the same time that the early research was being conducted, something else was going on in industry that contributed to fluoride's rise to fame. There was a crisis in the aluminum industry, with big companies such as Alcoa being sued for polluting and killing cattle and other livestock. Edward Bernays, one of the fathers of public relations, and a nephew of Sigmund Freud, came up with the idea of selling the public on the beneficial uses of fluoride, one of the dangerous byproducts of aluminum production. The economic motivation behind this sales effort, which was triumphantly successful, was not the millions of dollars that could be made by marketing fluoride products, but the billions that would be saved by industry if it did not have to clean up the fluoride it was putting into the environment.

TOXIC EFFECTS OF FLUORIDE The health hazards of fluoride are known, and have been for some time. In 1977, an executive of the National Cancer Society documented that there was a 5 percent increase in cancer in communities that began fluoridating their water. An even more notorious study and an attempt to suppress it involved Dr. William Marcus, a senior science advisor at the Environmental Protection Agency's Office of Drinking Water. He read a study that was done to test the dangers of fluoridation. It concluded that there was an increase of bone cancers in animals that were given fluorides. In April 1990, Dr.

Marcus went to a meeting where the National Toxicology Program was to review the study and found that the program's staff had downgraded every cancer reported. An investigation found that scientists at the program had been coerced into making these downgrades.

Dr. Taylor lists some of the ailments that may be caused or exacerbated by the accumulation of fluoride in the body; a depressed immune system, musculoskeletal problems, genetic damage, cancer, and kidney and thyroid problems. Other effects of fluoride include abdominal distress, tremors, convulsions, skin eruptions, headaches, increased thirst, and disturbances of calcium metabolism. Mottling of teeth, marked by white and brown patchy areas, also occurs.

HOW TO AVOID FLUORIDE To limit your exposure to fluoride, drink bottled or filtered water and use a nonfluoridated toothpaste. Dr. Breiner offers some additional recommendations. "As far as toothpaste, I like a toothpaste that has no fluoride in it and has natural ingredients. Same thing with the mouthwash. I like something called tooth and gum tonic, which is made without alcohol or any chemicals. It is an herbal product and has a number of really good ingredients such as echinacea, peppermint, thyme, and eucalyptus. This will also kill bacteria."

For a mouthwash, you can also use plain salt water. Dr. Breiner says, "Use nonfluoridated water and take some salt and swish that around your mouth. It is good for the gums. You can take some baking soda and mix that with a little peroxide and make your own toothpaste. You don't have to go to the store and buy something."

69

Skin Care

What goes in also comes out. The state of your body on the inside has a direct effect on the appearance and texture of your skin. Certain nutrients, foods, and herbs are important for healthy skin. Stephanie Tourles, a certified herbalist, aromatherapist, and reflexologist, and the author of *Naturally Healthy Skin*, tells us more.

"Nutrition is very important for skin care. I don't care what you put on the skin topically, if you are feeding yourself garbage, your skin is going to reflect that. What you eat is reflected on your face and body. In my daily quest for natural beauty and health and vitality, I am in awe of what Mother Nature has to offer us. She provides everything you need to encourage and support the healthy functioning of your skin, but it is up to you to partake of these offerings.

"My personal recommendation is that you try to eat a very balanced diet, preferably vegetarian with minimally processed whole foods in their natural state. Include approximately 40 to 60 percent complex carbohydrates, 20 to 30 percent lean proteins, and 10 to 20 percent fat. This all depends on your activity level and your state of wellness."

Tourles also recommends a number of essential vitamins, minerals, and fats.

Vitamins

She starts by describing five essential vitamins. "The five essential vitamins provide a potent combination of antioxidants and healing agents that boost your skin's ability to make you look your best. The first one is vitamin A or beta carotene. It is a fat-soluble antioxidant….Vitamin A is essential for growth and

---

maintenance of epithelial tissue, which is your skin tissue, and for the proper functioning of the mucous membranes. This vitamin helps prevent dry, rough skin, and premature aging. It speeds healing, especially of acne and impetigo, which is caused by Staph or Strep infection that result in pustules around the nose and mouth. Vitamin A also boosts your general immunity. Deficiency symptoms of this vitamin include premature wrinkles, acne, pimples, blackheads, cirrhosis, dry, rough, itchy, scaly, cracked skin especially on the feet and the hands and slowed healing. An early symptom of deficiency is what I call chicken skin, small raised bumps on the back of the neck, upper arms, back and the shoulder.

"The next vitamin group is the B complex vitamins. These are water-soluble nutrients and they are always grouped together in a complex when naturally occurring. You would never find just one of the B vitamins isolated like you see in the health food store. If you must supplement, this is my feeling, be sure that you take a supplement that supplies the entire complex. Outstanding vegetarian sources of this vitamin are brewer's yeast, whole grains, alfalfa, almonds, sunflower seed, all the soy products, green leafy vegetables, blue-green algae, fresh wheat germ (make sure you get it in the refrigerated section as it tends to go rancid rather quickly), molasses, peas, and beans. This is your antistress vitamin. It helps prevent premature aging and acne, and promotes healthy circulation and metabolism. It is very essential to wound healing such as sunburn, bruises, and infection. It aids in new cell growth and increases your vitality. Deficiency symptoms of this vitamin include a sore mouth and lips. Where your top and lower lip meet will get cracks and become red and very sore. Other deficiency symptoms are eczema, skin lesions, dandruff, a pale complexion, pigmentation problems, and premature wrinkling.

"The number three vitamin is vitamin C. This is a water-soluble antioxidant. Outstanding sources are rose hips, citrus fruits, fresh tomatoes, all kinds of berries, pineapples, apples and persimmons, anything that is green and leafy and especially your bell and hot peppers, and papayas. Vitamin C helps to produce collagen in your connective tissue. Collagen is what keeps your skin plump and firm and keeps you from getting wrinkles. Vitamin C also strengthens the capillary walls, speeds healing, and helps battle environmental stress and toxins. If you have a deficiency in vitamin C you will probably bruise more easily, your gums can become spongy, wrinkles form more quickly, you will notice sagging skin, premature aging, pyorrhea (which is a gum disease) and slowed healing.

"The last two vitamins that I recommend for skin care are vitamin D and vitamin E. Vitamin D is a fat-soluble nutrient. Most people think it has to come from milk or fish liver oils. These are good sources but vegetarian sources include fortified soy milk, alfalfa, watercress, and sunshine. Skin care benefits when you combine vitamin A and vitamin D to treat acne. It also treats herpes simplex, the little sores that show up around and just inside your lips. It helps slow premature aging and enhances bone mineralization and calcium absorption. This is great for your fingernails. Deficiency symptoms of vitamin D are a lack of vitality, very slow growth and bone problems.

"Vitamin E, our last vitamin, is a fat-soluble antioxidant. Outstanding sources are the cold pressed vegetable oils, not the vegetable oils you normally find in your grocery store. Those have been heated too high and heavily processed so you need to get the cold pressed oils. Whole grains, alfalfa, parsley, sprouted seeds, nuts, fresh wheat germ again and green leafy vegetables are good vegetarian sources. Skin care benefits for vitamin E are that it oxygenates the tissues and increases body stores of vitamin A, slows premature aging, helps to block the formation of tumors, speeds healing of severe burns and chronic skin lesions. It may also decrease scarring. Whenever I have gotten a burn I have always mixed vitamin E oil with rose hip seed oil and immediately put that on the sore place and I hardly ever have any scarring. It also promotes red blood cell formation. If you are deficient in vitamin E there will be a degeneration of epithelial cells, which are your skin cells in the organs, and skin germinating cells. This results in tissue membrane instability and collagen shrinkage, which leads to premature aging and the sagging of your skin. You skin can look very lackluster. You can be very tired because you are not getting the oxygen in your body. Remember I said vitamin E helps to oxygenate the tissues. You will also have an increased tendency to bruise as a result of the fragility of the red blood cells."

Minerals

"There are four minerals which I consider the building blocks of gorgeous skin," Tourles says. "The first one is iodine. Outstanding vegetarian sources for iodine are blue-green algae, sunflower seeds, kelp, iodized salt, and sea salt. If I use salt at all it is sea salt. Skin care benefits of iodine are that it aids in healing skin infections, increases oxygen consumption and the metabolic rate in the skin, and it helps prevent roughness and premature wrinkling. Deficiency symptoms of iodine include a slow growth in healing, a slow metabolism, very poor skin tone and dry skin. There is a contraindication for iodine: it may aggravate acne. Fish and shellfish are also great sources. If you have acne you may want to drastically decrease fish and cut down on your blue-green algae and maybe switch it over to barley grass instead. You may see good results by doing that.

"The next mineral is silicon. A good source for that is horsetail herb, a very good herb to combine with nettle and blue-green algae in capsule form. Echinacea root is very good, dandelion root, alfalfa, kelp, flax seed, barley grass, wheat grass, all varieties of apples and berries, onions, almonds, sunflower seeds and grapes are all good sources. Benefits of silicon are it aids in collagen formation, helping to keep the skin taut, tight, and uplifted. It helps to strengthen your bone and skin tissues and aids in wrinkle prevention. Deficiency symptoms include premature wrinkling, lack of skin tone, and sagging skin."

The third mineral is sulfur. "Sulfur can be found in turnip greens, dandelions, greens, radishes, horseradish, string beans, onions and garlic," Tourles says. "All of these foods have a strong flavor. Cabbage, celery, kale, soybeans, and asparagus are milder. Asparagus is particularly high in sulfur. Sometimes sulfur is called the beauty mineral. It really helps to keep the skin clear and smooth. Deficiency symptoms of sulfur include dry scalp, rashes, eczema, and acne."

"The last mineral is zinc. Good sources are blue-green algae and barley grass, alfalfa, yellow dock root, echinacea root, any of the sea weeds like kelp, fresh wheat germ, all variety of seeds, brewer's yeast, and all kinds of nuts and green leafy vegetables. Zinc aids in wound healing, promotes cell growth, and boosts immunity. It helps treat acne when combined with vitamin A and B. Deficiency of zinc includes slow healing, dandruff, and lowered resistance to infections."

Essential Fats and Fatty Acids

Tourles goes on to talk about the essential fats and fatty acids that are important for healthy skin. "Fat in the diet is very vital to your skin's health and beauty," she says. "Without fat your skin has no contour, no roundness. It cannot be beautiful without at least a thin layer of padding to support it and give it shape. Fat is a necessary requirement if you desire radiant and moisturized skin.

"As far as proper skin care goes there are two types of essential fatty acids that are greatly beneficial. These are omega-3 and omega-6 fatty acids. The first one is omega-3 and people usually think of coldwater fish such as blue fish, salmon, mackerel, or tuna as good source. If you want a vegetarian source, ground flax seeds or flaxseed oil. Flaxseed oil is sometimes called the vegetable alternative to fish oil. Walnuts and walnut oil, and Brazil nuts are other sources. The skin care benefits of omega-3 are it helps with proper wound healing, it is reported to relieve arthritis symptoms, it aids in healing eczema and cirrhosis, and it helps to balance the sebum or the oil production in the skin. A deficiency symptom of omega-3 is dry, scaly skin, eczema, inflammatory skin conditions, and slow healing.

"The main constituent in omega-6 is gamma linolenic acid or GLA for short. Good sources for this include evening primrose oil, borage oil, black currant seed oil, and blue-green algae. Skin care benefits are a smooth, healthy, moisturized skin and proper joint function and flexibility. Deficiency symptoms include dry and flaky skin, eczema, and painful stiff joints."

Herbal Formulas

HERBAL TEA Stephanie Tourles has formulated an herbal tea that is "a delicious way to boost your energy levels as well as your natural immunity. This tasty tea includes 2 tablespoons of lemon balm, 1 tablespoon of lavender flowers, 1 tablespoon of peppermint leaves, 1 tablespoon of chamomile flowers, 1 tablespoon of rose petals, 1 tablespoon of nettle, 1 tablespoon alfalfa, 1 tablespoon of rose hips, 2 teaspoons of dandelion leaves, 2 teaspoons of raspberry leaves, 1/2 teaspoon of ginger root (or you can substitute cinnamon bark). These last two ingredients are just to add a zingy flavor.

"Combine all of these herbs in a medium-sized bowl. Blend the ingredients and store this mixture in a tightly sealed tin, jar or plastic tub such as a Tupperware and store it away from light in a very cool, dry location. It is best if used within 6 months.

"I usually make three or four cups at a time so for each cup of tea you need 1 teaspoon of the dried herb. Bring a cup of water to boil in a small saucepan. Remove this from the heat and add 1 teaspoon of herbs. Cover this and allow it to steam for 10 or 15 minutes and strain before you drink it. You can add honey, lemon, cream, or maple syrup to enhance the flavor. This recipe yields approximately 30 cups of tea if you use 1 teaspoon of formula per cup."

SKIN OINTMENTS AND CLEANSERS Tourles describes an herbal ointment you can make yourself for soothing skin irritations, cuts and abrasions, and even for diaper rash. It has four simple ingredients: a half cup of vegetable shortening, preferably 100 percent hydrogenated soybean oil; 10 drops of colingela essential oil; 10 drops of everlasting or spike lavender essential oil; and 5 drops of orange or lemon essential oil.

"Start with the vegetable oil at room temperature and add all the essential oils all at once," Tourles says. "Whip all the ingredients together until thoroughly combined. It can be stored in a glass or plastic container with a tight lid and will keep, if refrigerated, for up to 1 year. To use, clean the infected area and apply the ointment and use as necessary to help heal and prevent infections. It is great for a nightly treatment for dry hands and feet and also as a cuticle treatment. It will have a beautiful orange color and it smells really nice, too."

Regular use of sunscreen is the most effective way to protect your skin from sunburn, aging effects, wrinkles, and cancer. Start with a sunscreen with an SPF or 15 or higher. SPF stands for sun protection factor. It means that you can stay out in the sun 15 times longer before burning that you can without sunscreen. Put it on your face, hands, and after your wash your hands. If you are older and beginning to see age spots, use an even higher SPF. Use it everyday all year round.

Psoralens are chemicals found in certain foods that make your skin more sensitive to the sun such that it burns more easily. Psoralens are found in foods like parsley, limes, and parsnips. Be sure to use a sunscreen with a high SPF if your diet includes a lot of psoralens.

Some perfumes cause age spots, especially those with musk or bergamot oil.

Small age spots can be bleached away with hydrogen peroxide. With a cotton swab use 30 percent hydrogen peroxide daily for several weeks. Another choice is hydroquinone, which interferes with your skin's production of melanin. It works very slowly but can fade age spots.

Tourles has another herbal formula for cleansing the skin. "I call it my Pure Cream Cleanser. This is great for all skin types except oily. It is a wonderful emollient, leaving skin soft and hydrated, and removes eye and lip makeup if you happen to wear those. It has only two ingredients: 1 tablespoon of heavy cream and 1 drop of carrot seed essential oil or rose essential oil. Rose oil can be very expensive. Mix the ingredients in a tiny bowl and apply the cream with a flannel cloth or a very soft washcloth in gentle circular motions over the entire face, neck, and chest. Rinse well, pat dry, and follow with your favorite herbal toner and moisturizer if you desire. There is so much fat in heavy cream that frequently you won't need an additional moisturizer unless it is the dead of winter and the air is very dry. This yields one or two treatments."

Cosmetic Laser Surgery

More and more people are lining up daily for cosmetic surgery. What are the pros and cons of the various procedures? Dr. Debra Sarnoff, a graduate of Cornell University and George Washington University's School of Medicine, is one of the premier laser surgery experts in North America, specializing in cosmetic dermatology and dermatological surgery.

Dr. Sarnoff sees lasers as a great new tool. "New methods and uses for laser surgery are emerging almost every month. Lasers can't do everything, but they have truly made a difference in cosmetic surgery, particularly in relation to what may seem minor problems, such as broken blood vessels on the face and around the nose, brown spots, age spots, liver spots, whatever you'd like to call them, on the tops of the hands or in the chest area." Lasers have proved helpful with problems such as removing tattoos. They are also useful for spider veins on the leg, acne scars, and wrinkles.

Lasers are essentially beams of light applied to the skin. Unlike a scalpel, which actually cuts the skin and causes some bleeding, a laser beam will pass through the skin without causing any bleeding. It has a particular target that it is trying to eradicate. There are certain problems that only lasers are capable of solving, just as there are certain problems only scalpel surgery can solve. For example, Dr. Sarnoff says, "There's no way that pulling and stretching and tightening the skin, through surgery, can change the quality of the skin. If your problem is that something is wrong with the quality of the skin, very often a laser can help that."

One cosmetic surgery procedure that can be done well with lasers is skin resurfacing. We all develop wrinkles as we get older. After smiling, laughing, and expressing ourselves with our faces for all these years, most of us develop lines around the eyes—crow's feet—as well as lines on the upper lip.

Dr. Sarnoff says that even the best face-lift in the world will not eradicate those lines. Something has to be done to resurface the skin. "In the old days, we used a machine called a dermabrader, which was like a little sanding machine that people used to try to peel off the top layers of the skin. In other cases, doctors used acid as a chemical peel. The theory was that when the skin healed, it would be much smoother and the wrinkles would not be as apparent.

Then, says Dr. Sarnoff, "Along came this generation of lasers. The laser can be used to peel off the top layers of skin as opposed to using a chemical or a dermabrading machine."

This procedure involves going to a reputable physician, preferably a dermatologist or plastic surgeon who is experienced in this technique, and having the top layers of skin removed in a controlled way with a laser. Healing will take at least 10 days, during which the recovering patient has to lie low. She will look like she had the worst sunburn ever. The skin will be red, moist, and chapped. She won't be able to put on makeup for at least 10 days.

The cost of resurfacing the entire face can be between $4,000 and $5,000. There may be some added costs for the operating room, as well as charges for anesthesia.

AGE SPOTS Many people have sunspots or age spots, what is called photodamage, from all those years of baking in the sun before we knew that ultraviolet rays are potentially harmful. Dr. Sarnoff explains, "A lot of that sun damage will be entirely reversible if the beam of light can be used to strip off those top layers of skin. That type of laser resurfacing is a fairly involved procedure that really takes a commitment and a healing time. It's not the kind of thing you just pop in to have as if you were going to the deli and do a little laser over your lunch break. That laser resurfacing is a bigger deal."

BROKEN BLOOD VESSELS, HAIR REMOVAL, TATTOO REMOVAL Dr. Sarnoff adds, "We are also using lasers now to help lighten stretch marks and to deal with birthmarks. The costs for these procedures are usually more in the hundreds of dollars. It depends on how large the discoloration or the tattoo is and how much time is required. For something like a tattoo, usually several visits are needed. They would be spaced about 6 to 8 weeks apart, and it would not be unusual to need up to eight treatments to clear a tattoo completely."

Procedures such as zapping broken blood vessels and removing little brown spots are simpler; the side effects are usually no more than a little bruising, crusting, or scabbing, something you might want to wear a small bandage over or apply a little antibiotic ointment to, but nothing that would keep you out of work or prevent you from functioning. Many times people have these procedures and go right back to work.

Lasers can also be an alternative to electrolysis for hair removal. The procedure can be done very rapidly, and the patient can immediately return to his or her activities.

KNOW WHAT TO ASK Dr. Sarnoff warns that a savvy consumer must ask the right questions. You must learn whether a procedure is a one-shot deal or will have to be repeated. And you should ask how long the improvement will last. Certainly you want something that is going to be cost-effective. Some laser treatments are really long-lasting. Laser removal for wrinkles has been around for about 5 years, and people who had the treatment when it was first introduced still look good. With hair removal, by contrast, very often the hair will grow back in a few months. Dr. Sarnoff stresses that you have to know that before you commit. "I think it is very important to ascertain ahead of time approximately how many treatments are needed and what you should expect."

KNOW THE RISKS There are risks, Dr. Sarnoff cautions. One is that you will pay good money and be disappointed because your underlying problem will still be there. "Something else that consumers have to be aware of is scarring. It's usually not the case that scars occur, and with a doctor who is well trained and experienced, I think that the technique is very safe. Nonetheless, it is a topic that definitely needs to be addressed before the procedure is done."

Sometimes there are some temporary changes in pigment. As the skin is healing, it can become a little darker or lighter than the surrounding skin. You must be aware how often this happens and know whether it is in fact only temporary or could be permanent.

There are very different types of lasers. Each beam of light accomplishes a different purpose, and the potential hazard from each is different. Still, there are some universal precautions that all competent laser providers follow. You need the correct eyewear, for example. Each laser is set at a very specific wavelength, and the protective eyewear needs to be specific to that wavelength.

Postoperative instructions make a difference, too. If you're removing tattoos or broken blood vessels, there is usually nothing else to do. However, with skin resurfacing, Dr. Sarnoff cautions that it is extremely important that patients follow the protocol afterward so that they do not get any kind of infection and heal properly.

LASERS AND RADIATION The number one fear people have about lasers is that they involve harmful radiation. But, as Dr. Sarnoff explains, the word "radiation" in the spelled-out version of laser actually refers to the verb "radiate," meaning "to give off light." Most of the beams of light used in lasers are in the visible light range. That is, they are part of normal light. The only unique thing about lasers is that they are monochromatic. You might have a red beam or a yellow or green one, as opposed to natural light, which is a blend of all the colors of the rainbow. Laser light is non-ionizing; it's basically safe, as opposed to x-rays or ultraviolet light from the sun, which are ionizing. Ionizing radiation may change our cells and damage our chromosomes. We can get in real trouble with that type of radiation; but most lasers are not in that part of the electromagnetic spectrum.

FINDING THE RIGHT PERSON TO DO THE PROCEDURE Another fear that people express to Dr. Sarnoff involves whether the specialist they are seeing is qualified. Physicians don't need any board certification to perform laser surgery and, in fact, one doesn't even have to have a medical degree to use lasers. Lasers are relatively new; many have been around only about 15 years. There are many wonderful doctors who trained at reputable universities and passed their boards in their respective fields, but the advent of lasers came after they graduated. Not every doctor has kept up with the technology and really understands it. A doctor might be board-certified in one particular field but know relatively little about laser techniques, but could get a laser this afternoon and start to do any of the procedures. Consumers have the right to know about the doctor's actual experience in laser surgery.

In Dr. Sarnoff's opinion, if you are considering cosmetic laser surgery, "The best thing to do is to ask around in your community. Start by asking your regular doctor, your neighbors, your friends, and anyone you know who might have had a laser procedure done similar to the type you are interested in. You can also call groups for a recommendation, such as the American Academy of Dermatology, the American Society of Plastic and Reconstructive Surgeons, or the American Society of Laser Medicine and Surgery."

She suggests that you make more than one consulting appointment. You want to meet the doctor and ask how many procedures like yours he or she has performed. Ask if you can see photos of the doctor's work. This may not be necessary for some of the minor procedures, but if you are thinking about resurfacing your face, it is very important to know that the doctor is experienced and is going to do it correctly.

70

Hair Care

A beautician who has treated hundreds of people's hair is asked whether she sees any connection between a person's diet and lifestyle on the one hand, and hair health on the other. She says, "Definitely, I see that when people eat well the hair is healthy looking. It's a reflection of what they eat and the habits they have. Everything is shown in the hair."

Another hairstylist adds, "Your hair is fed by the bloodstream so if there are any difficulties in that area it will be carried through into the hair and the skin. You could be losing your hair, it could be brittle or dull. Nutrition has an effect on everything in your body and so your hair is an appendage of what is going on. It is a reflection of who you are."

Nutritional Approaches to Better Hair Health

Dr. Danise Lehrer, a licensed acupuncturist and a doctor of homeopathy, confirms these common sense statements. She notes that in traditional Chinese medicine, hair health is viewed as a sign of the health of the kidneys, liver, and blood.

One clinical nutritionist tells us that for hair and overall body health, we should consume six freshly prepared green juices a day with organically grown vegetables. Increased circulation to the scalp is important so exercise should be part of any program. I recommend the following four stage program to provide increased vitality to your hair and scalp.

STAGE 1 DAILY PROTOCOL FOR THE FIRST THREE MONTHS

B complex (50 mg)
B$_{12}$ (100 mcg)
garlic (500 mg twice)
aloe (1 oz three times)
protein (9/10th g per kg of body weight)
6 glasses of dark green vegetable juice or 6 scoops of chlorophyll rich powder

STAGE 2 DAILY PROTOCOL FOR THE SECOND THREE MONTHS

sea vegetables (one serving)
flaxseed oil (1 tablespoon)
evening primrose oil (500 mg)
choline and inositol (500 mg twice)
PABA (100 mg)
folic acid (400 mcg)
biotin (500 mcg)

STAGE 3 DAILY PROTOCOL FOR THE THIRD THREE MONTHS

sea vegetables (1 serving)
zinc (50 mg)
L-cysteine (500 mg twice)
evening primrose oil (300 mg twice)
pantothenic acid (100 mg twice)
vitamin E (400 IU)
coenzyme Q10 (100 mg twice)
biotin (500 mcg)
choline and inositol (500 mcg)
B complex (50 mg of each)
B$_{12}$ (100 mcg)
silica (150 mg)
PABA (250 mg)
folic acid (800 mcg)
6 glasses of dark green vegetable juice, or 3 glasses dark green vegetable juice and 3 glasses of green plant extract, or 6 scoops of chlorophyll rich powder

STAGE 4 DAILY PROTOCOL FOR THE FOURTH THREE MONTHS

PABA (500 mg)
pantothenic acid (500 mg)
garlic (1,000 mg)
onion (1,000 mg)
sea vegetables (6 oz.)
biotin (500 mcg)
choline (1,000 mg)

inositol (1,000 mg)
niacin (250 mg)
borage oil (500 mg)
omega-3 oil (1,000 mg)
cayenne (5 mg)
protein (9/10th g per kg of body weight)
6 glasses of dark green vegetable juice, or 3 glasses dark green vegetable juice and
3 of green plant extract, or 6 scoops of chlorophyll rich powder

71

Natural Pet Care

We love our pets. They give us so much joy and happiness and unconditional love. Pet therapy, also known as Animal-Assisted Therapy, has become a well-known therapy for the emotionally disturbed, for children, in nursing homes, and in hospitals for cancer patients. How can we learn to treat our animals with as much respect as we treat each other? They certainly deserve it.

One alternative medicine group you should know about if you have a pet and want to provide it with holistic medicine is the American Holistic Veterinary Medical Association located in Bel Air, Maryland (410-569-0795).

Nutrition

Pat McKay, author of two books on this topic, has been studying nutrition and holistic health for animals for more than 30 years. She calls attention to the contents of commercial pet food. Produced in rendering plants, most people are probably not aware that road kill is put into the food.

"The average person doesn't have any idea what condition these animals are in. They can have anything from cancer, full of drugs, full of all types of bacteria, fungus. It's just unconscionable that we would put that type of food into a can or bag and call it any kind of food for animals. The food itself is not fit for any kind of consumption. When it says on the label 'For veterinary use only' they mean that people are not supposed to eat what is in the can. Why on earth would you feed it to your dog or cat?

"My suggestion is that you feed your pets 75 percent raw meat, 25 percent raw vegetables with a good organic calcium supplement. If you do you are going to have a very healthy dog or cat. I recommend that you feed the same proportions to dogs and cats. When they are in the wild they eat the same thing. They eat mice and lizards and small birds and rabbits. They are all eating the same things, so why we feel we have to have a dog food and a cat food is strictly commercial greed.

"To break down the food percentages even more: The meat should be 40 percent muscle meat and 20 percent organ meat; then 15 percent fat and 25 percent vegetable. But none of this is written in stone. You don't have to feed exactly those proportions every single day any more than you feed yourself and your children the exact amount of protein and carbohydrates every day."

Bach Flower Remedies

Rachelle Hasnas is a consultant and teacher of Bach Flower remedies and the author of *The Pocket Guide to Bach Flower Remedies*. She is very familiar with Dr. Bach's treatment principles and has used them with animals with amazing results.

Dr. Edward Bach was a British physician and medical researcher. As Rachelle Hasnas explains, "It was Dr. Bach's understanding that to truly cure a disease the treatment of symptoms was not adequate. For Dr. Bach the true cause of disease was located in the personality where emotional and mental disharmony are precursors of any illness. His new system of healing with flower remedies addressed all aspects of our being, body, mind and spirit. I would like to look at using Bach flower essences with animals. There have been some amazing results with animals and it seems they carry a lot less baggage than we humans do.

"The following examples are of the many stressful states that animals face. They can give you an understanding in selecting appropriate essences that treat these states in animals. All of us who have pets already know that pets certainly do have emotions. By being empathetic to their moods and emotional distress we can get a pretty good feeling as to what they may be suffering.

➤ "*Agrimony* assists with the torment many animals face when a wound or injury is slow to heal.

➤ "*Aspen* is great to help a very nervous and easily frightened animal.

➤ "*Century* aids the runt of the litter that always seems to be pushed by its bigger littermates.

➤ "*Cherry plum* is for the very aggressive animal that may threaten to bite and seems uncontrollable.

➤ "*Chestnut bud* is excellent in training a pet and it prevents the same mistakes being made.

➤ "*Chicory* assists with animals that demand a lot of attention and also those that are too possessive of their owners.

➤ "*Holly* assists with animals that seem jealous, lack trust and is also good for nasty temperaments.

➤ "*Large* is extremely effective for the animal that seems to lack self-esteem and is low in the pecking order.

➤ "*Mimulus* helps with fear as with thunderstorms and also for the timid and shy animal.

➤ "*Olive* is helpful after operations or an illness.

➤ "*Rockrose* treats panic and terror.

➤ "*Star of Bethlehem* is for any trauma, shock or grief an animal may experience and especially helpful with animals that have been victims of abuse.

➤ "*Vervain* and *impatiens* are both effective for the high strung and wired animal.

➤ "*Vine* is indicated for an animal that won't accept authority and is also the boss animal that dominates other animals.

➤ "*Walnut* is always indicated for any change taking place in the animal's life such as a move, new owner, new pet introduced to the home as well as a new child.

➤ "*Water violet* is indicated for the aloof animal that tends to be a loner as typified by the feline species.

➤ "*Wild rose* is effective for animals that appear listless.

➤ "*Willow* is excellent for feelings of resentment that crop up with a new pet in the home or the birth of a child.

➤ "*Rescue Remedy*. For all emergency crisis situations, Rescue Remedy is remarkable. When in doubt as to which individual essence to select, Rescue is always helpful."

Hasnas says that the dosage and frequency is the same for animals as it is for humans. She says, "Make a dilution bottle for your pet or place the concentrate directly in their food or water. The essences given by mouth directly from the concentrate have a high alcohol content and many pets will refuse the concentrate as they find the alcohol distasteful."

PART FOURTEEN
Selecting an Alternative Health Practitioner

U ltimately, you are responsible for your own well-being, Having access to
proper health care practitioners is an important element in health maintenance. Their educated guidance and treatment can be invaluable in times
of uncertainty and crisis, and for prevention and awareness-building.

Selecting the right health care professional can be an important decision
that will benefit you for the rest of your life. In the first chapter of this final section of the book, we provide an overview on how to go about finding and evaluating such a person. In the following chapter, you will find a comprehensive
Resource Guide listing the professional associations of many alternative medicine specialties, as well as the names and telephone numbers of hundreds of
practitioners organized by state. Many of those listed are the very same experts
who provided much of the information for this book.

72

General Guidelines

Alternative health practitioners can help define the weak links in your body's structure and function and then direct you toward optimal personal care. There are many different approaches, but some general guidelines are worth mentioning here.

Your Rights As a Patient

A good alternative medical practitioner will perform at least these three basic types of analysis before prescribing any treatment plan:

(1) take a detailed medical history; (2) perform a physical examination that goes beyond conventional methodologies; and (3) study carefully the results of appropriate laboratory tests taken at the time of the history taking and the physical examination.

In addition, you have the right to expect that the practitioner includes in his or her repertory, some or all of the following:

➤as many noninvasive diagnostic techniques as possible;

➤an awareness of the potential diagnostic value of even very minor signs and symptoms in the prevention of major dysfunction;

➤a preference for noninvasive over invasive techniques (for example, substances will be administered orally rather than intravenously, except when a condition calls for the more direct route);

➤a recognition of the importance of strengthening the body's resistive capacities and an interest, wherever possible, in attempting to repair any malfunctioning organ or gland;

➤a tendency, whenever possible, to treat the primary weak link first if more than one has been discovered (for example, if the stomach is producing insufficient hydrochloric acid, resulting in the malabsorption of calcium, among other substances, the resulting calcium deficiency could lead to osteoarthritis, periodontal disease, or skin problems; by treating the hydrochloric acid insufficiency, the physician would be treating the primary weak link);

➤an approach that treats the person as a whole person, not just a collection of ailing parts;the demonstrated ability to listen carefully and to skillfully classify any relevant symptoms to arrive at the best possible diagnosis;

➤an orientation toward optimal health and sensitivity to dysfunctions that signal an imbalance in the individual;

➤familiarity with a combination of approaches to help the person regain balance (for example, in addition to orthodox treatments, the physician's recommendations may include advice about stress reduction and lifestyle changes to reduce or eliminate causative factors in the environment);

➤a willingness to refer the individual, when the condition warrants, to other medical practitioners whose specialized knowledge in a given area may be necessary to provide the most valuable restorative program; and

➤a demonstrated awareness of the importance of the individual's own attitudes toward health and disease, and a willingness to communicate openly with the individual.

Your Role As a Patient

The alternative health practitioner should expect you to be an active, committed participant in the process, not a passive, disinterested patient who accepts everything the doctor recommends.

One form of this active participation may be the questions you ask with a view to getting the important information you need to help in your contributions to the healing process. Some examples are:

What, specifically, is being treated?

How do you know that that's the problem?

What are some realistic goals in my situation?

What is the time frame?

Does every individual with this condition get exactly the same tests and treatments?

What are my weak links?

Are these tests and this treatment relevant to my body and my condition?

The Importance of Commonplace Symptoms

Many people are living with symptoms that, because they are mild and do not constitute a full-blown disease state, are accepted, needlessly, as being an inevitable consequence of getting older. In fact, such people are often told by their conventional physicians: "Nothing is wrong with you. Everything is normal." And yet, the symptoms may be early warnings that something is out of balance. Gas in the lower bowel (flatulence), belching, heaviness in the stomach, heartburn, and bloating, for example, may all be indicators of a malfunctioning digestive system, depending on their frequency and severity. These conditions are not normal in a healthy state, and they often are correctable.

Similarly, many of the symptoms that accompany delayed allergic reactions (the masked, cyclical allergies) are widely accepted as normal, and therefore to be tolerated for no better reason than "that's the way it is." The failure to recognize a connection between these symptoms and allergies may be due to the fact that they do not appear for upwards of 30 hours after the ingestion of the offending food or chemical substance. Typical symptoms are headache, irritability, anxiety, sudden changes of mood, and excessive fatigue, as well as unexplained body aches and pains. These symptoms may not be severe enough to be labeled as disease states, so the underlying cause is repeatedly overlooked or denied by traditional practitioners. Even when the disorders are recognized, their true significance may still be missed by those who try to reverse the symptoms without addressing the underlying causes for their appearance.

Thus frequent colds, recurring infections, and fatigue are all part of the warning mechanisms used by the body to signal a malfunctioning immune system. But they are rarely recognized as such. The phenomenal sales of cold remedies, for example, reflect how little attention is paid to strengthening the immune system—an approach that would far more effectively reduce the incidence of these disorders.

Types of Therapies

It has never been my policy to make specific recommendations, to suggest to a person that a specific practitioner is the best doctor to see. The quality of a doctor's health care may depend on both the physician and the patient, as well as on their mutual compatibility. This is not something I, or anyone else, can predict in advance. But I still feel that people should be given some direction. So, what I have done here is supplied a directional guide. It is not meant to be a recommendation. Rather, I have offered some general guidelines.

ACUPRESSURE Acupressure, also known as shiatsu, is based on the principle that a vital energy, called *qi (chi)*, flows through the body. The primary cause of pain is an imbalance in this energy. The goal of the healer is to balance the client's energy so pain and discomfort do not manifest or, if they do appear, will be relieved.

The practitioner concentrates on certain pressure points that have metaphoric names that tell us something of what they do or how they are to be worked with. He or she uses thumbs, fingers, palms, forearms, elbows, and even knees to apply pressure to specified points in the body to modulate the flow of energy. During a treatment, the client lies on the floor on a comfortable padded surface, such as a futon, fully clothed or undressed to his or her level of comfort. What the client feels is pressure, which can be gentle or deeper at the places where the practitioner is working. As the pressure continues, the patient will generally feel relaxed and energized at the same time.

Acupressure is good for treating a variety of different pains. It is especially beneficial in combating chronic pain in the back, neck, or shoulders, but it has also proved effective in treating whiplash, herniated disk, and nervous problems, such as Bell's palsy.

ACUPUNCTURE Acupuncture sees pain as derived from blocked energy or *qi (chi)*. In treating this blockage, the practitioner has to determine whether it stems from an overabundance or deficiency in energy, so the treatment can be adjusted depending on whether it is necessary to strengthen or decrease *qi*. To accomplish this the acupuncturist will work to open blocked energy pathways, so healing energy can go directly to the point in the body where it is needed, thereby stimulating the body's natural healing capacities.

The acupuncturist first records the patient's medical history in the manner of a conventional doctor. Then, with the patient lying down or seated, depending on the area to be treated, fine-gauge, stainless steel needles are inserted into significant points and meridians (channels through which *qi* flows) to exert different physiological effects on the body and induce both relaxation and energization. The patient will remain in this position from 20 to 30 minutes, though an appointment with an acupuncturist may last up to an hour, since part of the time will be spent consulting about the employment of other traditional and herbal treatments that might be recommended. Bodywork and massage might also be included in the session.

According to Abigail Rist-Podrecca, a registered nurse, acupuncture works by "dilating the blood vessels, so that the vessels can open. You get more circulation, more of the nutrients, more oxygen flowing through the meridians."

Practitioners attend 3- to 4-year postgraduate-type programs. Schools are accredited for Master's degree programs through the National Accreditation Commission of Schools and Colleges of Acupuncture and Oriental Medicine. A certification examination is offered through the National Certification Commission for Acupuncture and Oriental Medicine. A minimum of 1,300 hours of training is required to sit for this exam. Medical doctors and dentists rarely require specialized training to perform acupuncture, although training is available through the American Academy of Medical Acupuncturists. (See the Resource Guide in the next chapter for information on how to contact these organizations.)

ALEXANDER TECHNIQUE Alexander technique is based on the concept that all of us know how to move comfortably as children but lose that natural flexibility over time. The teacher acts to help the student recapture this freedom and lightness of movement. Practitioners see themselves as teachers, and their sessions not as therapy but as teaching.

Each session is an experiential process in which the teacher guides the student with hands-on training to help her learn a new way of moving, by means of the teacher's hands stimulating the student's nervous system.

This technique can help mothers, for example, learn how to bend over and lift children in a new way that avoids stress on the back.

There are 10 affiliated societies for teachers of Alexander technique worldwide. Teacher certification requires 1,600 practical hours over a 3-year period.

ANTI-AGING MEDICINE Research over the last decade has given us a better understanding of the causes of aging. In particular, several theories have led to new therapies offering older people opportunities not only to improve their health but also to actually slow down the aging process.

Practitioners of anti-aging medicine challenge the view that aging inevitably means gaining weight, having high blood pressure, and succumbing to a variety of "age-related" diseases. They believe that aging well means being healthy and balanced from within. They start with a full spectrum of diagnostic tests, and then individualize treatments on the basis of a patient's specific profile, including hormone balance, vitamin and mineral levels, blood chemistry, cardiac and exercise capacities, memory capacity, and more. Many physicians, psychologists, and other health care professionals practice anti-aging medicine.

APPLIED KINESIOLOGY This discipline is related to Chinese acupuncture. Practitioners use it to determine which foods and herbs are best assimilated by the individual, in order to develop a healing diet and supplementation program that is finely calibrated to the person's own biology.

The patient extends her arm at shoulder level while holding a food or supplement in the other hand, and the practitioner pushes down on the extended arm. If the substance is appropriate for her, the arm will be strong and harder to force down. If the substance is not good for her, the arm will be weak. This is because the body can feel the value of the substance. Using various techniques, kinesiologists can study these reactions more precisely to determine proper individual diet.

AROMATHERAPY Aromatherapy depends on the therapeutic powers of essential oils. These oils are commonly used in skin and body care products in the United States, but their medicinal properties have long been accepted in other countries, particularly France, where, in many instances, their antimicrobial properties make them acceptable replacements for drug therapy. Pure essential oils can be used to cure cold and canker sores, calm the emotions, diminish joint swelling, clear the nasal passages and lungs, balance hormones, and for many other applications.

AYURVEDA Ayurveda means "the science of life." It is a system of medicine widely used in India for the past 4,000 years. Ayurveda believes that balance is the key to perfect health. It basically determines which of three body/mind types a person belongs to and, based on that type, helps people choose the type of foods they should eat and the type of exercise best for them. For more information, read *Perfect Health* and *Ageless Body, Timeless Mind* by Deepak Chopra.

BACH FLOWER REMEDIES The Bach flower remedies were developed by Dr. Edward Bach during the 1930s. They consist of 38 plant extracts that are used to treat physical and emotional problems. The extracts used in each case are selected according to the individual patient's personality. For instance, for a person who cannot say no, the suggested remedy derives from the beech tree. For some with an unhealthy fear of the unknown, a remedy derived from the aspen would be prescribed. Bach flower remedies are said to have positive effects on the psychological and emotional stresses that underlie many illnesses.

BIOFEEDBACK Biofeedback is a technique that teaches a person to consciously regulate normally involuntary bodily processes, such as heartbeats, brain waves, blood pressure, and muscle tension. The bodily process, such as heart rate, may be monitored by electronic equipment or by natural observation, such as holding a finger against an artery. With practice, the patient learns to slow down the heart rate, relax tension, and so on. Biofeedback is helpful for conditions such as migraines, tension headaches, digestive upsets, and any other disorders that are aggravated by stress.

Practitioner certification is recommended but not required. Practitioners are certified through the Biofeedback Certification Institute of America.

BODY ROLLING Body Rolling, a form of bodywork developed by Yamuna Zake, uses a 6- to 10-inch ball in a series of routines designed to elongate muscles and increase blood flow in all parts of the body. As the body weight presses into the ball, the ball applies pressure onto bone and creates traction that allows the entire length of a muscle to release. Body Rolling is useful to relieve pain and tension in many parts of the body.

CHELATION THERAPY Chelation therapy flushes toxins out of the blood. A synthetic amino acid, EDTA, is administered to the patient through an intravenous drip. The EDTA moves through the blood vessels and attaches itself to heavy metals in the blood such as mercury and lead, holding onto these substances until they are washed out of the body in the urine. Chelation therapy is being used increasingly to treat heart disease as well as other illnesses.

Protocols for the intravenous administration of EDTA are set by the American College for the Advancement of Medicine (ACAM) and require a prior medical examination

CHIROPRACTIC Chiropractic treatment involves the manual manipulation of vertebrae that have become misaligned, exerting pressure on nerves and blocking the flow of energy to various organs. The manipulation is called an adjustment. It involves the chiropractor's gentle and painless application of direct pressure to the spine and joints. The chiropractor may squeeze or twist the torso, pull or twist the limbs, or wrench the head or back. In this manner she or he is readjusting the spinal column to restore the normal relationship of one vertebra to another. This eliminates the body's energy blocks.

Chiropractic is effective in dealing with pain and as a preventive measure because it relieves nerve pressure as the spine is properly adjusted.

Despite the success that chiropractic has had in relieving pain and chronic disorders, for more than a quarter of a century the medical establishment has bullied this licensed profession into having to defend itself as if it were a subversive activity. The main reason for this attack appears to have been the desire to ensure the traditional medical doctor the top spot on the ladder of licensed healing professionals.

While chiropractic is still far from being accepted as a part of standard health care, it attracts more patients now than ever before and is more accepted than ever before by the mainstream medical community. There are now about 20 chiropractic colleges nationwide and chiropractors can get licensed in all 50 states. Some liberal arts colleges offer undergraduate degrees in chiropractic, and additionally, some facilities at member hospitals of the American Hospital Association have been opened to chiropractors. Now that chiropractic care finally seems to be on the verge of much broader acceptance than it has ever enjoyed in the United States, it is appropriate to consider more carefully how it can help in the treatment and prevention of various human ailments.

COLON THERAPY Colon cleansing refers to washing out the colon in order to remove toxic buildups. First the colon is irrigated with warm water, washing out encrustations and old fecal matter. Next, healing substances to reduce inflammation and strengthen the colon wall are infused.

CRANIOSACRAL THERAPY The sacral region is that at the bottom of the spine. Between that region and the head there should be maintained a balanced relation for the health of the organism. If a restriction is experienced at that point, pain will be felt and other problems may arise.

In craniosacral therapy, the practitioner places her or his hands on the patient's body in such a way as to bring the cranium and sacrum back into alignment and to reestablish a natural rhythm between them. Treatment usually centers on the head or lower back, although it may be done on many different parts of the body.

DENTISTRY, HOLISTIC Holistic dentistry, also known as biological dentistry and environmental dentistry, is a relatively new field that strongly emphasizes the symbiotic relationship between dental health and overall health. Body chemistry analysis and nutritional guidance are important components. Holistic dentists avoid materials and procedures they believe are toxic to the body. For example, they use porcelain, gold, or composite (plastic) restorations instead of mercury-based silver fillings. They use x-rays sparingly, not routinely. They avoid the use of fluoride. Among the broad-based treatment methods they favor are nutrition, homeopathy, and acupuncture.

There is no specific training program for holistic dentistry. Many dentists who adhere to the practice are members of a holistic dental organization (see the Resource Guide in the next chapter).

ENVIRONMENTAL MEDICINE Environmental medicine specialists, also known as clinical ecologists, see a strong association between overall health and exposure to allergens in the diet and environment. Over the past several decades they have found that thousands of substances in our food, water, and surroundings may be responsible for illnesses ranging from headaches and fatigue, to depression, digestive disorders, arthritis, and epilepsy. Environmental medicine differs from conventional medicine in that it does not simply try to identify and then suppress a symptom. Rather, it uses that symptom as a clue to determining the underlying causes of a problem.

The American Academy of Environmental Medicine is an organization of physicians who practice in this field.

ENZYME THERAPY Enzyme therapy uses enzymes to cure illness and enhance life. South American Indians used papaya as a healing agent, and medieval Europeans used the milky juice of plants of the spurge family for medical reasons. Today, many practitioners advocate enzyme supplementation to enable vitamins and other supplements, as well as food, to be properly absorbed.

There are many different types of enzyme therapy. One example is that which relies on the Wolfe and Benitez formulas, which combine animal and vegetable enzymes. The preparations are said to be powerful weapons against bacteria and other invasive microorganisms.

FELDENKRAIS Feldenkrais is a practice that helps eliminate poor movement habits and relieve chronic tensions. It uses very gentle movements that the student does herself, guided by the instructor, while lying on the floor. Alternatively the student lies on a massage table and the teacher uses a hands-on approach, taking the student through gentle movements to enable the student to let go of a chronic holding pattern.

The goal is to learn to differentiate between parts of the body that are relaxed and parts that are still tense. Thus the nervous system learns a new way of functioning.

GUIDED IMAGERY Guided imagery can be practiced either by an individual with a therapist or in a group setting. In the individual setting, the practitioner helps the client elicit her own mental images, which she then interacts with, perhaps in dialogue. For example, if the client is ill, she may call up images of the distressed part of her body and encourage it to heal through an imagistic interaction.

In a group, a facilitator helps the participants concentrate on building certain images whose healing power they can tap into. In this setting, the participant has the added benefit of being able to discuss the process with another participant afterward so as to further affirm and enrich the healing process.

HELLERWORK Hellerwork is a bodywork technique derived from Rolfing (see below). Both modalities work to improve body structure with deep tissue work, but Hellerwork, unlike Rolfing, is not painful. The practice has three components. In the first, hands-on part, the practitioner finds a misalignment in the body and works with the client to release it.

The second part is movement education. The practitioner analyzes the patient's posture and movements, then offers more relaxed and stressless ways to move. The third component is mind/body dialogue, whose purpose is to identify emotional patterns that underlie dysfunctional movement patterns.

HERBAL MEDICINE American interest in herbs has exploded in recent times. But herbal medicine is far from a new field, having been used worldwide for thousands of years. Herbs are plants or parts of plants, including leaves, flowers, stems, roots, and seeds. They contain active substances that have been found to enhance the immune system, detoxify the body, and fight insomnia, cancer, HIV, heart disease, and a host of other conditions. Herbs may be incorporated into foods or teas, taken in capsule or tincture form, or used as ointments on the skin. A number of different systems use medicinal herbs, including Western medicine, Traditional Chinese medicine, and Ayurvedic medicine.

There are no specific certification or licensing requirements for the practice of herbal medicine. Licensed naturopaths and acupuncturists are trained in using herbs, as are Ayurvedic doctors. The American Herbalists Guild is a membership organization of clinical herbalists.

HOLISTIC MEDICINE Holistic medicine is based on the belief that a person's health is affected by a wide range of factors, including genetics, diet and nutrition, physical activity, living conditions, and emotional well-being. Practitioners help patients establish healthy habits and take greater responsibility for achieving and maintaining their own good health. They use drugs and surgery when necessary, but place greater emphasis on disease prevention and treatment with less invasive modalities such as acupuncture, herbs, meditation, and relaxation.

Many physicians, psychologists, and other health care professionals practice holistic medicine.

HOMEOPATHY Homeopathy is based on the law of similars, the principle that what causes illness can also cure it. If a person has a head cold, you would give the person a substance that would cause cold symptoms in a healthy person, but in a sick person it helps to cure them. Homeopathy is limited in scope at this time in the United States, although 100 years ago it was the prevailing form of medicine—until allopathic medicine and the American Medical Association in particular launched an intensive drive against it, which culminated in its being virtually banned in this country.

Recently, there has been a renewed interest in homeopathy, and growing numbers of physicians are using its principles. Homeopathy is particularly effective in the treatment of fevers, bacterial infections, toxicity, and the cumulative effects of alcohol, drugs, tobacco, caffeine, or sugar. It is not recommended for cancer, AIDS, or heart disease.

HYDROTHERAPY In hydrotherapy, water is used to treat injury and disease. The water may be hot or cold, and applied either externally or internally. Among the many forms of hydrotherapy are herb and mineral baths, ice packs, rubs, compresses, steams, enemas, and colonic irrigations. Many physical therapists, naturopaths, and other alternative medicine practitioners believe that hydrotherapy has an important role to play in helping to treat aches, pains, colds and flus, as well as more serious conditions such as cancer, digestive disorders, and AIDS. Hydrotherapy may be performed in a clinical setting or at home.

HYPNOTHERAPY Hypnotherapy is the use of hypnosis—a temporary condition of altered attention—to enhance a person's physical and psychological health. Hypnotherapy can help to alleviate pain, control eating disorders, and stop addictions such as smoking, drinking, and drug abuse. It can be used in the treatment of psychological conditions such as anxiety, depression, phobias, and stress, as well as behavioral, learning, and sleep disorders. Hypnotherapy also can aid in the treatment of chronic illnesses such as arthritis, cancer, and multiple sclerosis.

Mental health professionals who may use hypnotherapy include psychiatrists, psychologists, and clinical social workers. The International Medical and Dental Hypnotherapy Association trains and certifies medical doctors, dentists, and hypnotherapists in the therapeutic use of hynposis. The National Guild of Hypnotists is another certifying body.

MAGNETIC FIELD THERAPY Magnets confer a wide range of health benefits because we are magnetic beings who derive energy from the earth's magnetic field. The earth has lost a good deal of its magnetism, which leaves the body in an unbalanced state and therefore vulnerable to disease. Magnets can help restore internal harmony. Susan Bucci, a holistically trained nurse, describes this therapy. "Magnets oxygenate tissues and allow cell walls to absorb more oxygen. They promote mental acuity and normalize pH balance by increasing alkalinity. Restorative sleep is enhanced. Therapeutically, they stop pain, fight infection, and reduce inflammation and fluid retention. Over time, fatty and calcium deposits dissolve and the circulatory system opens up."

MASSAGE THERAPY Massage therapy is used to treat a variety of ailments, including muscle spasm and pain, soreness, swelling and inflammation, temporo-mandibular joint syndrome, whiplash, headaches, and stress. It helps to release tension and enhance relaxation. It can help in detoxification. Some states require massage therapists to be licensed, others do not.

MEDITATION Meditation is a means of contemplation and reflection. It is commonly used to reduce stress and anxiety, and enhance a feeling of well-being. Other uses include alleviating pain, boosting immunity, battling alcohol and drug addictions, and managing high blood pressure and heart disease.

MIND-BODY MEDICINE Mind-body medicine seeks to balance the physical, mental, emotional, and spiritual aspects of a person's life. Practitioners believe that thoughts and emotions are vitally connected to overall health. They also contend that patients must be empowered to take greater control over the healing process. Among the therapies used by mind-body medicine are relaxation training, meditation, hypnosis, biofeedback, psychotherapy, guided imagery, and prayer. These therapies can be used in the home or in a variety of clinical or group settings.

MOVEMENT THERAPY Movement therapy is a form of psychotherapy that uses both creative and everyday movement to address a person's social, emotional, cognitive, and/or physical problems. Practitioners are trained in movement and psychology. They complete a master's degree in an approved program or an equivalent course of study approved by the American Dance Therapy Association (ADTA).

MYOTHERAPY Myotherapy is a physical treatment approach that involves applying pressure to localized trigger points to alleviate symptoms associated with muscle/joint pain and dysfunction. Trigger points are areas of circulatory, muscle and/or nerve abnormality. Myotherapy can help to restore the function of joints and muscles, improve range of range of movement, and reduce pain, spasm, and swelling.

NATURAL HYGIENE Natural hygiene is the practice of creating optimal conditions for the body and its constituent cells, tissues, and organs to pursue and sustain health. This means environmental purity of air, food, and water; a balanced primordial diet based on natural foods; and stress reduction and management. It precludes the use of most drugs, since they are antithetical to a modality that perceives illness to be due to inappropriate nutrition and toxic accumulations (drugs are usually toxic substances). Finally, it means a symbiotic relationship of all humankind and harmony with God and nature.

NATUROPATHY Naturopathic physicians can treat most conditions. They are not, however, allowed to perform major surgery (although they can perform minor surgery). Their very extensive background is centered in the botanical sciences, including the use of herbs and tinctures with a wide variety of natural immune-stimulating properties. Becoming a doctor of naturopathic medicine requires 4 years of graduate-level study in the medical sciences. The accrediting agency is the Council on Naturopathic Medical Education (CNME).

   The naturopath practices a natural form of health care whose traditions precede the advent of modern medicine. In this the naturopath resembles the traditional Tibetan physician, who must be able to identify nearly 1,000 different healing herbs, mineral sources, and animal sources. The naturopath has years of extensive study in the healing potential of such substances. He or she is also able to understand muscular and skeletal bodily adjustment. Naturopaths use a much broader basis for diagnosis than do conventional allopathic physicians.

NEURAL THERAPY In neural therapy, anesthetics are injected into nerves and other body tissues to restore the body's flow of energy and thereby relieve pain and illness. Many conditions respond well to neural therapy, including chronic pain, allergies, kidney disease, and prostate disorders. The American Academy of Neural Therapy provides information and referrals.

NURSE-MIDWIFERY Nurse-midwives provide obstetric and gynecologic care in birthing centers, hospitals, medical offices, and patients' homes. They view childbirth as a natural, normal process. Their focus is on helping families to have safe, satisfying birth experiences with as little medical intervention as possible. Most nurse-midwives only accept patients who are not considered high risk, i.e., those women who will probably have a normal delivery.

   Nurse-midwives are registered nurses who have been certified by the American College of NurseMidwives. In some states nurse-midwives must have a special license, while in others only a nursing license is required.

   In contrast to nurse-midwives, lay midwives have no formal training. Most lay midwives work in rural areas that do not have a lot of doctors. A few states license lay midwives.

NUTRITIONAL THERAPY Diet is vitally important to overall health. Certain vitamins and minerals are needed for energy, healing, and growth. Nutritional therapists address a range of conditions, including arthritis, asthma, fatigue, osteoporosis, heart disease, and psychological problems. They evaluate a person's diet and lifestyle, looking specifically at nutritional deficiencies, food allergies, and toxic exposures. Then they develop an individual program incorporating dietary changes, supplementation, and exercise.

ORTHOMOLECULAR MEDICINE Orthomolecular medicine is an alternative approach to mental and physical health whose goal is to identify and treat the root cause of disease. The objective is to balance and rebuild the whole body, not merely to mask or suppress symptoms. To do this, orthomolecular physicians try to establish an equilibrium among the essential nutrients that may be lacking, present in excess, or are being poorly absorbed. Orthomolecular physicians are conventionally trained medical doctors who feel that such an imbalance is often responsible for psychiatric as well as physical disorders.

The physician looks at diet, glandular function, glucose metabolism, and a host of other biochemical factors that may play a role in the patient's mental health. Imbalances in the body are corrected through judicious use of vitamins, minerals, amino acids, and other naturally occurring nutrients. Orthomolecular physicians frequently use a very high-dose vitamin regimen.

OSTEOPATHY Osteopaths are holistic doctors who combine conventional medicine with muscle and joint manipulation/realignment. They believe that good health requires restoring and maintaining the structural balance of the body. Also important are diet, lifestyle, and psychological well-being.

Doctors of osteopathy (D.O.s) can provide the same services that M.D.s can, including surgery and hospital admissions. D.O.s receive training similar to that of M.D.s. They are licensed throughout the United States as full physicians.

POLARITY THERAPY Polarity therapy is based on the belief that any stagnation or stopping of the natural flow of energy in the human body is the underlying cause of disease. The naturally occurring positive and negative energy fields of the body are in a polarity relationship with each other. However, when the energy is blocked, it turns neutral, and the surrounding tissues stagnate and become painful.

Practitioners use light forms of touch, gentle manipulation, and techniques such as rocking to restore the flow of energy, relieving stress and pain and encouraging healing. Polarity therapy is particularly useful for depression, anxiety, fatigue, headaches, fibromyalgia, and other conditions involving emotional blockages.

Standards of practice and a code of ethics are established by the American Polarity Therapy Association.

QI GONG The Chinese phrase *Qi gong* means air (considered the vital essence) and work. This traditional Asian practice utilizes aerobic exercise, meditation, relaxation techniques, and isometrics to control the vital energy of the body in the most efficient way. Like many Chinese practices, it emphasizes the unity of mind, spirit, and world.

The central practice is a combination of breathing, movement, and shallow meditation, in which the person is aware of what is going on but in a tranquil state in which positive images flow quietly through a relaxing mind. Once the person is in this state, the flow of the *qi* through the body is stimulated. This unobstructed flow will heal sickness or increase an existing sense of wellness.

RECONSTRUCTIVE THERAPY Reconstructive therapy, created in the 1920s by a pair of osteopathic physicians, works by stimulating the body's ability to heal itself. Substances that cause a slight irritation to tissues are injected into affected areas. Blood vessels grow into the region, bringing more oxygen, vitamins, and minerals, as well as fibroblast growth factor, into the cartilage, promoting tissue growth.

Dr. Arnold Blank, who has used reconstructive therapy to treat arthritis, describes how it works. "This therapy works best when the patients are in an optimal nutritional state. Vitamin and mineral levels are important in our healing response and ability. The injection consists of a variety of different liquids. Primary liquids I use are calcium, lidocaine, and saline. They take a moment and really aren't painful. The majority of patients feel improvement after the first three or four treatments, developing some strength and feeling less pain, even increasing the range of movement.

"The nutrients we may use, natural ones, include substances that have an anti-inflammatory effect, such as vitamin C, shark cartilage, sea cucumber, glutathione, and glucosamine sulfate. All these substances are used once reconstructive therapy has begun because the new blood vessels going to the tissues will enhance healing. These nutrients may not work well when there are no blood vessels going into the area, and so they should be administered after the therapy has begun its work."

REFLEXOLOGY Reflexology is based on the principle that people have reflex areas in their feet that correspond to every part of the body. The locations of the reflex points on the foot correspond to the way the organs and glands are distributed within the body. Massaging these specific areas on the feet thus helps to improve the functioning of particular organs and glands.

For example, the toes reflect the head area, the ball of the foot represents the chest area, and so on. The practitioner presses his or her fingers into the foot, using a variety of techniques, to massage and relax ill or stressed parts of the body.

REIKI Reiki is a type of massage therapy or bodywork in which pressure-point techniques are used to move energy through the body in order to create balance and harmony. The practice, Japanese in origin, teaches the student to attain an attunement with the universal energy.

Whereas many Asian techniques involve learning a discipline to guide the flow of energy, in Reiki the student attains attunement from a Reiki Master, who transmits it during a ritual process. This single attunement can never be lost, although with further attunements one can move to a higher spiritual level. There are schools of Reiki with three levels or "degrees" of proficiency.

ROLFING According to practitioners of Rolfing, pain is caused by chronic short-enings in the tissue. Correction of the pain can be accomplished by soft tissue manipulation. This manipulation creates order in the body so the client stands tall and free of restriction.

Rolfing is generally performed in a series of 10 sessions, designed to address all the shortenings in the structure systematically. Each session works in a different area. The basic goal of Rolfing is not pain relief per se; still it has been found useful for TMJ, frozen shoulder, carpal tunnel syndrome, tennis elbow, chronic hip problems, sciatica, cervical neuropathies, and knee, foot, and ankle problems.

The Rolf Institute of Structural Integration certifies Rolfers.

THERAPEUTIC TOUCH Therapeutic touch represents a reinvigoration of the old process of the laying on of hands, whereby the subtle touch of a healer on the patient's body will infuse her with positive energy. This therapy was originally developed by nurses and emphasizes the nurturing aspect of the practitioner.

A key ingredient of the practice is compassion for the patient being touched. Unlike most of the therapies reviewed here, this technique requires minimal training, which is why it is widely practiced by both professional medical practitioners and laypeople.

Nurse Healers Professional Associates is responsible for guidelines and curricula for teaching practitioners. There is no certification program. Therapeutic touch can be practiced by nurses after a 12-hour (or minimum 6-hour) program.

TRADITIONAL CHINESE MEDICINE Traditional Chinese medicine is based on ancient Taoist philosophy, which treats the whole person. The philosophy is that body and mind are one; there is no separation between the two. When *qi*, or universal energy, flows freely through the meridians, a person is healthy, but when *qi* is blocked or disrupted, the person develops pain or illness.

Practitioners begin by examining the patient to identify patterns of dishar-mony. They then prescribe herbal remedies based on these patterns.

TRAGER TECHNIQUE According to the theory behind Trager technique, pain is caused when someone frequently tightens her muscles in movement and posture. To correct this, the practitioner uses gentle motions to increase the patient's pleasure in the quality of her tissues and decrease the restriction and sense of holding. Gentleness is important, so that no message is sent to the body telling it that pain is on the way or causing the patient to tighten up.

The movement reaches into the central nervous system to convey the sensations of pleasure, lengthening, softening, and opening to the tissues and joints. This practice is used to relieve lower back, neck, and upper back pain; sciatica; migraines; TMJ disorders; carpal tunnel syndrome and other repetitive stress disorders.

The Trager Institute offers information, training, and certification in the Trager approach.

VISION CARE ANALYSIS Contrary to popular belief, eye problems are not an inevitable result of aging. Many eye diseases, including macular degeneration, cataracts, and glaucoma, can be prevented. Dr. Marc Grossman, an optometrist and licensed acupuncturist who lectures internationally on natural eye care, explains that it is not only the general public that has been misled.

"Eye care in this country is very symptom-oriented. In our training as eye doctors, we are taught that once something goes wrong with your eyes there is not much that we can do to try to improve it. We are not really taught much in school about prevention of eye problems. We are taught that eye problems are just a natural consequence of aging."

Dr. Grossman is among a small but growing group of vision care specialists who hold a different view. These practitioners treat eye diseases holistically, incorporating lifestyle, exercise, emotional well-being, nutrition, and herbs.

YOGA Yoga is an age-old system of mental and physical exercise that began in India. The goal of yoga is to bring the body, mind, and spirit into a state of harmony. The basis of yoga is breath and breathing practices, which help circulation and also help collect toxins so that they can be exhaled.

73

Resource Guide

The following list was supplied in part by the Alternative Medicine Yellow Pages (www.alternativemedicine.com). This list is intended for information purposes only. It is not meant to be an endorsement of a particular association or practitioner's services.

ACUPRESSURE

Acupressure Institute
510-845-1059

ARIZONA

Acu-Ki Institute
888-853-0646

CALIFORNIA

Nan Bakanjian
510-652-7957

Joseph Carter
510-524-4151

Maureen Chow Hicks
415-333-0376

Ellen Deck
415-381-1833

Roger Jahnke
805-682-3230

Marianne Lonergan
415-387-1674

Kathleen Moring
510-254-7643

FLORIDA

Aaron Applebaum
407-367-9009

Bodhi F. Kocica
305-666-2243

MASSACHUSETTS

Donald Cox
617-641-2728

C Tao Healthcare
617-846-9425

MICHIGAN

Joella Caskey
510-559-8874

John McDonald
616-429-7449

MINNESOTA

Sonmore
612-866-4000

NEW YORK

Sulvia Heyman
516-671-8864

Schaeffer
516-433-4536

WASHINGTON

Sandra B Golubinski
415-454-0135

ACUPUNCTURE—
CHINESE MEDICINE

Accreditation Commission for
Schools and Colleges of Acupuncture
and Oriental Medicine
8403 Colesville Rd, Ste 370
Silver Spring, MD 20910
301-608-9680

American Academy of Medical
Acupuncture
5820 Wilshire Blvd
Los Angeles, CA 90036
323-937-5514
www.medicalacupuncture.org

American Association of Oriental
Medicine
433 Front St
Catasauqua, PA 18032
610-266-1433
www.aaom.org

American Association of Acupuncture
and Bioenergetic Medicine
2512 Manoa Rd
Honolulu, HI 96822
808-946-2069
www.healthy.net

American College of Addictionology
and Compulsive Disorders
5990 Bird Rd
Miami, FL 33155-5202
305-661-3474

Council of Colleges of Acupuncture
and Oriental Medicine
1010 Wayne Ave, Ste 1270
Silver Spring, MD 20910
301-608-9175

National Acupuncture and Oriental
Medical Alliance
14637 Starr Rd Se
Olalla, WA 8359
253-851-6896
www.acuall.org

National Certification Commission
for Acupuncture and Oriental
Medicine
PO Box 97075
Washington, D.C. 20090-7075
Phone: 202-232-1404

ALABAMA

John L Stump
334-928-5058

ARIZONA

Bradley Kuhns
602-453-6245

CALIFORNIA

Linda Bienenfeld
310-477-8151

China Healthways Institute
800-743-5608

Henry Fusco
619-276-4188

Ira Golchehreh
415-485-4411

Caroline Heaviland
408-978-9851

Muffit Jensen
818-558-5613

Dina Jun
1-800-899-7277

David Katz
818-508-6188

Hung Lau Koon
415-697-8989

Randy W Martin
818-905-5755

Maoshing Ni
310-917-2200

Erik Nielsen
805-492-1811

Joel Penner
818-344-1983

Michael Tierra
408-429-8066

Janet Zand
310-457-7749

COLORADO

George H. Kitchie
303-584-9714

Le Victoria
303-322-8977

FLORIDA

Scott Beat
904-445-8003

Scott Beat
904-823-3351

Scott Beat
904-673-0400

Charlene Canali
305-667-8174

Paul Canali
305-667-8174

Joan Tirro
954-236-8685

Lydia Zaccaro
561-391-9280

ILLINOIS

Teena Akiyama
708-848-3526

Patricia D. Faivre
815-758-4494

Dan Plovanich
312-296-6700

Rebecca Qi
312-296-6700

KANSAS

Qizhi Gao
316-688-7154

KENTUCKY

James P. Odell
502-429-8835

LOUISIANA

Hether M. Churchill
318-269-0444

MAINE

Janet Allen
207-628-2582

MARYLAND

Zoe Dee Brenner
301-718-0953

MASSACHUSETTS

Donald Cox
617-641-0807

Maryann McCarthy
508-349-7592

NEW JERSEY

Dean Gallagher
908-291-5656

Su-Jung Shiuey
201-667-2394

NEW MEXICO

Diane H. Polasky
505-262-0555

Judith S. Caissie
505-988-7117

David Frawley
505-983-9385

Abbate Skya Gardner
505-988-3538

Thomas Pool
505-296-3340

Jonas R. Skardis
505-988-5551

NEW YORK

Alice S. Behr
212-995-5379

Julia Byrd
516-496-7766

Cindy Ehrich
914-478-1300

Guang Chen Guo
718-478-8828

Deborah Musso
212-995-5379

Prensky
212-861-9000

Strickler
212-772-2838

Christopher Trahan
212-714-0856

NORTH CAROLINA

Boyd Bailey
336-777-0037

OKLAHOMA

Ray Weathers
405-631-5450

OREGON

Joseph Kassel
503-935-3453

Benjamin Stott
503-488-3612

PENNSYLVANIA

Ming Ming Molony
215-964-2755

Ruey J Yu
215-628-9088

TENNESSEE

Tammy Naslund
615-298-2820

TEXAS

Sunny Chernly
817-461-6700

John A. Scott
512-444-6744

ALEXANDER TECHNIQUE

Alexander Technique International, Inc.
1692 Massachusetts Ave
Cambridge, MA 02138
617-497-2242

North American Society of Teachers of the Alexander Technique
PO Box 112484
Tacoma, WA 98411-2484
800-473-0620
www.nastat@ix.netcom.com

ALABAMA

Ron Dennis
205-322-6483

ARIZONA

Georgianne Y Farness
602-774-8056

Harriet Harris
215-985-1040

Lutey Layne Wilkey
602-423-9155

CALIFORNIA

Pamela Blanc
310-470-2628

Anne Bluethenthal
415-864-6683

Robert Britton
415-383-1934

Dale L Carolynne
310-827-0421

Ronit Corry
415-459-8820

Steven Corry
408-296-6960

Phyllis M. Gilmore
714-856-0809

Don Krim
310-550-0409

Raphael Morey
415-206-0920

Giora Pinkas
510-933-0602

Vittoria Segalla
916-345-7027

Shulamit Sendowski
818-886-4153

COLORADO

Alexander Technique Institute
303-449-4143

Colin Egan
303-449-4143

Anne Schwerdt
719-260-9506

CONNECTICUT

Rebecca Flannery
203-263-3544

Ilse R Giebisch
203-393-1663

Idelle Packer
203-661-8027

DELAWARE

Cynthia Morgan
302-737-7321

FLORIDA

James Franz
305-674-1124

Marja Scheeres
813-748-5754

GEORGIA

Ron Dennis
404-841-0386

HAWAII

Kevin Ahern
206-937-4518

Helen Higa
808-732-1180

Jill E. Togawa
808-396-9210

IDAHO

Linda Van Polen
208-883-4942

ILLINOIS

Edward Bouchard
312-935-7677

Rose Bronec
217-344-5274

Joseph Goldfield
217-367-6415

Nancy R Gootrad
312-822-0734

John Henes
708-475-7910

Azin Movahed
217-367-3172

Joan Murray
217-367-3172

Robert Resnick
618-457-7233

Philip Schalow
217-398-8466

INDIANA

Lawrence Webster
317-877-7486

LOUISIANA

Lemann C Coe
504-895-0304

Kate Vigneron
504-386-6579

MAINE

Judith Cornell
207-772-1984

Maria J Parker
207-729-0839

MASSACHUSETTS

Lawrence Carter
617-391-4025

Rivka Cohen
617-566-2218

Marie Gorst
413-584-1566

Meredith Osborn
413-247-5854

Christine Stevens
413-253-0677

Lawrence Young
508-741-0789

MICHIGAN

Jane R Heirich
313-761-2135

Stephen Hurley
313-577-3538

Elinore Morin
517-337-2390

MINNESOTA

Elizabeth Garren
612-375-9142

Mara Sokolsky
612-690-5559

MISSOURI

John Appleton
417-831-7131

Katherine Mitchell
314-726-1685

Patricia A Wilson
816-822-2865

MONTANA

Karla Booth
406-549-7308

NEW JERSEY

Pamela Anderson
201-744-7737

Lorna Faraldi
201-943-8741

Lauren Jones
609-466-1981

Jean McClelland
201-854-7483

Michael Protzel
908-459-5043

Esther Seligmann
609-921-1780

NEW MEXICO

Gayle Felbain
505-292-8005

Babette Markus
505-989-1552

Melissa Matson

NEW YORK

Wade Alexander
607-844-9300

Michele Arsenault
212-874-2530

Marilyn Barach
315-343-2947

Martha Bernard
212-924-1761

Alison Courtney
212-316-1891

Bill Cunnington
212-288-0818

Sara H Doran
718-768-8467

Marjorie Dorfman
516-385-4001

Fernande Girard
212-879-2862

Kim Jessor
212-925-1169

Jane Kosminsky
212-724-9755

Leslie Manes
914-967-8106

Janis Sharkey
914-232-8950

NORTH CAROLINA

Victoria M Hyatt
212-628-8583

NORTH DAKOTA

Daniel Halkin
701-235-4264

OHIO

Barbara Conable
614-299-3661

Helen Hobbs
216-291-4190

Neil Schapera
513-542-1010

OREGON

Alisa McMahon
503-357-7854

Jocelyn Parrish
503-223-1693

Rebecca Robbins
503-238-9861

PENNSYLVANIA

Lelis Calder
215-543-7789

Patricia Dressler
215-732-5799

Freyda Epstein
804-293-9930

Shelach Yael Lavi
412-682-1319

Pamela P Lewis
412-421-8409

Jeff Tessler
215-242-6346

RHODE ISLAND

Saura Bartner
401-751-6599

Carol G Malik
401-831-0542

Gerritsen H Robertson
401-831-4779

TENNESSEE

R Lee Joseph
800-484-7576

Joan Mercer
901-683-5137

Phyllis Richmond
615-373-1784

UTAH

Marjean Mckenna
801-537-1343

VERMONT

Rupa Cousins
802-387-5276

Kate Judd
802-257-1358

VIRGINIA

Buxton P Charmoy
804-741-0164

Chris Friedman
804-977-3432

Marian Goldberg
703-243-9465

Daria Okugawa
804-974-6418

Joy K Paoletto
804-741-3476

Constance Serchuk
212-677-1663

Frank Sheldon
804-971-7066

WASHINGTON

Jan B Jarvis
206-441-3270

Josette Pelletier
509-682-4577

Andrew Zavada
206-525-4405

WEST VIRGINIA

Jeff Goldman
804-353-6649

WISCONSIN

Chase Michael Johnson
414-963-9660

Babette Lightner
612-729-7127

WYOMING

Esther Seligmann
307-733-4441

ANTI-AGING MEDICINE

International College of Advanced
Longevity Medicine
1407-B N Wells St
Chicago, IL 60610
www.healthy.net

Jess Groesback, MD
Sacramento, CA 95814
916-441-4419

The Nevada Center of Alternative
and Anti-Aging Medicine
Reno and Carson City, NV 89703
775-888-4830

Martin C Simpson, MD, FACF
920-A Liverpool Circle
Lakehurst, NJ 08733

Stephen Pratt, MD
Southern Institute of Anti-Aging
Medicine and Research
Nashville, TN 37203
615-320-0433

Jess Groesback, MD
Mt. Vernon, WA 98274
360-424-0440

APPLIED KINESIOLOGY

ALABAMA

George Burroughs
205-476-9000

ALASKA

Sandra Vaisvil
907-561-3690

Craig B Hediger
907-376-4851

Gary L Webb
907-562-6181

ARIZONA

Charles B Boag
602-269-5717

Donald C Baker
516-785-8300

James D Reade
602-732-0911

John Brimhall
602-964-5107

John H Gelhot
602-994-4994

Lance J Morris
602-323-7133

CALIFORNIA

Carol Shwery
408-476-6906

Eve Campanelli
310-855-1111

Jan Dooley
707-822-9171

Janet E Green
510-653-0526

Kathleen M Power
818-793-7161

Mabel Chau
818-956-5165

Alan A Silverberg
916-877-1936

Bertrand Faucret
714-870-5036

Dan Dernay
510-682-1234

Eugene Charles
310-868-0100

Lee H Vagt
707-462-6684

Robert L Olson
714-526-2860

Warren B Friedman
415-459-2550

COLORADO

Gail Kuettel
303-351-6111

Mary Ann Testarmata
303-444-0422

Susan D Rivard
719-473-6963

David Walther
719-544-1468

Douglas P Brisson
303-678-8489

Kenneth H Koenig
303-476-1902

Roger Franz
303-425-0123

CONNECTICUT

Julius L Sanna
203-744-7440

Douglas J Koch
203-335-8293

Richard J Caskey
203-758-1765

Robert Porzio
203-756-7449

Roger A Yates
203-388-5781

FLORIDA

Barbara Bringas
305-385-1000

Connie D Steele
904-362-2411

Pamela D Greene
813-644-8451

Jack K Hendricks
813-294-3109

Alan M Shaff
407-495-4357

Frank Sivo
305-891-1210

Kevin M Usry
407-863-8779

Kirk Crist
813-262-0606

Terry Mcknight
813-786-1232

C Leslie Howard
407-768-0205

GEORGIA

Amy Stevens
404-998-8844

Jane Saadeh
404-297-0022

Virginia S Mayo
404-297-0022

Jay Hammer
404-872-8779

Larry K Haberski
404-294-5050

Robert G Robideau
404-740-8244

Ronald A Weinstein
404-593-4357

Gurusahay S Khalsa
404-843-3400

HAWAII

Karl Hynes
808-329-6888

Gerald J Felcher
808-828-6844

Robert Klein
808-959-4588

ILLINOIS

Amelia W Case
312-266-9090

Laurie A Krzynowek
708-885-2580

Carl J Destefano
708-858-9780

Craig Hilgendorf
708-668-9626

Jerold Morantz

Mark W Terry
618-532-5929

Stephen W Boudro
708-544-2700

INDIANA

Bernard M Nonte
812-482-2923

Don Danklefsen
219-347-1637

Steven C Mangas
317-247-1717

IOWA

Don E Miller
319-393-6530

Forrest J Heise
319-754-5751

James D Hogg
309-786-2747

Mark Knutson
319-266-1838

KANSAS

Evan Mladenoff
913-491-1071

Milton E Dowty
316-684-0550

KENTUCKY

Bruce Jackson
317-827-0393

John T Hughes
606-329-9311

Sean P Brady
502-458-6165

LOUISIANA

Sylvia Beaumont
504-861-8000

Richard Guidry, Jr
318-981-2937

MARYLAND

Constance A Dale
410-687-4270

Robert A Ozello
301-279-0950

Robert B Lawrence
410-838-5131

MASSACHUSETTS

Antonia Orfield
617-868-8742

Margot R Barnet
508-752-3404

Conrad Henrich
413-525-6293

David A Newton
617-235-5962

George A Debs
508-755-2125

Lawrence Bronstein
413-528-2948

Norman C Levesque
413-737-1636

MICHIGAN

Linda S Sayer
313-677-1900

Nancy Heacock
616-345-3660

Allan Zatkin
313-881-0662

Bruce Deboe
517-684-3993

Charles M Lietz
616-530-3333

Emil Morlock
616-532-5291

James J Beno
616-347-4445

William D Ryckman
810-653-0602

MINNESOTA

C Robert Nelson
612-922-0616

Shapiro V Harvey
218-722-4845

Tatiana Riabokin
612-935-9360

MISSOURI

Dolores P Grebe
314-351-7771

Shauna Mathis
501-855-4739

Bert Hanicke
314-991-5655

David G Trybus
417-869-2066

Gary E Anderson
816-425-6311

MONTANA

Gary A Strong
406-252-1221

Robert T Hager
406-755-1722

NEBRASKA

Steven W Engen
308-237-2891

NEVADA

Dale Anderson
702-458-1181

John J Ediss
702-882-7085

Randall W Robirds
702-646-1150

Timothy D Francis
702-221-8870

NEW HAMPSHIRE

Paul J Loch
603-772-7888

Vincent P Procita
603-924-3777

A Douglas Nicoletti
603-898-5500

NEW JERSEY

Annalee Kitay
201-325-0065

Barbra F Gibbons
201-887-0860

David A Cheetham
609-547-2965

Edward M Burstein
908-665-0770

Jeffrey Horning
609-778-8688

John N Kane
201-744-4904

Michael L Smith
908-591-0070

Paul D Lauria
609-266-1557

NEW MEXICO

Patricia A Sheppard
505-982-2797

Frank M Ninos
505-334-3633

Jimmie McClure
505-989-9561

NEW YORK

Christine M Gizoni
516-589-7814

Diane J Reppert
607-272-4290

Glenda R Rose
716-754-9039

Mary E Olsen
516-421-1248

Anthony Leroy
914-354-0005

Bruce S Cooperstein
914-232-9497

Jaime S Warren
516-599-0010

Ora Golan
718-846-0886

Richard Bloom
914-425-9575

Salvatore Cordaro
718-325-8162

Thomas A Rogowskey
212-645-1961

Vincent Esposito
718-627-1127

NORTH CAROLINA

Lorraine Dumas
813-485-8721

David B Dauphine
704-295-9896

Edward E Flaherty
919-776-4304

John R Schmitt
919-847-3555

Mark Diener
704-554-1141

Samuel F Yanuck
919-942-8516

William E Sisson, Jr
910-392-3770

NORTH DAKOTA

Darrel Hestdalen
701-227-1104

Derryl Moon
701-474-5948

OHIO

Cecilia A Duffy
216-466-1186

Rebecca L Hartle
513-748-0940

Bruce Hartle
513-748-0940

Mark G Duckwall
513-767-7251

OKLAHOMA

John F Demackiewicz
405-364-1244

Paul E Plowman
405-840-5600

Victor L Gdanski
405-335-5112

OREGON

Carol Cooper
503-393-6071

Donald E Vradenburg
503-754-0325

John D Palmer
503-378-0068

Nick Friedman
503-668-3604

Steven McClure
503-254-1522

PENNSYLVANIA

Carole Sgrillo
215-343-3658

Janet Calhoon
717-566-3245

Alex P Karpowicz
717-342-0767

Dennis T Rehrig
215-566-9040

Glenn G Bloom
412-731-9441

Robert Rabenau
717-464-2719

Stephen D Smith
215-647-2755

RHODE ISLAND

Clive W Bridgham
401-245-7010

Gary J Post
401-789-5008

Roger Redleaf
401-944-6582

SOUTH CAROLINA

Lewis R Hinson
803-599-9255

TENNESSEE

Sara E Windham
615-584-0479

Barry W Sunshine
615-984-6850

Ben Markham
615-622-6007

William S Brennion
615-356-0876

Stephen R Cobble
615-691-2910

TEXAS

Len Lopez
972-458-0099

Alfred B Colwell
713-351-7343

Alvin R Mauldin
512-447-3332

James S Jackowski
214-368-8977

Mark Schulz
713-541-4402

Arvel F Huneycutt
817-645-3996

UTAH

Karl Hawkins
801-268-0100

Korin A Branham
801-268-8090

VERMONT

Kimberly O'Boyle
802-877-3567

Kurt Vreeland
802-649-3122

William J Schenck
802-878-8330

VIRGINIA

Bonnie Shapiro
703-642-8527

Catherine K Carson
703-273-6106

Rose M Julian
703-689-2300

Alan S Weinstein
703-379-2225

James M Taylor
804-520-7246

Richard A Mowles
703-989-4584

WASHINGTON

Frank Y Kitamoto
206-842-4772

John Stoutenburg
206-483-5041

Michael C Taggart
206-821-1101

A Gordon Green
206-483-2320

WEST VIRGINIA

E Morgan Jones
304-636-3570

WISCONSIN

Gabrielle Laden
608-257-7212

Jan M Jensen
414-645-1616

Gene Vradenburg
715-723-2696

Herbert Kuehnemann
414-447-6062

WYOMING

Paul White
307-358-5066

AROMATHERAPY

National Association for Holistic
Aromatherapy
2000 2nd Ave Ste 206
Seattle, Washington 98121
800-ASK-NAHA
www.naha.org

ARIZONA

Anna Marie Fritsche
602-494-7332

Ann Kane
602-934-7929

Teri Magyar
602-963-7644

Anthony Addesso
602-843-9249

CALIFORNIA

Annemarie Buhler
818-300-8096

Helen Thomas
707-527-7313

Linda Anne Kahn
619-457-0191

John Steele
818-986-0594

Michael J Grossman
714-770-7301

Yugal K Luthra
916-442-4945

Claudia Zdral
510-522-0998

FLORIDA

Arlene Carr
407-649-8162

Cynthia J Kratz
407-835-6821

Harriet D Costa
813-584-7246

IDAHO

Annette Davis
208-232-5250

ILLINOIS

Marianne Steenvoorden
312-296-6700

MASSACHUSETTS

Janet Beaty
508-772-0222

John Lentz
413-548-9763

NEW JERSEY

Elisabeth Lindberg
201-934-1751

PENNSYLVANIA

Bonita Cassell
215-398-9642

WASHINGTON

Elise Contento
206-283-2819

AYURVEDIC MEDICINE

American School of Ayurvedic
Sciences
10025 NE 4th St
Bellevue, WA 98004
206-453-8022

Ayurvedic Institute
11311 Menaul Ne Ste A
Albuquerque, NM 87112
505-291-9698

Maharishi Ayur-Ved Products
PO Box 49667
Colorado Springs, CO 80949-9667
800-843-8332

BIOFEEDBACK TRAINING

Association for Applied
Psychophysiology and Biofeedback
10200 W 44th Ave Ste 304
Wheat Ridge, CO 80033
303-422-8436
www.aapb.org

Biofeedback Certification Institute of
America
10200 West 44th Ave, Ste 304
Wheatridge, CO 80033
303-420-2902

CHELATION THERAPY

American Board of Chelation
Therapy
70 W Huron St
Chicago, IL 60610
312-266-7246

American College for Advancement
in Medicine
23121 Verdugo Dr
Laguna Hills, CA 92653
www.acam.org

ALABAMA

Gus J Prosch, Jr
205-823-6180

ALASKA

Robert Martin
907-376-5284

Robert Rowen
907-344-7775

ARIZONA

Gordon H Josephs
602-778-6169

William W Halcomb
602-832-3014

Stanley R Olsztyn
602-954-0811

ARKANSAS

Norbert J Becquet
501-375-4419

William Wright
501-624-3312

CALIFORNIA

Joan M Resk
714-842-5591

Pamela S L Nathan
619-755-3340

David A Steenblock
714-770-9616

Eugene D Finkle
707-984-6151

Julian Whitaker
714-851-1550

Murray Susser
310-477-8151

T Gilford
408-433-0923

COLORADO

James R Fish
719-471-2273

Terry S Friedmann
602-381-0800

DELAWARE

George Yossif
302-856-5151

FLORIDA

Bach McComb
941-957-0200

Herbert Slavin
954-748-4991

Gary L Pynckel
813-278-3377

Martin Dayton
305-931-8484

Donald J Carrow
813-832-3220

Ricardo V Barbaza
407-335-4994

Ray Wunderlich
813-822-3612

GEORGIA

Bernard Mlaver
404-395-1600

William E Richardson
404-607-0570

C Lee Ralph
404-423-0064

Terril J Schneider
912-929-1027

HAWAII

Clifton Arrington
808-322-9400

IDAHO

Stephen Thornburgh
208-466-3517

Charles T Mcgee
208-664-1478

K Peter McCallum

ILLINOIS

Phillip P Sukel
708-253-0240

Terry W Love
815-434-1977

Hugh A Jenkins
312-445-6800

Paul J Dunn
708-383-3800

Thomas Hesselink
708-844-0011

INDIANA

Harold T Sparks
812-479-8228

Norman E Whitney
317-831-3352

George Wolverton
812-282-4309

IOWA

Horst G Blume
712-252-4386

KANSAS

Terry Hunsberger
316-275-7128

Roy N Neil
913-628-8341

Stevens B Acker
316-733-4494

KENTUCKY

John C Tapp
502-781-1483

Kirk Morgan
502-228-0156

LOUISIANA

Felix K Prakasam
318-226-1304

Joseph R Whitaker
318-467-5131

MAINE

Joseph Cyr
207-868-5273

MARYLAND

Christopher C Brown
410-268-5005

Paul Beals
301-490-9911

Health Management Institute
301-816-3000

MASSACHUSETTS

Michael Janson
617-661-6225

Richard Cohen
617-829-9281

Ruben Oganesov
617-254-2500

MICHIGAN

Cal Strecter
219-924-2410

Grant Born
616-455-3550

William M Bernard
313-733-3140

Lovell L Farris
313-861-2100

Vahagn Agbabian
810-334-2424

MINNESOTA

Jean R Eckerly
612-593-9458

Keith J Carlson
507-247-5921

Steven E Klos
612-929-4568

MISSISSIPPI

James H Sams
601-327-8701

James H Waddell
601-875-5505

Robert Hollingsworth
601-398-5106

MISSOURI

Charles J Rudolph
816-453-5940

Clinton C Hayes
314-583-8911

James Rowland
816-361-4077

William C Sunderwirth
417-837-4158

Simon M Yu
314-721-7227

MONTANA

Timothy A Binder
406-363-4041

NEBRASKA

Otis W Miller
308-728-3251

NEVADA

Robert Vance
702-385-7771

Terry Pfau
702-258-7860

NEW JERSEY

Allan Magaziner
609-424-8222

Gary Klingsberg
201-585-9368

Charles Harris
908-506-9200

Eric Braverman
609-921-1842

Gennaro Locurcio
908-351-1333

NEW MEXICO

Annette Stoesser
505-623-2444

Jacqueline Krohn
505-662-9620

W J Shrader
505-983-8890

NEW YORK

Serafina Corsello
516-271-0222
212-399-0222

Christopher Calapai
516-794-0404

Kenneth A Bock
914-876-7082

Michael B Schachter
914-368-4700

Richard N Ash
212-628-3133

Robert C Atkins
212-758-2110

Ronald Hoffman
212-779-1744

Savely Yurkovsky
516-334-5926

NORTH CAROLINA

John L Laird
704-252-9833

John L Wilson
704-252-9833

Bhaskar D F Power
919-535-1411

NORTH DAKOTA

Richard H Leigh
701-775-5527

Brian Briggs
701-838-6011

OHIO

David D Goldberg
513-277-1722

Ernest F Shearer
614-262-1308

John Baron
216-642-0082

Ted Cole
513-779-0300

OKLAHOMA

Gaylord D Snitker
918-749-8349

Charles D Taylor
405-525-7751

Howard Hagglund
405-329-4457

OREGON

Robert Sklovsky
503-654-3938

John E Gambee
503-686-2536

Ronald L Peters
503-482-7007

PENNSYLVANIA

Sally Ann Rex
215-866-0900

Robert H Schmidt
215-437-1959

Roger Stewart
412-322-1945

Donald Mantell
412-776-5610

Mura Galperin
215-677-2337

Von Kiel
215-776-7639

SOUTH CAROLINA

Theodore C Rozema
803-796-1702
800-992-8350

SOUTH DAKOTA

Theodore Matheny
605-734-6958

TENNESSEE

James Carlson
615-691-2961

Stephen Reisman
615-356-4244

TEXAS

Gerald Hall
915-598-0601

Herbert Carr
210-787-6668

John L Sessions
409-423-2166

Francisco Soto
915-534-0272

Robert Battle
713-932-0552

Vladimir Rizov
512-451-8149

UTAH

Dennis Harper
801-288-8881

Cordell Logan
801-562-2211

D Remington
801-373-8500

VERMONT

T Lee Alan
802-524-1062

VIRGINIA

Aldo Rosemblat
703-241-8989

WASHINGTON

Paula Bickle
360-253-4445

Burton B Hart
509-927-9922

Jonathan Wright
206-631-8920

WEST VIRGINIA

Albert V Jellen
304-242-5151

Steve M Zekan
304-343-7559

WISCONSIN

Alan W Spaeth
414-463-1956

Timoteo L Galvez
608-238-3831

Heyden Richard L Vander
414-435-5915

CHIROPRACTIC

American Chiropractic Association
1701 Clarendon Blvd
Arlington, VA 22209
703-276-8800
www.amerchiro.org

International Chiropractors
Association
1110 N Glebe Rd
Arlington, VA 22201
703-528-5000

American College of Addictionology
and Compulsive Disorders
5990 Bird Rd
Miami, FL 33155-5202
305-661-3474

ALABAMA

George Burroughs
334-476-9000

William Cargile
334-626-2588

John Stump
334-928-5058

ALASKA

Christine J Miller
907-235-7212

Craig B Hediger
907-376-4851

Mark Munson
303-321-4977

ARIZONA

Jan Viafora
602-284-9550

Lorayne M Christensen
612-488-9417

Gerald Jursek
602-997-7607

Greg Muchnij
602-491-6331

Sheldon Deal
520-323-7133

Thomas G Maday
520-886-2875

ARKANSAS

Beverly Foster
501-371-0152

CALIFORNIA

Kenneth A. Thomas
650-738-2225

Alexandra Pettis
818-243-4353

Doralee Jacobson
805-569-2001

Jane Guttman
909-337-0434

James Daris
310-478-1006

John D Nikolatos
415-552-6662

Jud Surai
818-766-0111

Kenneth L Eckhardt
707-762-1895

Peter de Armas
619-755-8055

COLORADO

Barbara Stokoe
303-440-4880

Catherine C Mcguire
719-481-3394

Catherine J Lyon
303-444-1212

Pamela J Corson
970-224-2282

Pamela L Hart
303-449-2225

Alan R Messer
303-776-6110

Dan L Langolf
303-237-6170

Glenn A Johnson
303-772-4544

Jack Zellner
303-444-7524

Michael R Daws
303-973-2777

CONNECTICUT

Joyce Schumann
203-227-6211

Lou Soteriou
203-598-3113

Julius L Sanna
203-744-7440

Roger A Yates
203-388-5781

William P Trebing
203-625-0307

DELAWARE

Larry Zaleski
302-368-0124

Melvin Rosenthal
302-322-3030

Roger Allen
302-734-9824

FLORIDA

Charlene Canali
305-667-8174

Connie D Steele
904-362-2411

Jan E Jensen
904-222-2952

Nancy Soliven
407-622-4706

Aaron Applebaum
407-367-9009

Edward Douglas
813-763-4320

Michael O Daniel
407-567-7590

Norman Gibson
407-996-7105

Robert E Walsh
305-525-2225

William W Griffin
813-758-2827

GEORGIA

Frances C Cavaliere
404-320-1500

Jane Saadeh
404-297-0022

Gregory B Talley
404-892-8191

Kenneth S Feder
404-252-0050

Nelson D Bulmash
404-499-9650

Gurusahay S Khalsa
404-843-3400

HAWAII

Janet Lindsay
808-533-1181

Karl Hynes
808-329-6888

Robert Klein
808-959-4588

Russell Rosen
808-244-6100

Miggins Larry
808-242-8508

IDAHO

Ann Raymor
208-882-3723

Annemarie Swenson
612-483-3963

Kathy Bennett
208-454-9000

Brad Egbert
208-356-8818

Charles Wilcher
208-336-0000

David Long
208-736-1976

James Hollingsworth
208-375-4415

John Whalen
208-345-3632

Jon Harmon
208-345-5588

Suneil P Polley
208-788-5092

Verdean Fulton
208-939-9195

ILLINOIS

Elizabeth Erkenswick
312-943-5433

Elizabeth Erkenswick
708-869-1313

Karen Berk
312-761-5401

Laurie A Krzynowek
708-885-2580

Carl J Destefano
708-858-9780

Craig Hilgendorf
708-668-9626

Daniel Shain
312-296-6700

David Buck
708-475-2993

Michael Luban
312-553-2020

Michael D Henry
217-544-5446

Paul G Varnas
312-525-0007

Stephen W Boudro
708-544-270

INDIANA

Jean C Squire
317-251-3018

Dexter A Nardella
317-284-6720

Steven C Mangas
317-247-1717

Debra R Cummings
319-752-4544

Honey L Heber
319-728-2359

IOWA

Anthony J Bart
712-757-0102

Brett M Medhus
515-752-1642

Brian C Nook
712-275-4790

Dale L Anliker
319-752-5743

Dean Jacobs
319-337-3856

James A Passick
515-576-6857

Jay Jerald Bleil
319-323-3652

Michael S Sellz
319-354-1166

Ronald D Pehl
515-232-3374

Thomas J Desalvo
319-285-4803

KANSAS

Evan Mladenoff
913-491-1071

Milton E Dowty
316-684-0550

KENTUCKY

Marcia K Segura
606-441-6058

Sylvia Beaumont
504-861-8000

Bruce Jackson
317-827-0393

John T Hughes
606-329-9311

LOUISIANA

Jewell Warren
504-355-3741

Patricia Skergan
504-926-2273

Randall Hirsack
504-924-2979

MAINE

Roger B Nadeau
207-284-7760

MARYLAND

Constance A Dale
410-687-4270

Douglas Beech
301-469-6700

Robert B Lawrence
410-838-5131

Ronald Parks
410-486-5656

MASSACHUSETTS

Paul J. Giordano
508-324-9999

Barbara S Silbert
508-465-0929

Deborah S Miller
617-661-1450

Sally Atkinson
413-527-8630

Conrad Henrich
413-525-6293

Erin Dwyer
617-254-8670

Kevin Lowey
508-255-5866

Stephen Stern
617-444-4163

MICHIGAN

Ardell J Weissert
517-427-5551

Dawn A Lancaster
313-595-8203

Joyce C London
616-754-9172

Nancy Heacock
616-345-3660

Aaron Blossom
517-484-3615

Dennis L Bloom
313-561-2199

John L Dallas
517-882-0251

Robert P Radtke
313-258-3244

Thomas A Clark
313-379-3346

MINNESOTA

Ann Ivey
612-588-4618

Carol Lipschultz
612-644-9691

Judy Lemieux
218-879-3951

Susan L Clarke
612-227-8776

Bernard E Williams
612-251-2600

Brian Hilbert
612-255-5188

David C Giliuson
612-423-5050

Gary Lawrence
612-464-3395

Jeff Brist
612-546-9151

John Lambert
612-228-1900

Timothy Sheehan
612-485-2380

MISSOURI

Dolores P Grebe
314-351-7771

John M Bott
314-962-1116

Robert Nagy
314-339-0220

Ronald L Schippers
515-842-5583

MONTANA

Linda Baldwin
406-721-4590

Lynn M Butler
406-728-5114

Douglas Smithson
406-251-4473

NEBRASKA

Brook Bowhay
308-632-7094

Faye Jones
402-426-4443

Gayle Beach
402-592-7686

Gordon Kuether
402-426-3663

Steven Shockley
402-334-0840

Geanne Grimes
402-564-2622

NEVADA

Craig Dabci Roles
702-451-0480

Dale Anderson
702-458-1181

Fred L Stoner
702-259-0030

Randall W Robirds
702-646-1150

Timothy D Francis
702-221-8870

Darwyn Grierson
702-645-8222

NEW HAMPSHIRE

Joel S Shrut
603-742-3270

Paul J Loch
603-772-7888

NEW JERSEY

Barbra F Gibbons
201-428-8264

Benjamin N Loparo
201-825-8884

Bill Dixon
201-825-8884

David S Rosenstein
201-666-6844

James Cameron
908-479-1180

Thur Sprieser
201-334-6053

NEW MEXICO

Carol Rosen
505-268-1845

Gretchen Silver
505-268-1845

Frank M Ninos
505-334-3633

Harold J Kieffer
505-884-0044

Youn T Bak
505-751-3063

NEW YORK

Beth John
516-249-2310

Carol L Goldstein
212-489-9396

Carolyn H Friedman
914-362-1680

Christa L Rivelli
518-453-9252

May E Zawacki
516-739-0075

Susan Aberle
718-832-1830

David Breitbach
718-832-1830

Ingeborg Eibl
716-271-7856

Jaime S Warren
516-599-0010

Samuel R Anteby
718-963-3103

Stanley A Wieczorek
716-637-2133

Wayne Batterman
516-569-0401

NORTH CAROLINA

Julianne Bruskewicz
919-755-0024

Lorraine Dumas
813-485-8721

David B Dauphine
704-295-9896

Edward E Flaherty
919-776-4304

Eldon L Clayman
704-437-5462

John R Schmitt
919-847-3555

NORTH DAKOTA

Robert L Thomsen
701-845-2481

Timothy M Olson
701-234-0028

William C Swanson
701-748-2136

OHIO

Cecilia A Duffy
216-466-1186

Rebecca L Hartle
513-748-0940

Bruce A D Hartle
513-748-0940

David A Freland
419-474-1553

James C Kreger
419-841-4207

James P Powell
216-494-5533

OKLAHOMA

Gaylord D Snitker
918-749-8349

John F Demackiewicz
405-364-1244

Victor L Gdanski
405-335-5112

OREGON

Carol Cooper
503-393-6071

Joyce Patten
541-488-5828

Shelley Simon
503-287-9849

Brian Buttler
503-829-2297

David Wheeler
503-235-4413

John M Kalb
541-482-0625

Nick Friedman
503-668-3604

Signy Erickson
541-549-3583

PENNSYLVANIA

Donna Funk
215-630-0270

Janet Calhoon
717-566-3245

Renee Sexton
215-364-7737

Anthony V Fasano
215-657-4464

Dennis T Rehrig
215-566-9040

Glenn G Bloom
412-731-9441

Robert Rabenau
717-464-2719

RHODE ISLAND

Clive W Bridgham
401-245-7010

Roger Redleaf
401-461-2125

SOUTH CAROLINA

Linda Lorenzo
803-272-1015

Monica L Kemp
803-292-3291

James R Deason
803-439-1713

Roger S Jaynes
803-232-0082

SOUTH DAKOTA

Alan Juel
605-348-5134

Roger Van Riper
605-285-1677

TENNESSEE

Keith South
615-298-2820

Norma J Fisher
615-443-0523

Sara E Windham
615-584-0479

TEXAS

Louise Nadeau
214-739-0191

Mary K Osborn
512-327-6101

Susan Harding
512-479-0771

Clifford Mullins
903-581-6766

Dale K Sandvall
817-861-9400

Michael A Kapsner
512-441-1240

Thomas Matts
214-520-1137

Tim McCullough
713-451-6722

UTAH

Kevin Morgan
801-583-0900

Korin A Branham
801-268-8090

VERMONT

Louis Vastola
802-362-3633

Kimberly Boyle
802-877-3567

Kurt Vreeland
802-649-3122

Randal Schaetzke
508-255-8489

William J Schenck
802-878-8330

VIRGINIA

Barbara F Sikes
812-422-7972

Bonnie Shapiro
703-642-8527

Rose M Julian
703-689-2300

Joseph M Skinner
703-356-8887

Philip Newman
703-659-2273

Thomas Roselle
703-698-7117

WASHINGTON

Lisa Polec
206-726-0630

Anthony Calpeno
206-565-2444

Carl James Savard
503-221-1441

John D Kojis
360-254-8866

Joseph Dispenza
206-446-3151

Vincente O Saraco
360-671-0696

WEST VIRGINIA

E Morgan Jones
304-636-3570

WISCONSIN

Cheryl C Folstad
608-372-2747

Jan M Jensen
414-645-1616

Linda Capra
715-235-7333

Herbert Kuehnemann
414-447-6062

Mark Bergquist
715-392-4078

Orval Hidde
414-261-5607

William Borrmann
414-725-4918

WYOMING

Lisa Brady
307-739-0553

COLON THERAPY

American Colon Therapy Association
11739 Washington Blvd
Los Angeles, CA 90066
310-390-5424

American Association of
Naturopathic Physicians
2366 Eastlake Ave Ste 322
Seattle, WA 98102
206-323-7610
www.naturopathic.org

ARIZONA

Jeffrey Feingold
602-945-8773

CALIFORNIA

Robert L Garabedian
209-229-6553

Lawrence F Schnell
619-741-8155

Beth Marx
510-834-1557

Delores Hepburn
415-333-3303

Denise Wilson
408-358-2537

Doug Lynner
213-462-4578

Rubio Geronimo
800-388-1083

Skinner
310-518-4555

COLORADO

Jackie Parker
303-920-4666

CONNECTICUT

Rajesh P Vyas
203-259-2700

Vishvanath
203-259-2700

GEORGIA

Yakov Koyfman
Tucker, GA 30084

NEW HAMPSHIRE

Jack M Larmer
603-595-7755

ILLINOIS

Hugh Jenkins
312-445-6800

NEW JERSEY

Ursula Szpryt
908-613-4961

Faina Munito
201-736-3743

NEW YORK

Tovah Finman
914-921-5433

The Natural Alternative Center
212-580-3333

PENNSYLVANIA

P Jayalashmi
215-473-4226

OHIO

Robert C Angus
419-358-4627

OKLAHOMA

Bruce A Frye
918-250-1072

OREGON

Alex Serkalow
503-588-2333

Andrew Perry
503-364-1441

TEXAS

Tam Phan
409-833-6097

Looney
409-863-7445

Wilson
409-863-7445

WASHINGTON

Amy Lind
206-938-1393

Richard Marshall
206-457-1515

The Hope Clinic
206-527-1366

DENTISTRY, HOLISTIC

American Academy of Biological
Dentistry
PO Box 856
Carmel Valley, CA 93924
408-659-5385

Environmental Dental Association
9974 Scripps Ranch Blvd
San Diego, CA 92131-1825
800-388-8124

Holistic Dental Association
PO Box 5007
Durango, CO 81301
www.holisticdental.org

ALASKA

Burton A Miller
907-277-2600

Charles T Connell
907-562-7909

ARIZONA

Cecil C Barton
602-990-9544

Stan Farnum
602-721-7874

A J Ayers
602-881-8585

ARKANSAS

John H Sinclair
501-741-2254

CALIFORNIA

Carl K Colbie
916-343-5571

Edward M Arana
408-659-5385

Frederick W Howe
916-334-1730

Gary M Verigin
209-838-3522

George Schuchard
714-628-4783

Marvin Prescott
310-476-8302

Robert L Olson
714-526-2860

Timothy A Kersten
916-335-5491

COLORADO

Robert E Mcferran
303-237-3306

Scott Mcadoo
303-393-0039

Stephen M Koral
303-443-4984

CONNECTICUT

Morris Sunshine
203-374-5777

Stephen S Baer
203-227-6338

FLORIDA

James A Harrison
407-965-9300

James Hardy
407-678-3399

GEORGIA

Ronald M Dressler
404-349-2088

IDAHO

James E Pfost
208-375-7786

ILLINOIS

Daniel R Dieska
708-429-4700

John A Rothchild
708-884-1220

Phillip P Sukel
708-253-0240

KANSAS

William M Payne
316-241-0266

MARYLAND

Eugene A Sombatoro
410-964-3118

MASSACHUSETTS

Bruce M Sorrin
914-338-7200

MICHIGAN

David W Regiani
810-627-4934

John Lielais
810-642-5460

MINNESOTA

Gary J Olin
612-770-8982

MONTANA

Duane E Christian
702-882-4122

NEW JERSEY

John J Tortora
908-721-0210

NEW MEXICO

Chris Norton
505-988-1616

NEW YORK

David L Lerner
914-265-9643

Donald R Barber
716-632-7310

Jay Dooreck
516-621-2430

OHIO

Richard J Chanin
513-729-2800

William A Westendorf
513-923-3839

OKLAHOMA

Paul E Plowman
405-840-5600

OREGON

Dick W Thom
503-526-0397

Jeffrey A Williamson
503-684-4174

PENNSYLVANIA

Alan D Krausz
215-668-2330

Som N Gupta
412-828-1920

Gerald H Smith
215-968-4781

Owen Rogal
215-545-2104

Ronald Niklaus
717-737-3353

SOUTH DAKOTA

Larry Lytle
605-342-0989

TEXAS

Jack B Snowden
817-275-2633

UTAH

Joseph Hansen
801-753-2322

VIRGINIA

Wayne L Whitley
703-371-9090

WASHINGTON

Frank Y Kitamoto
206-842-4772

George J Grobins
206-564-2722

Mitchell L Marder
206-367-6453

Robert B Stephan
509-325-2051

Ruos Borneman
206-293-8451

WISCONSIN

Allen C Owen
414-421-1700

Douglas L Cook
414-842-2083

DETOXIFICATION THERAPY

American Association of
Naturopathic Physicians
2366 Eastlake Ave Ste 322
Seattle, WA 98102
206-323-7610
www.naturopathic.org

American Board of Chelation
Therapy
70 W Huron St
Chicago, IL 60610
312-266-7246

American College for Advancement
in Medicine
23121 Verdugo Dr
Laguna Hills, CA 92653
www.acam.org

American Natural Hygiene Society
11816 Race Track Rd
Tampa, FL 33626-3105
813-855-6607

ALASKA

John D Walsh
907-258-1390

Robert Rowen
907-344-7775

ARIZONA

John R Prentice
206-338-2702

Paul Deloe
602-886-9988

CALIFORNIA

Marilyn Snow Jones
818-222-2080

Eve Campanelli
310-855-1111

Mark Holmes
310-271-6467

Robert Broadwell
714-965-9266

Roger Jahnke
805-682-3230

Richard A Kunin
415-346-2500

COLORADO

Ruth Adele
719-636-0098

CONNECTICUT

Joseph Reneson
203-347-8894

FLORIDA

Martin Dayton
305-931-8484

Leonard Haimes
407-994-3868

GEORGIA

Stephen Edelson
404-841-0088

HAWAII

Paul Kenyon
808-591-2872

ILLINOIS

Frank Yurosek
708-319-0192

Hugh Jenkins
312-296-6700

INDIANA

David Darbro
317-913-3000

KANSAS

Dorothy Emery
913-682-4848

KENTUCKY

Mary Broeringmeyer
800-626-3386

MASSACHUSETTS

Janet K Beaty
508-772-0222

MICHIGAN

David W Regiani
810-627-4934

MINNESOTA

Thomas Stowell
612-644-4436

MISSOURI

Simon M Yu
314-721-7227

MONTANA

Michael Lang
406-752-0727

NEW JERSEY

Faina Munito
201-736-3743

NEW MEXICO

Willard H Dean
505-983-1120

NEW YORK

Kenneth A Bock
914-876-7082

Michael B Schachter
914-368-4700

Jennie Kramer
516-271-0222

Joyce St Germain
516-271-0222

Serafina Corsello
516-271-0222

Scott Gerson
212-505-8971

Richard N Ash
212-628-3133

NORTH DAKOTA

Brain Briggs
701-838-6011

OHIO

Heather Morgan
513-439-1797

OREGON

Elaine Gillaspie
503-224-8083

Rita Bettenburg
503-252-8125

Alex Serkalow
503-588-2333

Leia Melead
503-282-1224

Prafulla Morris
503-699-2547

Skye Weintraub
503-345-0747

PENNSYLVANIA

Roger Stewart
412-322-1945

P Jayalashmi
215-473-4226

SOUTH DAKOTA

Larry Lytle
605-342-0989

WASHINGTON

Cheryl L Wood
206-778-5673

Magda Mische
206-376-5454

Lynda S Hamner
509-548-7090

David B Wood
206-778-5673

Michael G Lamarche
206-334-4087

Ruos Borneman
206-293-8451

ENVIRONMENTAL MEDICINE

American Academy of Environmental
Medicine
7701 E Kellogg
Wichita, KS 67207-1705
www.healthy.net

ALABAMA

Andrew M Brown
205-547-4971

Morton Goldfarb
205-252-9236

C Orian Truss
205-328-6481

Humphry Osmond
205-759-0416

ALASKA

F Russell Manuel
907-562-7070

ARIZONA

Gene D Schmutzer
602-795-0292

William W Halcomb
602-832-3014

Kent L Pomerory
602-391-0141

Ralph F Herro
602-266-2374

Stanley Olsztyn
602-945-4501

ARKANSAS

Laura Koehn
501-521-3363

Harold Hedges
501-664-4810

William Wright
501-624-3312

G Howard Kimball
501-269-4301

Aubrey M Worrell
501-535-8200

CALIFORNIA

Marlene Lehr
510-838-4180

Susan Kuss
510-676-9293

Betty Stratford
510-837-3911

Chuck Rudy
415-924-6852

Richard P Plant
619-942-8610

Bryan Bouch
707-778-3171

John Henderson
619-293-7745

Murray Susser
310-477-8151

Peter Madill
707-823-3312

Richard A Kunin
415-346-2500

Zane R Gard
619-571-0300

Elson Haas
415-472-2343

COLORADO

Linda C Wright
303-440-5588

Del Stigler
303-831-7335

Kendall Gerdes
303-377-8837

Marshall Mandell
203-838-4706

Peter D'Adamo
203-661-7375

Ehrico Liva
203-347-8600

DELAWARE

Jerome E Groll
302-645-2833

ILLINOIS

Norene B Hess
708-446-1923

Pauline Harding
708-653-9900

Hamid Mahmud
618-548-4613

Mohammad T Ghani
708-344-3550

Theron Randolph
708-844-9898

Thomas Hesselink
708-844-0011

Walt Stoll
606-233-4273

INDIANA

Myrna D Trowbridge
219-462-3377

Frederick H Simmons
317-662-6950

Lawrence S Webster
317-877-7486

Robert M Armer
317-846-7341

Julie Larson
219-422-1643

IOWA

Martin G Meindl
515-424-0640

Robert W Soll
515-247-8750

Nyle D Kauffman
319-338-7862

KANSAS

Dorothy Emery
913-682-4848

Charles Hinshaw
316-262-0951

Joseph Shaw
913-235-6221

KENTUCKY

John H Parks
606-254-9001

Kirk Morgan
502-228-0156

Nanine Henderson
502-893-5422

LOUISIANA

Stephanie F Cave
504-767-7433

Thomas J Callender
318-233-6022

MAINE

Christiane Northrup
207-846-6163

Bruce W Kenney
207-774-9668

Maurice C Hothem
207-797-4148

David Getson
207-775-7433

MARYLAND

Barbara A Solomon
301-668-5611

Neil Solomon
301-337-2707

Arnold Brenner
410-922-1133

Paul R Cook
410-337-2707

Richard E Layton
410-337-2707

MASSACHUSETTS

Myra B Shayevitz
413-584-4040

Ralph Palombo
617-593-0180

Joseph P Keenan
413-568-2304

Michael Janson
617-661-6225

N Thomas La Cava
508-829-5321

R Gopal Malladi
413-536-2978

Svetlana Kaufman
508-453-5181

MICHIGAN

Ruth Walkotten
616-733-1989

Paula Davey
313-662-3384

Kenneth Ganapini
313-733-3140

William M Bernard
313-733-3140

Edward Linker
313-973-1010

Harry R Butler
313-676-2800

Dahagen Agbabian
313-334-2424

Silver J Tulin
810-932-0010

MINNESOTA

Jean R Eckerly
612-593-9458

Edward Sweere
507-345-3323

Keith Sehnert
612-920-0102

John L Wilson
612-679-1313

MISSISSIPPI

Thomas Glasgon
601-234-1791

Madeline Permutt
314-997-2111

MISSOURI

Albert Nehl
314-837-1141

Doyle B Hill
417-926-6643

James Rowland
816-361-4077

John T Schwent
314-937-8688

William L Traxel
314-686-2411

Tipu Sultan
314-921-7100

MONTANA

Sylvia Seymour
406-222-0300

Catherine H Steele
406-727-4757

Charles H Steele
406-727-4757

Curt G Kurtz
406-587-5561

NEBRASKA

Roy Donovan
308-327-4703

Otis W Miller
308-728-3251

NEVADA

Eunice Tang
702-826-9500

Terry Pfau
702-258-7860

David F Charles
702-388-7337

Michael L Gerber
702-826-1900

Reed W Hyde
702-731-3117

Ji-Zhou J Kang
702-798-2992

NEW HAMPSHIRE

Michele C Moore
603-357-2180

NEW JERSEY

Constance Alfano
201-444-4622

Allan Magaziner
609-424-8222

Phillip Bennet
609-737-2700

Eric Braverman
609-921-1842

Michael Burnhill
908-463-1966

Richard Podell
908-464-3800

NEW MEXICO

Jacquelyn A Krohn
505-662-9620

Shirley B Scott
505-966-9960

Joseph Collins
505-434-4699

Norman Harrison
505-522-1988

Harold A Cohen
505-898-7115

D Klinghard
505-988-3086

NEW YORK

Marjorie S Siebert
718-386-2020

Doris J Rapp
716-875-5578

Christopher Calapai
516-794-0404

Alfred V Zamm
914-338-7766

Kenneth A Bock
914-876-7082

Louis Perrish
212-737-3636

Martin Feldman
212-744-4413

Michael B Schachter
914-368-4700
914-358-6800

Miklos L Boczko
914-949-8817

Morton M Teich
212-988-1821

Neil L Block
914-359-3300

Paul Cutler
716-284-5140

Richard Izquierdo
718-589-4541

Richard N Ash
212-628-3113

Ronald Hoffman
212-779-1744

I-Tsu Chao
718-998-3331

Kalpana D Patel
716-883-2611

Savely Yurkovsky
516-334-5926

NORTH CAROLINA

John L Laird
704-252-9833

Logan Robertson
704-235-8312

Phillip Bickers
919-573-9228

Walter A Ward
910-760-0240

Bhaskar D Power
919-535-1411

NORTH DAKOTA

Eugene B Byron
701-780-6000

Galen J Each
701-234-3610

Richard H Leigh
701-775-5527

OHIO

Heather Morgan
513-439-1797

John Baron
216-642-0082

Ted Cole
513-779-0300

Arthur Gardikes
513-434-0555

Arturo Bonnin
513-435-8999

Donald S Nelson
216-836-3016

Richard F Bahr
513-299-8788

Escarlito U Sevilla
216-792-1956

Stoyan P Daskalov
216-823-3219

OKLAHOMA

Donald M Dushay
918-744-0228

Howard E Hagglund
405-329-4458

Jerald M Gilbert
405-789-9500

V J Conrad
405-341-5691

OREGON

Judy Peabody
503-324-1616

James Wm Fitzsimmons
503-474-2166

Robert Sklovsky
503-654-3938

Donald C Mettler
503-228-9497

Joseph T Morgan
503-269-0333

Paul E Dart
503-484-7202

Ronald L Peters
503-482-7007

Arn Strasser
503-223-6414

PENNSYLVANIA

Christiane M Siewers
412-782-2992

Helen F Krause
412-366-1661

Harold E Buttram
215-536-1890

Howard Lewis
412-531-1222

Leland J Green
215-855-9501

Sidney P Lipman
814-452-2405

K R Sampathachar
215-473-4226

Leander T Ellis
215-477-6444

RHODE ISLAND

Albert Puerini
401-943-6910

Mary Radio
401-353-5888

SOUTH CAROLINA

Allan D Lieberman
803-572-1600

Anthony E Harris
803-648-7897

Rocco D Cassone
803-536-5511

Maartin Zwerling
803-648-9555

TENNESSEE

William Neely
615-929-Well

Calvin P Bryan
615-821-1177

Richard G Wanderman
901-683-2777

William G Crook
901-423-5400

TEXAS

Vickey C Halloran
713-440-0800

Alfred R Johnson
214-368-4132

Billy G Mills
214-279-6767

Gerald Parker
806-355-8263

John L Sessions
409-423-2166

Robert R Thoreson
512-258-8729

Constantine A Kotsanis
817-481-6342

Everett P Stewart
806-793-8963

Jacob Siegel
713-973-8832

William Rea
214-368-4132

UTAH

David Harbrecht
801-292-8303

Dennis Remington
801-373-8500

Robert Payne
801-269-8817

Dennis Harper
801-288-8881

VERMONT

Charles E Anderson
802-879-6544

T Lee Alan
802-524-1062

VIRGINIA

Susan Zimmer
703-364-2045

Keith Jassy
804-379-1145

Henry J Palacios
703-356-2244

Roger D Neal
703-628-9547

Sohini Patel
703-941-3606

WASHINGTON

Jennifer Huntoon
206-632-8804

Lora Shelton
206-734-1560

Joseph Dispenza
206-446-3151

Murray L Black
509-966-1780

Walter ND Crinnon
206-747-9200

Albert G Corrado
509-946-4631

Elmer M Cranton
360-458-1061

Ralph Golan
206-324-0593

WEST VIRGINIA

Michael Kostenko
304-253-0591

Albert V Jellen
304-242-5151

Prudencio Corro
304-252-0775

WISCONSIN

David L Morris
608-782-2027

Eleazar M Kadile
414-468-9442

T Galvez
608-238-3831

Vijay K Sabnis
608-782-2027

ENZYME THERAPY

Don Barber
Pensacola, FL
901-285 6775

Carolyn Bormann
Twin Peaks, CA
909-337-3671

Kimberly Kelly
Seattle, WA
206-281-9047

Nancy Hancock
New York, NY
212-758-2110

Jonathan Collin
Kirkland, WA
206-820-0547

Stephen Edelson
Atlanta, GA
404-841-0088

F Soto
El Paso, TX
915-774-9996

R Evers
El Paso, TX
915-774-9996

R James
El Paso, TX
915-774-9996

Rubio Geronimo
San Diego, CA
800-388-1083

Donohoe
Medford, OR
503-770-5563

Skinner
Torrance, CA
310-518-4555

FELDENKRAIS METHOD

Feldenkrais Guild
3611 SW Hood Ave
Portland, OR 97201
800-775-2118
www.feldenkrais.com

ALASKA

Gail Nolan
907-424-3503

Gail Pettengill
907-276-3414

Henry Cloud
907-235-6472

ARIZONA

Judith K Geis
602-625-5904

Ken Largent
503-223-1665

Lindley H Silverman
602-287-3024

Steve Streeter
602-628-8183

CALIFORNIA

Andrea Wiener
619-281-5575

Bobbie J Veronda
707-745-4399

Carol Lessinger
801-364-8090

Carol Pinto
213-663-6093

Marcia Margolin
408-688-0216

Alan Sheets
415-459-6795

Bob Schulenburg
213-666-3873

Howard Bornstein
415-328-9181

Rukmini J Oribello
510-654-1897

Sachiye Nakano
310-544-1624

COLORADO

Charlotte Watership
303-756-8101

Emily N Dangel
303-771-8809

Ginger Mitchell
303-861-3818

Jennifer L Merrall
303-782-4779

Jack Heggie
303-449-8100

Bethany Cobb
303-722-1740

CONNECTICUT

Louise Larcheveque
203-633-9506

Marjorie Hutensky
203-644-4038

Rona Klein
802-253-4165

Avram J Hellerman
203-281-7919

Rahina S M Friedman
203-322-7961

William J Massir
203-776-5734

FLORIDA

Carol Phillips
904-378-7891

Deborah Vukson
305-534-8832

Emma S Johnson
305-763-3832

Bill Mott
305-764-2894

Henry Revich
305-667-4576

Angele Dibenedetto
305-661-5227

Sandy Burkart
304-293-3610

GEORGIA

Therese E Stogner
404-325-2211

HAWAII

Maryann Gianantoni
808-531-5604

Jerome Karzen
808-572-8554

Jerry Shapiro
808-324-1761

IDAHO

Robert L Spencer
208-342-5141

Jim Chubb
208-726-0710

ILLINOIS

Myra Ping
312-878-8700

Susan Alberts
708-328-8817

Thomas Hanley
414-273-6066

Harvey Arkin
312-296-6700

John Palumbo
312-327-1988

Stephen R Duke
815-756-6033

Steve Corrick
808-879-1190

IOWA

Sheilah Manley
515-263-2660

KANSAS

David Moses
415-861-5520

KENTUCKY

Joann Stickler
606-269-2243

LOUISIANA

Ellen Soloway
504-895-5196

MAINE

Jane Burdick Scholz
207-594-7746

MARYLAND

Donna H Blank
301-365-2450

Lucy M Rouse
410-433-1079

Miriam U Nanartowich
303-987-3410

Aliza Lidovsky Stewart
410-358-6725

J Kelly Russell
301-587-7287

MASSACHUSETTS

Joyce Kegeles
508-791-8389

Sally Schmidt
413-747-9819

Suzanne Oppenheim
617-868-1840

Barry S Levine
617-566-4330

Josef Dellagrotte
508-874-2398

Needham J McCoy
508-689-3003

MICHIGAN

Jill Whelan
616-526-2879

Joann Serota
313-651-2009

Liz Dickinson
517-355-2363

Nancy Denenberg
313-761-1514

Rebecca Malm
313-642-6560

Meena Narula
810-853-5853

MINNESOTA

Marjorie Moore
612-331-9155

MISSOURI

Barbara Anderson
816-363-5253

Nancy Schumacher
816-931-5781

MONTANA

Mary Easton
303-447-8853

Jerome Karzen
406-721-7038

NEBRASKA

Nancy F Williamson
402-488-3331

NEW HAMPSHIRE

Barbara Levin
603-679-1817

Raymond H Rosenstock
603-924-7401

NEW JERSEY

Jacqueline Wollins
908-545-5744

Judie Fujita
201-783-3379

Edward Feldman
908-247-6890

Lawrence Phillips
609-683-4433

NEW MEXICO

Felicia N Trujillo
505-984-8775

Katrin Smithback
505-983-3919

Lucretia Weems
505-989-8933

Lynn Godwin
301-680-0853

NEW YORK

Alicia Fortinberry
914-245-8348

Alta A Morris
212-473-4899

Amber B Grumet
212-242-2309

Carol Mcamis
607-274-3426

Jill Dorfeld
607-962-3099

Joan Pfitzenmaier
212-496-5703

Katherine Fan
914-762-4181

Lisa Wiener
718-855-9347

Lisa C Nathanson
516-431-1383

Frederick Onufryk
716-275-9675

NORTH CAROLINA

Annette A Johannesen
919-697-1050

Dianne Postnieks
704-377-4735

Joanne Dahill
305-444-6714

Joy Eudailey
704-326-3880

OHIO

Dorthea J Morton
513-836-5382

Rose M Zucker
216-543-4655

Jonathan Smith
216-795-1330

OKLAHOMA

Robert Gross
918-496-9401

OREGON

Bonnie R Humiston
503-926-6625

Pamela S Lewis
503-345-0775

John B Chester
503-399-9129

PENNSYLVANIA

Andrea Lewandowski
800-783-1008

Anna Smukler
215-242-6667

Cheryl Hertzog
215-933-8095

Jim Stehens
215-456-9130

Terry Hemlock
814-724-1765

David Zemach Bersin
510-549-9140

RHODE ISLAND

Carol J Ricci
401-934-2707

Elyse Landesberg
401-596-3699

Laura C French
401-783-4714

Richard Rogers
401-625-1128

SOUTH CAROLINA

Jane-Ella M Taylor
803-271-9552

Cathi Siebert
512-328-4015

Marta R Welch
915-751-9690

Peggy Mckinley
512-696-4179

Patrick F Siebert
512-328-4015

Ross M Stewart
214-385-4555

UTAH

Jill F Fuchs
801-486-2096

Maralee Platt
801-485-9864

VERMONT

Bradley Poster
802-257-7410

Mischul Brownstone
802-425-3355

VIRGINIA

Carla O Reed
602-957-8736

Joan Frain
703-979-7953

Maureen Mchugh
703-841-9359

Phyllis H Herman
703-522-7126

John P Link
703-204-2914

Gerta K Goldberg
703-527-3749

WASHINGTON

Ann Hart
206-527-8760

Juliann W Walter
206-821-0321

Linda Creech
206-871-3508

Mary R Hudak
509-493-1223

Robert Macdougall
206-323-1400

WEST VIRGINIA

Allison Rapp
304-291-1509

William T Stauber
304-599-6059

WISCONSIN

Pamela Kihm
708-272-8709

David Laden
608-257-7212

Chase Michael Johnson
414-963-9660

FLOWER REMEDIES

CALIFORNIA

Daniel Beilin
831-685-1400

Jeffrey Garson Shapiro
661-291-1166

Deborah Davis
805-969-1992

Kathleen Connell
408-425-3320

Tim Moore
209-229-8202

CONNECTICUT

Paul Cunningham
203-454-4485

FLORIDA

Alicia Sirkin
888-875-6753

HAWAII

Jacqueline Carson
808-934-3233

KENTUCKY

Mary Broeringmeyer
800-626-3389

MINNESOTA

Robert Gallagher
612-824-3157

NEW JERSEY

Irene Osten
908-382-1245

John J Tortora
908-721-0210

OHIO

Wm A Westendorf
513-923-3839

PENNSYLVANIA

Kathryn Strick
814-835-2241

Roger Stewart
412-322-1945

WASHINGTON

Lynda Hamner
509-548-7090

Frank Y Kitamoto
206-842-4772

Robert Jongaard
206-321-6470

GUIDED IMAGERY

Academy for Guided Imagery
PO Box 2070
Mill Valley, CA 94942
800-726-2070

International Association of
Interactive Imagery
PO Box 124
Vila Grande, CA 95486
www.iaii.org

American Holistic Medical
Association
6728 Old Mclean Village Dr
Mc Lean, Va 22101-3906
919-787-5181
www.holisticmedicine.org

American Holistic Nurses Association
PO Box 2130
Flagstaff, AZ 86003-2130
1-800-278-AHNA
www.ahna.org

ALASKA

Dee Ashington
907-277-5353

ARIZONA

Anne Zell
602-955-6883

Joyce McRae
602-885-2745

Ruth Unger
602-296-6604

Marnel Plutchok
602-990-2766

Paula L King Kennedy
602-957-2368

CALIFORNIA

Ann Swallow
916-542-9114

Audrey Kinser
805-395-1068

Carol Aronoff
415-454-7154

Stephen G Venanzi
714-651-1393

Terry Miller
415-696-5388

Alan Matez
619-455-5911

Terry Schenk
714-582-8606

Thomas Holloway
916-961-4540

William Collinge
707-829-6813

Arthur F Levit
510-596-6351

COLORADO

Patricia Pike
303-839-9900

Ruthann Balas
303-925-9252

Barry E Fields
303-920-2067

Raymond Hill
719-548-8118

FLORIDA

Cynthia J Kratz
407-835-6821

Margot Escott
813-774-2360

Henry N N Merritt
904-771-8934

Robert D Willix
407-362-0724

GEORGIA

Marc Eaton
912-283-6629

HAWAII

Pamela Mckenna
808-885-7111

IDAHO

Marlys M Borreson
208-368-7800

David Edgerly
208-385-7461

ILLINOIS

Janet Pence
815-455-3081

Michael Greenberg
708-364-4717

INDIANA

Vanessa Leon Roth
317-251-1607

IOWA

David Wenger Keller
319-372-6280

KENTUCKY

Barbara Miller
502-852-6127

LOUISIANA

Claudio Guillermo
504-532-5092

MARYLAND

Judith Wa
617-932-9003

MINNESOTA

Paula Forte
612-471-0045

Jann Fredickson
612-457-4872

MISSOURI

John R Price
816-531-2325

M Christine Mcinturff
314-949-8555

MONTANA

Renee Berglund
208-523-3895

Sandra Mckee
406-252-6674

NEBRASKA

Patricia Trowbridge
609-461-1825

NEW MEXICO

Norma Leib
505-344-8010

NEW YORK

Janice P Stefanacci
516-496-7766

Allan Warshowsky
516-488-2877

Joanne Coewy
212-675-1682

NORTH CAROLINA

Randall Maynard
910-766-4023

OHIO

Katherine Lindberg
216-262-1390

Judith Spater
614-587-3670

OKLAHOMA

Dee Dutt
405-743-2419

OREGON

Diane M Mason
503-488-5436

Jan L Ferguson
503-636-4774

Patricia Pingree
503-221-4970

Jack Hegrenes
503-494-8304

Rod Newton
503-482-0670

Daru Maer
503-620-6699

PENNSYLVANIA

Joseph O'Donnell
800-392-1475

Pamela Magerle
814-838-0123

PA Society of Behavioral Medicine
215-848-2297

SOUTH CAROLINA

Thomas H Grady
803-571-6200

TEXAS

Barbara Cavanagh
512-467-7010

Beverly Mcgregor
214-480-9355

Charlene Strawn
409-696-3307

Lou Diekemper
806-762-4186

UTAH

Paula Swaner
801-277-8339

Lavon Mceveny
801-466-4664

WASHINGTON

Betty Darby
206-525-1595

Josephine Fletcher
206-537-6301

Katy Murray
206-438-0306

Leonard Goodman
206-524-2113

Bill Womack
206-526-2164

Charles Buser
206-426-9717

HELLERWORK

Hellerwork, Inc.
406 Berry St
Mt. Shasta, CA 96067
800-392-3900
www.hwork@snowcrest.net

Hellerwork International
3435 M St
Eureka, CA 95503
1-800-392-3900
www.hellerwork.com

ARIZONA

Monica Balog
818-502-1188

Bob Elkins
602-629-9205

Brugh Joy
602-636-5579

ARKANSAS

Jane P Roark
501-666-2442

Duane Hall
501-575-0807

James Rule
501-664-1170

CALIFORNIA

Ana Viren
805-964-9055

Judy Frankel
510-849-4207

Kay Hogan
408-438-4503

Sharon Keane
415-365-1242

Sherry Little
714-562-6747

Dan Bienenfeld
310-477-8151

Fred Borenstein
213-654-1125

John Lefan
415-861-1302

Marion Klein
310-477-6987

Scott J Henderson
310-398-3990

Stephen J Bulger
619-259-9132

COLORADO

Valerie Van Zyl
303-666-7133

Dan Buscarello
303-986-6761

Marcus Morrissey
303-986-6761

Paul Tepley
303-444-7945

CONNECTICUT

Hedda Leonard
203-262-1483

Jacqueline Entwistle
203-245-9110

FLORIDA

Eleanor King
407-694-0450

Fred Covan
305-294-7522

GEORGIA

Jane Farrell
404-292-8403
404-256-6397

HAWAII

Alan H Beer
415-780-4320

Darri Heller
808-575-2981

Geordie Thorpe
808-572-1657

INDIANA

Patrick Vonderau
219-486-1253

LOUISIANA

Mary E Woosley
318-598-3401

MASSACHUSETTS

Duane Hall
508-624-4801

D Anca Norma
617-646-1974

MICHIGAN

Anne Carbone
313-662-5770

MISSOURI

Roger Weinerth
314-821-0646

Carmelita Beets
816-453-2041

MONTANA

Paula Johnson
206-435-5744

NEVADA

P Tanzy Maxfield
702-355-1617

NEW JERSEY

Debbie Clydesdale
201-612-9683

Frances C Ogden
201-731-8634

Karen Murphy
609-683-9121

Susan Belfiore
609-924-5474

Seth Klevans
609-924-6250

Kate Appel
609-683-4377

NEW MEXICO

Fred Borenstein
505-471-3663

NEW YORK

Diane T Peri
212-861-3451

Jeanne Muscarella
212-495-6220

Teresa Piacentini
718-832-6715

Bill A Nselmo
212-532-2207

Jay Cardinale
718-965-9192

Ron Feinman
516-944-7459

Stuart Bell
914-232-3122

OHIO

Judy Harlan
216-562-6788
216-360-0836

Howard Rontal
614-764-9167

Bethany Hrbek
216-751-8653

PENNSYLVANIA

Barbara Hopkins
215-249-0672

Becky Debus
215-666-0411

Cathy Stoops
215-625-0769

Bernard Shanfield
215-626-2744

Gene Miller
215-432-2641

TEXAS

Linda Kay Kanelakos
713-972-1717

Shirley Norwood
713-520-6905

James Rule
214-522-6638
817-732-4614

Sharrin Michael
408-475-0315

VERMONT

Susan Clarke
802-295-3309

D Anca Norma
802-658-9590

VIRGINIA

Cindy Brown
804-530-5148

Margaret Hyer
703-777-3670

WASHINGTON

Diane Naismith
206-632-1160

Donna Bajelis
206-784-8504

Janice K Alt
206-547-5356

Lynn M Cosmos
509-452-2961

Don St John
206-632-1160

Robert Donovan
360-647-5158

HERBAL MEDICINE

American Herbalists Guild
PO Box 70
Roosevelt, UT 84066
435-722-8434
www.healthy.net

Herb Research Foundation
1007 Pearl St Ste 200
Boulder, CO 80302-5124
800-748-2617
www.herbs.org

American Association of
Naturopathic Physicians
2366 Eastlake Ave Ste 322
Seattle, WA 98102
206-323-7610
www.naturopathic.org

ALABAMA

Healthy Way
205-967-4372

ARIZONA

Paul Deloe
602-886-9988

Silena Heron
520-282-6909

Lila Flagler
602-721-8821

Samuel Flagler
602-721-8821

CALIFORNIA

Ira Golchehreh
415-485-4411

Deborah Davis
805-969-1992

Elisabeth Sandler
310-339-1362

Kathi Head
619-236-8285

Linda S Nelson
707-447-2556

Teresa Gentile
818-707-3126

Don Canavan
510-524-8652

Erik Nielsen
805-492-1811

Gregory Alexander
415-383-7224

Matthew D Bauer
909-599-2347

Robert J Broadwell
714-965-9266

Roger Jahnke
805-682-3230

Skip Shoden
310-451-4419

William Zhao
707-445-2290

COLORADO

Ruth Adele
719-636-0098

Andrew Lange
303-443-8678

Mary Goodrich
303-927-9617

CONNECTICUT

Gabriele Kallenborn
203-454-5989

Jacqueline Germain
203-347-8600

Jeffrey J Klass
203-481-5219

Ronald Schmid
201-227-0887

Ehrico Liva
203-347-8600

Keli Samuelson
203-347-8600

FLORIDA

Harvey Kaltsas
813-955-4456

Luis Pagani
305-868-6801

Robert D Willix
407-362-0724

Ember Carianna
407-835-6821

Joya L Schoen
407-644-2729

Jay Holder
305-661-3474

ILLINOIS

Mary Ellen Marino
312-296-6700

INDIANA

Joy L Martin
812-425-5811

Frank Jacques
317-856-5211

Ronald Porks
410-486-5656

MARYLAND

Zoe Dee Brenner
301-718-0953

Douglas Beech
301-469-6700

MASSACHUSETTS

Barbara S Silbert
508-465-0929

Catherine M Umphress
508-371-1228

Shivanatha Barton
617-277-4150

MICHIGAN

Carl Bayha
616-668-4730

MINNESOTA

Andrew Lucking
612-924-8112

Robert Gallagher
612-824-3157

Thomas Stowell
612-644-4436

MISSOURI

Dorothy Kanion
816-779-4844

MONTANA

Sarah B N Lane
406-726-3000

NEVADA

Lynn Schwartzman
702-435-7501

NEW JERSEY

Peter Kadar
201-984-2800

Charles H Mintz
609-825-7372

NEW YORK

Ellen Kamhi
800-829-0918

Karen Fuller
212-932-8442

Nancy Hancock
212-758-2110

Richard M Chin
212-686-9227

Scott Gerson
212-505-8971

Chi Chow
516-496-7766

James Strickler
212-772-2838

NORTH DAKOTA

Brian E Briggs
701-838-6011

OKLAHOMA

Bruce A Frye
918-250-1072

OREGON

Carol Petherbridge
503-770-5563

Kathleen German
503-635-6643

John G Collins
503-667-1961

Mitchell B Stargrove
503-526-0397

Ray Wood
503-249-2957

Robert Sklovsky
503-654-3938

PENNSYLVANIA

Cara Frank
215-438-2977

Roger Stewart
412-322-1945

Donald Mantell
412-776-5610

Harold E Buttram
215-536-1890

TEXAS

Gilbert Manso
713-840-9355

UTAH

William Nunn
801-265-0077

K Brent Jamison
801-467-3007

UTAH

School of Natural Healing
800-372-8255

WASHINGTON

Debra Clapp
206-299-9038

Jill Stanbury
206-687-2799

Ursula Hall
206-581-0408

Linda Chiu Hole
509-747-2902

Karl Mincin
206-853-7610

Donald Brown
206-623-2520

Larry Siegler
206-885-5400

Robert Jongaard
206-331-6470

Jonathan Collin
206-820-0547

School of Herbal Medicine
206-697-1287

WEST VIRGINIA

Albert V Jellen
304-242-5151

HOLISTIC MEDICINE

American Holistic Medical
Association
6728 Old Mclean Village Dr
McLean, Va 22101-3906
919-787-5181
www.holisticmedicine.org

American Holistic Nurses Association
PO Box 2130
Flagstaff, AZ 86003-2130
1-800-278-AHNA
www.ahna.org

ALASKA

Robert Martin
907-376-5284

Torrey Smith
907-277-0932

ARIZONA

Gene D Schmutzer
602-795-0292

Gordon H Josephs
602-778-6169

Lloyd D Arnold
602-939-8916

William W Halcomb
602-832-3014

ARKANSAS

John L Gustavus
501-758-9350

William Wright
501-624-3312

CALIFORNIA

Elsa H Con
408-622-9114

Carol A Shamlin
408-378-7970

Terri Su
707-571-7560

Carl K Colbie
916-343-5571

Robert L Olson
714-526-2860

Thomas A Sult
916-542-4181

William C Kubitschek
619-744-6991

Charles A Moss
619-457-1314

Charles B Farinella
619-324-0734

Charles E Law
818-761-1661

Claude Marquette
415-964-6700

Mohamed Moharram
805-965-5229

Philip C Stavish
714-722-0175

COLORADO

George J Juetersonke
719-596-9040

Terry S Friedmann
602-381-0800

Aspen Chiropractic & Holistic
303-920-1247

CONNECTICUT

Amalia J Punzo
203-792-6003

Paul Epstein
203-853-6800

Marshall Mandell
203-838-4706

Sidney Baker
203-287-1800

Ananais Hasan
203-243-5055

DELAWARE

Jerome E Groll
302-645-2833

FLORIDA

Hana T Chaim
904-672-9000

Kathyrn Price
305-292-7282

Gary L Pynckel
813-278-3377

Joseph G Godorov
305-595-0671

Alfred S Massam
813-773-6668

Donald J Carrow
813-832-3220

Harold Robinson
813-646-5088

Ricardo V Barbaza
407-335-4994

Travis L Herring
904-775-0525

William Watson
904-623-3836

Eteri Melnikov
813-748-7943

H Lee Eugene
813-251-3089

GEORGIA

Oliver L Gunter
912-336-7343

Terrill J Schneider
912-929-1027

C Lee Ralph
404-423-0064

G Hugh Johnson
912-272-8494

HAWAII

Clifton Arrington
808-322-9400

Wismer Clark
808-941-0522

IDAHO

Frankie Avalon Wolfe
208-343-3482

Charles T Mcgee
208-664-1478

ILLINOIS

Pauline Harding
708-653-9900

Peter Senatore
708-872-8722

Terrill K Haws
708-577-9451

Hamid Mahmud
618-548-4613

John R Tambone
815-338-2345

Laurence S Webster
217-877-7486

Richard E Hrdlicka
708-232-1900

INDIANA

Alan W Sidel
219-484-8545

George Wolverton
812-282-4309

Thomas G Goodwin
219-980-6117

KANSAS

Stevens B Acker
316-733-4494

John Gamble
913-321-1140

KENTUCKY

Kirk Morgan
502-228-0156

Stephen S Keteck
606-677-0459

LOUISIANA

Stephanie F Cave
504-767-7433

James P Carter
504-588-5136

Joseph R Whitaker
318-467-5131

Adonis J Domingue
318-365-2196

MAINE

Bruce W Kenney
207-774-9668

Joseph Cyr
207-868-5273

MASSACHUSETTS

Carol Englender
617-965-7770

Jeanne T Hubbuch
617-965-7770

Michael Janson
617-661-6225

MICHIGAN

Albert Scarchilli
313-626-7544

Grant Born
616-455-3550

James Ziobrn
313-779-5700

Kenneth Ganapini
313-733-3140

Marvin D Penwell
313-735-7809

Paul A Parenta
810-626-7544

Robert N Israel
517-782-5700

MINNESOTA

Keith J Carlson
507-247-5921

Michael Dole
612-593-9458

John L Wilson
612-679-1313

MISSISSIPPI

James H Sams
601-327-8701

Robert Hollingsworth
601-398-5106

Thomas S Glasgow
601-234-1791

Pravinchandra Patel
301-622-7011

MISSOURI

Clinton C Hayes
314-583-8911

Edward W Mcdonagh
816-453-5940

John T Schwent
314-937-8688

Ralph D Cooper
417-624-4323

Ronald H Scott
314-468-4932

William C Sunderwirth
417-837-4158

Bruce A Stayton
816-836-5010

MONTANA

Micheal Lang
406-752-0727

Curt G Kurtz
406-587-5561

NEBRASKA

Otis W Miller
308-728-3251

NEVADA

Daniel F Royal
702-732-1400

Ji-Zhou J Kang
702-798-2992

NEW HAMPSHIRE

Michele C Moore
603-357-2180

NEW JERSEY

Richard B Menashe
908-906-8866

Walter Burnstein
201-584-4947

Charles H Mintz
609-825-7372

Eric Braverman
609-921-1842

Ivan T Krohn
908-367-2345

Marc J Condren
908-469-2133

Rodolfo T Sy
908-738-9220

NEW MEXICO

Daniel Bruce
505-757-2156

Gerald Parker
505-271-4800

John T Taylor
505-271-4800

Nightsky Laser
505-982-4744

NEW YORK

Christopher Calapai
516-794-0404

Michael B Schachter
914-358-6800

Mitchell Kurk
516-239-5540

Neil L Block
914-359-3300

Richard Izquierdo
718-589-4541

Richard J Ucci
607-432-8752

Robert Snider
315-764-7328

Ronald Hoffman
212-779-1744

Tsilia Sorina
718-375-2600

NORTH CAROLINA

Francis M Carroll
910-654-3143

John L Laird
704-252-9833

Keith E Johnson
919-281-5122

NORTH DAKOTA

Brian E Briggs
701-838-6011

OHIO

Heather Morgan
513-439-1797

Charles S Resseger
419-668-9615

David D Goldberg
513-277-1722

Jack Slingluff
216-494-8641

John Baron
216-642-0082

Charles W Platt
513-526-3271

Don K Snyder
419-399-2045

Richard Sielski
614-653-0017

OKLAHOMA

Charles D Taylor
405-525-7751

Howard Hagglund
405-329-4457

Jerald M Gilbert
405-789-9500

John W Ellis
405-749-0193

Robert E Farrow
918-689-7705

V J Conrad
405-341-5691

OREGON

Leslie D Elder
503-669-2766

Paul E Dart
503-484-7202

Ronald L Peters
503-482-7007

Terence H Young
503-371-1558

PENNSYLVANIA

Bill Illingworth
814-623-8414

Robert H Schmidt
215-437-1959

David M Schultz
814-274-7450

Harold E Buttram
215-536-1890

Norman E Wenger
717-222-9595

Ralph A Miranda
412-838-7632

RHODE ISLAND

Carol L. Thomas
401-521-0912

Richard Picard
401-942-6967

TENNESSEE

Calvin P Bryan
615-821-1177

Fred M Furr
615-693-1502

Matt Hine
719-635-6553

Richard G Wanderman
901-683-2777

TEXAS

Billy G Mills
214-279-6767

Gary H Campbell
817-457-8992

Gerald Parker
806-355-8263

Harlan Wright
806-792-4811

Howard J Lang
817-268-1171

Michael E Truman
817-281-0402

Andrew Campbell
713-497-7904

Everett P Stewart
806-793-8963

UTAH

Dennis D Harper
801-373-8500

D Remington
801-373-8500

VERMONT

Charles E Anderson
802-879-6544

VIRGINIA

Peter C Gent
804-744-3551

Harold Huffman
703-867-5242

Scott V Anderson
703-941-3606

Floyd Herdrich
703-978-4956

WASHINGTON

Murray L Black
509-966-1780

David Buscher
206-453-0288

Elmer M Cranton
360-458-1061

Randall E Wilkinson
509-453-5506

Richard S Wilkinson
509-453-5506

WISCONSIN

Sandra A Herbage
608-246-9070

Jerry Yee
414-258-6282

HOMEOPATHY

American Institute of Homeopathy
1585 Glencoe
Denver, CO 80220
303-898-5477

Homeopathic Academy of
Naturopathic Physicians
PO Box 69565
Portland, OR 97201
503-795-0579

Council for Homeopathic
Certification
PO Box 157
Corte Madera, CA 94976

Council on Homeopathic Education
801 N Fairfax
Alexandria, VA 22314
703-548-7790

Homeopathic Educational Services
21224 Kittredge St
Berkeley, CA 94704
510-649-0294

International Foundation for
Homeopathy
2366 Eastlake Ave E, Ste 325
Seattle, WA 98102
206-304-8230

National Center for Homeopathy
801 N Fairfax Ste 306
Alexandria, VA 22314
703-548-7790
www.healthy.net

North American Society of
Homeopaths
10700 Old County Rd
Minneapolis MN 55441
612-593-9458

ALASKA

Mary Minor
907-563-8180

Scott Jamison
907-586-6810

Torrey Smith
907-277-0932

ARIZONA

Ilene M Spector
602-293-2218

Louise Gutowski
602-443-1600

Jeffrey H N Feingold
602-945-8773

Mark James
602-774-1770

Stephen M Davidson
602-246-8977

CALIFORNIA

Jeffrey Garson Shapiro
661-291-1166

Dr. Meenaksh Bhargava
408-402-0303

Brenda Beeley
415-459-5430

Cathleen Rapp
408-358-7797

Christine P Civerella
510-524-3117

Elisabeth Sandler
310-339-1362

Wendy Brajkovich
805-772-5807

Eliza Ladyzhensky
909-736-8185

Linda C Johnston
818-776-8040

Sandra N Kamiak
408-741-1332

David R Riley
619-462-7890

David Warkentin
415-457-0678

Harry Swope
818-786-9627

Hollis King
619-587-1822

Kevin Laporta
707-445-0586

Joseph Sciabbarrasi
310-477-8151

Joseph M Helms
510-841-7600

Hiten Shaw
714-783-2773

Ifeoma Ikenze
415-258-9600

COLORADO

Glenn D Nagel
406-728-8544

Jacob J Schor
303-355-4547

Dennis H Kay
303-290-9401

Nicholas Nossaman
303-388-7730

Andrew Lange
303-443-8678

Nancy Rao
303-449-8581

CONNECTICUT

Amy B Rothenberg
203-763-1225

Gabriele Kallenborn
203-454-5989

Nancy A Mazur
203-676-2240

Harold M Ofgang
203-798-0533

Paul Herscu
203-763-1225

Stephen Tobin
203-238-9863

Thomas Livingstone Jr
203-824-0751

Jose M Mullen
203-537-3699

Ronald A Grant
203-227-2402

DELAWARE

David Ehrenfeld
302-994-2582

FLORIDA

Mary Lee Tupling
954-567-4449

Gayle Fuqua
904-760-7799

Mary Lee Tupling
305-566-6203

Henry Merritt
904-771-8934

Mark B Frank
813-788-0496

Peter Fishman
305-975-7246

Robert R Karman
800-753-9792

William C Blecha
407-878-1790

Travis L Herring
904-775-0525

GEORGIA

Jane Saadeh
404-297-0022

Michelle Tilghman
404-498-5956

Rosalyn Miller
404-636-7222

Virginia S Mayo
404-297-0022

Newton Laboratories
800-448-7256

HAWAII

Anne L Maguire
206-776-6085

Jacqueline Carson
808-934-3233

Jeff Baker
808-878-6660

IDAHO

Brent Mathieu
208-338-5590

Stephen Thornburgh
208-466-3517

Todd Schlapfer
208-664-1644

ILLINOIS

Ruth Martens
708-668-5595

Clifford Kearns
708-307-8585

Mark H Labeau
312-266-8620

Michael Luban
312-553-2020

Luc Maes
312-296-6700

IOWA

Daniel Dixon
515-472-0332

KENTUCKY

Victoria Snelling
502-426-4325

MAINE

Mary L Garner
207-772-9812

MARYLAND

Christina B Chambreau
410-771-4968

Monique Maniet
301-270-4700

Anthony M Aurigemma
301-495-3060

Carvel G Tiekert
410-569-7777

Romi Scavullo
410-367-3429

MASSACHUSETTS

Barbara S Silbert
508-465-0929

Christine Luthra
617-524-3892

Lisa A Harvey
413-586-4551

Larry L Raffel
617-484-2544

Robert G Sidorsky
413-625-9517

Robert I Orenstein
508-362-8188

Shivanatha Barton
617-277-4150

MICHIGAN

Nancy Eos
810-231-2193

David A Epstein
810-757-0010

Jerome L Dylewski
616-663-8422

Dennis K Chernin
313-973-3030

Edward J Linkner
313-973-1010

Robert N Israel
517-782-5700

Gregory Kruszewski
313-752-7241

MINNESOTA

Valerie O Hanian
612-593-9458

Andrew Lucking
612-924-8112

Eric Sommermann
612-593-9458

Gary J Olin
612-770-8982

MISSOURI

F Carmain Dutton
816-252-5147

NEBRASKA

Randall S Bradley
402-391-6714

NEBRASKA

Joanne Stefanatos
702-735-7184

Daniel F Royal
702-732-1400

Duane E Christian
702-882-4122

Fuller Royal
702-732-1400

NEW HAMPSHIRE

Jack M Larmer
603-595-7755

Naturopathic Clinic of Concord
603-228-0407

NEW JERSEY

Jane Cicchetti
201-402-8510

James F Claire
609-627-5600

Paul Gilbert
908-254-7946

Gennaro Locurcio
908-351-1333

Pratap Singhal
201-759-2241

NEW MEXICO

Mary Alice Cooper
505-266-6522

Larry Marrich
505-889-3333

David Riley
505-989-9018

NEW YORK

Karen Fuller
212-932-8442

Therese A Osborne
518-274-2276

Edwin Schwarz
914-268-7887

George P Najim
518-647-5150

Gregory R Gumberich
516-294-9494

Harold Ofgang
212-684-2290

Michael Glass
607-589-7220

Michael B Schachter
914-368-4700

Paul Scharff
914-356-8494

William L Bergman
212-684-2290

Prestas Iris Ramirez
607-659-4220

Wu Mei Hsu
315-652-6168

NORTH CAROLINA

Nancy Toner
516-567-1706

Susan Delaney
919-929-1132

Todd A Smith
910-760-9355

John Koontz
919-471-1579

OHIO

Kevin K Granger
614-864-3888

Michael Somerson
513-667-2222

Michael C Garn
216-920-8009

OREGON

Carol Petherbridge
503-770-5563

Mary F Caselli
503-224-7224

Adam Ladd
503-252-8125

Andrew Elliott
503-343-0571

James Massey
503-292-1895

Larry Herdener
503-434-6170

Stephen A Messer
503-343-2384

PENNSYLVANIA

Lucy Nitskansky
215-698-1042

Clyde D Shick
814-756-3648

George H Hopkins
215-688-8808

Donald Mantell
412-776-5610

Philip L Bonnet
215-321-8321

C Edgar Sheaffer
717-838-4879

Deva K Khalsa
215-493-0621

SOUTH CAROLINA

Jeanne Demyan
803-834-7334

Roger Jaynes
803-232-0082

SOUTH DAKOTA

Gregg Zike
605-245-2383

TENNESSEE

Victoria Snelling
901-357-9696

Corinne Rovetti
615-428-2186

TEXAS

Osa J Okundaye
214-255-1114

Alan Levine
415-861-0168

Karl Robinson
713-526-1625

Lawrence M Cohen
210-733-0990

Robert E Hazelwood
512-479-0101

UTAH

Vaughn Cook
801-944-4070

Cordell E N Logan
801-562-2211

VERMONT

John R Roos
802-864-7967

Julian Jonas
802-869-2883

VIRGINIA

Richard D Fischer
703-256-4441

Richard M Evans
703-569-2963

Frank W Gruber
804-498-8700

George Guess
804-295-0362

WASHINGTON

Barbara Kreemer
206-281-4282

Krista Heron
206-522-0488

Bruce Milliman
206-525-8015

Richard S Wilkinson
509-453-5506

Kaiten Rivers
509-576-0811

WISCONSIN

Sandra A Herbage
608-246-9070

Alice Lipscomb
414-351-2340

Mike D Kohn
608-255-1239

HYDROTHERAPY

International Association of Colon
Hydrotherapy
PO Box 461285
San Antonio, TX 78246-1285
210-366-2888
www.healthy.net

Kathi Head
San Diego, CA
619-236-8285

Teena R Armstrong
La Palma, CA
310-402-9042

Doug Lynner
Los Angeles, CA
213-462-4578

Terry S Friedmann
Denver, CO
602-381-0800

Sarah Cole
Kenner, LA
504-461-5478

Bruce Milliman
Snoqualmie, WA
206-888-9408

Doug Lewis
Seattle, WA
206-525-8078

HYPNOTHERAPY

National Guild of Hypnotists
PO Box 308
Merrimack, NH 03054
603-429-9438

International Medical and Dental
Hypnotherapy Association
4110 Edgeland Ste 800
Royal Oak, MI 48073
800-257-5467

ARIZONA

Richard Corvino
602-881-1530

CALIFORNIA

Daniel Sosa
661298-0835

Janet Long
510-531-3267

Joella Mcgonagle
818-986-5704

Lila Berkheim
213-650-7344

Suzanne Marie Angelus
510-631-0360

Teresa R Achuff
619-546-1449

COLORADO

Shari Akers
816-361-2752

John H Altshuler
303-740-7771

FLORIDA

Henry Merritt
904-771-8934

ILLINOIS

Eleanor Laser
841-677-7334

Georgia Hayden
708-428-1332

Janet Pence
815-455-3081

Wendell Loder
309-794-9688

IOWA

David S Strawn
319-366-3182

LOUISIANA

Sarah Cole
504-461-5478

MICHIGAN

Anne H Spencer
810-549-5594

MINNESOTA

Janet M Johnson
612-235-3396

James Baltzell
218-829-1845

MISSISSIPPI

Bonnie Miller
601-795-6109

MISSOURI

Irene Hickman
816-665-1836

Hermann Witte
314-851-6054

NEBRASKA

Michael Braunstein
402-551-5810

NEVADA

Michael Maglione
702-451-4544

NEW JERSEY

John Gatto
908-964-4467

NEW MEXICO

Joleen Streit
505-892-1313

Roy L. Streit
505-975-7777

NEW YORK

Janice P Stefanacci
516-496-7766

Maurice Kouguell
516-868-2233

S Alexander Weinstock
212-534-8224

NORTH CAROLINA

Randall Maynard
910-766-4023

OHIO

Patty McCormick
513-426-3797

James A Ward
513-831-3600

PENNSYLVANIA

David Frederick
717-560-5609

Francis J Cinelli
215-588-4502

Norbert Bakas
412-931-5602

TEXAS

Ed Martin
713-359-7284

JUICE THERAPY

Wood
Phoenix, AZ
602-298-6061

Rubio Geronimo
San Diego, CA
800-388-1083

Blackway
Huntington Bh, CA
714-840-8661

Marino
Placentia, CA
714-993-7757

Rosche
Palo Alto, CA
415-856-3151

Rinder
Littleton, CO
303-979-5498

Battista
Fort Myers, FL
813-433-3738

Wa
Woburn, MA
617-932-9003

Ndman
Rockford, MI
616-874-8920

Margolius
Mt Pleasant, SC
803-792-4612

Zimberoff
Issaquah, WA
206-525-5025

MAGNETIC FIELD THERAPY

Charles T Connell
Anchorage, AK
907-562-7909

Lloyd D Arnold
Glendale, AZ
602-939-8916

Charles A Moss
La Jolla, CA
619-457-1314

Michael Rosenbaum
Corte Madera, CA
415-927-9450

Mary Broeringmeyer
Murray, KY
502-753-2962

Wm A Westendorf
Cincinnati, OH
513-923-3839

Roger Stewart
Pittsburgh, PA
412-322-1945

Don Fountain
Pullman, WA
509-332-1435

MASSAGE THERAPY

American Massage Therapy
Association
820 Davis St Ste 100
Evanston, IL 60201
874-864-0123

ALASKA

Christine J Miller
907-235-7212

ARIZONA

Corrine W Larson
602-471-7344

Patrick Fitch
602-955-2677

Lila Flagler
602-721-8821

Samuel Flagler
602-721-8821

CALIFORNIA

Penny Layne
323-664-7788

Coralie Jenner
707-552-5992

Carol Carpenter
415-547-6442

Ellen Mastros
408-275-9451

Lucie Batbeau
510-549-1222

Maryann Zimmermann
619-488-1921

Nancy Sarrat
916-587-7746

Michael R Gach
510-845-1059

Neil Levinson
310-967-3489

E W Mueller
619-291-9811

COLORADO

Gail Kuettel
303-351-6111

Ruth Marion
303-443-5131

Mark Akers
816-361-2752

Togi Kinnaman
719-685-5431

Timothy A Binder
303-786-8116

CONNECTICUT

Paul Cunningham
203-454-4485

Rajesh P Vyas
203-259-2700

K Pramica Vishvanath
203-259-2700

DELAWARE

Melvin J Rosenthal
302-322-3030

Enhancement Wellness
302-629-4665

FLORIDA

Ann L Mcalhaney
305-273-9282

Cynthia J Kratz
407-835-6821

Elizabeth Heller
305-742-8399

Geri Parsons
407-365-9283

Daniel A Ulrich
813-287-1099

Neal Heller
305-742-8399

Paul Davenport
904-378-7891

GEORGIA

Leticia Allen
404-454-7167

Philip A Hurd
404-455-6767

Farra Allen
404-454-7167

HAWAII

Kathryn J Robinson
808-733-0000

Laura L Conti
808-328-8106

Susan Fitzgerald
808-879-4327

IDAHO

Brent Mathieu
208-338-5590

ILLINOIS

Hilda Allen
312-296-6700

Patricia D Faivre
815-758-4494

Allen Uretz
312-296-6700

James M Hackett
312-477-9444

Frank O Yurosek
708-319-0192

INDIANA

Jann Thomas
812-471-0161

Joy L Martin
812-425-5811

Rose M Lewis
219-962-9640

Ruthann Hobbs
317-724-7745

IOWA

Ruth A Carlson
319-363-5831

KANSAS

Stanley Beyrle
316-687-0035

Integrative Body Works
316-688-3308

MAINE

Mary L Garner
207-772-9812

Nancy W Dail
207-832-5531

MARYLAND

Jacob E Teiterbaumm
410-224-2222

Royal Schomp
301-946-5457

Therapies Integral
207-257-2964

Carol A O'Toole
410-820-7545

MASSACHUSETTS

Harriet W Wells
508-465-5618

Janet K Beaty
508-772-0222

Ben E Benjamin
617-576-1300

Donald Cox
617-641-0807

Frank Bialosiewicz
413-247-9322

Steven Tankanow
508-757-7923

Wenjing Ding
617-472-8428

MICHIGAN

Lynne Piekins
313-667-9453

Michael J Gonzalez
517-355-7994

Robert D Rousseau
313-642-5460

Sandy Fritz
313-667-9453

MINNESOTA

Sally N Petersburg
612-379-3822

Steve Sonmore
612-825-6510

Scott M Ross
612-863-4700

MISSISSIPPI

Denise Johnson
228-386-0835

MONTANA

Michael Lang
406-752-0727

NEW HAMPSHIRE

Patrick Cowan
603-882-3022

NEW JERSEY

Arleen Lapalermo
708-705-1955

Carolyn Storey
609-795-5469

Elisabeth Lindberg
201-934-1751

Ramona H Henry
201-837-1388

Ursula Szpryt
908-613-4961

Michael Brofman
908-747-2874

NEW MEXICO

Carol Maxson
505-255-4064

Connie Mattox
505-982-8398

Charles T Brown
505-268-6870

Lonnie Howard
505-982-8398

Harold A Cohen
505-898-7115

NEW YORK

Ellen Goldsmith
212-274-8217

Felicia Fussichen
516-261-0343

Laurie Towers
718-837-0545

Linda Kruger
212-717-1393

Sarah Brown
716-248-0690

Adam Brown
212-627-5073

Robert J Hoffman
516-922-4606

NORTH CAROLINA

Andrea Knapp
919-933-2212

Nancy Toner
516-567-1706

Sharon King
919-967-2639

Rick Rosen
910-376-9696

OHIO

Judith Spater
614-587-3670

Sharon Barnes
513-932-8712

C D Thompson
614-841-1122

Alan Hundley
513-281-8606

OREGON

Elaine Gillaspie
503-224-8083

Jeanne Pace
509-486-2585

Sally Lamont
503-636-2734

Gregory Garcia
503-228-6959

Noel Peterson
503-636-2734

PENNSYLVANIA

Claudia Ireman
215-997-2548

Katherine H Stewart
717-737-5299

Suzanne Miller
215-282-2110

Harry J Lynd
215-657-7514

Shirley Dillard
615-848-1040

TENNESSEE

Darren Williams
615-298-2820

TEXAS

Charlotte Small
817-498-0716

Dee Dee Viator
409-738-3439

Linda Kay Kanelakos
713-972-1717

Hervey H Perez
214-669-3246

Sharla Taylor
214-480-9355

Renee Bork
Bryan, Tx
409-775-4595

UTAH

Norman Cohn
801-521-3330

Vaughn Cook
801-944-4070

William Nunn
801-265-0077

VIRGINIA

Laurie Blackwood
804-270-1053

J Joseph
804-488-7883

WASHINGTON

Cheryl L Wood
206-778-5673

Patty J Kruschke
509-586-6434

Brian Utting
206-292-8055

Don Fountain
509-332-1435

J Douwe Rienstra
206-385-5658

WISCONSIN

Marlis Moldenhauer
414-223-3416

MEDITATION

ARIZONA

Marnel Plutchok
602-990-2766

CALIFORNIA

Jeanette Applegate
408-458-5530

Judie Gold
213-937-0223

James E Duval
714-960-0357

Roger Jahnke
805-682-3230

Anu De Monterice
707-795-2141

COLORADO

Barry E Fields
303-920-2067

CONNECTICUT

Roberta K Tager
203-226-4548

FLORIDA

David Perlmutter
813-262-8971

Powell
813-693-7450

ILLINOIS

Shelly Amdur
312-296-6700

Luc Maes
312-296-6700

MAINE

Eileen Fingerman
207-737-4359

MARYLAND

Douglas Beech
301-469-6700

MASSACHUSETTS

Don L Goldenburg
617-527-7485

L Divya Shinn
508-544-2851

NEW JERSEY

Irene Osten
908-382-1245

Kim Peralta
201-595-8720

John Gatto
908-964-4467

NEW YORK

Richard M Chin
212-686-9227

Allan Warshowsky
516-488-2877

Scott Gerson
212-505-8971

OREGON

James Massey
503-292-1895

PENNSYLVANIA

A David Dimmack
215-843-6534

SOUTH CAROLINA

Thomas H Grady
803-571-6200

TEXAS

Anil Gupta
214-644-5823

WASHINGTON

Christine Chmielewski
206-361-4700

Joan Sanabend
206-682-1425

Don Fountain
509-332-1435

Reed S Johnson
206-361-4700

MIND-BODY MEDICINE

Association for Applied
Psychophysiology and Biofeedback
10200 W 44th Ave Ste 304
Wheat Ridge, CO 80033
303-422-8436
www.aapb.org

CALIFORNIA

Cathie A Lippman
213-653-0486

Priscilla Slagle
310-826-0175

Bernard Rimland
619-281-7165

Jack Loskiu
213-342-1338

John Ackerman
805-682-1011

Phillip H Taylor
818-889-8249

Fawn Christianson
408-257-3313

COLORADO

Carole Sgrillo
215-343-3658

Nanna Bolling
719-475-0952

CONNECTICUT

Amalia Punzo
203-343-8509

Paul Epstein
203-853-6800

FLORIDA

Kenneth W Hoover
407-679-0662

Jay M Holder
305-661-3474

Harriet Costa
813-584-7246

GEORGIA

Amy Stevens
404-998-8844

Stan Dawson
404-993-9820

Milton Fried
404-451-4857

C Lee Ralph
404-423-0064

ILLINOIS

Eleanor Laser
708-677-7334

August Alonzo
312-296-6700

Philip J Berent
708-459-1003

Lal Archana
312-296-6700

KANSAS

Daryl Pokea
913-256-6189

KENTUCKY

John C Tapp
502-781-1483

John H Parks
606-254-9001

LOUISIANA

Claudio Guillermo Jr
504-532-5092

MAINE

Conrad R Wurtz
207-782-1035

MARYLAND

Douglas Beech
301-469-6700

Arnold Brenner
410-922-1133

MASSACHUSETTS

Abby Seixas
617-891-8450

Deb Murray
508-897-5250

Laura F Lubin
617-964-6849

Catherine M Umphress
508-371-1228

Gary L Whited
617-354-6420

MICHIGAN

Maram Hakim
313-285-9456

MINNESOTA

William Brauer
612-871-2611

MISSISSIPPI

David Penton
601-497-6000

MISSOURI

Hermann Witte
314-851-6054

Integrative Wellness Systems
816-361-2752

NEW HAMPSHIRE

Naturopathic Clinic of Concord
603-228-0407

NEW MEXICO

Carol Maxson
505-255-4064

NEW YORK

Janice P Stefanacci
516-496-7766

Karen Fuller
212-932-8442

Katharine Fryer
212-808-4940

Michael Glass
607-589-7220

Michael B Schachter
914-368-4700

Richard Ribner
212-246-7010

Scott Gerson
212-505-8971

Jose Yaryura-Tobias
516-487-7116

OHIO

Judith Spater
614-587-3670

Francis McCafferty
216-835-3892

Ronan M Kisch
513-293-9113

OKLAHOMA

Charles D Taylor
405-525-7751

OREGON

Joy Craddick
503-488-0478

Karl E Humiston
503-967-9390

Prafulla Morris
503-699-2547

PENNSYLVANIA

Lance Wright
610-461-6225

Philip L Bonnet
Leander T Ellis
215-477-6444

Matthew & Ellen Cohen
215-667-2204

RHODE ISLAND

David S Elliott
401-831-5251

SOUTH CAROLINA

Thomas H Grady
803-571-6200

VIRGINIA

Catherine K Carson
703-273-6106

WASHINGTON

Donald McCabe
206-331-4424

Bebe Keown
503-485-5263

Diana Sill
206-547-1471

WEST VIRGINIA

Tara C Sharma
304-523-8800

Deleno Webb
304-525-9355

WISCONSIN

Eleazar M Kadile
414-468-9442

MOVEMENT THERAPY

Corrine W Larson
Rio Verde, AZ
602-471-7344

Shelia M Johnson
Mill Valley, CA
415-332-7559

Sue Unger
Calistoga, CA
707-942-0464

Cynthia Christy
Orlando, FL
407-332-3391

Diane Elliot
Minneapolis, MN
612-724-6773

Ilene Watrous
Princeton Jct, NJ
609-799-5204

Roger Tolle
New York, NY
212-787-5167

Laurie Blackwood
Richmond, VA
804-270-1053

Center Inner Dance
Seattle, WA
206-527-9553

David Laden
Madison, WI
608-257-7212

MYOTHERAPY

ARIZONA

Enid Whittaker
602-529-3979

Sandra Dirks
602-529-3979

Michael Haines
602-529-3979

Ron Sacco
602-277-6859

CALIFORNIA

Debbie Grace
805-928-3296

Lori Drummond
714-497-4243

COLORADO

Judith Gearhart
303-776-8853

CONNECTICUT

Christine W Godfrey
203-521-5320

Pat Shriner
203-255-0005

INDIANA

Terry L Huff
317-642-0529

KENTUCKY

Susie Kalz
606-679-1655

MASSACHUSETTS

Betsy T Wilkes
617-942-0840

Claire Naylor
413-528-5600

Dee Winslow
413-253-3209

Mary A Cernak
413-529-0223

MARYLAND

Jan Stoughton
301-258-0205

MICHIGAN

Patricia Isaacson
313-887-9880

Robert W Howell
313-443-0796

MINNESOTA

Thomas G Benson
612-755-1366

MONTANA

Glenn Wilcox
406-862-1104

NEW HAMPSHIRE

Jane Sawyer
603-532-7318

NEW JERSEY

Joan A Colombo
201-641-5438

NEW YORK

Marilyn B Hilly
914-723-1119

PENNSYLVANIA

Nancy L Bleam
215-867-8886

VERMONT

Marilyn B Hilly
802-496-2550

NATUROPATHIC MEDICINE

American Association of
Naturopathic Physicians
2366 Eastlake Ave
Seattle, WA 98102
206-323-7610
www.naturopathic.org

American Naturopathic Medical
Association
PO Box 96273
Las Vegas, NV 89193
702-897-7053
www.anma.com

Canadian Naturopathic Association
PO Box 4520, Sta C
Calgary, Alberta T2T 5N3
403-244-4487

Council on Naturopathic Medical
Education
PO Box 11426
Eugene, OR 97440-3626
503-484-6028

Institute for Naturopathic Medicine
66 1/2 N State
Concord, NH 03301-4330
603-225-8844

National College of Naturopathic
Medicine
11231 SE Market St
Portland OR 97216
503-255-4860

ALASKA

Hope Wing
907-561-2330

Mary Minor
907-563-8180

Cary Jasper
907-276-4611

John Soileau
907-451-7100

Patton Pettijohn
907-276-5077

ARIZONA

Stacey Kargman
520-293-5400

Dana Myatt
602-955-0551

Louise Buratovich
602-831-0717

Clark Hansen
602-991-5092

Konrad Kail
602-493-2273

Autumn Holder
520-323-7133

Jorge Badillo Cochran
520-323-7133

CALIFORNIA

Tara Levy
925-602-0582

Bonnie Marsh
619-436-3455

Janet Zand
310-457-7749

Katherine Tsoulas
408-629-6079

Harry Swope
818-786-9627

Ian Mussman
310-313-7824

James Mally
916-782-1275

Marcua Laux
310-391-7744

Hung Lau Koon
415-697-8989

COLORADO

Ellen Dale
303-526-0217

Ruth Adele
719-636-0098

Charles Cropley
303-449-1295

Johannah Reilly
303-541-9600

CONNECTICUT

Amy B Rothenberg
203-763-1225

Gabriele Kallenborn
203-454-5989

Loretta Osik
203-792-3187

Michelle J Pouliot
203-482-4730

Eugene R Zampieron
203-598-0400

Jeffrey J Klass
203-481-5219

Peter D'Adamo
203-661-7375

DELAWARE

Diane Newman
302-655-7841

FLORIDA

Debra Gibson
305-783-0544

David Eaton
813-321-4286

James Mckee
407-628-2603

Michael Dappalonia
407-898-8929

Ralph Helland
813-626-9341

Carl Yaeger Jr
305-759-6689

Eteri Melnikov
813-748-7943

GEORGIA

Albert Nehl
404-336-5521

HAWAII

Anne L Maguire
206-776-6085

Diane Ostroff
808-947-1315

Jack Burke
808-537-4345

Jonathan Mather
808-885-7711

Collon Brayce
808-242-6787

IDAHO

Brent Mathieu
208-338-5590

Elwin C Klein
208-743-1168

Milton Nelson
208-624-4661

Samuel Wagner
208-263-2328

Todd Schlapfer
208-664-1644

ILLINOIS

Shelia Leidy
312-296-6700

Hugh Jenkins
312-296-6700

John R Tambone
815-338-2345

IOWA

Daniel Dixon
515-472-0332

Ed Wallace
819-643-2035

Roy Sumpter
319-385-6339

KANSAS

Natural Medical Care
785-749-2255

KENTUCKY

John C Tapp
502-781-1483

MAINE

Mary L Garner
207-772-9812

Miranda Marland
207-781-7600

MASSACHUSETTS

Paul J Giordano
508-324-9999

Janet K Beaty
617-863-0598

Barry Taylor
617-254-7700

James M Lemkin
413-268-3500

Shivanatha Barton
617-277-4150

MICHIGAN

John Mcdonald
616-429-7449

Stephen D Nugent
810-557-1776

Susan Kroes
616-722-0398

MINNESOTA

Helen C Healy
612-644-4436

Robert Gallagher
612-824-3157

Amrit Devgun
612-227-8776

Bruce Boraas
612-721-5882

MISSOURI

Albert Nehl
314-837-1141

MONTANA

Amy G Haynes
406-728-2415

Elisabeth Kirchof
406-586-8244

Nancy Aagenes
406-723-6609

Michael Bergkamp
406-442-2091

Medicine Tree Clinic
406-745-3600

NEBRASKA

Randall Bradley
402-391-6714

NEVADA

Terry Pfau
702-258-7860

Michael L Gerber
702-826-1900

Lynn Schwartzman
702-435-7501

NEW HAMPSHIRE

Pamela Herring
603-228-0407

Leon Hecht
603-427-6800

Devra Krassner
603-433-3212

NEW JERSEY

Jack Larmer
201-385-7106

NEW MEXICO

Joan Kirk
505-758-9704

Linda Showler
360-385-1145

Marianne Calvanesse
505-294-4505

Don Leathers
505-986-0919

Govindha Mcrostie
505-988-4210

NEW YORK

Karen Fuller
212-932-8442

Victoria Zupa
718-622-7800

Daniel Squillanty
718-729-1417

Michael B Schachter
914-368-4700

Shoshana Margolin
212-961-1378

NORTH CAROLINA

Susan Delaney
919-929-1132

Gilbert Alvarado
919-933-7373

Stephen Barrie
704-253-0621

OHIO

Donna Church
1-614-895-3216

David Sukalac
216-942-7130

OREGON

Edythe Vickers
503-233-1324

Hilary Farberow
503-232-1100

Mary F Caselli
503-224-7224

Dick W Thom
503-526-0397

Edward Geller
541-772-2787

Gregory Garcia
503-624-1321

Ravinder Sahni
503-641-8503

PENNSYLVANIA

Ella Mcelwee
814-766-3643

Brian Freeman
717-730-9066

Gerald Reisinger
717-283-5194

Lance Wright
610-461-6225

Michael Dipalma
215-345-0731

Howard J Miller
814-274-7070

SOUTH DAKOTA

Lauri Aesoph
605-339-3645

TENNESSEE

Eddy Boyd
615-298-2820

Stephen L Reisman
615-356-4244

TEXAS

Julia Trick
214-923-3195

Stephen Sporn
510-524-5477

James F Jennings
210-340-1717

William I Fox
915-672-7863

Michael McCann
409-798-9103

UTAH

Cordell Logan
801-562-2211

VERMONT

Mary L Bove
802-254-9332

Molly Fleming
802-863-7099

William Warnock
802-985-8250

VIRGINIA

Christy Teter
540-432-9855

Claire Zieman
804-623-0814

Dwight Zieman
804-623-0814

WASHINGTON

Andrea Black
509-422-5700

Cindy Beck
360-330-0562

Letitia Watrous
509-327-5143

Linda Costarella
802-254-9332

Bruce Milliman
206-888-9408

Carlo Calabrese
206-523-9585

Esteban Ryciak
206-682-6314

Leyardia Black
206-468-3714

Littlebrave Beaston
206-527-2176

WISCONSIN

Karen Kunkler
608-241-1911

Jerold Grotzinger
541-485-4548

NEURAL THERAPY

ALABAMA

Gus Prosch
205-823-6180

Robert E Mcalister
205-285-7808

ARIZONA

Lawrence Pollack
406-848-7896

CALIFORNIA

Linda Forbes
310-453-1918

Carl K Colbie
916-343-5571

Gary Emmerson
714-836-4553

George Schuchard
714-628-4783

Bernard Mcginity
916-485-4556

Soram Khalsa
310-652-6100

COLORADO

Jean Rowe
303-771-1594

Linda C Wright
303-440-5588

DELAWARE

Eugene Godfrey
302-734-5600

FLORIDA

Donald Wagner
813-654-8908

Douglas Phillips
407-848-1711

Sandford Pollak
904-292-3080

IOWA

Horst G Blume
712-252-4386

LOUISIANA

Edna Doyle
504-456-5160

Felix K Prakasam
318-226-1304

NEVADA

Bob Vance
702-385-7771

NEW JERSEY

Gennaro Lucurcio
908-351-1333

NEW MEXICO

Dietrich Klinghart
505-988-3086

NEW YORK

Richard N Ash
212-628-3133

OKLAHOMA

Robert Talley
405-321-8030

John Merriman
918-744-5959

PENNSYLVANIA

Owen Rogal
215-545-2104

Ronald Niklaus
717-737-3353

TEXAS

Allen Sprinkle
817-267-8810

John Baldwin
713-622-7777

Ben Thurman
915-653-3562

Philip O'Neill
915-332-2673

VIRGINIA

Aldo Rosemblat
690-6030

WASHINGTON

Jeff Harris
206-517-4748

NURSE-MIDWIFERY

American College of Nurse Midwives
818 Connecticut Ave NW
Washington, DC 20006
202-728-9860
www.acnm.org

NUTRITIONAL THERAPY

American College for Advancement
in Medicine
23121 Verdugo Dr
Laguna Hills, CA 92653
www.acam.org

American Preventive Medical
Association
9912 Georgetown Pike
Po Box 458
Great Falls, VA 22066
800-230-APMA
www.healthy.net

ARIZONA

John Dommisse
520-577-1940

Gordon H Josephs
602-778-6169

William W Halcomb
602-832-3014

Stanley R Olsztyn
602-954-0811

ARKANSAS

John L Gustavus
501-758-9350

Aubrey M Worrell
501-535-8200

Norbert J Becquet
501-375-4419

CALIFORNIA

Kenneth A. Thomas
650-738-2225

Nancy Mullan
818-954-9267

Bridget Frank
805-389-0749

Joan M Resk
714-842-5591

Doug Lynner
213-462-4578

Erik Nielsen
805-492-1811

Jack Alpan
213-383-3833

John P Toth
510-682-5660

Lucien Martin
310-392-8184

Roger Jahnke
805-682-3230

Skip Shoden
310-451-4419

Victor Molinari
213-723-1994

William C Kubitschek
619-744-6991

Murray Susser
310-477-8151

Sean Degnan
619-320-4292

William J Goldwag
714-827-5180

COLORADO

Dionne Reid
970-963-3458

Ruth Adele
719-636-0098

Linda C Wright
303-440-5588

Glen Nagel
406-728-8544

Michael Malmgren
303-782-9277

Stephen M Koral
303-443-4984

John Altshuler
303-740-7771

CONNECTICUT

Jeffrey J Klass
203-481-5219

DELAWARE

George Yossif
302-856-5151

FLORIDA

Len Warner
Don Barber
901-285 6775

Elizabeth Rohack
407-278-8358

Marla Russell
813-593-5933

Gary L Pynckel
813-278-3377

Herbert Pardell
305-922-0470

Herbert R Slavin
305-748-4991

Bruce Dooley
305-527-9355

Harold Robinson
813-646-5088

James Parsons
407-784-2102

Neil Ahner
407-744-0077

Travis L Herring
904-775-0525

William Post
305-977-3700

Calderon C Ramirez
305-441-6669

GEORGIA

David Epstein
404-525-7333

Bernard Mlaver
404-395-1600

William E Richardson
404-607-0570

Terril J Schneider
912-929-1027

Young S Shin
404-242-0000

Oliver L Gunter
912-336-7343

HAWAII

Helen Joseph
808-737-3077

Clifton Arrington
808-322-9400

Wismer Clark
808-941-0522

IDAHO

Brent Mathieu
208-338-5590

Todd Schlapfer
208-664-1644

Peter McCallum
208—263 K -5456

ILLINOIS

Judith Wiker
312-296-6700

Jim Foster
217-344-1188

Peter Senatore
708-872-8722

Terrill K Haws
708-577-9451

Terry W Love
815-434-1977

Paul J Dunn
708-383-3800

Richard E Hrdlicka
708-232-1900

Walt Stoll
708-233-4273

Razvan Rentea
312-583-7793

INDIANA

George Wolverton
812-282-4309

Barbara F Sikes
812-422-7972

KANSAS

John Gamble Jr
913-321-1140

Terry Hunsberger
316-275-7128

Stevens B Acker
316-733-4494

KENTUCKY

Stephen S Kiteck
606-677-0459

LOUISIANA

Christy Graves
504-646-4415

James P Carter
504-588-5136

Joseph R Whitaker
318-467-5131

Phillip Mitchell
318-357-1571

Adonis J Domingue
318-365-2196

Saroj T Tampira
504-277-8991

MAINE

Joseph Cyr
207-868-5273

MARYLAND

Eugene A Sombatoro
410-964-3118

Harold Goodman
301-565-2494

Christopher C Brown
410-268-5005

Paul Beals
301-490-9911

Ronald Parks
410-486-5656

MASSACHUSETTS

Carol Englender
617-965-7770

Daniel A Kinderlehrer
508-465-6077

Michael Janson
508-362-4343

Richard Cohen
617-829-9281

Thomas N La Cava
508-854-1380

Barbara Silbert
508-465-0929

MICHIGAN

Cary Wolf
248-737-0802

James Ziobrn
313-779-5700

Kenneth Ganapini
313-733-3140

Paul A Parenta
810-626-7544

Thomas A Padden
810-473-2922

Leo Modzinski
517-785-4254

Seldon Nelson
517-349-2458

MINNESOTA

Jean R Eckerly
612-593-9458

Michael Dole
612-593-9458

Steven E Klos
612-929-4568

MISSISSIPPI

James H Sams
601-327-8701

James H Waddell
601-875-5505

Robert Hollingsworth
601-398-5106

Pravinchandra Patel
301-622-7011

MISSOURI

Dorothy Kanion
816-779-4844

Charles J Rudolph
816-453-5940

Clinton C Hayes
314-583-8911

John T Schwent
314-937-8688

Lawrence Dorman
816-358-2712

William C Sunderwirth
417-837-4158

Tipu Sultan
314-921-7100

MONTANA

Sarah Lane
406-726-3000

NEBRASKA

Otis W Miller
308-728-3251

NEVADA

Robert Vance
702-385-7771

Steven Holper
702-878-3510

NEW JERSEY

Arnold J Susser
800-526-4240

Constance G Alfano
201-444-4622

Allan Magaziner
609-424-8222

Gary Klingsberg
201-585-9368

Charles H Mintz
609-825-7372

Rodolfo T Sy
908-738-9220

Majid Ali
201-586-4111

NEW MEXICO

Joan Kirk
505-758-9704

Shirley B Scott
505-966-9960

Gerald Parker
505-271-4800

NEW YORK

Shari Lieberman
212-929-3152

Serafina Corsello
212-399-0222

Christopher Calapai
516-794-0404

Gregory R Gumberich
516-294-9494

Maxwell Owusu
718-842-0828

Robert Newman
516-368-6320

Allan Warshowsky
516-488-2877

Bob Snider
315-764-7328

Miklos L Boczko
914-949-8817

Neil L Block
914-359-3300

Paul Cutler
716-284-5140

Richard Izquierdo
718-589-4541

Richard N Ash
212-628-3133

Reino Hill
716-665-3505

Tsilia Sorina
718-375-2600

NORTH CAROLINA

Sophie A Johnson
888-802-6862

William D Roberts
828-648-1278

John L Wilson
704-252-9833

Keith E Johnson
919-281-5122

NORTH DAKOTA

Brian E Briggs
701-838-6011

OHIO

L Terry Chappel
419-358-4627

Jeffrey Smith
440-439- 6819

Ronald Ruscitti
216-536-2123

William D Mitchell
614-761-0555

Derrick Lonsdale
216-835-0104

Don K Snyder
419-399-2045

OKLAHOMA

Bruce A Frye
918-250-1072

Charles H Farr
405-691-1112

Leon Anderson
918-299-5039

Charles D Taylor
405-525-7751

Howard Hagglund
405-329-4457

V J Conrad
405-341-5691

OREGON

Bev Fisk
541-386-3780

Terence H Young
503-371-1558

Bruce A Dickson
503-434-6515

PENNSYLVANIA

Monica Ziegler
814-234-0785

Sally Ann Rex
215-866-0900

Bill Illingworth
814-623-8414

Paul M Kosmorsky
215-860-1500

Robert H Schmidt
215-437-1959

Frederick Burton
215-844-4660

George C Miller
717-524-4405

Steven C Halbert
215-886-7842

Chandrika Sinha
412-349-1414

Mura Galperin
215-677-2337

SOUTH CAROLINA

Theodore C Rozema
803-457-4141

TEXAS

Linda Martin
214-985-1377

Jim P Archer
210-697-8445

John L Sessions
409-423-2166

Michael Samuels
214-991-3977

Thomas E Reeves
713-977-0005

Francisco Soto
915-534-0272

John P Trowbridge
713-540-2329

Vladimir Rizov
512-451-8149

Elisabeth-Anne Cole
409-548-8610

UTAH

Dennis C Harper
801-288-8881

D Remington
801-373-8500

VERMONT

Charles E Anderson
802-879-6544

VIRGINIA

Susan Zimmer
703-364-2045

Peter C Gent
804-744-3551

Harold Huffman
703-867-5242

Scott V Anderson
703-941-3606

Vincent Speckhart
804-622-0014

Sohini Patel
703-941-3606

WASHINGTON

Tamara Payne
206-838-2620

Linda Chiu Hole
509-747-2902

Karl Mincin
206-853-7610

Burton B Hart
509-927-9922

George J Grobins
206-564-2722

Richard Marshall
206-457-1515

The Hope Clinic
206-527-1366

WEST VIRGINIA

Tara C Sharma
304-523-8800

Steve M Zekan
304-343-7559

Prudencio Corro
304-252-0775

WISCONSIN

Sandra Herbage
608-246-9070

Jerry N D Yee
414-258-6282

William J Faber
414-464-7680

ORTHOMOLECULAR MEDICINE

International Society for
Orthomolecular Medicine
16 Florence Ave
Toronto, Ontario, Canada M2N 1E9
416-733-2117
www.orthomed.org

ALABANA

Humphry Osmond
205-759-0416

ARIZONA

John Dommisse
520-577-1940

Aubrey Worrell
501-535-8200

CALIFORNIA

Nancy Mullan
818-954-9267

Priscilla Slagle
310-826-0175

Bernard Rimland
619-281-7165

Jeffry L Anderson
415-927-7140

John Ackerman
805-682-1011

Murray Susser
310-477-8151

Robert Buckley
510-886-7002

Ro Waiton
408-354-2300

FLORIDA

Albert F Robbins
407-395-3282

IDAHO

K Peter McCallum
208-263-5456

KENTUCKY

John H Parks
606-254-9001

MAINE

Conrad R Wurtz
207-782-1035

MARYLAND

Arnold Brenner
410-922-1133

MASSACHUSETTS

Carol Englender
617-965-7770

MINNESOTA

William Brauer
612-871-2611

MISSISSIPPI

David Penton
601-497-6000

NEW JERSEY

Walter Burnstein
201-584-4947

NEW YORK

Serafina Corsello
212-399-0222

Jose Yaryura-Tobias
516-487-7116

Katharine Fryer
212-808-4940

Terence Dulin
516-293-4276

Charles Biller
914-834-2185

Richard Ribner
212-246-7010

Richard Schwimmer
718-252-3622

OHIO

Francis McCafferty
216-835-3892

PENNSYLVANIA

Ella Mcelwee
814-766-3643

Paul M Kosmorsky
215-860-1500

David M Goldstein
412-366-6780

Philip L Bonnet
215-321-8321

Ralph A Miranda
412-838-7632

TEXAS

Harlan Wright
806-792-4811

UTAH

Dennis Remington
801-373-8500

VIRGINIA

Henry J Palacios
703-356-2244

WASHINGTON

Donald McCabe
206-331-4424

WEST VIRGINIA

Deleno H Webb
304-525-9355

WISCONSIN

Robert S Waters
800-200-7178

Eleazar M Kadile
414-468-9442

OXYGEN THERAPY

ARIZONA

Gene Schroeder
602-445-4390

CALIFORNIA

Carolyn Bormann
909-337-3671

James Walkenbach
310-473-8298

Michael Carpendale
415-750-2133

COLORADO

Zachary Brinkerhoff
303-237-1530

FLORIDA

Alfred S Massam
813-773-6668

Leonard Haimes
407-994-3868

Richard Worsham
904-791-3234

Eteri Melnikov
813-748-7943

INDIANA

Thomas M Mcnaughton
813-365-6273

KANSAS

Stanley Beyerle
316-687-0035

MARYLAND

Paul Beals
301-490-9911

MISSOURI

Charles J Rudolph
816-453-5940

John Moreshead
703-885-2304

NEVADA

Steven Holper
702-878-3510

NEW YORK

Mitchell Kurk
212-517-4414

NORTH DAKOTA

H Leigh Richard
701-775-5527

OHIO

James P Frackelton
216-835-0104

James Ventresco Jr
216-792-2349

OKLAHOMA

Nita Mcneill
405-376-4556

Gaylord D Snitker
918-749-8349

Charles D Taylor
405-525-7751

OREGON

James Wm Fitzsimmons
503-474-2166

TEXAS

Elizabeth Cole
512-548-8610

Francisco Soto
915-534-0272

Jerome L Borochoff
713-461-7517

VIRGINIA

Elizabeth Davidson
703-352-5200

Richard D Fisher
703-256-4441

WASHINGTON

Jeff Harris
206-517-4748

WISCONSIN

Eleazar M Kadille
414-468-9442

OSTEOPATHY

American Academy of Osteopathy
3500 DePauw Blvd, Ste 1080
Indianapolis, IN 46268-1136
317-879-1881

American Osteopathic Association
142 E Ontario St
Chicago, IL 60611
312-280-5800
www.healthy.net

QI GONG

Qi Gong Institute of East West
Academy of Healing Arts
450 Sutter Pl, Ste 2104
San Francisco CA 94108
415-788-2227

American Foundation of Traditional
Chinese Medicine
505 Beach St
San Francisco, CA 94133
415-776-0502

Susan Arima
Santa Monica, CA
310-453-4339

Hamilt
San Jose, CA
408-223-0911

Lehrer
Santa Monica, CA
310-397-9525

Roger Jahnke
Santa Barbara, CA
805-682-3230

Luis Pagani
Miami, FL
305-868-6801

Qizhi Gao
Wichita, KS
316-688-3308

Romi Scavullo
Baltimore, MD
410-367-3429

Alan Stolowitz
Chappaqua, NY
914-923-1984

Guo-Guang Chen
Elmhurst, NY
718-478-8828

Weathers
Tulsa, OK
918-836-5454

Perrault
Boyertown, PA
215-369-5567

Christine Chmielewski
Seattle, WA
206-361-4700

RECONSTRUCTIVE THERAPY

Kent L Pomerory
Scottsdale, AZ
602-391-0141

Norbert J Becquet
Little Rock, AR
501-375-4419

Martin Dayton
N Miami Beach, FL
305-931-8484

Michael Ziff
Orlando, FL
407-293-3185

Joseph Cyr
Van Buren, ME
207-868-5273

Christopher C Brown
Annapolis, MD
410-268-5005

Gennaro Locurcio
Elizabeth, NJ
908-351-1333

Marjorie S Siebert
Flushing, NY
718-386-2020

L Terry Chappel
Bluffton, OH
419-358-4627

James Carlson
Knoxville, TN
615-691-2961

Prudencio Corro
Beckley, WV
304-252-0775

REIKI

Reiki Alliance
PO Box 41
Cataldo, ID 83810-1041
208-682-3535

Reiki Outreach International
PO Box 609
Fair Oaks, CA 95628
916-863-1500

Davena Amick-Elder
Tucson, AZ
520-574-7854

Penny Layne
Los Angeles, CA
323-664-7788

Cynthia Laureano
Buena Park, CA
714-523-5719

James Walkenbach
Los Angeles, CA
310-473-8298

Susan M Pataky
Bridgeport, CT
203-255-8914

Katharine King
West Palm Beach, FL
561-684-6820

Jann Thomas
Evansville, IN
812-471-0161

Peggy Horne
Columbia, MD
909-336-3637

Rosemary Ratzin
Frostburg, MD
301-689-1794

Elisabeth Lindberg
Ramsey, NJ
201-934-1751

Carol Sokolow
Patchogue, NY
516-758-4105

Nilsa Vergara
Jackson Hts, NY
718-651-2260

Jonna Alexander
Portland, OR
503-256-0931

Kathryn Strick
Erie, PA
814-835-2241

Marion Yaglinski
Media, PA
610-566-5669

Catherine K Carson
Fairfax, VA
703-273-6106

ROLFING

International Rolf Institute
PO Box 1968
Boulder, CO 80306
303-449-5903

ALABAMA

J Thomas West
205-539-0641

ALASKA

Barbara Maier
907-562-0926

Jodi Miller
907-235-4393

David Brickell
907-479-3709

Gwin A Moerlein
907-349-3739

ARIZONA

Linda K Collier
602-745-1570

Mary Agneessens
602-266-5055

Patti A Selleck
602-277-8066

Jim D Asher
602-622-4201

Matthew Oren
602-954-7171

William L Scurlock
602-282-1497

ARKANSAS

Tara Detwiler
501-666-6800

CALIFORNIA

Barbara Anderson
714-962-5951

Bridget Beck
707-575-6852

Cheryl Whyatt
415-668-5332

Evelyn D Lehner
213-394-0198

COLORADO

Hannah Pierce
303-449-8664

Jane Harrington
303-447-2760

Joy Ptasnik
303-789-0494

Suzanne Picard
303-494-3281

Victoria Cashman
303-530-1325

Roger T Jordan
303-449-2788

Larry B Ybarra
303-499-8858

Paul Reynolds
303-670-1814

Gael Ohlgren
303-385-5031

CONNECTICUT

Anne Dahlberg
203-767-0070

Mary C Staggs
203-522-4008

Sharon Sklar
203-233-8437

Craig Swan
203-629-2620

Crancoise L Brunette
203-868-1723

DELAWARE

Ellen Halligan
302-798-6308

FLORIDA

Candace Cressor
813-446-4290

Patricia Nelson
305-929-9739

Janis G Davis
813-896-8807

David Clark
813-933-6229

Gary Robb
407-783-2029

Jeff Reisman
305-352-1626

Pulitzer H King
813-467-4627

GEORGIA

Caroline Widmer
404-266-1992

Elizabeth A Eason
404-662-6155

Les Kertay
404-636-0785

HAWAII

Barbara D Leach
808-732-4828

Gladys Man
808-955-2494

Marjorie O'Neill
808-883-9477

Charles Winchell
808-822-7663

Gene R Sage
808-875-4409

James Lawson
808-262-9017

IDAHO

Christa B Valentin
208-344-8296

John C Valentin
208-344-8296

ILLINOIS

Edward Spencer
312-275-9940

Michael Blackburn
212-724-6677

Robert G Ahrens
708-328-7174

Sol Arkov
312-642-3804

Thomas Earnest Jr
708-394-9257

Karen Giles
708-769-0470

INDIANA

Dan Dyer
317-253-7639

John Maurer
812-339-2784

Simeon Rodgers
812-332-0184

IOWA

Judi Clinton
319-338-2556

Ron Petit
515-752-6255

Ralph Bianco
515-472-9048

KANSAS

Elaine Brewer
913-749-2740

Larry Redding
913-841-8481

Brian Anson
816-931-0944

KENTUCKY

John Maurer
502-895-2230

LOUISIANA

Kathy Rooney
504-488-6174

John H Schewe
504-488-6174

John R Demahy
504-488-7555

MAINE

Lily Hill
207-763-3811

Paul Ma Gordon
207-439-8522

Noel Clark
207-582-4580

Michael Mathieu
207-465-3009

Judi Clinton
207-772-9812

Thomas Myers
207-772-9812

MARYLAND

Holly Howard
301-269-6032

Holly Howard
410-997-5673

Joy Belluzzi
301-654-5025

Larry Kofsky
301-356-5937

Michael R Feldman
410-280-6488

Steve Hancoff
301-929-2579

Francis Wenger
301-867-2742

Tessy Brungardt
301-239-7360

MASSACHUSETTS

Betty J Wall
508-540-1079

Ellen Landauer
413-339-8527

Lydia Gadman
508-465-9770

Charles Maier
413-339-8527

Dennis S Bailey
617-834-0748

Eric Jacobson
617-643-6874

Richard Shaw
413-586-8252

MICHIGAN

Kathleen L Strauch
517-351-9240

Kim Tillen
313-421-0991

Theresa A Pearce
906-337-3113

Anthony Zimkowski
313-856-6806

Jeff Belanger
313-973-6898

Jim Z Tavrazich
313-548-5240

Karen Parker
313-652-9330

MINNESOTA

Tom Gustin
612-871-2181

Wayne Henningsgaard
Sandy Henningsgaard
612-331-3530

Siana Goodwin
612-379-3895

MISSOURI

Deborah A Nuckolls
816-753-4888

Marilyn F Beach
816-753-4888

Tara Detwiller
417-261-2393

Mark Cook
816-363-0615

MONTANA

Michael C Stabile
406-586-7295

Robert K Murray
406-782-8550

NEVADA

Kim I Webster
702-348-1488

Lorna Benedict
702-322-7438

David Macdonald
702-825-8444

Peter Levine
702-329-9282

Wolfgang Baumgartner
702-324-3323

NEW HAMPSHIRE

Ticia Agri
603-778-6247

Kevin Frank
603-968-9585

NEW JERSEY

Ruth Solomon
908-821-6868

Chuck Carpenter
908-422-8029

Ron Spechler
201-767-9251

Steven Glassman
201-816-8333

William Harvey
609-397-2500

NEW MEXICO

Jan Henry Sultan
505-983-8847

Kristen Kuester
505-989-7529

Linda Holley
505-880-1558

Brian Fahey
505-243-7458

Dean Rollings
505-989-9050

Andree Neumeister
505-982-1368

NEW YORK

Beth Ullmann
212-243-3644

Dorothy Hunter
212-724-6677

Judith Roberts
212-724-6677

Lisa Tackley
617-266-8584

Don Van Vleet
212-369-8038

Gary Robb
716-877-0676

John Botsford
607-272-5980

Paul Zimmerman
716-682-9720

NORTH CAROLINA

Jennette M Presnell
919-821-3760

Kathy Rooney
919-852-7315

Brian D Hopkins
919-286-5877

Cameron Nims
919-929-4111

Gray Kimbrell
704-344-8124

Janice Presnell
704-586-3433

OKLAHOMA

Dan Gentry
405-749-1363

Erik Dalton
405-728-7711

Kay Lewis Blanchard
918-749-4559

Diane L Sullivan
541-388-4167

Karen Lackritz
541-345-2926

Paul Brown
503-227-6309

PENNSYLVANIA

Linda Grace
215-985-1263

Rebecca Carli
215-848-4739

Helmut M Maul
215-649-3205

Thomas Droege
412-321-2851

William Harvey
215-438-3773

Matthew & Ellen Cohen
215-667-2204

RHODE ISLAND

Elaine Haire
401-941-7625

Joe Wheatley
401-397-4428

Steve Cavanagh
401-294-9660

SOUTH DAKOTA

Charlie Evander
703-523-6355

TENNESSEE

Allison Hubbard
615-383-7716

Charlie Evander
615-968-9109

Gregory Schaller
615-584-4714

Randy Mack
615-383-7716

TEXAS

Dena Roberts
512-327-2928

Kathleen Mcbride
713-488-4553

Patty Sanders
512-459-4402

Robert W Pittman
915-544-9355

Sam Johnson
214-360-0624

UTAH

Aline Newton
801-484-6569

Nancy E Stotz
415-398-2625

David Keffer
801-484-6569

Judah R Lyons
801-355-6363

Iginia V Boccalandro
801-355-6363

VERMONT

Jeffry H Galper
802-865-4770

Iginia V Boccalandro
802-524-4468

VIRGINIA

Rose Huzdovich
703-707-9489

Viki Van Wey
804-422-0774

G Cosper Scafidi
703-998-0474

Eva Jo Wu
703-989-1617

WASHINGTON

Ellen D Madsen
206-753-8095

Sarah Emory
206-781-9656

Sherri Cassuto
206-633-2612

Allan M Kaplan
206-548-9165

Gonya W Klein
206-285-6471

WISCONSIN

Patrice A Naparstek
608-246-0628

Suzanne E Filut
414-255-5445

Brian Moore
414-961-2210

David Laden
608-257-1144

Gregory Persick
414-797-7867

THERAPEUTIC TOUCH

Nurse Healers Professional Associates
1211 Locust St
Philadelphia, PA 19107
215-545-8079

TRAGER TECHNIQUE

Trager Institute
21 Locust Ave
Mill Valley, CA 94941
415-388-2688
www.trager.com

ARIZONA

Corrine W Larson
602-471-7344

Peggy Richards
602-990-0450

Marnel Plutchok
602-990-2766

CALIFORNIA

Alicia L Gates
619-543-0144

Carol Campbell
408-429-8216

Joellen Larsen
714-240-4954

Sandra Golden
619-283-9008

Gary Brownlee
310-546-3144

Mark Bauman
415-324-1824

Fawn Christianson
408-257-3313

COLORADO

Ann Jones
303-972-4316

Marian D Whitney
303-422-2323

Sally Goddard
303-963-9165

Jacque Jackson
303-973-0410

John Pagano
203-294-0465

Carolea Burgess
203-429-4420

FLORIDA

Ann L Mcalhaney
305-273-9282

Celia R Cassiano
305-891-4720

Elizabeth E Rohack
407-278-8358

Regina Kujawski
305-491-8519

Susan V Rubin
407-367-9009

HAWAII

Laura L Conti
808-328-8106

Wendy Rundel
808-885-7383

INDIANA

Elizabeth Moreland
317-926-5108

Jann Thomas
812-471-0161

Annie Carpenter White
317-254-9989

IOWA

Betty R Krueger
515-472-8371

MAINE

Carla S Keene
207-647-5364

Christie Lyons
207-985-9135

Lucy Viele
207-967-3794

MARYLAND

Karen Roberts
410-750-7543

MASSACHUSETTS

Diane Allen
508-649-6960

Holly Chaplin
617-899-4769

Penelope Pureheart
508-544-6851

Ken Wieder
413-274-6089

Martin Anderson
617-738-0091

L Divya Shinn
508-544-2851

T Lee Robin
301-428-8146

NEW JERSEY

Ilene Watrous
609-799-5204

Irene Darpino
609-451-3970

Maxine Guenther
908-741-5447

NEW MEXICO

Carol Maxson
505-255-4064

Ellen Verkerke
505-982-0841

Ruth Alpert
505-982-6377

Jean Hopkins
505-262-0847

NEW YORK

Sarah Brown
716-248-0690

Clifford Shulman
212-724-9755

Robert Brown
716-248-0690

Roger Tolle
212-787-5167

Sharmila Cohen Gold
516-725-4995

NORTH CAROLINA

Sharon King
919-967-2639

OHIO

Judith Spater
614-587-3670

Alan Hundley
513-281-8606

Carrissa Fitzsimons
513-324-3439

OREGON

Jeanne Pace
509-486-2585

PENNSYLVANIA

Katherine H Stewart
717-737-5299

Monique Perrault
215-369-5567

Suzanne Miller
215-282-2110

David Haines
717-397-9007

A David Dimmack
215-843-6534

TEXAS

Charlene Strawn
409-696-3307

Vanita Garner
817-694-6405

UTAH

Mary C Redmond
801-596-0629

VERMONT

Jan Sandman
802-229-4671

WASHINGTON

Christine Chmielewski
206-361-4700

Reed S Johnson
206-361-4700

Beth Cachat
206-822-7781

Wimsey Cherrington
206-233-8620

Amy Heiland
206-528-8496

WEST VIRGINIA

John W Riffe
304-296-2357

WISCONSIN

Emily Meyer
608-249-1206

Leslie Hutchins
608-256-0079

VETERINARY MEDICINE

American Holistic Veterinary
Medicine Association
2218 Old Emmorton Rd
Bel Air, MD 21015
410-569-0795
www.altvetmed.com

VISION CARE ANALYSIS

Suzanne J Young
Fremont, CA
510-657-8973

Moses Albalas
Los Angeles, CA
213-306-3737

Richard Stanley
Daly City, CA
415-992-4640

Suzanne Skinner
Torrance, CA
310-518-4555

Antonia Orfield
Cambridge, MA
617-868-8742

Ray Gottlieb
Madison, NJ
201-377-6556

Marc Grossman
New Paltz, NY
914-255-3728

YOGA

International Association of Yoga
Therapists
109 Hillside Ave
Mill Valley, CA 94941
415-383-4587

ALASKA

Phyllis Plondee
907-346-1857

Tammy R Moser
907-745-5248

Nirvair Khalsa
907-345-3841

ARIZONA

Carol Mitchell
602-840-1166

Desiree Rumbaugh
602-954-3331

Padmini Ann Higgins
602-779-3450

Priscille Potter
602-323-1222

Sami Mahatarananda
602-323-1222

CALIFORNIA

Ana T Forrest
310-453-5252

Estelle Jacobson
310-301-3917

Katherine Rabinawitz
707-942-5862

Kelly Piper
310-553-0583

Mara Carrico
619-942-4244

Andrew J Kerr
714-497-5245

Frederick Fulmer
310-827-5144

Gary Majchrzak
213-243-8527

Lenny Norton
408-426-9642

Siri D Galliano
310-278-5483

Swami Premananda
213-255-5345

Swami Vignanananda
707-445-8368

Tomino Uwate
310-698-8690

COLORADO

Barbara J Maroney
303-766-1394

Delores Pluto
719-475-0269

Kathryn C Warner
719-636-0093

Lee Shar
303-772-8259

CONNECTICUT

Christine Rosow
203-231-9642

Ellie Brawn
203-599-3373

Marleen Salko
203-254-2434

Alan J Franzi
203-799-9642

John Grasso
203-452-1619

Janaki Pierson
203-263-2254

Nidrahara K Rhodes
203-348-1721

DELAWARE

Kathleen Wright
302-656-6983

DISTRICT OF COLUMBIA

Ravi Singh
202-475-0212

FLORIDA

Andrea Weiss
305-945-7399

Anita Simons
813-922-0549

Cheryl Kostoris
813-855-9747

Denise Brittain
813-823-3882

Elizabeth B Russell
305-667-8787

Maria Lentine
407-276-7596

Ronny Dubinsky
305-292-1854

Tony Luttenberger
305-296-3010

Guru S Mata
407-856-9408

GEORGIA

Susan Kolb
770-457-4677

Deborah Timberlake
404-378-7072

Linda Deicarlo
408-874-7813

Jack Kennard
404-266-8383

Roger Gatlin
404-767-1016

HAWAII

Caroline Muir
Charles Muir
808-572-8364

Sandra Joran
808-373-3447

Lake Garren
808-732-4589

Meenakshi Honig
808-879-9324

Swami Swaroopananda
808-879-9324

ILLINOIS

Beatrice Briggs
312-868-0400

Hilda Allen
312-296-6700

Kay Clay
312-963-4252

Susan Witz
312-944-0855

Ed Schwartz
312-327-0434

Michael Larocca
708-388-3397

Arlene Capron
708-452-5119

INDIANA

Lorrie Collins
317-257-4165

Marsha Wenig
219-872-9611

Chester Bentley
317-773-2504

Don Wenig
219-872-9611

Darrian C Merritt
812-332-8029

Sharon Rose Haq
812-288-0979

IOWA

Jacqueline Modak
319-243-9936

Jan Mitchell
515-432-8566

Jo Bartruff
515-472-4971

KANSAS

Ant Carver
913-272-8423

Dana Riffel
316-945-8188

KENTUCKY

Amanda M Smith
606-624-0413

Judi R Ice
502-241-4307

Nancy L Bloemer
606-261-0394

Morgan S Goddes
812-288-5044

Thangam Rangawamy
502-589-2212

MAINE

Barbara Lyon
207-941-2344

Elaine Mcgillicuddy
Francis Mcgillicuddy
207-797-5684

Jennifer Cooper
207-775-0975

Linda B McCart
207-725-6370

Roseanna R Rich
207-288-3022

MARYLAND

Carol Cavanaugh
301-649-6265

Danielle L Alvares
617-354-2113

Helen Heffer
410-740-2337

Suzie Hurley
301-890-1993

Bob Glickstein
410-720-4340

John Schumacher
301-656-8992

Stan Andrzojewski
410-357-4110

MASSACHUSETTS

Carolyn Kildegaard
508-627-8007

Dorothy Kerzner
508-750-6722

Nancy Paglia
413-367-9487

Arthur Kilmurray
617-643-0117

David King
617-847-0617

Phil Milgrom
508-952-3057

MICHIGAN

Addie Emmons
616-372-7011

Betty J Alexander
Davisburg, Mi 48350-0173

Jo Ann Reis
313-547-3893

Karen L Ufer
313-769-4228

David Ivory
517-823-8352

Jonathan Kest
313-680-3414

Ronald J Chalfant
517-787-5002

MISSOURI

Cynthia Gage
Livingston, Mo
406-333-4478

Lou Ann Freeman
Springfield, Mo
417-885-4450

Mary A Taylor
314-227-0603

Sharon B Womack
314-469-3200

Roger Bruce
314-773-3940

MONTANA

Judith L Landecker
406-449-2205

Lora Sinisi
406-585-8151

Charles Landecker
406-449-2205

Charles Udell
406-449-2205

NEBRASKA

Karin Parkerson
402-346-8367

Miriam Ben Yaacou
402-333-1115

NEVADA

Aileen E Ignadiou
702-870-6192

Sherry Russell
702-362-6174

Claude Cooke
702-384-1188

Sasi Velupillai
702-578-8893

NEW HAMPSHIRE

Cynde Denson
603-436-7194

Doreen Schweizer
603-448-1706

Gloria J Wheeler
603-673-8658

Rosemary T Cloug
603-886-7308

Tom Sherman
603-863-5791

NEW JERSEY

Christina Kuepper
201-612-8844

Ginny St Clare
908-906-9705

Kathleen Caputo
201-857-8772

Stacey Ackerman
201-644-0468

Constance Alfano
201-444-4622

Joseph Zamarelli
908-789-9147

Judah Roseman
609-424-7501

Richard Cicchetti
201402-8510

Swami D Saraswati
201-836-6975

NEW MEXICO

Deborah Bristow
505-989-3626

Fern S Ward
505-258-3399

Susan Voorhees
505-474-3537

Michael Hopp
505-988-3330

Lad Vasant
505-292-7268

NEW YORK

Beryl Bender
212-661-2895

Elizabeth K Sheffield
516-922-5280

Francie Ricks
914-941-3469

Ingrid Schiavone
718-667-7380

Jean Aronoff
516-674-0656

Jeanette Miller
212-666-6294

Judith Deluca
716-343-8403

Robyn Ross
212-864-2399

Suzanne Hodges
718-834-0105

Lenny Markowitz
718-543-8982

Stephen J Gitto
914-782-7991

Thom Birch
212-661-2895

Jourdan Arpelle
212-505-0751

Rama Patella
212-787-4908

NORTH CAROLINA

Joy Doherty
919-231-9424

Louisa Klein
919-768-3770

Mary Lou Buck
704-525-2293

Tom Thompson
919-692-4854

OHIO

Bobbi Holliday
216-333-2944

Carol Williams
216-235-5914

Dayle Hails
614-753-1070

Karen S M Holby
216-533-0162

Suzanne B Stichtenoth
513-874-8671

Devhuti Milcetich
216-678-5370

OKLAHOMA

Annette Clifton
405-528-6834

Wilma H Miles
405-478-1550

OREGON

Barbara Jensen
503-287-1087

Jean Harkin
503-385-0929

Mari G Ayatri
503-482-4799

Susan Curington
503-299-1310

Petrini J York
503-471-6132

Dan Mcleod
503-363-6408

Ken Rowlett
503-345-4388

Lilijoy Rothstein
503-292-5740

Shan Ma Titus
503-683-1873

RHODE ISLAND

Suzanne Newton
401-454-5026

Maureen R Gordon
401-751-2001

Ross Labossiere
401-783-1377

Stephen Fortunato
401-737-7200

SOUTH CAROLINA

Mary-Ellen Lefort
803-639-2583

TENNESSEE

Andrea Cartwright
615-584-0109

Jan Campbell
615-383-0785

Louise Hoyt
901-681-0009

Robbie Williams
615-373-8210

Bill Buckler
615-254-0631

TEXAS

Abigail Kaehler
512-854-8750

Diana Lyons
713-468-3633

Karen Korras
214-696-6250

Fred Dowd
214-352-2039

George Purvis
713-468-3633

Walter Reece
817-756-2228

Anil Gupta
214-644-5823

UTAH

Charlotte Bell
801-355-2617

Jay Jones
801-363-3696

Mary Wilson
801-649-9415

Mark Maura
801-649-9415

VERMONT

Martha Whitney
802-862-5118

Penelope Hoiden
802-658-6410

Susan Wahlrab
802-223-3364

Thea Lloyd
802-644-8246

Dean C Orcoran
802-748-1516

Jyoti Hansa
802-785-4711

VIRGINIA

Betsey Downing
703-435-1571

Debbie R Stevens
703-343-7706

Lois Williams
703-370-0617

Ray Torber
804-422-1164

Uma M Nolen
804-353-0252

WASHINGTON

Gayle Knoepfler
206-646-9661

Theresa Elliot
206-781-4990

Richard Schachtel
206-526-9642

Vijay Elarth
206-527-0975

WISCONSIN

Margot Snowdon
307-733-9260

Nancy D Siewart
414-453-4407

Chris Saudek
608-788-7258

Cheri Krey
414-248-3202

Marti Marino
414-961-1440

Index

About the Author

GARY NULL, PH.D., is one of America's leading health and fitness writers and alternative practitioners. Trained as a nutritionist, he is the author of dozens of books and hundreds of medical articles. His one-hour health radio program airs daily on WBAI in New York City, and is carried weekly on 32 stations nationwide over the Virtual Radio Network. Null is a former faculty member at the New School for Social Research and a National TAC Master Champion Racewalker. Among his many bestselling books are *For Women Only!: Your Guide to Health Empowerment, The Food-Mood-Body Connection,* and *Gary Null's Ultimate Anti-Aging Program.* He lives in New York City and Naples, Florida.